DUPLEX SCANNING IN VASCULAR DISORDERS

DUPLEX SCANNING IN VASCULAR DISORDERS

THIRD EDITION

D. EUGENE STRANDNESS, JR., M.D.

Professor
Department of Surgery
University of Washington
Department of Surgery, Vascular Division
University of Washington Medical Center
Seattle, Washington

LIPPINCOTT WILLIAMS & WILKINS
A **Wolters Kluwer** Company
Philadelphia · Baltimore · New York · London
Buenos Aires · Hong Kong · Sydney · Tokyo

Acquisitions Editor: Beth Barry
Developmental Editor: Selina M. Bush
Production Editor: Elaine Verriest McClusky
Manufacturing Manager: Colin Warnock
Cover Designer: Mark Lerner
Compositor: Lippincott Williams & Wilkins Desktop Division

© 2002 by Lippincott Williams & Wilkins
530 Walnut Street
Philadelphia, PA 19106 USA
LWW.com

Printed in China

Library of Congress Cataloging-in-Publication Data

Strandness, D. E. (Donald Eugene), 1928-
    Duplex scanning in vascular disorders / D. Eugene Strandness, Jr.–3rd ed.
      p. ; cm.
    Includes bibliographical references and index.
    ISBN 0-7817-2631-X
      1. Duplex ultrasonography.   2. Blood-vessels—Ultrasonic imaging.   3.
    Blood-vessels—Diseases—Diagnosis.   I. Title.
      [DNLM: 1. Vascular Diseases—ultrasonography.   2. Ultrasonography,
        Doppler, Duplex.   WG 500 S897d2001]
    RC691.6.D87 S77 2001
    616.1'307543—dc21
                                                                    2001029924

                          10 9 8 7 6 5 4 3 2 1

CONTENTS

CONTRIBUTING AUTHORS

Michael Bertoglio, B.A., R.D.M.S., R.V.T. Clinical Diagnostic Sonographer, University of Washington, Vascular Diagnostic Service, Seattle, Washington

Kirk W. Beach, Ph.D., M.D. Research Professor, Department of Surgery; and Adjunct, Departments of Bioengineering and Electrical Engineering, University of Washington, Seattle, Washington

Kim Cantwell-Gab, B.S.N., R.N., R.V.T., C.V.N., R.D.M.S. Vascular Surgery Nurse Specialist, Department of Surgery, Division of Vascular Surgery, University of Washington Medical Center, Seattle, Washington

Karen A. Gates, B.A., R.V.T. Research Vascular Technologist, Department of Surgery, Division of Vascular Surgery, University of Washington Medical Center, Seattle, Washington

Richard Manzo, B.S., C.C.V.T., R.V.T. Vascular Technologist, Vascular Diagnostic Service, University of Washington Medical Center, Seattle, Washington

Bridget A. Mraz, B.S., R.D.M.S., R.V.T. Registered Vascular Technologist, Vascular Diagnostic Service, University of Washington Medical Center, Seattle, Washington

Kari A. Olmsted, B.S., R.V.T. Registered Vascular Technologist, Vascular Diagnostic Service, University of Washington Medical Center, Seattle, Washington

Jean F. Primozich, B.S., R.V.T., F.S.V.T. Senior Vascular Research Technologist, Department of Surgery, University of Washington, Seattle, Washington

Watson B. Smith, B.A., R.D.M.S., R.V.T. Registered Vascular Technologist, Vascular Diagnostic Service, University of Washington Medical Center, Seattle, Washington

Molly J. Zaccardi, B.A., R.V.T. Manager, Vascular Diagnostic Laboratory, University of Washington Medical Center, Seattle, Washington

PREFACE TO THE FIRST EDITION

In order to properly treat disorders of the vascular system, it is necessary to make a correct diagnosis and precisely define the location and extent of involvement. The traditional history and physical examination are often followed by some form of angiography, which provides confirmation of the diagnosis and a precise delineation of the disease and its extent. This information is essential, particularly if some form of interventional therapy is planned. It is this approach that remains the mainstay of cardiovascular diagnosis.

While the invasive diagnostic methods provide important data, they do have serious drawbacks. They may produce discomfort to the patient and in some cases may be the cause of serious complications. More important, the information obtained tells us very little about the functional effects of the observed lesions. In addition, angiography is unable to provide information concerning the natural history of the disease. Due to the need for additional information, considerable effort has been expended in the development of suitable noninvasive methods that could provide both anatomic and functional information on the effects of vascular disorders. Most of the methods in current use do not provide precise information on the exact location and status of the disease. Nonetheless, the information on limb blood pressure and volume changes and flow has given us considerable insight as to how diseases of the vascular system affect function. The introduction of ultrasound as an imaging method and the employment of the Doppler principle to assess flow velocity began to change the field. While imaging and Doppler techniques have serious limitations when used separately, together the techniques overcome many problems. After the concept of duplex scanning was introduced in 1974, the entire field of noninvasive diagnosis took on new dimensions.

In one instrument—the ultrasonic duplex scanner—we now have the capability of examining every major artery and vein that is commonly affected by disease. This remarkable method is rapidly becoming the most commonly used diagnostic system in laboratories devoted to the study of vascular disease.

This book is a review of my approaches to the evaluation of vascular disease and the way in which duplex scanning plays a role in that evaluation. It is not intended to be an encyclopedia of past or present progress in the field. Since my experience has spanned the development and application of both the indirect and direct diagnostic methods, I am in a rather unique position to write on this subject. I was privileged to play a part in the development and testing of many of the methods in common use today. This is an exciting time for the physicians and technologists who work in this field. We not only have the ability to define vascular disease in more precise anatomic and physiologic terms, but we can also study the problem over time. It is no longer necessary to wonder if the treatment works; we can find out. In addition, the natural history of the diseases we treat can be studied for the first time.

This book will be of particular interest to vascular surgeons, radiologists, and those technologists who perform the tests. For residents and fellows with an interest in the vascular system, it should provide an overview of the diagnostic approaches that are available and are in use. While the views expressed are largely my own, I hope the content of this book will be of use to the reader.

D. Eugene Strandness, Jr.

PREFACE

This third edition has been considerably expanded to include the words and practice of my technologists at the University of Washington. Although my chapters relating to the applications of duplex scanning methods cover much of the background and progress in the field, I believe we all realize that this progress is only possible because of the technologists' excellent efforts. Just as a good surgical scrub nurse should hand the surgeon the correct instruments, the technologist must give the correct information to the referring physician. This is being accomplished in my laboratory because of the devotion of my technologists. I have often commented on the extraordinary role they play in our health care system. In fact, I cannot think of anyone not possessing a medical degree who has the same amount of responsibility to the patient, whose welfare and often whose outcome from an illness depend on the accuracy of the studies being done. This enormous responsibility is handled well by our technologists who willingly spend the necessary time to get the studies done accurately.

Progress continues on several fronts as evidenced by the new material in this book. Duplex scanning continues to make inroads on invasive tests, which, as will be shown, are now often avoided entirely, even to the point of taking the patient to the operating room on the basis of duplex scanning alone. This has been one of the major accomplishments in my lifetime and something only dreamed of when I started in this business.

Another major advance is the information that we can provide the patient. We no longer have to answer "I don't know" to a lot of questions. For example, based entirely on the long-term studies done with duplex scanning, we can now counsel patients on the risk of stroke depending on the degree of involvement found. We can tell them what the risk of stroke is likely to be and how often we should monitor the status of their disease. It is remarkable that in 1984 we knew—based on follow-up duplex studies—that a greater than 80% stenosis of the carotid bulb was particularly dangerous. The skeptics did not trust the data, but, 17 years later, they have to admit that the studies done with duplex in the long-term turned out to be correct!

We are moving forward in many areas as evidenced by this volume. I hope that the detailed information provided by the technologists will complement my contributions and make this a useful bible for the vascular laboratory. Watching the technology grow and the technologists mature with these advances has been a great experience. What of the future? It is clear that quantitative three-dimensional imaging is going to play a key role in many areas. For example, with the advent of endovascular grafting of aortic aneurysms, the need for inexpensive long-term quantitative studies of outcome are essential. The need for this is obvious given the reports of spontaneous rupture in patients who were thought to have been successfully treated. We now have the capability of evaluating many aspects of these grafts and the changes that occur, not only with the grafts themselves, but with the native aorta as well. The future will indeed be exciting for this field.

D. Eugene Strandness, Jr.

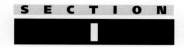

SECTION

I

BACKGROUND

VASCULAR STUDIES: PAST AND PRESENT

HISTORICAL ASPECTS

The impetus for the development of noninvasive testing methods resulted from the fact that data other than those available by angiography were insufficient to document many aspects of arterial and venous disease. Although progress in the therapy of arterial occlusive disease in the 1950s to the 1970s was rapid, the development of new methods for studying the vascular system lagged far behind. A good deal of the early work was carried out in the research setting, where physiologists began to examine the effects of vascular disease on function. Problems arose when attempts were made to transfer this information and the methods used to obtain it to clinical practice. There was considerable resistance to noninvasive methods because these methods did not seem to modify or improve the way in which patients were diagnosed or treated. As history has shown, this impression was incorrect.

The earliest developments relied entirely on indirect measurements of the effects of vascular disease on function. Although they were of interest, these developments did not penetrate the "black box" to provide the kind of information that physicians felt they needed. The techniques were largely indirect until ultrasound became available. It was with the marriage of Doppler methods with imaging that the field rapidly took off and became accepted. Even today, however, there are those who maintain that angiographic methods alone remain the gold standard. We now have variants on the "angiographic scene," such as spiral computed tomography scanning and magnetic resonance imaging methods that are being touted as major advances. Yet, in terms of their output, these systems still suffer from the same problems that angiography does, with the exception of safety. The transition from the use of invasive studies alone to those available in the vascular laboratory has occurred rapidly since the early 1990s. Although in the past the vascular laboratory was used only by interested vascular surgeons, it has now come to occupy a key place in the practice of medicine. It is fair to say that the modern hospital cannot function well without such a facility.

Before the availability of the vascular laboratory, the physician had to rely entirely on three types of information:

the nature of the patient's presenting complaint, the demonstration of bruits and/or pulse deficits, and the disease location as verified by arteriography. The surgical procedures devised to correct the abnormality were based on the location and extent of the disease. The initial results were often spectacular, with the restoration of flow to the ischemic tissues. Verification of the surgical results appeared to be simple, by noting a return in pulses in the involved limb and the patient's report of the relief of symptoms.

My appearance on this scene was during the time of rapid growth in the field in both the application of arteriography and the perfection of surgical approaches. It was during my first year in the research laboratory that I was faced with the realities of atherosclerosis and the frustrations of trying to obtain quantitative information on the disease and on its functional impact on the circulation. My early attempts to study atherosclerosis were made difficult by the lack of suitable study methods that could provide hemodynamic data on the effects of the disease. Although arteriography was sufficient to localize the disease, one had to infer from the pictures its hemodynamic impact. In addition, arteriography was not suitable for long-term follow-up studies. Finally, the traditional chart review approach to the evaluation of therapeutic results with multiple observers and entries, which varied in their accuracy and content, was a further source of difficulty. I soon recognized that the status of pulses noted by one observer was not often verified by another. Who was right?

The frustration of this experience led to a search for better methods that, by necessity, had to be noninvasive. One of the early works that seemed to hold promise was the observation of Winsor in 1950 (1) that measurements of limb blood pressure could be useful in assessing the effects of arterial obstruction. By using a pneumoplethysmograph as the sensor, he developed methods of measuring systolic blood pressure at all levels of the limb. The principles seemed simple. If an arterial lesion was sufficient in its extent to interfere with perfusion and call into play the available collaterals, the blood pressure distal to such sites had to be reduced. Conversely, if a surgical procedure could either remove or bypass the sites of obstruction, the distal pressure had to increase (2).

Surprisingly, even this simple concept was not readily accepted. This was because most physicians thought that such testing was irrelevant, given the perceived accuracy of a well-performed physical examination. This attitude was so common that it held the field of noninvasive testing hostage for many years. Nonetheless, the concept of noninvasive testing was so important that it could not be held back. I began to apply it in a comprehensive manner—to both the preoperative and postoperative evaluation of patients with peripheral arterial disease. It quickly became obvious that the simple method of measurement of limb systolic blood pressure could be used to determine whether a surgical procedure was successful. In addition, it provided a baseline value that could be used for natural history studies, regardless of what was done to the patient (3,4). It is now accepted that a change in ankle systolic pressure defined in relation to arm systolic pressure (the ankle/brachial index) should be a routine measurement.

Blood pressure is but one element of the physiologic assessment; hence, it has some limitations. What about blood flow and its measurement? In the past, the most widely applied method for measuring flow used primarily by physiologists was venous occlusion plethysmography (5). This method could be used to measure flow at the level of the digits, the forefoot, and the calf but was cumbersome to use. It soon became apparent that these measurements had some serious limitations and that flow information was not as useful clinically as the assessment of systolic pressure, which was much easier to achieve. Why? We quickly learned that, because arterial obstruction developed gradually, the collateral circulation was usually sufficient to maintain resting blood flow levels distal to an obstruction in a normal range, even with advanced disease (6,7). For example, it soon became clear that it was possible to have a very ischemic foot and in some cases actual gangrene with normal levels of blood flow in the calf.

What was needed was a method that would allow the examination of blood flow patterns directly from the arteries at any desired site of the circulation. The first glimmer of hope was the observation by Satomura in 1959 (8) that ultrasound waves could be transmitted through the intact skin to derive information on the velocity of flow by using the Doppler effect. This observation by Satomura seemed important, and it was vigorously pursued by me and my colleagues.

THE CONTINUOUS WAVE DOPPLER

The ability to transmit ultrasound waves through the skin to detect blood flow by the Doppler effect was undoubtedly the greatest advance made in the late 1950s. Although the continuous wave (CW) Doppler had to be applied "blindly" in a sense, it was possible to use one's knowledge of anatomy to guide the examination and determine what vessels were being insonated. Dr. Robert Rushmer, one of the early physiologists with an interest in this field, was able to predict its potential for use in humans (9). He applied the terminology *nondestructive testing* (10).

When the first transcutaneous CW Doppler system was developed at the University of Washington, there were two applications that appeared worthy of further research. The first and simplest was its use for the detection of fetal life. The second, and the one that began the research that ultimately led to the development of duplex scanning, was its use in the arterial system (11). The first device ever sold in the United States was the result of this effort and was called the Doptone (11,12). This device was marketed by Smith Kline Instrument Company in Philadelphia and consisted of a single transducer coupled with a loudspeaker to provide only audible output of the Doppler-shifted frequencies (Fig. 1.1).

When it was used for the detection of fetal life, the endpoint was simple: finding the fetal heartbeat, which was obviously faster than that of the mother. The problems associated with its use in the arterial system were much more complex. Although it soon became apparent that there were audible Doppler-shifted frequencies that could be recognized as normal or abnormal, this was not enough. In fact, if the only information conveyed to the observer were this subjective, it would be of limited value for both screening and long-term follow-up studies. One of the major problems was the lack of a good analog display of the arterial velocity patterns. This remained a problem in the field from its inception until the introduction of fast Fourier transforms (FFT) spectrum analysis (Fig. 1.2).

Early in its application, it was obvious that if the CW Doppler system could be developed to sense the direction

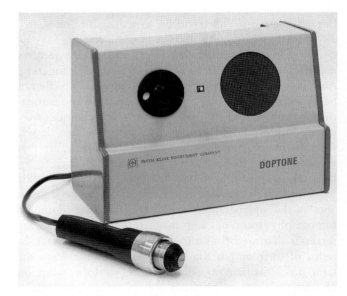

FIGURE 1.1. This was the first continuous wave Doppler system marketed in the United States and produced by Smith Kline Instrument Company of Philadelphia. The unit consisted of the transducer, which contained the electronics, and a speaker. It was not possible to obtain analog recordings of the Doppler data, although with this system, the audio output could be recorded for off-line audiospectrum analysis of the Doppler-shifted signals. (From Strandness DE Jr, Schultz RD, Sumner DS, et al. Ultrasonic flow detection: a useful technique in the evaluation of peripheral vascular disease. *Am J Surg* 1967;113:311–320, with permission.)

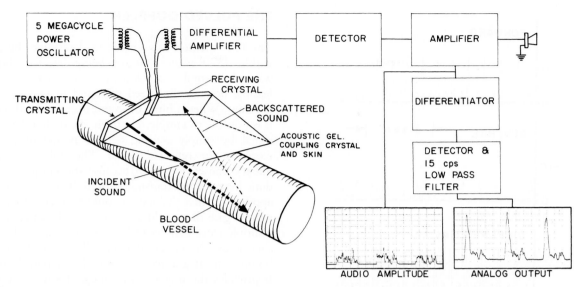

FIGURE 1.2. Block diagram of the original continuous wave Doppler system developed at the University of Washington for investigation of peripheral arteries and veins. The initial method of analog signal processing used with this system was a differentiator that did not faithfully reproduce all the information with regard to the Doppler-shifted signal. This system was nondirectional. (From Strandness DE Jr, McCutcheon EP, Rushmer RF. Application of a transcutaneous Doppler flowmeter in evaluation of occlusive arterial disease. *Surg Gynecol Obstet* 1966;122: 1039–1045, with permission.)

of flow, it would be indispensable in evaluating peripheral vascular disease. It was clear from studies using electromagnetic flowmeters in animals that arterial flow in peripheral arteries had complex forward–reverse flow changes occurring within a single heart cycle (Fig. 1.3). For example, in the lower limbs, there was the prominent forward-flow component that was followed by a brief period of reverse flow. Depending on the resistance of the vascular bed, this would be followed by another short, but definite, period of forward flow.

McLeod in 1969 (13) took advantage of the fact that there were positive and negative frequency shifts associated with a change in direction of flow. He was able to separate the two by the use of a circuit that introduced a phase shift before detection, permitting a recording of the changes either as a composite analog waveform or on separate channels. This was an important development, further perfected by Nippa and colleagues in our laboratory in 1975 (14). Now, in addition to being able to characterize the phasic nature of flow, we could accurately determine its direction. This development became essential for many of the clinical applications that were to follow (Figs. 1.4 and 1.5).

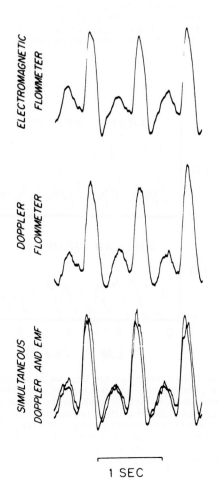

FIGURE 1.3. The upper tracings were made from the femoral artery of a dog using an electromagnetic flowmeter. The complex waveforms seen and their changes over a single heartbeat are evident. When continuous wave Doppler is used at the same site to make a recording, the similarity is obvious. (From Strandness DE Jr, Sumner DS. Measurement of blood flow. In: *Hemodynamics for surgeons.* New York: Grune & Stratton, 1975:3:31–46, with permission.)

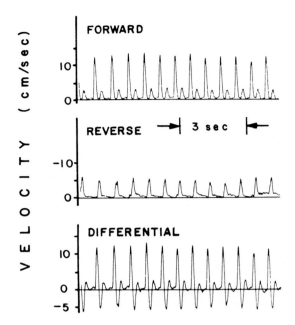

FIGURE 1.4. By separating the positive and negative Doppler shifts associated with changes in the direction of blood flow, it is possible, by using a zero-crossing detector, to display the directional changes. As noted from this recording from a peripheral artery, it is feasible to display the directional changes on two channels or to present them as a differential display. (From Nippa JH, Hokanson DE, Lee DR, et al. Phase rotation for separating forward and reverse blood velocity signals. *IEEE Trans Sonics Ultrasonics* 1975;SU-22:340–346, with permission.)

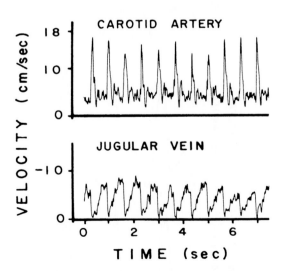

FIGURE 1.5. The continuous wave Doppler beam was directed at both the carotid artery and the jugular vein, where flow is going in opposite directions. By complete separation of the positive and negative Doppler shifts, it is possible to record velocity signals from two vessels unambiguously. (From Nippa JH, Hokanson DE, Lee DR, et al. Phase rotation for separating forward and reverse blood velocity signals. *IEEE Trans Sonics Ultrasonics* 1975;SU-22:340–346, with permission.)

THE PULSED DOPPLER

The CW method was unable to determine the exact site within tissues where flow was being detected; therefore, it was only natural to develop a pulsed system (15). This was feasible because the speed of sound in tissue is relatively constant. When a burst of sound is transmitted into tissue, it is possible to sample selectively the desired backscattered signal by simply waiting a fixed period of time before receiving the reflected signal. The pulse repetition frequency chosen is critical because the sampling has to be done between the transmit periods. The beauty of such an approach is that the system could be used either with one sample gate that could be moved by the operator or with multiple gates that could sample simultaneously at several sites across the vessel's diameter. The pulsed Doppler has become an integral part of all duplex systems in use today. It provides the user the advantage of selectively sampling blood flow from any point site within the artery.

THE ARTERIAL WALL AND ATHEROSCLEROSIS

During the time we were beginning to use Doppler methods as a technique for the study of arterial and venous problems, an interest developed in the use of echo-ranging devices for visualizing tissues and their structure. This raised the question as to the degree to which the atherosclerotic plaque could be distinguished from the normal wall based on its ultrasonic characteristics. If it were possible to use the imaging capabilities of ultrasound to evaluate the arterial lesions so commonly encountered, this would be a major advance that could have a major impact on how the disease could be studied. To study this systematically, we used arterial segments removed during autopsy to examine the role of ultrasound in detecting atherosclerotic plaques.

These initial studies were designed to measure how atherosclerosis affected the transmission of ultrasound and to relate these changes to the histologic characteristics of the arterial wall at the sites of measurement (16). This was done by opening the arterial segments longitudinally and mounting them in a holder that could be moved in a horizontal direction in a water tank through a sound beam directed at them (Fig. 1.6). To measure the attenuation of ultrasound, the reflections from a small target were obtained as the specimen was moved in front of it. The attenuation due to the artery wall was measured by inserting or removing known amounts of electrical attenuation required to keep the echo from the rod at a constant amplitude as the tissue was inserted or removed. The ultrasound source used was pulsed at 5 MHz.

To represent the data systematically, the attenuation plots were made on an X-Y recorder before and after decalcification (Fig. 1.7). In this manner, it was possible to local-

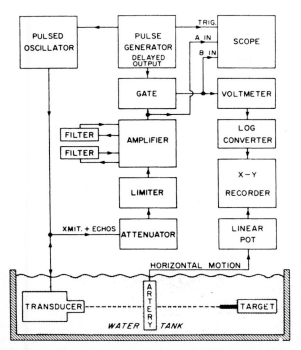

FIGURE 1.6. Block diagram of the mapping system used to document the amount of attenuation of the transmitted sound beam when passed through human arterial tissue. The positions of the transducer, the artery, and the target rod are shown. (From Hartley CJ, Strandness DE Jr. The effects of atherosclerosis on the transmission of ultrasound. *J Surg Res* 1969;9:575–582, with permission.)

ize areas of attenuation and relate them to x-rays of the specimen and the histologic sections that were prepared (Fig. 1.8). The study showed that the major factor in the diseased arterial wall that led to the attenuation of ultrasound was the presence of calcium. For example, calcified areas attenuated the ultrasound in the range of 30 to 40 dB, as compared with 0 to 5 dB in the noncalcified areas. Most important, it was noted that even microscopic deposits of calcium could produce significant attenuation of the sound beam. This study emphasized the importance of calcium in the arterial wall and how it interfered with the transmission of ultrasound. On the negative side, it did not appear that other materials within the plaque had much more effect on sound transmission than the normal wall.

This study led to the development of a real-time compound ultrasonic scanning device to produce either a longitudinal or cross-sectional view of the artery. The system at this stage did not include Doppler because we were interested only in displaying the geometric changes produced by the atherosclerotic plaque.

The prototype system consisted of a scanhead that contained three transducers in a rapidly rotating head. One transducer was placed vertical to the surface, with the other two at an identical angle off the vertical. The purpose of the three transducers was to permit visualization of the entire cross-section of the vessel without creating distortion of the portrayal of the vessel (Fig. 1.9).

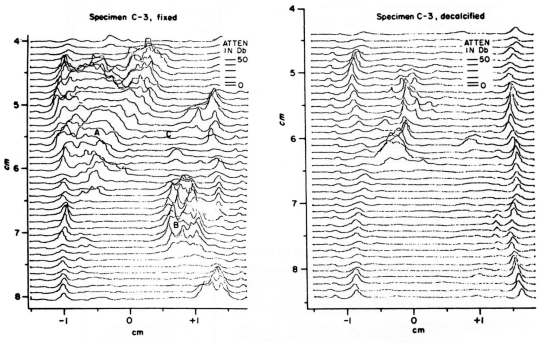

FIGURE 1.7. Attenuation maps of an arterial specimen before and after decalcification. The "mountainous" areas represent those segments of the specimen with attenuation of the intensity of the sound beam. After decalcification, much of the attenuation is no longer present. The remaining changes represent the edge effects where there was distorted geometry. (From Hartley CJ, Strandness DE Jr. The effects of atherosclerosis on the transmission of ultrasound. *J Surg Res* 1969;9:575–582, with permission.)

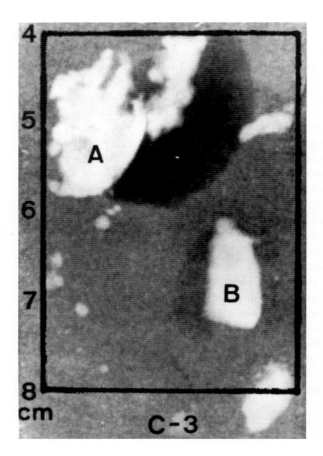

FIGURE 1.8. The areas of calcification (*A* and *B*) that led to the marked attenuation of the transmitted sound beam shown in Figure 1.10 are noted on the x-ray of the specimen. (From Hartley CJ, Strandness DE Jr. The effects of atherosclerosis on the transmission of ultrasound. *J Surg Res* 1969;9:575–582, with permission.)

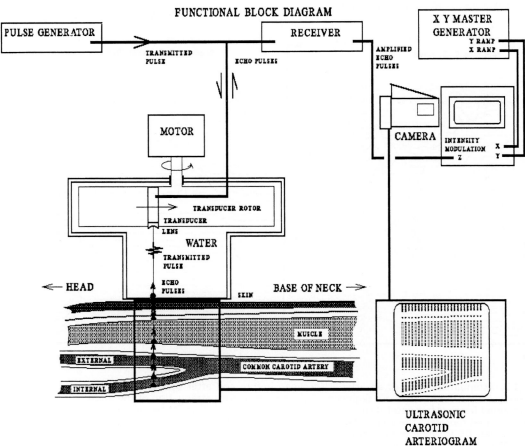

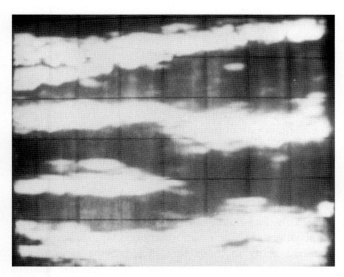

FIGURE 1.10. The crude image obtained of the carotid bifurcation with the system shown in Figure 1.12 was interpreted as showing a patent internal carotid artery. Using arteriography, the artery was found to be occluded.

The images created by this system were crude but did allow us to apply the device clinically and to begin the study of patients with carotid artery disease. One of the first patients evaluated is shown in Figure 1.10, which shows a longitudinal display of the carotid artery, with both the internal and external carotid arteries in view. In examining the image, it appeared that both the internal and external carotid arteries were patent. However, when an arteriogram was done, it was noted that the internal carotid artery was occluded. Obviously, the material that was occluding the vessel had similar acoustic properties as blood and could not be detected on the basis of image alone.

This failure of the B mode to detect a thrombus in the internal carotid artery represented a major problem that would have to be solved. From a clinical standpoint, it was not so important to know exactly what the material was; rather, it was important to know whether the vessel was open or occluded.

The most direct solution to the problem appeared to integrate the B-mode image with a Doppler system used as a flow detector to assess vessel patency. At this stage, we did not intend to use the Doppler for any other purpose. For this to work effectively, the Doppler would have to be incorporated into the system and not used as a stand-alone device. This single-patient study pointed out the need to combine imaging with Doppler, leading to the development of duplex scanning. These early results with duplex scanning were published by Barber and associates in 1974 (17,18). The concept was sim-

ple, but the integration of the two ultrasound modalities into a clinically usable transducer was a formidable problem that took considerable time and effort to solve.

After several methods were tested to integrate the two systems, it was elected to use a single-gate pulsed Doppler with the imaging component. With the single-gate system, the operator had sufficient liberty to assess flow velocity at any desired site within the vessel being interrogated.

FLOW VISUALIZATION AND VELOCITY PATTERNS

During the same time that the B-mode imaging and the embryonic duplex systems were being developed, we began working on a new concept of arterial visualization that we termed *ultrasonic arteriography*. The concept was simple and was based on the premise that, by using a pulsed Doppler system in conjunction with a position sensing arm, it should be possible to generate images of the interior of arteries at all points where flow was occurring (19,20) (Fig. 1.11). In practice, the user would be able to generate images of the arterial lumen by scanning an area of interest, such as the carotid bifurcation. An example of a normal carotid bifurcation is shown in Figure 1.12. This was an exciting development because it was the first time that the generation of images very similar to those seen on conventional arteriography was possible (Fig. 1.13).

When this type of system was developed, it was possible to generate additional data about the flow characteristics at the point in the artery being sampled. For example, the user had available the audio output to monitor the changes in flow as the transducer and the sample volume of the pulsed Doppler were moved within the vessel. This was important because, as areas of narrowing were encountered, the user could tell by the change in the frequency of the return signal where to direct his or her attention. Another advantage of the system was that the signal could also be recorded, providing a hard copy of the velocity pattern at the site of detection.

During the course of these studies and those with CW Doppler, we soon became aware of the fact that there were velocity patterns characteristic of various vascular beds that were of considerable interest. Many of these changes were characterized by McDonald in 1960 (21), whose landmark book *Blood Flow in Arteries* not only addressed the types of velocity patterns that could be expected but also dealt with the factors responsible for the changes that were noted in the flow to the different organs and vascular beds. For example, it was clear that, in vascular beds with a relatively high resistance under resting conditions (such as the legs),

FIGURE 1.9. This block diagram shows the prototype B-mode scanner that was built to provide information on the nature of the carotid arterial wall and changes that might have occurred secondary to atherosclerosis.

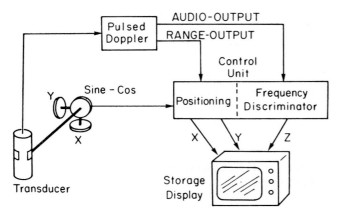

FIGURE 1.11. Block diagram of an ultrasonic arteriography system designed to use the Doppler effect together with a pulsed system to generate images of flow occurring within a vessel. (From Mozersky DJ, Hokanson DE, Sumner DS, et al. Ultrasonic visualization of the arterial lumen. *Surgery* 1972;72:253–259, with permission.)

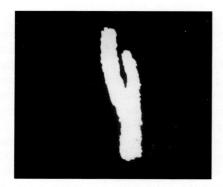

FIGURE 1.12. Ultrasonic arteriogram of a normal carotid bifurcation.

the velocity patterns routinely showed a triphasic flow response (Fig. 1.14). It was also clear that the waveform shape and its phasic characteristics could quickly be affected by a change in peripheral resistance. For example, in cases with a decrease in peripheral resistance, the reverse-flow component is lost and returns only when peripheral resistance returns to baseline levels (Fig. 1.15). For organs with low resistance at all times (brain, liver, kidney, and spleen), there is no reverse-flow component at any time in the heart cycle. This low resistance is accompanied by a high-volume flow rate and a high end-diastolic frequency in the velocity waveform (Fig. 1.16).

Many of these facts were appreciated early in our experience with ultrasound, but we did not have a good way of displaying the Doppler information. Our own experience spanned many methods that included the zero-crossing detector and off-line ultrasonographic spectral analysis (10,11). The most widely available method was the zero-crossing detector, which was inexpensive and could be used with most recording systems to portray the shape and directional characteristics of the velocity waveforms. It had so many disadvantages that it was a poor method to use (22). It required a very good signal-to-noise ratio, the output was amplitude dependent, and it often missed high-frequency, low-amplitude signals (Fig. 1.17). In addition, with mixed arterial and venous signals, the exact source of the signal could often be confusing.

Off-line spectral analysis was available in the 1970s and did provide additional information that was interesting but also confusing (10) (Fig. 1.18). Most of our early experience was with the Kay ultrasonograph, which permitted an off-line analysis of only a few heartbeats of information. As

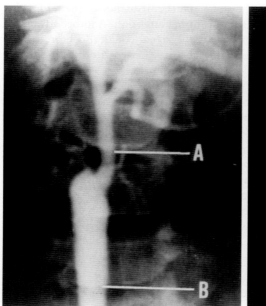

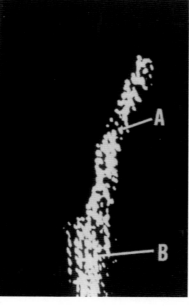

FIGURE 1.13. Ultrasonic arteriogram of an occluded internal carotid artery compared with the arteriographic appearance. (From Mozersky DJ, Hokanson DE, Sumner DS, et al. Ultrasonic visualization of the arterial lumen. *Surgery* 1972;72:253–259, with permission.)

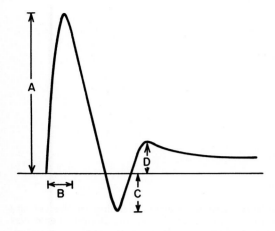

FIGURE 1.14. Diagrammatic representation of a velocity waveform with reverse diastolic flow, which is the type of waveform seen in vascular beds with a high resistance. Peak systolic velocity *(A)*, rise time *(B)*, diastolic reverse flow *(C)*, and diastolic forward flow *(D)*. (From Nicholls SC, Kohler TR, Martin RL, et al. Use of hemodynamic parameters in the diagnosis of mesenteric insufficiency. *J Vasc Surg* 1986;3:507–510, with permission.)

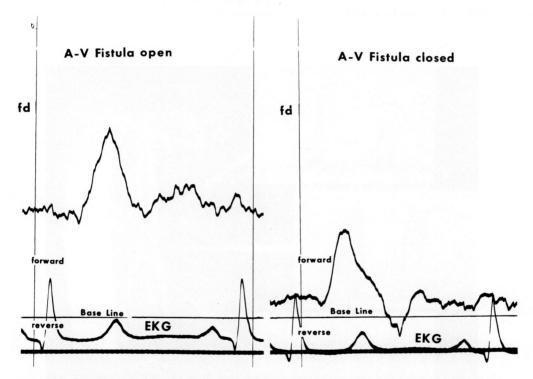

FIGURE 1.15. The velocity waveform on the *left* was taken proximal to an arteriovenous fistula showing the very high end-diastolic frequency. When the fistula is occluded, the high resistance to flow returns, and the waveform has the same characteristics as shown in Figure 1.14.

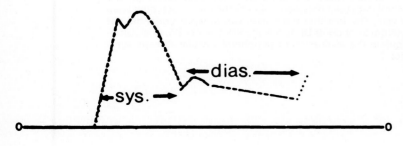

FIGURE 1.16. Diagrammatic representation of the type of velocity waveform pattern seen in arteries supplying organs of low resistance (e.g., brain, liver, kidney). Flow above the zero line occurs throughout the cardiac cycle, with high diastolic forward-flow velocities (e.g., carotid, celiac, renal arteries). Dias., diastole; sys., systole. (From Nicholls SC, Kohler TR, Martin RL, et al. Use of hemodynamic parameters in the diagnosis of mesenteric insufficiency. *J Vasc Surg* 1986;3:507–510, with permission.)

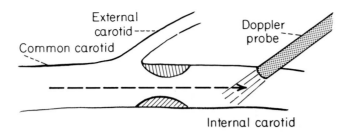

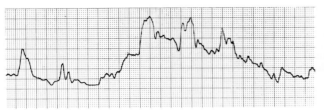

Velocity across the stenotic segment

FIGURE 1.17. A zero-crossing detector recording of the velocity changes seen at the time of operation as the Doppler beam was moved across the area of stenosis. The increase in velocity is noted, but a great deal of important information is lost with the zero-crossing detector method. This technique was clearly not suitable for velocity recordings.

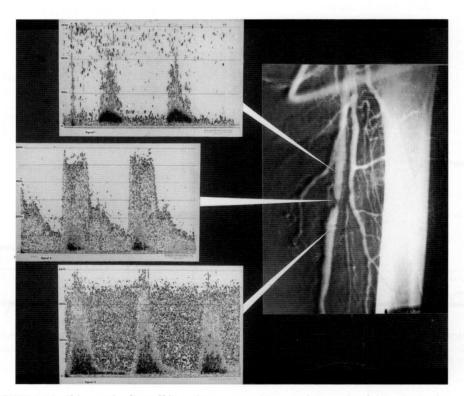

FIGURE 1.18. This was the first off-line ultrasonographic recording made of the velocity changes proximal to, in, and distal to a site of stenosis. These recordings were made on audiotape and were analyzed at a later time. The spectral data seen between pulses in the lower recording were undoubtedly the flow in the femoral vein. The fact that the system was nondirectional did not permit separation of the two signals. (From Strandness DE Jr, Schultz RD, Sumner DS, et al. Ultrasonic flow detection: a useful technique in the evaluation of peripheral vascular disease. *Am J Surg* 1967;113:311–320, with permission.)

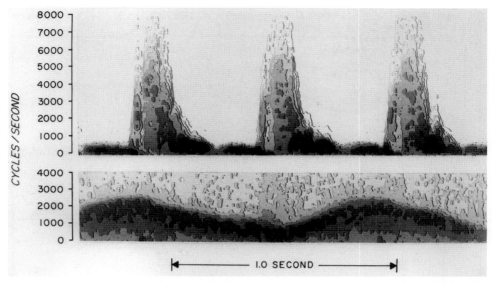

FIGURE 1.19. The ultrasonographic recordings were taken at different times from the femoral artery *(top)* and femoral vein *(bottom)*. The system could not be used to display directional information. This method had to be done off-line and could analyze only 2 seconds of data.

noted in Figure 1.19, there was a considerable amount of data portrayed over a dynamic range of 42 dB. It was not directional but did faithfully reproduce the contour of the waveform and its relationship to times in the cardiac cycle. The wide dynamic range provided a great deal of information, but we did not know what to make of it at the time. This was well before we were aware of the concept of spectral broadening and its significance.

Thus, when ultrasonic arteriography and the earliest phases of duplex scanning development were underway, the processing of the Doppler signal presented us with our biggest problems. We did not have an accurate and reproducible way of displaying all the information available in the velocity data we could obtain.

DEVELOPMENT OF THE FAST FOURIER TRANSFORMS METHOD

Once the feasibility of combining B-mode with pulsed Doppler became a reality, progress was rapid in the technologic phases of the electronics and transducer development. It then became possible to begin applying the device to patients (Fig. 1.20). The major advance in the signal processing was possible because of the assistance of the Honeywell Corporation. Dr. Ira Langenthal and Mr. James Gessert were able to develop for our use a real-time and online fast Fourier transforms (FFT) spectrum analyzer that could be adapted to the output of the pulsed

Doppler in the duplex scanner (23,24). This device was able to provide a total of 10 kHz of frequency shift data (7 kHz for the forward-flow and 3 kHz for the reverse-flow components) from the backscattered signal. For the first time, we had accurate displays of the Doppler data, and we were also able to begin to relate the velocity changes to the status of the arterial circulation at the sites

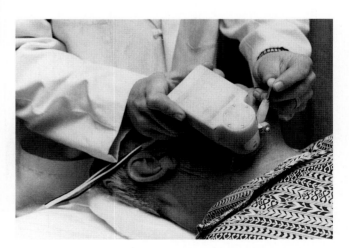

FIGURE 1.20. This was the scanhead used for the first prototype duplex scanner suitable for the study of large numbers of patients with carotid disease. The transducer was quite large, making it difficult to display the internal carotid artery high in the neck.

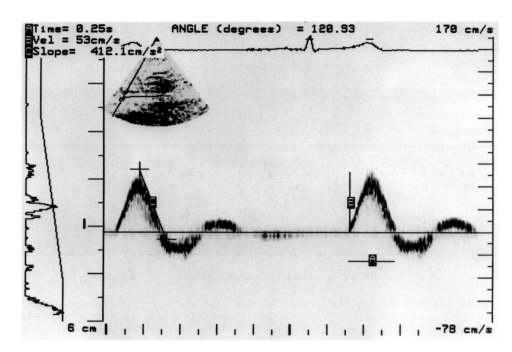

FIGURE 1.21. These velocity patterns were analyzed by the first fast Fourier transforms spectrum analyzer available for this purpose. This system was developed by James Gessert of Honeywell Corporation.

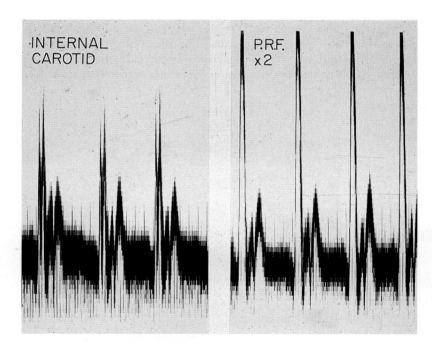

FIGURE 1.22. Fast Fourier analyzed spectra from the common carotid artery, demonstrating aliasing. On the left, there is foldover of the peak frequencies that is eliminated by doubling the pulse repetition frequency of the system. (From Strandness DE Jr. Doppler ultrasonic techniques in vascular disease. In: Bernstein EF, ed. *Noninvasive diagnostic techniques in vascular disease.* Vol. 2. St. Louis: CV Mosby, 1982:13, with permission.)

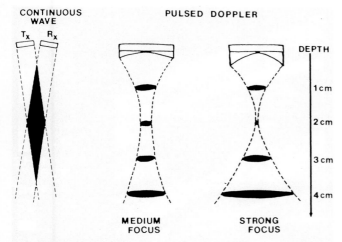

FIGURE 1.23. Diagram illustrating the areas that are insonated when one is using continuous wave (CW) and pulsed Doppler systems. A large sample volume may, in effect, act as a CW system if it is large enough to encompass the entire vessel lumen. For the carotid artery, as small a sample volume as possible should be used. (From Knox RA, Phillips DJ, Breslau PJ, et al. Empirical findings relating sample volume size to diagnostic accuracy in pulsed Doppler cerebrovascular studies. *J Clin Ultrasound* 1982;10:227–232, with permission.)

of interrogation. Some examples of these early outputs are shown in Figure 1.21.

Additional problems that were not immediately recognized needed attention and solutions. The dual capacity of the pulsed Doppler in both transmitting and receiving placed limits on the frequencies that could be displayed. With a pulsed system, the maximal frequency that can be displayed is less than half the pulse transmitting frequency. This is referred to as the *Nyquist limit*. If the peak frequencies encountered exceed that limit, they "flip over" and are displayed on the reverse-flow side of the spectral display. This is referred to as *aliasing*. If this fact is not recognized, it can be confusing to the user. An example is shown in Figure 1.22.

Another problem that caused us a great deal of difficulty until we recognized it and its importance was related to the shape and size of the sample volume produced by the pulsed Doppler (25). If one is interested in examining very discrete areas within an artery, the sample volume size should be as small as possible (26). For example, if the sample size is the same as the width of the vessel being examined, the data obtained would be the same as those obtained using a CW Doppler. Early in our work, we found that, for discrete measurements such as in the carotid artery, a sample volume size of 3 mm³ was adequate to describe the important local velocity changes in arriving at accurate information with regard to spectral broadening at the site of interrogation (Fig. 1.23).

COLOR DOPPLER DUPLEX SCANNING

One of the major disadvantages of standard "black and white" duplex scanning is that the lumen of the vessel and its course may often be difficult to identify in some locations and under some circumstances. For example, if the carotid artery was always parallel to the skin and followed a prescribed anatomic direction, the problem would be simple. However, it is well known that the extracranial carotid artery may follow an unusual course, with a bulb that varies in size and configuration. In addition, there is always the possibility that the internal carotid artery may have a kink or loop that is difficult to follow by the image alone. The experienced technologist who is aware of this fact can use the pulsed Doppler to aid in the search, but it is often difficult.

The problem can be even more difficult for vessels that are deeply placed, and image quality is less than that obtained from those vessels that are more superficially placed. Examples are found in the abdomen, where localization of arteries such as the celiac, superior mesenteric, and renal may be difficult to separate from echoes arising from surrounding soft tissue. In these cases, exact localization of the arteries may require considerable searching using the knowledge concerning their location and the pulsed Doppler to identify flow.

To overcome some of these difficulties, several approaches have been used. The first, as noted earlier, was to generate an "image" of flow by generating dots within the lumen at every point where the velocity shift exceeded a certain preset limit. This was done using both CW and pulsed Doppler systems. One of the first to generate a flow image using color was the CW system developed and employed by Curry and White (27). In this system, normal velocities were portrayed in one color, with the moderate and high velocities coded in two different colors. This had the advantages of not only seeing where flow was occurring but also providing information on how fast the blood was moving and the sites where narrowing had developed. One of the drawbacks of that approach was the fact that the scanning procedure had to be done manually in the manner required for the ultrasonic arteriography method developed by Mozersky and associates (19) mentioned earlier in this chapter. These systems filled an important role at the time but are no longer in use.

What was needed was a method that would display in real-time the flow within the vessel in color. The credit for developing the first (1978) color systems that took advantage of combining B-mode imaging and flow goes to Brandestini and Forster (28). Their multichannel system displayed velocity information in the B-mode field of data. This was used later by Eyer and coworkers (29) in a duplex system. The first commercial system to accomplish this was produced by the Quantum Corporation of Issaquah, Washington. This system generated the real-time monochrome B-mode display in a conventional manner by amplitude detection of returned echoes from tissue (30). This would generate a gray-scale value for the amplitude of the return echoes.

The color flow component of the system worked by analyzing the phase changes between echoes from each ultrasound scan line. About 10 pulses are required to obtain one line of color flow information. The axial resolution of the color flow information is the same as that obtained for the B-mode information. The hue and intensity of the color are determined by the direction and magnitude of the Doppler-shifted signal. In practice, flow receding from the transducer is assigned the color red, with that occurring toward the transducer appearing blue. The choice of colors is arbitrary, but because arteries are red and veins are blue by convention, this is employed in all color systems on the market. The B-mode and Doppler information are updated about 18 times per second, giving the impression of a real-time display (Fig. 1.24).

In addition to color-coding the magnitude and direction of the velocity changes, it is possible to record the absolute frequency shifts or angle-adjusted velocity by using the standard single-sample volume approach used in the conventional scanners. It is important that the measurement of the velocity patterns be done with the FFT spectrum analyzer because the use of color alone tends to underestimate the magnitude of the frequency shift. With the color display and analysis method used, the rapid return and display of the velocity data do not permit the use of the FFT method of spectral analysis. Autocorrelation is used most commonly, whereby each echo is compared with the one from the preceding pulse. This determines the motion of the sampled red blood cells that has occurred within the sample interval. At least three pulses are needed to determine the direction and magnitude of the velocity change. From this, a value for mean flow is produced but will be lower than that seen by FFT analysis of the same signals (31).

The major use of color is as a pathfinder for the technologist. It tells the examiner exactly where the flow stream is and where suspected areas of narrowing might be located. The advantages of color flow can be summarized as follows (32):

1. Color flow provides an immediate presentation of the location, direction, and "apparent" velocity of flow.
2. The color flow image tells the examiner where to place the sample volume for precise determination of the velocity change to be recorded.

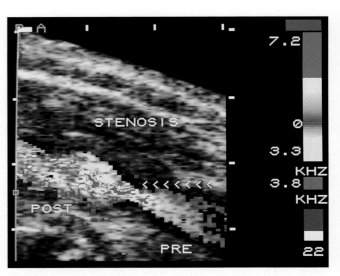

FIGURE 1.24. Color display of a tight stenosis in the internal carotid artery. In the stenotic segment, the velocity is increased and marked with a green tag, signifying that the velocity has exceeded 3.8 kHz. In the poststenotic region, there is an admixture of colors, suggesting poststenotic turbulence.

3. Color flow provides an appreciation of flow disturbances and perhaps a qualitative estimate of their magnitude.

Some limitations of the color flow method are extremely important to recognize. These can be summarized as follows (32):

1. Color flow images have a relatively low spatial resolution as compared with gray-scale presentations.
2. The frame rate is relatively low.
3. Averaging is done to increase the frame rate.
4. Aliasing occurs at relatively low pulse repetition frequencies. This may be difficult for the inexperienced operator to recognize immediately in the real-time display. An example of aliasing in a color display is shown in Figures 1.25 and 1.26.
5. Some degradation of the B-mode imaging is necessary to optimize the color display.
6. The velocity changes demonstrated by the hue of the colors tend to underestimate the actual velocity changes that are taking place.
7. The power requirements are higher than those needed for gray-scale presentations.

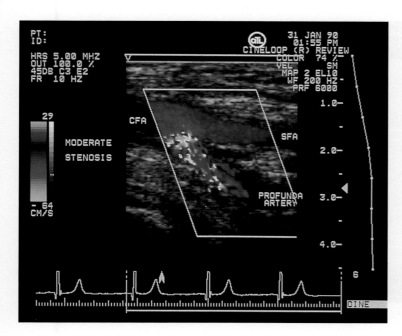

FIGURE 1.25. In this example of a stenosis in the profunda femoris artery, it appears that flow in the jet is moving in a reverse direction by the blue color displayed. This is not the case, but it clearly illustrates how aliasing can develop in a color display.

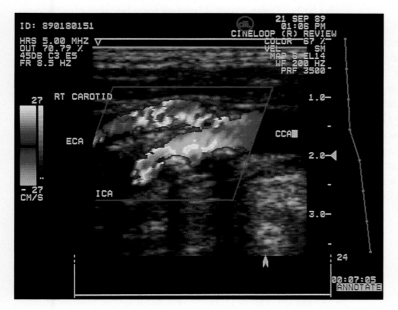

FIGURE 1.26. Aliasing is clearly seen in this scan showing stenoses of both the internal and external carotid arteries.

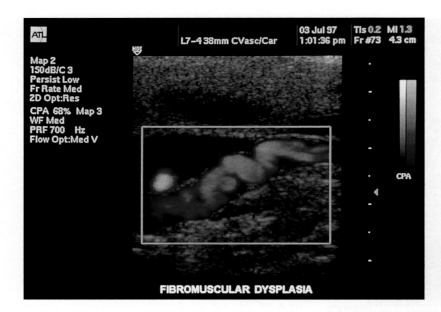

FIGURE 1.27. Power Doppler display of fibromuscular dysplasia of the renal artery. The string of beads, which is characteristic of this disease, is demonstrated clearly in this example. However, it is not often possible to get this type of display.

POWER DOPPLER

The ability to display the integrated power of the Doppler signal resulted in a display that was independent of angle and not effected by aliasing. Examining organ perfusion in organs such as the kidney and liver also became possible. This new power Doppler display has the potential for higher sensitivity to flow, better edge detection, and better depiction of the continuity of flow (Fig. 1.27). Although it has not resulted in a major advance in the diagnostic capability of ultrasonic duplex scanning, it has proved to be a very useful addition to the application of color Doppler. There are circumstances covered in this book in which it has provided very useful additional information (32–35).

CLINICAL APPLICATIONS

When duplex scanning was first developed, it was designed for use only in the carotid circulation for the following reasons: (a) the carotid artery was of major clinical importance and accessible to ultrasound imaging methods because of its close proximity to the skin surface, (b) all the details with regard to the transmitting frequency used (5 MHz) were designed for vessels close to the skin, and (c) arteriographic confirmation of the results with the duplex scanner was readily available. We would, on occasion, attempt to investigate other vessels, such as the femoral artery, but a serious look at other vascular beds had to await improvements in transducer design and the availability of a range of transmitting frequencies. The remaining chapters of this book deal with the specific applications as they have evolved since the 1980s as the technology has improved and as the vascular beds of great clinical interest have become more accessible to this form of energy.

It is apparent that the application of duplex ultrasonic methods has far exceeded any of our early expectations. There are no blood vessels of clinical interest that cannot now be reached. The vascular laboratory is now the first stop for nearly all suspected vascular problems and the final stop when the results of therapy need to be assessed. In addition, the method can now provide natural history data that were not available in the past.

REFERENCES

1. Winsor T. Influence of arterial disease on the systolic blood gradients of the extremity. *Am J Med Sci* 1950;220:117–126.
2. Strandness DE Jr, Bell JW. Peripheral vascular disease: diagnosis and objective evaluation using a mercury strain gauge. *Ann Surg* 1965;[Suppl]:61.
3. Yao JST, Hobbs JT, Irvine WT. Ankle systolic pressure measurements in arterial disease affecting the lower extremities. *Br J Surg* 1969;56:676–679.
4. Strandness DE Jr. The role of physiologic testing in postoperative evaluation and follow–up. In: Strandness DE Jr, ed. *Peripheral arterial disease.* Boston: Little, Brown, 1969:163–193.
5. Whitney RJ. The measurement of volume changes in the human limbs. *J Physiol (Lond)* 1953;121:1–27.
6. Sumner DS, Strandness DE Jr. The relationship between calf blood flow and ankle blood pressure in patients with intermittent claudication. *Surgery* 1969;65:763–771.
7. Barendsen GJ. Plethysmography. In: Verstraete M, ed. *Methods in angiology.* The Hague: Martinus Nijhoff, 1980:38–92.
8. Satomura S. Study of flow patterns in peripheral arteries by ultrasonics. *J Acoust Soc Jpn* 1959;15:151–158.
9. Rushmer RF, Baker DW, Stegall HF. Transcutaneous Doppler

flow as a nondestructive technique. *J Appl Physiol* 1966;2: 554–566.

10. Strandness DE Jr, Schultz RD, Sumner DS, et al. Ultrasonic flow detection: a useful technique in the evaluation of peripheral vascular disease. *Am J Surg* 1967;113:311–320.

11. Strandness DE Jr, McCutcheon EP, Rushmer RF. Application of a transcutaneous Doppler flowmeter in evaluation of occlusive arterial disease. *Surg Gynecol Obstet* 1966;122:1039–1045.

12. Strandness DE Jr, Sumner DS. Measurement of blood flow. In: *Hemodynamics for surgeons*. New York: Grune & Stratton, 1975: 3:31–46.

13. McLeod FD Jr. Progress report, directional Doppler blood flow meter. May 1969, NRG 33-010-074, Cornell University.

14. Nippa JH, Hokanson DE, Lee DR, et al. Phase rotation for separating forward and reverse blood velocity signals. *IEEE Trans Sonics Ultrasonics* 1975;SU-22:340–346.

15. Baker DW. Pulsed ultrasonic Doppler blood flow sensing. *IEEE Trans Biomed Eng* 1970;17:170–185.

16. Hartley CJ, Strandness DE Jr. The effects of atherosclerosis on the transmission of ultrasound. *J Surg Res* 1969;9:575–582.

17. Barber FE, Baker DW, Nation AWC, et al. Ultrasonic duplex echo Doppler scanner. *IEEE Trans Biomed Eng* 1974;21: 109–113.

18. Barber FE, Baker DW, Strandness DE Jr, et al. Duplex scanner II for simultaneous imaging of artery tissues and flow. *Ultrasonics Symposium Proc IEEE* 1974;74CH0896-ISU.

19. Mozersky DJ, Hokanson DE, Baker DS, et al. Ultrasonic arteriography. *Arch Surg* 1971;103:663–667.

20. Mozersky DJ, Hokanson DE, Sumner DS, et al. Ultrasonic visualization of the arterial lumen. *Surgery* 1972;72:253–259.

21. McDonald DA. *Blood flow in arteries*. Baltimore: Williams & Wilkins, 1960.

22. Reneman RS, Spencer MP. Local Doppler audio spectra in normal and stenosed carotid arteries in man. *Ultrasound Med Biol* 1979;5:1–11.

23. Phillips DJ, Powers JE, Eyer MK, et al. Detection of peripheral vascular disease using the duplex scanner III. *Ultrasound Med Biol* 1980;6:205–218.

24. Strandness DE Jr. Doppler ultrasonic techniques in vascular disease. In: Bernstein EF, ed. *Noninvasive diagnostic techniques in vascular disease*. Vol. 2. St. Louis: CV Mosby, 1982:13.

25. Knox RA, Phillips DJ, Breslau PJ, et al. Empirical findings relating sample volume size to diagnostic accuracy in pulsed Doppler cerebrovascular studies. *J Clin Ultrasound* 1982;10:227–232.

26. Breslau PJ. *Ultrasonic duplex scanning in the evaluation of carotid artery disease*. Thesis. University of Maastricht, The Netherlands, 1981:46–50.

27. Curry GR, White DN. Color coded ultrasonic differential velocity scanner (echoflow). *Ultrasound Med Biol* 1978;4;27–35.

28. Brandestini MA, Forster FK. Blood flow imaging using a discrete-time frequency analyzer. *Ultrasonics Symp Proc IEEE* Ch 1344 SU, 1978:287–293.

29. Eyer MK, Brandestini MA, Phillips DJ, et al. Color digital echo/Doppler image presentation. *Ultrasound Med Biol* 1973;7;21–31.

30. Zierler RE, Phillips DJ, Beach KW, et al. Noninvasive assessment of normal carotid bifurcation hemodynamics with color-flow ultrasonic imaging. *Ultrasound Med Biol* 1987;13:471–476.

31. Beach KW. 1975-2000: A quarter century of ultrasound technology. *Ultrasound Med Biol* 1992;18:377–388.

32. Hamper UM, DeJong MTR, Caskey CI, et al. Power Doppler imaging: clinical experience and correlation with color Doppler US and other imaging modalities. *Radiographics* 1997;17:499–513.

33. Steinke W, Reis S, Artemis N, et al. Power Doppler imaging of carotid artery stenosis: comparison with color Doppler imaging and arteriography. *Stroke* 1997;10:1981–1987.

34. Mariinoli C, Pretolesi F, Crespi G, et al. Power Doppler sonography: clinical applications. *Eur J Radiol* 1998;2:133–140.

35. Nicholls SC, Kohler TR, Martin RL, et al. Use of hemodynamic parameters in the diagnosis of mesenteric insufficiency. *J Vasc Surg* 1986;3:507–510.

2

TRADITIONAL METHODS OF PATIENT EVALUATION

Patients traditionally enter the health care delivery system because of a set of symptoms and signs that seem serious enough to them to warrant further evaluation. When the patients appear in the physician's office, they are questioned and examined, with the results determining the ultimate course of events. In some cases, a brief examination provides enough information to dictate a further course of action, but many times, more data are required to make that decision.

Physicians are taught to recognize patterns that not only suggest which organ system is involved but also indicate the potential gravity of the situation. Vascular disease produces problems caused by an interference with either delivery of blood to tissue or its return to the right side of the heart. In some cases, such as with aneurysms of the abdominal aorta or the peripheral arteries, the symptoms and signs may be related to either the aneurysm itself, disruption of the wall, sudden thrombotic occlusion, or embolization of its contents to the lower limb. Finally, the clinical presentation may be dictated by an event at a site removed from the disease itself. This is most clearly evident in the case of emboli to the brain with carotid artery disease and pulmonary emboli from sites within the deep venous system—usually the leg.

Before performing any of the duplex scanning testing procedures, it is important to review the presenting complaints and to include that information with the written assessments of the test results. This is an important and necessary exercise because it provides a basis for the test being done and its proper interpretation. The first encounter with the patient is usually the essential step that will determine outcome. An error made at this time may be catastrophic if it leads to the wrong diagnosis, workup, and treatment.

In this chapter, the major factors we consider when evaluating patients to determine the diagnosis and treatment are reviewed. At the same time, the limitations of the history and physical examination are stressed. Those situations are emphasized in which more information is essential for both the diagnosis and management. To separate the entities in a reasonable and practical manner, acute situations are presented first and the chronic conditions later.

ACUTE VASCULAR EMERGENCIES

What is a vascular emergency? Simply defined, it is a situation the outcome of which can be reasonably defined in terms of the time required to correct the situation before irreversible tissue changes will occur. One would think that these instances would be instantly recognized and acted on, but such is not always the case. Delays in recognition and treatment are more common than we would like to see, often with a disastrous outcome. In the following sections, our approaches to these problems will be reviewed. Emphasis is placed on those situations in which immediate action is required, the types of tests that may be warranted to make the diagnosis, and the importance of the diagnosis in terms of management.

ACUTE ARTERIAL OCCLUSION

Acute arterial occlusion occurs by three mechanisms: embolism, thrombosis, or mechanical injury of the vessel. The cause of the interruption in flow becomes important in the diagnostic tests used and in the management, but not in the recognition of the ischemia and its potential gravity.

When the physician first sees the patient, there are only two basic questions that need an immediate answer: Is there acute arterial occlusion? Is limb viability in question? If the answer to both questions is yes, then time is of the essence because immediate correction of the occlusion becomes absolutely essential if the limb is to be preserved.

The ischemic limb is usually described in terms of the five "Ps": pallor, pain, paresthesias, pulselessness, and paralysis. I should like to add another "P," which is the physician, the critical person in arriving at the correct appreciation of the presenting complaints. By definition, the onset is abrupt, with the patient noting a change from a previous state dramatic enough to warrant a visit to the physician. The site at which the symptoms are first noted is the most distal part of the limb. This is because the point farthest away from the source of the blood—the heart—is the first to suffer when the arterial supply is suddenly interrupted.

Subjectively, the patient will first note the appearance of pain, coldness of the foot or hand, and paresthesias. When this occurs, the blood flow drops to such a low level that the foot or hand becomes pale.

If the pain persists, this is a favorable sign, indicating that the nerves supplying the distal limb are still capable of providing the warning messages to the brain. If the nerve function is preserved, this is certain evidence that the tissue subserved by these nerves is also viable. If the pain disappears, it has two meanings, one ominous, the other favorable. If the nerves have lost their ability to transmit the ischemic stimuli to the brain, it means they must have their blood supply restored, and quickly, if the other tissues are to survive. The time interval during which limb viability begins to be irreversibly lost is in the range of 4 to 6 hours. If the blood flow is not restored within this time frame, tissue loss will be almost certain, the extent of which will depend on the level and extent of the occlusion. It is important to emphasize that the limb dies from the inside out—the nerves, then the muscle, and finally the skin.

The pain immediately experienced may also disappear because of the opening of the collateral circulation and restoration of blood flow, albeit at reduced levels, yet sufficient to maintain tissue viability. If this is, in fact, the case, time may not be such an important element in deciding what course of action should be taken.

At this stage, the physical examination will provide supporting evidence for the diagnosis and estimation of the gravity of the situation. Limbs that are immediately threatened are cold, pale, and unable to appreciate light touch in the ischemic areas. Pulse deficits are invariably present with one important exception. This is when there have been extensive microemboli to the distal foot or hand. In this circumstance, the major arteries are usually patent and serve as conduits for the atheroemboli that usually arise from ulcerated plaques or areas of thrombosis at some point proximal to the foot and toes (1) (Fig. 2.1).

Major pulse deficits provide information only on the most proximal site of the occlusion. They provide no information on the possible distal extension of the thrombotic process.

A detailed history with regard to the status of the other limb is important. If the patient gives a history of intermittent claudication and this can be verified by a pulse deficit, this is suggestive evidence that the patient has chronic occlusive arterial disease, with the current acute episode representing an acute thrombosis in the region of a high-grade stenosis. In the course of the physical examination, it is always important to look for the presence of a popliteal aneurysm that can thrombose and release emboli, which can be a cause of acute ischemia.

In patients who have palpable pulses to the level of the foot and appear to have microemboli as the cause of the ischemia, it is very important to look for bruits from the level of the abdominal aorta to the popliteal fossa. Very few

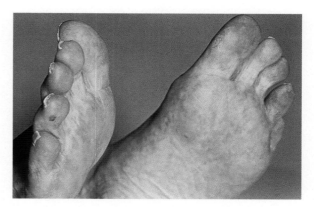

FIGURE 2.1. When patients develop microemboli that pass to the plantar and digital arteries, the appearance of the foot may be a useful clue. The patient in this figure had embolized cholesterol crystals in both feet. He presented with pain, coolness, and the very prominent livido reticularis pattern. Transmetatarsal amputations were required to control the pain. The cholesterol crystals seen by polarized light were the cause of the arterial occlusion and ischemia.

physicians regularly listen over the superficial femoral and popliteal artery for bruits, and this is a mistake. The presence of a bruit provides the following information: (a) the location of an area of narrowing, (b) the patency of the vessels distal to the site of the bruit (bruits are transmitted downstream from their site of origin, not upstream), and (c) possibly the site of an ulcerated plaque that is the source of the microemboli.

The causes of acute ischemia in the upper extremity are similar to those found in the leg. However, there are obvious differences that need to be remembered, particularly in terms of etiology. Atherosclerosis of the arteries supplying the arm is very rare, except for the first part of the subclavian followed by involvement of the innominate artery. Thus, acute ischemia secondary to thrombosis of an atherosclerotic plaque is very unusual. The principal causes of acute ischemia are secondary to emboli, which most often arise from the chambers on the left side of the heart. Another infrequent cause is release of emboli from a damaged subclavian artery at the thoracic outlet. Chronic compression of the subclavian artery can lead to intimal damage with subsequent thrombosis and release of emboli. In our institution, this is seen about once or twice a year. These events most typically occur in younger patients who are in good health. Thus, in any patient who suddenly develops acute ischemia of the hand, damage to the subclavian artery from repeated compression injury must be kept in mind.

Other causes of acute hand ischemia are to be found with those disorders that produce Raynaud's syndrome. These include Buerger's disease, scleroderma, and mixed connective tissue disorders. These patients give a history of sensitivity to cold with the typical triphasic color response on exposure to cold. The fingers turn white (the "dead fin-

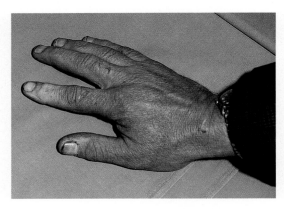

FIGURE 2.2. This patient had the secondary form of Raynaud's syndrome with the ischemia confined to one finger secondary to digital artery occlusion. In the primary form of the disorder, the cold sensitivity is found in all 10 fingers.

ger"), followed by cyanosis, which terminates in the fingers turning red (Fig. 2.2). Although this clinical syndrome is usually a chronic problem, there are cases in which acute thrombosis of the digital and palmar arteries can lead to acute ischemia and gangrene. The most common condition in my experience that leads to this problem is scleroderma (Fig. 2.3).

In addition to the history and physical examination, a survey with the continuous wave (CW) Doppler followed by duplex scanning can be very useful in determining the site of the occlusion. The survey must include the examination of the axillary, brachial, radial, and ulnar arteries. It is also useful to listen to the pads of the fingertips because this may provide a clue as to the extent of the occlusion and its effects on both collateral inflow to the hand and the extent of the perfusion to the fingers themselves. It is very important to listen to the flow patterns from comparable sites in the other arm and hand. This provides information on the nature of the velocity patterns and the extent to which flow may be reduced. It is very important to measure the digit

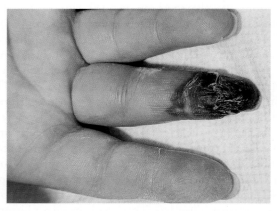

FIGURE 2.3. Patients with scleroderma may develop spontaneous gangrene of a portion of fingers or toes. This is a result of extensive thrombosis of the digital arteries.

systolic pressure. If signals are heard at the tip of the finger, the CW Doppler can be used. If no signals are heard, the photoplethysmograph (PPG) will have to be used. This is very important baseline information to follow the outcome of therapy.

Diagnostic and Therapeutic Strategies

Limb-threatening Ischemia: Lower Extremity

Under these circumstances, it is absolutely necessary to move with dispatch and not waste time trying further to evaluate the location and extent of the arterial occlusion. It is imperative that the occlusion be corrected as soon as possible. Any further diagnostic testing must be done without delaying the patient's trip to the operating room. This means, of course, that, as soon as the diagnosis of limb-threatening ischemia is made, a vascular surgeon must be notified promptly and the patient prepared for immediate transfer to the operating room, where the occlusion can be corrected.

The only noninvasive testing that should be carried out at this time is a survey with the CW Doppler and measurement of the ankle systolic blood pressure. How should this be added to the examination, and what information can be obtained (2)?

The arterial velocity patterns should be noted at the same sites on both limbs and include the common femoral artery, proximal to distal superficial femoral artery, the popliteal artery, and the tibial arteries at the ankle. There are three findings of value:

1. The finding of a triphasic signal indicates that the arterial inflow to this level is normal.
2. The presence of a monophasic signal signifies the presence of significant arterial disease proximal to the examination site.
3. The absence of a velocity signal has different potential meanings, depending on the site. If there are no detectable flow signals from the major proximal arteries (popliteal to the external iliac), this is almost certain evidence that these arteries are occluded. The failure to detect flow from the tibial and peroneal arteries at the level of the ankle must be interpreted in a different manner. Although they may in fact be occluded, the collateral input around more proximal occlusions may be so poor that the flow is below the detectable limit of the CW velocity detector (the lower limit of detectable flow is about 4 cm/sec).

The presence of detectable blood flow at the level of the ankle from the tibial-peroneal arteries signifies that the collateral circulation is generally adequate to maintain perfusion to the foot. As might be expected, the amount contributed by the collateral circulation varies and cannot be quantified. The absence of detectable flow may be a more ominous finding. Even if the foot appears viable under these circumstances, it warrants very close watching over the ensuing several hours. If flow returns to the tibial arteries during this period, the collateral circulation is improving.

If the ankle systolic pressure can be measured, the absolute value is of importance in assessing the status of the collateral circulation. In this circumstance, a pressure above 50 mm Hg is reassuring because it signifies that the collateral circulation is adequate and will tend to improve. Systolic pressures below this level should be considered warning signs that perfusion is marginal, and the limb should be considered in the potentially threatened category.

Finally, what about arteriography in the radiology suite? This should not be done in the patient with limb-threatening ischemia. All it accomplishes in this setting is to delay the patient's trip to the operating room. The surgical approach will be dictated by the highest level of occlusion and its possible etiology. Furthermore, an arteriogram can be done in the operating room without delaying the restoration of flow. The actual strategies used by vascular surgeons in restoring flow are beyond the scope of this volume.

Limb-threatening Ischemia: Upper Extremity

Many of the principles relating to the evaluation of acute ischemia of the hands are similar to those employed for the lower limb. The interpretation of the symptoms of pain, paresthesias, pallor, pulselessness, and paralysis requires the same vigorous and rapid evaluation. The finding of normal Doppler signals at the level of the wrist indicates that the cause of the ischemia is likely to be found in either the palmar or digital arteries. The presence of abnormal signals in either the radial or ulnar arteries is certain evidence of a proximal stenosis or occlusion. However, the presence of flow at that level of the circulation indicates that the collateral circulation may be adequate for limb survival but tells the examiner little about the extent to which function would be impaired if nothing further is done. In general, if one finds flow in the arteries at the level of the wrist during the acute episode, it is likely that with time, the circulation will improve even further. However, one must not use these findings to propose nonoperative therapy unless there are coexisting medical problems that make this an undesirable approach. In cases in which nonoperative therapy is chosen, it is important to follow the course of collateral development by the measurement of either wrist or finger blood pressures. As the collateral circulation improves, the systolic pressure will increase.

In cases with severe ischemia in which time is of the essence, one may proceed directly to the operating room, particularly if the etiology of the acute occlusion is thought to be secondary to emboli from a cardiac source. On the other hand, if the cause is thought to be secondary to emboli from the subclavian artery at the thoracic outlet, arteriography at some stage in the workup may be neces-

sary. Duplex scanning is good for detecting stenotic or occluded subclavian arteries but may not be good enough to show small areas of intimal injury that may be present. In this setting, the surgical correction of the problem may be in two stages. The first is to remove the occluding thrombi from the brachial, radial, and ulnar arteries, which may be followed at a later time with repair of the subclavian artery at the site of chronic injury.

Non–Limb-threatening Ischemia

By definition, the limbs in this category will survive, even if nothing is done to correct the occlusion that brought the patient to the hospital. This does not, of course, mean that nothing is to be done. It simply means that we are no longer working against the clock in terms of restoring flow. In this circumstance, it is often important to obtain as much information as possible before instituting therapy. Because time is not as critical, it may be possible to consider forms of therapy other than surgery, such as fibrinolytic therapy, to remove the offending occlusion.

Traditionally, other than the use of the CW Doppler as indicated previously, arteriography is generally considered the next step. This permits an accurate delineation of the site of occlusion and may direct the treating physician to the form of therapy to be used. Duplex scanning is becoming the next study, because in most cases, it dictates the type of therapy to be employed.

With the greater application of cardiopulmonary bypass and the use of intraaortic balloon pumping, we are seeing more patients with ischemic limbs, for which the exact underlying cause may not be clear. Because these patients are very ill, arteriography is usually not feasible. In this setting, duplex scanning can be of great value. It may be possible to find the cause of the ischemia without resorting to arteriography. The types of situation in which duplex scanning may be of great value include the following:

1. It is possible with the balloon pump in place to survey not only the iliac arteries but also those distal to the inguinal ligament. If, before insertion of the balloon pump, ankle/arm indices (AAIs) had been measured, they can be remeasured to give objective evidence of what transpired leading to the acute change in perfusion.
2. False aneurysms are becoming an important complication of not only coronary arteriography and angioplasty but can also be observed after removal of the balloon pump. In this circumstance, it is possible not only to make the diagnosis by duplex scanning but also to use duplex scanning as a form of therapy. Many of these lesions can be injected with thrombin under ultrasound guidance to thrombose the aneurysm.
3. Because the status of the runoff arteries below the knee may be the key to success or failure of any therapeutic

attempt, knowledge of their status is of great importance. Duplex scanning can be of great assistance in these cases.

CHRONIC (NON–LIMB-THREATENING) ISCHEMIA

Lower Limb

Patients with chronic ischemia of the lower limb are by far the most common and constitute the major referrals to the vascular laboratory. They generally present with exercise-induced leg pain of varying severity. The most common patients are those with intermittent claudication, but an increasing number of patients with nonvascular causes of leg pain are also referred for evaluation. These latter patients are generally lumped into the category of the "pseudoclaudication" syndrome, with the cause of their leg pain due to neural and orthopedic problems.

The history given by the patient in most cases may be sufficient to make the diagnosis. The patient who has true intermittent claudication will have a walk-pain-rest cycle that is constant from day to day (3). The walking distance required to bring on the pain and the time required for it to disappear are consistent every time the patient tries to walk. The pain is never brought on by standing or sitting, and the patient never has to lie down to obtain pain relief. In addition, the pain is brought on much sooner by any activity that increases the workload. For example, walking up a hill or stairs is always more difficult.

The patient who has nonvascular causes for the leg pain will have a walk-pain cycle that is not constant from day to day (4). The patient will have good days and bad days. In addition, it is not unusual for the pain to be brought on by standing or sitting for prolonged periods of time. The patient may also have to lie down to obtain complete relief.

The major items to be looked for on the physical examination are bruits and pulse deficits, which are the hallmarks of arterial stenosis and occlusion. It should be noted that the level of the pulse deficits might provide an important clue to the basis of the leg pain. In my practice, I use the following guidelines in evaluating a patient:

1. The most common site for pain to develop with exercise is in the calf muscles. This is true even when the level of disease is proximal to the major muscle groups of the thigh and buttock.
2. When the pain develops at other sites, it is usually similar to pain in the calf.
3. The level of pulse deficit is a good marker for the most proximal level of involvement but little else. For example, if there is a normal femoral pulse, but nothing distal to that point, one can be certain that the superficial femoral artery is narrowed or occluded, but it tells one nothing about the status of the arterial system distal to that level.

4. Bruits, when detected, radiate downstream from their origin and not proximally. It is good practice to listen not only over the abdominal aorta, iliac, and common femoral arteries but also over the superficial femoral and popliteal arteries.
5. A patient who has a good history of intermittent claudication and has normal foot pulses invariably has a stenotic lesion, which is usually found in the iliac artery. The clue is, of course, the presence of a bruit, which is usually elicited at rest and may be accentuated after exercise when flow is increased through the area of narrowing (5).
6. When the disease is confined to the arteries below the knee, the claudication that may occur is generally very mild.
7. When the patient complains of instep claudication, it is nearly always secondary to Buerger's disease. This symptom is very rarely seen with chronic occlusive disease secondary to atherosclerosis.

Guidelines for Severity

When a patient appears with true intermittent claudication, it is important to determine how severe the problem is and the impact it is having on the patient's life. This is quite simple in two situations—when walking even short distances is a problem, and when the claudication interferes with one's occupation. These situations are usually quite clear because the patient will often go to great lengths to get improvement, which may include agreeing to have surgery performed to correct the abnormality.

The most commonly used term to define severe claudication is *lifestyle limiting*, which covers nearly all bases. Let me illustrate this with an example. I was asked to see an executive of a large manufacturing firm for the problem of bilateral calf claudication. The workup showed that the basis for the leg pain was bilateral superficial femoral artery occlusions. Because the patient's job did not involve a great deal of walking, this posed no problem for a period of 10 years before retirement. During this time, the disease had not progressed; however, within 6 months of retiring, the patient was back to see me, literally demanding that something be done. Now, because of his need for more exercise and his love of doing it, his claudication had become an important issue. Because of his insistence, above-the-knee bilateral vein grafts were done, which gave him immediate relief and a good long-term result. If, during his time of employment, he had been a postman, it is very likely that these operative procedures would have been done much sooner to permit him to continue working.

As one will immediately note, these are, in many respects, very subjective criteria that do not lend themselves to critical analysis. They depend on the patient's perception of the problem and its impact on his or her life.

Methods of Assessment

As with every other patient problem dealing with the arterial circulation, there is a hierarchy of tests that is used to fit the needs of the patient and the physician for the particular condition being evaluated. Using them in a structured fashion will be necessary to approach the problem at hand.

We always measure the AAI at the time the patient is first seen. This not only confirms our suspicion but also provides an objective baseline reading for comparison during the time of follow-up, when repeat studies are done. The guidelines for interpretation are as follows:

1. What is normal? In general, any AAI must be equal to or greater than 1.0 to be considered normal. Because there is some variability in the measurement, we consider a value of greater than 0.95 as being normal. However, there is a small subset of patients who have normal pressures at rest but still have arterial disease as the cause of their claudication (6). As noted earlier, these patients have some stenotic segment in or proximal to the popliteal artery as the cause of the symptoms. As will be noted shortly under resting flow conditions, there is not a pressure drop, but a gradient will develop during exercise.
2. An AAI of greater than 0.5 is most commonly found in patients with single-segment disease of the more proximal arterial system (popliteal to aorta).
3. When the AAI is below 0.5, this is usually a sign that the occlusion involves more than one arterial segment. The most common example of this is with combined aortoiliac and superficial femoral involvement.
4. In some diabetic patients, it may not be possible to measure the ankle systolic pressure owing to medial calcification. This most commonly involves the tibial-peroneal trunks but can, in rare situations, also involve the popliteal and superficial femoral arteries. However, this process is in no way related to atherosclerosis; in fact, the two may exist independently of each other. What is the magnitude of the problem? In vascular clinics, up to 14% of diabetic patients (primarily type II diabetes) have this problem. In these cases, it is often necessary to measure the systolic pressure at the level of the toes, where the digital arteries are rarely calcified. For further information on this subject, one should consult the review by Carter (5). In general, the toe systolic pressure should be greater than 70% of the systolic pressure recorded at the arm level.
5. It has to be emphasized that, when the pressures are measured and an AAI is calculated, the arm systolic blood pressure should also be measured using CW Doppler. This method provides the sharpest and most accurate endpoint for systolic pressures that can be obtained. Another error that is commonly made is to determine the systolic pressure during cuff inflation and not during deflation from suprasystolic levels. As Carter

(5) has shown, this can produce significant errors in the measurement.

Exercise testing has become an integral part of the evaluation process because it provides information on several important aspects of a patient's ability to perform (7). The important data that can be obtained include the following:

1. The distance the patient can walk under controlled conditions. Although there may be variations on how this test is performed, we prefer to use a treadmill that is set at 2 mph on a 12% grade. This speed and elevation can be handled by most patients but can be altered if they appear to represent too much stress for the patient. Although cardiac stress testing requires pushing the patient to his or her limit, this is not necessary for testing the peripheral circulatory response. We arbitrarily limit the walking time to 5 minutes, which is adequate to elicit the necessary hemodynamic response. In addition, any patient who can walk this duration has very minimal claudication and is generally not considered a candidate for intervention.
2. It is important to note the time of onset of the pain, its location, and the maximal distance the patient can walk. We have also found that it is important to note the walking pattern because this may provide clues to the etiology of the patient's problem. In general, if the cause of the pain is not vascular, the walking time before the symptoms appear is very short (often less than 1 minute). The location of the pain is often different than is most commonly seen when vascular disease is the cause.
3. An important additional bit of information that is of use is the development of cardiorespiratory problems during walking. It is not at all unusual to find that shortness of breath and angina pectoris occur in some patients. These often point the diagnosis in a different direction that may be of more immediate consequence than the claudication. We have not, as a routine, monitored the patient's electrocardiogram during walking and have not seen any reason to do so. We have never had a serious adverse event on the treadmill that would suggest we change this practice. However, when patients develop chest pain or shortness of breath during the walking period, the test is promptly stopped.
4. The ankle blood pressure response to exercise is an important part of the evaluation. If a patient has true vascular claudication, the ankle pressure will fall after exercise and will require several minutes for recovery to the preexercise level (6,7). The one fact that is of great importance is that true claudication does not occur without a significant drop in ankle pressure. The normal limits for the pressure changes after exercise have been defined as a less than 20% fall in pressure with a recovery time of less than 3 minutes. When the patient is stopped because of ischemia to the exercising muscles,

the pressure drops are usually large—often to 0—with a very prolonged recovery time that may in some cases be longer than 20 to 30 minutes. It is not necessary to calculate the AAIs after exercise because this is not relevant to the hemodynamic response. It is well known that the arm systolic pressure will rise after exercise in direct relationship to the work that has been accomplished. We do not measure the arm pressure after the exercise test has been completed because it adds nothing to the interpretation of the test results. I realize that some laboratories continue this practice, but it is not necessary.

5. The exercise test is particularly important in the evaluation of patients with pseudoclaudication. If the ankle blood pressure response to exercise is normal, one must look for causes other than the vascular system. What of the patient who has both arterial disease and neuromuscular causes for the pain? When this occurs, it is usually the nonvascular problems that stop the patient first, which is nearly always within the first minute on the treadmill. In addition, the ankle blood pressure response, although abnormal, is not of the type and severity seen with vascular claudication. For example, if the vascular disease is so severe that the patient can walk only a minute or less, the ankle pressure fall will be far greater than 20% from baseline, with a recovery time to the pre-exercise level that is well in excess of 3 min.

After this type of evaluation combined with the clinical presentation has been completed, it are possible in nearly all cases to decide whether further studies are needed. In many cases, it is not necessary to proceed further with duplex studies or arteriography. The patient may then be counseled with regard to conservative measures and placed in a long-term follow-up program.

On the other hand, if the patient is considered a candidate for interventional therapy, be it balloon angioplasty or surgery, a preliminary duplex scan can be of great value in selecting the proper form of therapy.

Upper Limb

In contrast to the lower limb, patients presenting with exercise-induced pain in an arm are rare. This might seem surprising because narrowing and occlusion of the subclavian artery is a common finding, particularly in elderly patients with atherosclerosis elsewhere in the arterial system. There are probably several reasons for this. First and foremost, the arms are not exercised to the same extent as the legs, thus reducing the amount of blood flow that is required for usual activity. The other reason relates to the role of the vertebral artery as an effective input collateral to the arm. Although difficult to prove because of the small number of cases, the only cases of true claudication of the arm that I have seen are those in which the vertebral artery on the side of the subclavian disease has an anomalous origin from the arch of the aorta. In this setting, the collateral vessels available to the arm are smaller, providing much higher resistance to flow. Most of the referrals to the vascular diagnostic center for the evaluation of the arm circulation are patients who present with symptoms suggestive of problems involving the posterior circulation to the brain—the *subclavian steal syndrome*. In theory, exercise of the arm on the side of the subclavian artery occlusion might siphon enough blood away from the posterior circulation to produce symptoms of dizziness, syncope, and drop attacks. This is an uncommon event even in cases with subclavian artery occlusion.

The most common referrals to the vascular diagnostic laboratory are patients who develop intermittent digital ischemia when the hands are exposed to cold (Raynaud's phenomenon). There are two varieties of the syndrome—primary and secondary. In the primary form, which is benign, the palmar and digital arteries remain patent without any demonstrable structural abnormality. The secondary form is much more serious because it is associated with a long list of systemic diseases, of which the collagen vascular diseases are the most common, with scleroderma leading the list. The syndrome can also occur secondary to repetitive trauma (air hammer disease and the hypothenar eminence syndrome), Buerger's disease, and the monoclonal gammopathies. It has also been observed that occlusive lesions in the arm, palmar, and digital circulation, regardless of the etiology, can lead to the development of the syndrome.

In the course of the evaluation, the prime role of the vascular laboratory is to determine the anatomic status of the circulation to the digits and assess their response to cold exposure. The physical examination is usually not helpful unless digit ulceration is noted. When this is seen, the diagnosis is the secondary form of the syndrome because patients with primary Raynaud's disease never develop enough digital ischemia to lead to tissue loss.

The diagnostic approach should include the following:

1. The measurement of arm, wrist, and digit blood pressures. This can be done with a PPG, strain gauge plethysmograph, and CW Doppler. Doppler can be used for this purpose only if signals are audible at the fingertip. Normally, the systolic pressure at the level of the fingers must be more than 80% of that recorded from the upper arm. Values below this level signify arterial obstruction at some point proximal to the recording site. In practice, the plethysmographic methods should be employed to make the measurements.

2. If a proximal site of obstruction such as in the subclavian, axillary, or brachial arteries is suspected, this can be confirmed by the arm pressure measurements and a duplex evaluation. It is always important to examine identical sites in both arms. Normally, the velocity patterns in the upper extremity are biphasic or triphasic.

3. The final test of value in being certain that true cold sensitivity is the diagnosis is to measure the digit blood

pressure response to cooling. The test is done by measuring the digit systolic pressure before briefly immersing the hands in ice water. Normally, the finger pressure will stay the same or increase. With true cold sensitivity, the finger blood pressure will often fall to unrecordable levels.

If, by any of the above tests, it can be shown that palmar or digital artery occlusion is present, the patient has the secondary variety of the syndrome. All of the systemic diseases that are associated with the development of cold sensitivity have digital or palmar artery occlusion as a part of their progression. The finding of normal digit blood pressures, volume pulse waveforms, and normal velocity signals at all levels of the arm makes the diagnosis of primary Raynaud's disease a certainty. In this case, it is not necessary to embark on an extensive and costly workup looking for a systemic cause for the problem.

ACUTE VENOUS THROMBOSIS

It is well known that acute venous thrombosis of the deep venous system is the most common vascular disorder that develops in the course of hospital treatment. This is because it can occur in any patient who is ill and is required to remain in bed for prolonged periods of time. The disorder has been with us since antiquity and continues to plague us. Its consequences are severe and can be divided into those that are life threatening and those that lead to a lifelong disability secondary to the postthrombotic syndrome.

What is the magnitude of the problem, in terms of both mortality and long-term sequelae? Exact figures for the annual numbers of deaths from pulmonary emboli are difficult to obtain because they come largely from autopsy statistics and individual institutions. However, it is a fair estimate that between 100,000 and 150,000 deaths occur every year, with a much larger number having the event but surviving it (8). If we estimate that those who survive are double that number, the survivors will remain at risk for the long-term sequelae. This, of course, underestimates the total number of patients who are at risk for postthrombotic syndrome because most patients who develop deep venous thrombosis will never have pulmonary emboli as a complication. This total number has been estimated to be in the range of 850,000 patients annually (9,10). Although we do not have accurate figures on its current incidence, it is unlikely that acute venous thrombosis is decreasing. This is because, as we continue to treat patients with advanced and complicated illnesses, the very settings in which it is most likely to occur will continue to be commonplace. At this stage, it is important to emphasize that I am referring to deep venous thrombosis and that the following discussion does not apply to the entity of superficial thrombophlebitis, which, in my view, is an entirely separate process. The involvement of the superficial venous system is truly an inflammatory disorder that rarely extends into the deep venous system. Although it is not usually bacterial in origin, it does have all the hallmarks of an inflammatory response, with marked local tenderness, hyperemia, and pyrexia. Although the same terminology (thrombophlebitis) is commonly applied to the deep venous system even today, it should not be used in this fashion because deep venous thrombosis is rarely associated with a significant inflammatory response (11).

The etiology of deep venous thrombosis remains a mystery in terms of the actual events that take place, but it appears that the three major elements of Virchow's triad—stasis, hypercoaguability, and endothelial damage—remain the key factors (12). For those interested in the diagnostic approaches to this disorder, it is important to understand where it occurs in the deep venous system because the diagnostic steps used for its discovery will have to address each of these segments if the methods are to be clinically useful.

Commonly Involved Venous Segments

Our knowledge of the localization of deep venous thrombi came about because of two major factors—the use of venography and ^{125}I-labeled fibrinogen. The classic studies of Bauer in 1940 (13) clearly outlined all the roentgenographic signs associated with deep venous thrombosis. The technique has been refined to make it possible to evaluate the entire venous system from the level of the foot to the inferior vena cava (14).

The introduction of labeled fibrinogen by Hobbs in 1962 (15) led to the widespread use of this method for studying the natural history of venous thrombosis from its inception. The elegant studies of Kakkar and associates (16) and Nicolaides and colleagues (17) clearly showed that, after operation, venous thrombi may develop in the first few days, with the most common site of origin being in the sinuses of the soleus muscle. It soon became apparent that most of these thrombi remained confined to this area even without therapy, with about 20% propagating to the popliteal vein.

Venographic studies tend to give a different picture for the following reasons. Venography is rarely done in the very early phases of deep venous thrombosis. It is most commonly performed when symptoms and signs develop that indicate involvement of the larger, more proximal veins. In addition, unless the venogram is carefully done with the intent of also visualizing the soleal sinuses, the earliest developing thrombi are often missed.

As a result of the use of labeled fibrinogen and venography, there have developed two schools of thought with regard to the natural history of deep venous thrombosis. The first, arrived at by the users of ^{125}I-labeled fibrinogen, is that most, if not all, thrombi have their origin in the calf, with the involvement of the larger veins occurring by extension (17). The second view is that thrombi can occur *de novo* in venous segments at points removed from the calf and without evidence of extension from that site (18).

Where, then, do thrombi occur, and what is their significance in terms of diagnostic approaches? In general, venous thrombi occur in three major areas of the deep venous system:

1. There is little doubt that the soleal sinuses are the most common site. When the venous thrombi remain confined to this area, they rarely produce symptoms and do not cause pulmonary emboli of any significance.
2. Another common site of involvement is in the sinus of the venous valve. If confined to this area, thrombi are rarely detected because they are rarely the cause of symptoms and signs. However, it is well known that the base of the thrombus in the sinus may be the scaffold from which the thrombus may grow in size, extending into the lumen of the vein and ultimately occluding it.
3. The final and very important areas are the proximal veins (popliteal to the inferior vena cava). Iliofemoral venous thrombosis is at least two times as common on the left side (19). These larger venous segments are of great importance because of the potential for thrombi in these areas becoming serious and, on occasion, fatal pulmonary emboli.

The importance of the localization of venous thrombi will become more evident when we discuss the diagnostic tests that are used for its detection.

There are few areas in vascular medicine in which there have been more mistakes made than in the diagnosis of acute deep venous thrombosis. This is because most patients do not present with a set of symptoms and signs that are, in and of themselves, diagnostic of the underlying condition. The reason for this confusion may rest with two major elements that have led to this problem. The first is the terminology used in describing the entity. It is still common for physicians to refer to the process as thrombophlebitis, which implies that the thrombotic event is either secondary to or associated with an inflammatory response. This is clearly not the case for the involvement of the deep veins and is only true for the cases of superficial venous involvement, which clearly appears to have an inflammatory component. Thus, the term *phlebitis* should be used only in describing the superficial venous disease commonly seen. In addition, there is no evidence that the underlying cause of the two processes is the same.

The other diagnostic maneuver that continues to be used by the medical community is Homans' sign, either to rule in or rule out the presence of deep venous thrombosis. This test is done by dorsiflexing the foot and noting whether there is associated pain in the calf of the leg. This test is so nonspecific that it should be discarded. A positive test can occur because of a wide range of conditions involving the soft tissues of the calf. A negative test does not rule out the diagnosis.

Symptoms and signs include the presence of pain, which is often quite subtle. This may or may not be associated with limb swelling. In some instances, there may be an increase in the temperature of the limb, but this is extremely variable. It has been shown that even an experienced physician will be accurate only 50% of the time in making the correct diagnosis when the clinical presentation and the physical findings alone are used to arrive at this diagnosis (20).

There is only one situation in which the clinical presentation is, in and of itself, adequate to arrive at a diagnosis. This is with the problem of iliofemoral venous thrombosis (phlegmasia cerulea dolens). This process involves extensive thrombosis of the iliac, common femoral, and superficial femoral veins. When this occurs, the entire limb becomes acutely swollen, with associated severe pain and cyanosis of the limb. No other entities produce this symptom complex.

Given the difficulties of arriving at a clinical diagnosis of acute deep venous thrombosis, what should be the strategy of the physician? It is now clear that an objective and non-invasive test should be done immediately to verify the diagnosis of venous obstruction. The most commonly used test is ultrasonic duplex scanning. The CW Doppler can be used as a preliminary screening method, but it is very operator dependent (21). Today, most patients are sent directly for a duplex scan because it is currently the gold standard.

The venogram has been and even today remains the gold standard in some situations, but it does have the liability of all invasive tests. It is painful and can lead to undesirable sequelae, with a small number of patients actually developing a chemical phlebitis from the hyperosmolar contrast material. Although the nonionic contrast materials may reduce the risk of developing phlebitis as well as the discomfort associated with the test, it is expensive to use. Another major drawback is that venography is a test that is used only once to arrive at the diagnosis. It is rarely done a second time to document the course of therapy and its outcome.

Duplex scanning is proving to be the best method of establishing the diagnosis of deep venous thrombosis and also of documenting the natural history of the disorder. It is now possible not only to monitor the fate of the thrombus but also to assess the role of the patient's intrinsic fibrinolytic system in lysing the thrombus and its effect on subsequent valve function.

UPPER EXTREMITY VENOUS THROMBOSIS

There are two problems that are seen that the vascular diagnostic service is called on to evaluate. The first is effort thrombosis, and the second is a result of the placement of venous catheters used for hyperalimentation or infusion of chemotherapeutic agents. In both situations, the arm becomes swollen with prominent veins around the shoulder that are the collaterals bypassing the area of occlusion. Effort thrombosis is a problem of the thoracic inlet, where chronic compression is thought to be the inciting factor leading to intimal damage and subsequent thrombosis. The diagnosis is suspected by the presenting complaints of pain and swelling. The cause can often be verified by a duplex study. When this is done, it is important to examine identical sites from both arms, comparing the velocity patterns that are observed. Flow in veins distal (toward the hand) to the site of occlusion often exhibits a continuous flow pattern that is not affected by respiratory events.

POSTTHROMBOTIC SYNDROME

The most important structure in the deep venous system that permits normal function is the venous valve. These remarkable structures are found at strategic points in the venous system. Their major function is to ensure antegrade flow and prevent the reversal of flow during activation of the calf muscle pump. They are found in the superficial veins, the perforating components, and at all levels of the deep venous system up to and including the iliac veins in some people. Normally, the flow of blood from the lower leg is from the superficial veins to the deep system. When the valves become incompetent, however, the effect depends on the site involved.

For example, if the valves in the calf veins become incompetent, flow with calf muscle contraction will be bidirectional, creating hypertension in the distal veins and reversal of flow in the perforating veins (22). This is often referred to as a *high-pressure leak* and subjects the subcutaneous tissues of the lower leg to marked swings in pressure. These perforating veins are mainly located along the course of the posterior tibial vein, which may explain the frequent occurrence of the pigmentation and ulceration in this area.

From a clinical standpoint, it is well known that a previous episode of deep venous thrombosis may lead to the development of chronic venous insufficiency. On the other hand, a most disturbing fact is that up to half of patients with the syndrome may never give a history of such an event (23). This suggests that there may be other causes, or that the episode of deep venous thrombosis that led to the damage was not recognized or was forgotten by the patient.

Patients with postthrombotic syndrome present with one or more complaints—chronic swelling, pain, hyperpigmentation, and, in late cases, ulceration. The swelling is always at the level of the ankle and may extend further up the limb, depending on the extent of the damage to the valves of the deep venous system. If the edema involves the dorsum of the foot, this is only seen when there is lymphatic obstruction. This is mentioned because it is not uncommon to have patients referred to the vascular laboratory for venous studies when the underlying etiology is involvement of the lymphatics. The pigmentation will involve the lower medial side of the calf and ankle, where the perforating veins are normally found. The same pertains to the location of the ulcers when they occur.

A less commonly recognized complication of postthrombotic syndrome is venous claudication (24). This occurs when there is chronic proximal venous obstruction (iliofemoral) in a patient who is very active physically. The patient notes with increasing exercise the development of severe thigh and occasional calf pain that is described as bursting. The pain usually requires the patient to lie down and elevate the limbs to obtain relief. The reason it has not been commonly recognized in the past is that most patients with chronic venous obstruction do not exercise enough to develop the pain.

This complaint occurs because of the chronic venous obstruction and is not due to chronic valvular incompetence. Although the venous collaterals are adequate to maintain the limb free of edema most of the time, the marked increase in flow that occurs with exercise cannot be accommodated, and the venous volume increases to the point of producing the pain. It is only when the volume of blood on the venous side decreases that the pain will go away. Patients will find this out early, which is why they find elevation of the limb beneficial in relieving the discomfort.

How should patients who potentially fall into the category of chronic venous insufficiency be evaluated? From a clinical standpoint, the history combined with simple inspection of the limb is usually sufficient to make the diagnosis. However, when one is considering the therapy to be used, it is important to establish the location and extent of the venous involvement. This can be done by carrying out a duplex scan.

Varicose Veins

A common problem seen in the vascular clinic is the patient who presents with varicose veins. If the patient has a strong family history and the varicosities involve the greater or lesser saphenous systems, one is tempted to label the patient as having primary varicose veins, which means that the deep venous system is competent (25). Another clue to the diagnosis of primary varicose veins is the lack of significant discomfort, edema, or pigmentation. It is generally accepted that primary varicose veins do not lead to the development of pigmentation and ulceration, which, again, emphasizes the importance of the valves in the deep venous system in protecting the lower limb.

To be certain of the diagnosis, it is important to assess the location and extent of the valvular incompetence and chronic obstruction that may be present. There are several ways that this can be accomplished noninvasively, including CW Doppler, photoplethysmography, and duplex scanning (26,27). For most purposes, it is a simple matter to establish this at the time of the clinic visit as long as the physician is aware of the problems involved. Although duplex scanning can be shown to be the best method of studying venous function, it is not practical to do so for every patient unless surgery is being planned. If this is the case, a complete duplex scan should be done, mapping all sites of valvular incompetence in the superficial venous system. This is done so that the operation can be tailored to fit the patient's disease. This is a major advance for the field of venous surgery.

The examination recommended in the clinic at the time of the first visit is to evaluate the venous system with the CW Doppler. It is important that the examination be done in a systematic manner to establish the level and extent of the valvular incompetence. This is done beginning at the level of the common femoral vein and working down the leg to the level of the ankle. To ensure maximal venous filling, the patient should be examined in a −10 degrees Trendelenburg's position.

The procedure and the pitfalls of the examination are as follows:

1. At the level of the common femoral vein, incompetence can be established only by the performance of Valsalva's maneuver. It must be recognized, however, that, if there are valves in the iliac veins and they are competent, it may not be possible to establish the competence of the veins from that point to the level of the transducer. However, in clinical practice, this does not appear to be a significant problem.
2. If the transducer is moved to the level of the superficial femoral vein, it may be possible to determine the competence of the valves in the superficial femoral vein as long as the valves proximal to this point are incompetent. If there are competent valves in the common femoral or iliac veins, it will be impossible to establish the presence or absence of competence in this vein.
3. The same reasoning applies to the popliteal and posterior tibial veins. It should be noted that if reflux is noted with Valsalva's maneuver at these levels, all valves proximal to this point are incompetent.
4. When the greater and lesser saphenous veins are examined, the same methods are applied with the same interpretation as given previously.

Because the CW Doppler examination is used only for preliminary screening test, the duplex scan should be done to study both the superficial and deep venous systems. The use of duplex scanning for the evaluation of venous disease is covered in Chapter 28.

Extracranial Arterial Disease

One of the most important functions of the vascular laboratory is the investigation of the carotid and vertebral arteries. Stroke remains the third most common cause of death in the Western world, with atheroembolism from the carotid artery accounting for as many as half of all these events. These patients are first seen both as inpatients and outpatients. The need to pursue a duplex scanning is largely based on historical events, with the physical examination playing a minor role. If one has symptoms or signs of ischemic cerebrovascular disease, then a duplex scan is mandatory. On the other hand, many patients are referred for study after a bruit is found on physical examination. The bruit is only a marker and cannot be used to determine the severity of the underlying arterial narrowing.

It is important to measure the blood pressure in both arms at the time the patient is first seen because one possibility might be the presence of the subclavian steal syndrome. In this setting, a high-grade stenosis or occlusion of the subclavian artery may result in reversal of flow in the vertebral artery, leading to posterior circulation symptoms. However, it must be pointed out that reversal of flow in the vertebral artery in and of itself is nearly always a benign finding. The results of the randomized clinical trials showing a benefit for endarterectomy make duplex scanning even more important. As will be noted in this book, the duplex scan results in and of themselves may be all that is needed for the patient to undergo carotid endarterectomy.

REFERENCES

1. Kempczinski RF. Atheroembolism. In: Kempczinski RF, ed. *The ischemic limb*. Chicago: Year Book Medical Publishers, 1985: 81–94.
2. Strandness DE Jr. Noninvasive tests in vascular emergencies. In: Bergan JJ, Yao JSt, eds. *Vascular surgical emergencies*. Orlando: Grune & Stratton, 1987:103–111.
3. Strandness DE Jr. Intermittent claudication. In: Brest AN, ed. *Peripheral vascular disease*. Philadelphia: FA Davis, 1971:53–63.
4. Goodreau JJ, Greasy JK, Flanigan DP, et al. Rational approach to the differentiation of vascular and neurogenic claudication. *Surgery* 1978;84:749–757.
5. Carter SA. Role of pressure measurements in vascular disease. In: Bernstein EF, ed. *Noninvasive diagnostic techniques in vascular disease*. St. Louis: CV Mosby, 1985:513–544.
6. Carter SA. Response of ankle systolic pressure to leg exercise in mild or questionable arterial disease. *N Engl J Med* 1972;287: 578–582.
7. Strandness DE Jr, Zierler RE. Exercise ankle pressure measurements in arterial disease. In: Bernstein EF, ed. *Noninvasive diagnostic techniques in vascular disease*. 3rd ed. St. Louis: CV Mosby, 1985:575–583.
8. Silver DS. Pulmonary embolism: prevention, detection and nonoperative management. *Surg Clin North Am* 1974;54:1089–1106.
9. Coon WW, Willis PW. Deep venous thrombosis and pulmonary embolism: prediction, prevention and treatment. *Am J Cardiol* 1959;4:611–621.
10. McLachlin AD. Venous disease of the lower extremities. *Curr Probl Surg* 1967;Jan:3–44.
11. Beckering RE, Titus JL. Femoropopliteal venous thrombosis and pulmonary embolism. *Am J Clin Pathol* 1969;52:530–537.
12. Virchow R. Neuer Fall von todtlicher Embolie der Lungenarterien. *Arch Pathol Anat Physiol* 1856;10:225–228.
13. Bauer G. A venographic study of thromboembolic problem. *Acta Chir Scand* 1940;84[Suppl 61]:1–75.

14. Rabinov K, Paulin S. Roentgen diagnosis of venous thrombosis in the leg. *Arch Surg* 1972;104:134–144.
15. Hobbs JT. External measurement of fibrinogen uptake in experimental venous thrombosis and other local pathological states. *Br J Exp Pathol* 1962;43:48–58.
16. Kakkar VV, Howe CT, Flanc C, Clarke MB. Natural history of deep vein thrombosis. *Lancet* 1969;2:230–232.
17. Nicolaides AN, Kakkar VV, Renney JTG. Soleus sinuses and stasis. *Br J Surg* 1971;58:307(abst).
18. Mavor GE, Galloway JMD. Iliofemoral venous thrombosis: pathological considerations and surgical management. *Br J Surg* 1969;56:45–59.
19. Cockett FB, Lea-Thomas M. The iliac compression syndrome. *Br J Surg* 1965;52:816–821.
20. Haeger K. Problems of acute deep venous thrombosis: the interpretation of signs and symptoms. *Angiology* 1969;20:219–235.
21. Barnes RW. Doppler ultrasonic diagnosis of venous disease. In: Bernstein EF, ed. *Noninvasive diagnostic techniques in vascular disease*. St. Louis: CV Mosby, 1985:452–458.
22. Arnoldi CC, Linderholm H. On the pathogenesis of venous leg ulcer. *Acta Scand Chir* 1968;134:427-440
23. Cockett FB, Jones DFE. The ankle blow-out syndrome: a new approach to the varicose ulcer problem. *Lancet* 1953;1:17–23.
24. Killewich LA, Martin R, Cramer M, et al. Pathophysiology of venous claudication. *J Vasc Surg* 1984;4:507–511.
25. Gundersen J, Hauge M. Hereditary factors in venous insufficiency. *Angiology* 1969;20:346–355.
26. Kohler TK, Strandness DE Jr. Noninvasive testing for the evaluation of chronic venous disease. *World J Surg* 1986;10:903–910.
27. Killewich LA, Martin R, Cramer M, et al. An objective assessment of the physiologic changes in the postthrombotic syndrome. *Arch Surg* 1985;120: 424–426.

3

HEMODYNAMICS OF THE NORMAL ARTERIAL AND VENOUS SYSTEM

For the accurate detection and understanding of the major diseases that affect the arterial system, it is necessary to appreciate some elementary and basic facts as they relate to pressure and flow within these vessels. For diagnostic purposes, most of our observations are made on large and medium-sized vessels. These are defined as vessels with proper names. Although there are vascular disorders that involve the microcirculation, these must be examined by indirect physiologic testing procedures. Most of the disorders seen in the vascular laboratory are at the macro level. Unless you have an appreciation for the physiology involved, you will not be able to do the best job in carrying out the testing procedures outlined in this book. This is where imaging alone falls down because one has to infer from what is seen what the consequences might be. This has been and remains a problem when the physiologic aspects are not appreciated or are simply ignored.

In the Western world, atherosclerosis is the most important disease we encounter and is the one that we will spend a good deal of time discussing in this book. To appreciate how it distorts the normal physiologic functions of the system, it is important to review briefly its localization within the arterial system and the basic changes it produces in the arterial wall. The only other major arterial disorder that is commonly confused in terms of its localization in the arterial system is Buerger's disease (thromboangiitis obliterans).

ATHEROSCLEROSIS: PATHOLOGY AND LOCALIZATION

Little is known about the sequence of events that finally leads to the development of the arterial lesion, which, in turn, leads to the development of symptoms and signs; however, some features of the disease are well recognized and should be known to those who work in the area of diagnostic methods designed to detect it.

The earliest lesion found in the arterial system is the lipid streak. This can be seen even in infancy and consists of subintimal collections of fat that, in and of themselves,

never cause problems. Because these are often found in the same locations as the far-advanced lesions, they are often considered to be their true precursors. This is only a theoretic consideration because the actual transition to the complicated plaque has never been documented in humans.

Those lesions of concern are the fibrous and complicated plaques. The fibrous plaque is a relatively uniform lesion that is characterized by abundance of smooth muscle and fibrous tissue. It is also characterized by having a smooth surface and by the lack of calcification. It is doubtful that the fibrous plaque is a cause of problems, other than the fact that it is most likely the precursor of the more advanced complicated plaque commonly associated with clinical events.

The complicated plaque is recognized by its several features. The features themselves point to the reasons this lesion is potentially very dangerous. In its earliest forms, when its presence does not lead to an increased risk, is when it possesses a fibrous cap that shields the underlying material from the circulation. When the integrity of the cap is lost, several events can occur, the consequence of which is entirely dependent on the location of the plaque. This exposes the subendothelial collagen, which renders this area more "thrombogenic," becoming a site where platelets may accumulate, forming a nidus of material that may become embolic. Intraplaque hemorrhage is also common and is thought by some to be the mechanism behind the sudden increase in the size of the lesion. This is an attractive hypothesis, but we do not believe it actually happens as postulated. Other features include the development of necrosis, calcification, and varying degrees of infiltration with inflammatory cells. There is also an accumulation of lipid within the lesion itself; this may be important in terms of plaque growth by its effect on clinical outcome.

It is important to understand these changes in the lesions because, as the resolution of ultrasonic imaging has improved, more attempts are being made to characterize them by duplex scanning. This is being done to develop criteria that might be useful in predicting which patients are at risk for the development of ischemic events.

For unknown reasons, atherosclerosis tends commonly to involve some areas of the arterial circulation and regularly to spare others. Some arterial segments are very susceptible to the development of the disease, whereas others are not. A good example of the latter is the arteries of the arm distal to the origin of the subclavian artery. It is rare to have these arteries develop the complicated plaques, with one exception: Patients with chronic renal failure who are on dialysis may develop lesions in the arteries of the arm.

It has been noted that, in general terms, atherosclerosis can be described as a disease of branch points and bifurcations. This is generally true because every radiologist and vascular surgeon knows and permits the use of many of the reconstructive procedures designed to correct the narrowing and occlusions that can result.

The more common examples of such localization are important to those interested in the application of duplex scanning because they provide information on where to concentrate our efforts. The more clinically important are as follows:

The carotid bifurcation. It is now well recognized that this unique bifurcation (the bulb) is a common site for the disease to occur. We know from clinical studies and those by Zarins and colleagues (1) that the disease first starts in the posterolateral aspect of the bulb. In its earliest form, it is a fibrous plaque that has a uniform and smooth covering. As the lesion progresses, it does so circumferentially, ultimately involving the entire bulb and the origin of the external carotid artery as well. By the time the plaque involves the entire bulb, it is nearly always the complicated type, with the frequent appearance of calcification. Thickening of the arterial wall is almost universally seen proximal to the bulb and extends down to the origin of the common carotid arteries. On the other hand, the disease rarely extends beyond the distal margin of the bulb itself. This is the only reason that an operation, such as endarterectomy, can be used to remove the lesion. In recent years, it has been recognized that the single most predictive factor for the development of a transient ischemic attack or stroke is the degree of stenosis at the level of the bulb. The high-grade lesions are the most dangerous and are the ones that we must be able to detect with a high degree of accuracy. A key question relates to why high-grade lesions are the cause of problems and not those with minimal to moderate narrowing of the bulb. Our current thinking is that it relates to the integrity of the fibrous cap. It would appear that as long as the fibrous cap remains intact, there is little chance that an event might occur. This is true even if the lesions become hemodynamically significant in the carotid artery because the collateral circulation via the circle of Willis is usually good enough to maintain perfusion at normal levels. As will be pointed out shortly, similar degrees of narrowing a peripheral artery would lead to the development of symptoms.

The aortic bifurcation. The distal aorta and common iliac arteries are a common site for developing the complicated lesions that frequently progress to produce high-grade stenoses and total occlusions. The aortic wall proximal to this area is frequently thickened as well. The external iliac artery, which is relatively short and straight, does not have the same high incidence of involvement.

Branch points. Wherever there is a major branch point, the complicated lesions can commonly be found. The more notable are the renal arteries, the celiac and superior mesenteric arteries, the profunda femoris artery, and the proximal superficial femoral artery. When the plaques develop here, it is nearly always near the orifice and at most the first 1 or 2 cm that are involved. The arteries beyond that point are commonly spared. It is for this reason that, in the course of duplex scanning, it is important to concentrate on these areas to detect the stenotic lesions.

Exceptions. There are some areas that would appear to deviate from these generalizations. The most prominent is the adductor hiatus (Hunter's canal) in the midthigh, where there is a high incidence of involvement. It is of interest that the popliteal artery is much less commonly involved, a fact known to vascular surgeons who frequently use this vessel as a point to insert bypass grafts when treating femoral artery obstruction. The arteries below the knee have not been as well characterized, but it is known that the distal posterior tibial artery and the anterior tibial artery at its origin are commonly the sites of involvement. There do not appear to be any specific patterns of involvement for the peroneal artery.

The role of type II diabetes. There are disorders, such as diabetes, that change some of the considerations noted previously. For reasons that are not understood, the atherosclerosis that occurs with this disease is more extensive and has a different distribution than seen in the nondiabetic patient with atherosclerosis. These differences are important, clinically and from the standpoint of duplex scanning. The differences in the distribution of the disease explain many of the reasons for the higher rate of limb loss. Type II diabetic patients account for more than half of all amputations in the United States, yet constitute only about 3% of our population.

The type II diabetic patient has a lower incidence of involvement of the aortoiliac segment than the nondiabetic patient. With regard to the femoropopliteal segment, the extent of involvement in the two populations is the same. It is the most common site for occlusive lesions, particularly in the adductor canal. However, the diabetic patient has a much higher incidence of occlusive lesions in the three medium-sized arteries below the knee (2,3). The disease appears to be the same histologically in the diabetic patient. Thus, in scanning the limbs of patients with diabetes, the observer should be aware of the different patterns of involvement.

GENERAL HEMODYNAMIC CONSIDERATIONS

With the heart as the propelling force, the arterial system consists of a series of branching conduits, the physical characteristics of which are suited for optimal delivery of blood to the tissues with a minimum of energy loss. Their entire purpose is to deliver oxygenated blood to the tissues along with the necessary nutrients to maintain optimal function. The amount of blood an organ or tissue receives depends on its level of metabolism and the varying demands placed on its function. As is well known, some organs, such as the brain, kidneys, and liver, demand large quantities of blood at all times during the day and are generally classified as low-resistance organs. On the other hand, organ systems, such as the small bowel and musculature of the arms and legs, have extremely variable demands. These are classified as variable-resistance tissues, the functional activity of which must be known at the time of the study. Another tissue that has extremely wide demands is the skin, where flow can vary greatly depending on environmental factors. As will be shown, this type of information is useful from a diagnostic standpoint when applying duplex scanning to a variety of organ systems.

The venous circulation is, in many respects, more complex than its arterial counterpart, owing to several factors that are important to recognize. These include some of the following: (a) the veins are collapsible, in contrast to the arteries, which are not; (b) the veins contain valves located at strategic points in the system to prevent reversal of flow and to protect the tissues against the large swings in pressure that can occur with muscular activity; (c) the venous system is a low-pressure system, as compared with its arterial counterpart; (d) the effect of gravity is very important in determining its volume and function; and (e) the events associated with respiration and the contractions of the right side of the heart are important in determining its function.

INTRAVASCULAR PRESSURE

With each contraction of the heart, the two ventricles of the heart expel the necessary volume of blood to supply the lungs and the systemic circulation. The volume of the output of the two sides of the heart must be closely matched and at the same time meet the needs of the organs, which vary widely. The major arteries that carry the blood to the systemic circulation must do this efficiently without a great deal of energy loss. This is accomplished in the normal person with a minimal pressure loss from the level of the aortic root to the small, unnamed arteries that are prearteriolar. The normal drop in the mean pressure is only about 10 mm Hg over this large distance, further supporting the minimal resistance changes that occur to this level of the circulation (4). This situation is drastically changed at the

level of the arterioles, where the largest drop in pressure normally occurs. These microscopic vessels are the "gatekeepers," in a sense, and not only protect the organism against large drops in driving pressure but also control the volume of blood the tissue needs to support its activities at the moment.

It is important to understand the dynamics of the arterial pressure because this information serves as the basis for the use of pressure as a method of detecting the presence of arterial disease and estimating its extent. It is clear that the best method of estimating the presence of arterial narrowing and determining its hemodynamic significance is to measure the pressure gradient from above to below areas of suspected narrowing.

The actual shape of the generated waveform is determined by the strength of the myocardial contraction, the viscoelastic properties of the receiving vessels, the resistance of the vascular beds, and reflections that occur from branch points and bifurcations. The wall of the arteries consists of elastin, collagen, and smooth muscle. In the central aorta, elastin predominates, but, as one moves peripherally, the amount of smooth muscle and collagen increases. In the arteries below the groin, the ratio of collagen to smooth muscle increases, and the arteries become progressively stiffer.

The change in the properties of the arteries has a dramatic effect on the shape of the arterial pressure waveform. In the central aorta, it is triangular in shape, with a dicrotic notch noted after peak systole. As one moves farther down the arterial system, there is a gradual increase in the systolic pressure, with a transformation in the shape of the waveform. The dicrotic wave becomes more prominent in late diastole, so that, by the time we reach the level of the distal arteries, two distinct components are seen (Fig. 3.1). While the systolic pressure gradually increases, there is a corresponding decrease in the mean pressure, which is, of course, necessary to maintain flow in the proper direction. Given these considerations, this is why the systolic pressures recorded at the level of the ankle are normally higher than those recorded at the level of the arm.

One of the remarkable features of veins is their capacity to undergo great changes in volume, with only slight changes in transmural pressure. It is this fact that explains the capacitance function of the venous system that is so essential for its proper performance. The venous wall is, on average, about one third to one tenth as thick as the systemic arteries. The media of the vein is largely smooth muscle, with very little elastin present. Because of gravitational effects, the percentage of smooth muscle varies, depending on the location of the vein. In the veins of the foot, the percentage of muscle is between 60% and 80%, as compared with about 5% for the axillary vein (5). The smooth muscle is arranged in a helical fashion and is most prominent in those vessels subjected to the greatest hydrostatic pressures. It is not commonly appreciated that the materials compos-

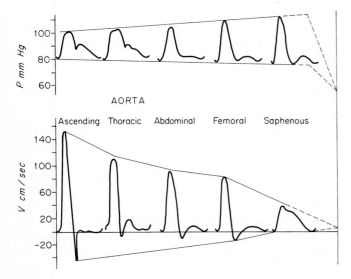

FIGURE 3.1. Diagrammatic representation of the pressure and velocity changes that occur in arteries of the dog from the level of the thoracic aorta to the periphery. As noted, there is a progressive increase in the level of the systolic pressure and a decrease in the peak systolic velocities. The velocity change shown in the saphenous artery of the dog is not seen in humans. Velocity recordings taken from human tibial arteries are nearly identical to those shown for the femoral artery of the dog. (Redrawn from McDonald DA. *Blood flow in arteries.* Baltimore: Williams & Wilkins, 1960, with permission.)

ing the wall are stiffer per unit of cross-section than arteries at the same distending pressures. The stiff nature of the vein should be expected, because of the relative paucity of the elastin and the prominent adventitia, which consists largely of collagen. We showed that the pressure-strain elastic modulus of the human saphenous vein at systemic arterial pressures corresponds closely to that of the arteries (6,7).

Flow in the venous system varies widely, depending on many factors that are difficult to consider without knowing the precise interacting events that may be operating at the time. For example, it is known that, under resting conditions in the supine position, flow in the veins of the lower leg is determined by the pressure changes in the abdomen that occur with the movement of the diaphragm during breathing. With descent of the diaphragm, the pressure increases, and venous flow ceases temporarily.

Because venous pressure varies so much with change in body position, respiratory activity, and contractile events on the right side of the heart, the conditions under which it is measured must be precisely known if any sense is to be made of it. The relationships between the mean pressures recorded in the arterial and venous system in upright and supine humans are shown in Fig. 3.2.

The pressures shown in Fig. 3.2 are affected by the action of the heart, the body position, and the resistance across the arterioles at the time of measurement. It should be noted that the gradient from the arterial to the venous circulation is the same, regardless of the position. However, as noted with the arm extended above the head, the negative effects of gravity are clearly illustrated. The arm pressure falls by 64 mm Hg, and the venous pressure is zero as the veins collapse. Thus, the blood flow to the hand in this position decreases (8).

In contrast to the arterial circulation, measurement of pressures in the veins under resting conditions is of little value from a diagnostic standpoint. This is true regardless of the status of the veins, with the possible exception of acute venous thrombosis, in which the venous collaterals have not yet developed. Even here, the measurement of venous pressure has been of little diagnostic value.

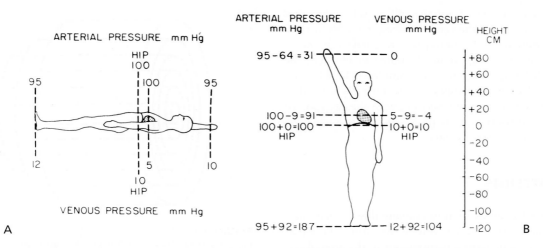

FIGURE 3.2. Intravascular pressures in the supine **(A)** and upright **(B)** human. See text for explanation. (From Strandness DE Jr, Sumner DS. *Hemodynamics for surgeons.* New York: Grune & Stratton, 1975:120–160, with permission.)

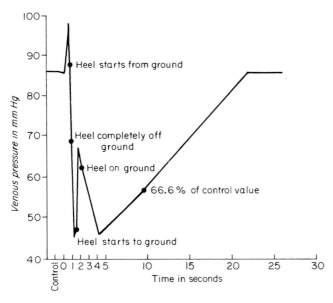

FIGURE 3.3. Average venous pressures recorded from a superficial vein on the dorsum of the foot during a single step. (Redrawn from. Pollack AA, Wood EH. Venous pressure in the saphenous vein at the ankle in man during exercise and changes in position. *J Appl Physiol* 1949;1:649–662, with permission.)

The estimation of venous pressure has found its greatest value in assessing the status of the venous valves. As noted earlier, the valves have one function only: to assist in the antegrade motion of blood when the muscle pumps have been activated. Thus, they play a very small role when the person is standing quietly or is in the recumbent position (9). In the quiet standing position, Ludbrook (9) found the pressures in the superficial and deep veins to be essentially the same. Arnoldi (10) found the pressure in the posterior tibial vein to be about 1 mm Hg higher, which he thought would keep the valves in the perforating veins closed in the quiet standing position.

Because it is the activity of the calf muscle pump that activates the closure of the venous valves, it is only natural that the measurement of venous pressure distal to the valves of interest would be important. As noted in Fig. 3.3, the changes with a single step are very complex (11). They are characterized by several changes of note. First, there is a dramatic fall in venous pressure. Second, with the cessation of the step, the recovery time is prolonged. This is changed with damage to the venous valves.

FLOW PATTERNS

Because Doppler can be used to evaluate flow velocity patterns, it is necessary to review briefly the normal flow patterns as they exist in various components in the arterial system. The flow within the arterial system is determined by many factors, some of which are as follows:

- Nature and strength of myocardial contraction
- Status of the cardiac valves, particularly the aortic valve
- Compliance characteristics of the arteries themselves
- Presence of branch points bifurcations and curvatures
- Viscosity of the blood
- Resistance to flow offered by the tissues and organs being perfused

In the discussion that follows, the assumption will be that the cardiac performance, including the aortic valve, is normal. With regard to the compliance of the arteries, this is determined primarily by the mix of collagen, elastin, and smooth muscle found in the media of the arteries. Arteries tend to get stiffer as one proceeds down the arterial tree. This is because the ratio of collagen to elastin changes. For example, in the thoracic aorta, elastin is more abundant than collagen. This reverses as one goes distal to the inguinal ligament. These changes are important and affect both intraarterial pressure and the velocity patterns that are recorded. Yet these changes are not the dominant factors that determine the flow patterns that are observed.

Flow is generally classified as laminar, disturbed, and turbulent. Laminar flow is present when the velocity profile is parabolic (Fig. 3.4). Flow velocity is maximal at the center of the artery but zero at the wall. This is also referred to as fully developed flow. When found, the mean velocity is equal to one half the peak. The extent to which flow becomes truly laminar depends on the location at which the measurement is made referable to its origin or source, which is the heart. In most flow models, true laminar flow is present if one is 200 diameters distal to the flow source. It should be clear that in humans, these conditions are not often found. For example, the velocity profile seen in the common carotid artery is not parabolic but is blunt. This is what one would expect given its short distance from the flow source. The one artery where flow tends to be para-

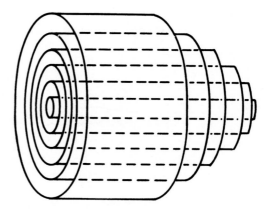

FIGURE 3.4. With laminar blood flow, the flow velocity is maximal in center stream with a gradual and symmetric reduction toward each wall. (From Strandness DE Jr, Sumner DS. *Hemodynamics for surgeons.* New York: Grune & Stratton, 1975:120–160, with permission.)

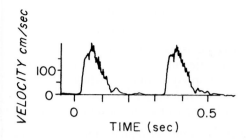

FIGURE 3.5. Velocity of blood flow in the ascending aorta of the dog. Note that there is a brief period of disturbed flow when peak systole is reached, which continues during diastole. Flow is stable during acceleration of the blood. (From Strandness DE Jr, Sumner DS. *Hemodynamics for surgeons.* New York: Grune & Stratton, 1975:120–160, with permission.)

bolic is in the superficial femoral artery, which is straight, long, and relatively constant in diameter.

The transition from true laminar flow to disturbed and turbulent flow is dependent on several factors. The major determinants of these changes can be estimated from the Reynolds number (Re). This is determined by the tube diameter (d), the mean velocity (V), the specific gravity of blood (Π), and fluid viscosity (v), as follows:

$$Re = dV\Pi/v$$

When the Reynolds number exceeds 2,000, the inertial forces may disrupt the laminar flow and lead to fully developed turbulence. In the normal arterial circulation, fully developed turbulence will not be found, but disturbed flow may commonly be seen, particularly at and just after peak systole. This is a transient phenomenon and can often be seen in Doppler velocity tracings (Fig. 3.5). It should be noted that disturbed flow will be seen just after peak systole when the spectral width is noted to be wider than that seen during the acceleration phase, during which flow is stable and the width of the spectrum is narrow. True turbulence has a blunt velocity profile and marked spectral broadening.

In this setting, the red blood cells are no longer moving at similar speeds during the major portion of the heart cycle (Fig. 3.6).

A major factor that determines the flow patterns that are observed is the geometry of the arterial system. This dominates the velocity profile that develops and the direction of the velocity vectors. For example, in the case of the arch of the aorta, the velocity vectors are not parallel to the walls, and helical flow patterns are observed. At the site of bifurcations, boundary layer separation is found to varying degrees. The presence of this phenomenon is most prominent in the carotid bulb, which will be reviewed shortly. Other areas where it has been postulated to occur are at the bifurcation of the abdominal aorta, at major visceral branches, and in the proximal profunda femoris artery (Fig. 3.7). It is important to be aware of this because it can be easily recognized by the use of Doppler techniques, in particular with color Doppler. In fact, the demonstration of boundary layer separation at key bifurcations is a good index of normality.

Another major factor that determines the flow patterns observed is the resistance of flow offered by the tissues being supplied by the artery. In the normal arterial circulation, the organs that have a consistently low resistance to flow are the brain, the liver, and the kidney. The remaining major tissues supplied that are of interest from a diagnostic standpoint are generally considered to be high-resistance tissues when they are in a resting metabolic state. These include the muscles and the intestine. However, as their metabolic activity increases, requiring more blood for proper function, the resistance to flow diminishes markedly.

The velocity patterns of all low-resistance tissues can be characterized by the presence of end-diastolic flow that is always above zero (Fig. 3.6). For high-resistance organs and tissues, the velocity patterns show a triphasic response, which is forward–reverse–forward flow. However, as the resistance to flow decreases to increase flow, the reverse flow component disappears, and the end-diastolic flow is above

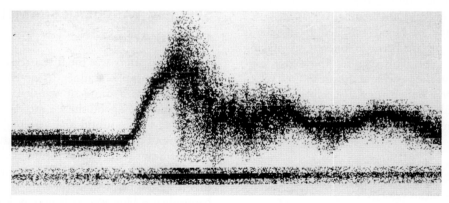

FIGURE 3.6. The ensemble average of several heartbeats taken from the internal carotid artery display, the spectral broadening that occurs after peak systole. This undoubtedly represents the helical flows that are generated by the dilatation of the carotid bulb.

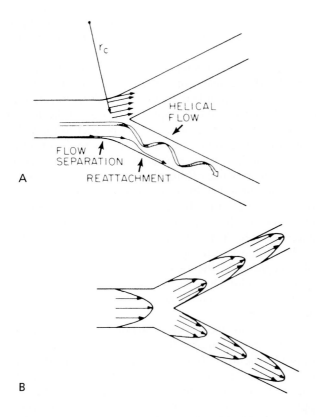

FIGURE 3.7. Flow patterns from a bifurcation. These schematic representations were from flow models. **A:** Flow separation will be noted in the lateral angle with helical flow developing in the branch; *rc* is the radius of curvature at the bifurcation. **B:** Velocity profiles at a bifurcation. (**A** adapted from photographs in Ferguson GG, Roach MM. Flow conditions at bifurcations as determined in glass models with reference to the focal distribution of vascular lesions. In: Bergel DH, ed. *Cardiovascular fluid dynamics.* Vol 2. London: Academic Press, 1972; **B** suggested by Texon M, Imparato AM, Lord AW Jr. The hemodynamic concept of atherosclerosis. *Arch Surg* 1960;80:47–53. Both **A** and **B** were adapted from the work listed above, in Strandness DE Jr, Sumner DS. *Hemodynamics for surgeons.* New York: Grune & Stratton, 1975:120–160, with permission.)

zero. This is seen in the legs during and after exercise and in the superior mesenteric artery after eating.

Because the volume of blood supplied to tissues is important, there has always been an interest in making measurements of this type. This requires knowledge concerning the diameter of the vessel and the mean flow velocity; hence, it would seem only natural that duplex scanning might play a role in this regard. Unfortunately, the problem is not as simple as it might seem.

$$Q = A \cdot V$$

where Q = volume flow
A = cross-sectional area
V ± mean velocity

If one is using an ultrasonic method to assess volume flow, the variables that need to be assessed are as follows:

$$Q = \frac{A \cdot \Delta f \cdot C}{2fo \cdot \cos\Theta}$$

where A = cross-sectional area
Δf = frequency shift
C = speed of sound in tissue
fo = transmitting frequency
Θ = angle of sound beam to velocity vectors

From an ultrasonic standpoint, the variables that have to be known are the diameter of the artery, the frequency shift, and the cosine of the angle of the incident sound beam with the artery. The transmitting frequency of the system and the speed of sound in tissue are known. Small errors in the diameter measurement result in large errors in the calculation of cross-sectional area. Another potential source of error that is well known is the angle of the sound beam with the artery. Even errors as small as 5 degrees can result in errors as high as 10% in the velocity determination. This is even assuming that the flow is laminar and the velocity profile is parabolic. However, one error that has not been fully appreciated is the fact that flow may not be laminar and the flow vectors may not be parallel to the wall (Fig. 3.7). This would, of course, make the relationship between the angle of the beam and the velocity vectors even more uncertain. All of these factors make the measurement of volume flow quite uncertain unless all of the potential variables can be estimated with some precision. The development of the vector Doppler may correct the problem of nonaxial velocity vectors, but this is still in the experimental stage and requires further work to find its true value.

Another fact that is often forgotten is that the range of normal values for volume flow is quite large. In addition, it is well known that if the collateral circulation is good, the total perfusion to the organ, even in the presence of a total occlusion, may remain in a normal range. This factor has largely obviated the use of volume flow estimates for both diagnostic purposes and follow-up studies. We have not found that volume flow measurements play a role in the clinical evaluation of peripheral arterial disease.

SPECIFIC VASCULAR SEGMENTS

Carotid Artery

The carotid artery was the first arterial segment to be studied with the duplex scanner. Its closeness to the skin and its importance as a cause of transient ischemic events and strokes made it a good site for the initial application of this technology. The carotid and vertebral arteries provide the major input to the brain under normal circumstances. They communicate at the base of the brain via the circle of Willis, which is, in theory, the ideal communicating network in that it should be possible for a single vessel to supply both hemispheres. However, as is now well known, the circle of Willis may not be functionally complete in up to half of the population. This has an important impact on who may suffer an ischemic event when the internal carotid artery is acutely occluded.

The brain is a low-resistance organ demanding a high-volume flow rate at all times. As will be shown, this is important in dictating the types of velocity patterns that can be observed with the pulsed Doppler systems used with the duplex scanner. The common carotid artery supplies two beds of varying resistance. The face is a variable resistance bed that has many characteristics of the patterns seen in the upper and lower extremity. Thus, flow in the common carotid is split between the brain, which normally receives 70% to 80% of the flow, and the external carotid artery.

The flow velocity patterns seen in the common carotid and vertebral arteries are often referred to as being "quasi-steady," which simply means that the flow at all times in the pulse cycle is above zero. In this regard, this end-diastolic flow velocity is the best indicator of the resistance to flow offered by the organ in question. As noted in Fig. 3.8, the normal common carotid velocity waveform has a clear window beneath the systolic peak and an end-diastolic velocity above zero. In the case of the external carotid artery, the velocity pattern is seen to be more pulsatile, with the prominent late systolic incisura and an end-diastolic level that is much closer to zero.

The clear systolic window reflects the point of sampling in the center of the artery and the size of the sample volume used for the measurement. In our practice, we believe it is important to use a very small sample volume (3 mm^3) for

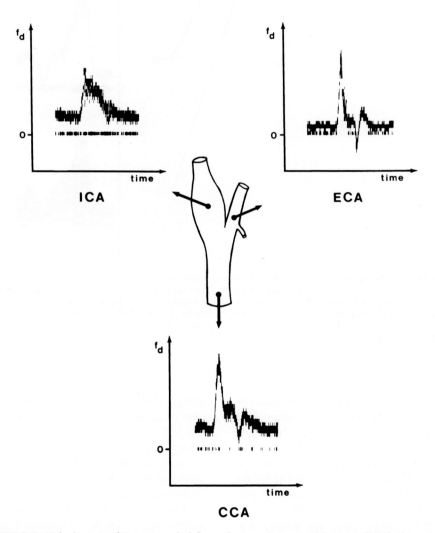

FIGURE 3.8. Velocity waveforms recorded from the common carotid artery *(CCA)*, the external carotid artery *(ECA)*, and the internal carotid artery *(ICA)* near the flow divider of a normal person. See text for explanation. (From Langlois YE, Roederer GO, Strandness DE Jr. Ultrasonic evaluation of the carotid bifurcation. *Echocardiography* 1987;4:141–159, with permission.)

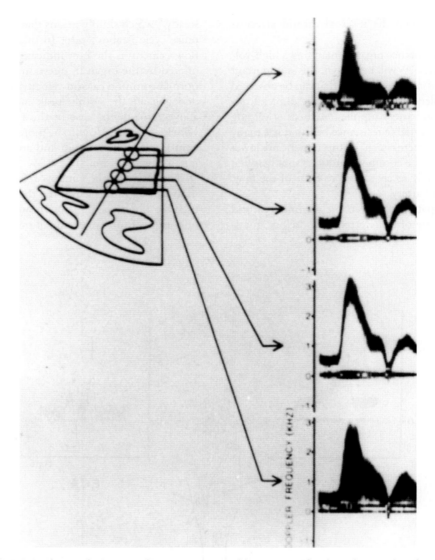

FIGURE 3.9. These velocity recordings are an ensemble average of 16 heartbeats taken from the sites indicated in the common carotid artery of a normal person. Note that, with the sample volume placed near the two walls of the vessel, marked spectral broadening is present as a result of the steep velocity gradients at this site. (From Phillips DJ, Greene FM, Langlois Y, et al. Flow velocity patterns in the carotid bifurcations of young presumed normal subjects. *Ultrasound Med Biol* 1983;9:19–49, with permission.)

studies of the carotid artery. This is because, if the measurement also were to include the flow near the wall where there is a very steep velocity gradient, spectral broadening would be noted (Figs. 3.9 and 3.10). It is now known that the velocity profile in the common carotid artery is blunt and not parabolic (Fig. 3.10). The velocity distributions for the bulb and the internal carotid artery are more complex, particularly for the posterolateral aspect of the bulb.

The bulb region forms a unique geometric arrangement that greatly complicates the flow patterns that occur. It is the only region in the body where there is a prominent dilatation in an arterial segment. This has, of course, led to the termi-

nology that is in common use, that is, the carotid bulb. It is also of interest that, when atherosclerosis occurs, it occupies the bulb itself, with little extension into the internal carotid artery. In fact, the work of Zarins and colleagues (1) clearly showed that the earliest lesions developed in the posterolateral aspect of the bulb, the site of some prominent flow changes unique to this region of the arterial circulation.

During our early studies of the carotid bifurcation, we did not appreciate the complexity of the flow patterns in the normal carotid bulb. There was an area of boundary layer separation with reversal of flow that was not recognized as being a normal finding. This led to many errors, particu-

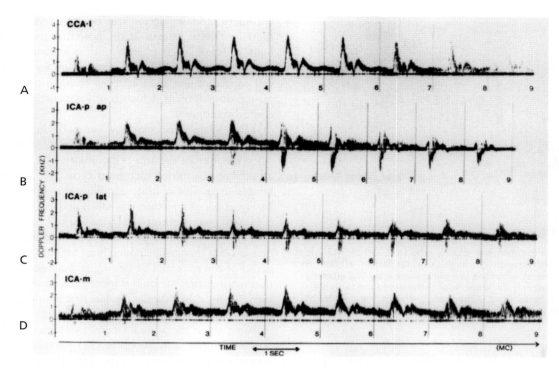

FIGURE 3.10. Flow velocity profiles generated at different anatomic positions of the carotid artery system of a normal person. The sites examined were low common carotid artery **(A)**, proximal internal carotid artery (bulb region) from the anteroposterior approach **(B)**, proximal internal carotid artery from the lateral approach **(C)**, and the mid-internal carotid artery **(D)**. The sample volume was stepped across the lumen of the artery in 1-mm increments. (From Ku DN, Giddens DP, Phillips DJ, et al. Hemodynamics of the normal human carotid bifurcation: in vitro and in vivo studies. *Ultrasound Med Biol* 1985;11:13–26, with permission.)

larly in calling normal subjects abnormal, thus giving us a poor specificity for the test. However, as we became more aware of the situation, it became apparent that the presence of such flow patterns could be useful for classifying the carotid bulb as normal (13).

Some of the early studies that characterized the flow across such a bifurcation were completed in scaled models of the normal carotid configuration (14–16). These model studies done with both steady and pulsatile flow clearly

defined some of the time-varying flow changes that can occur. An example of such flow changes that occur after peak systole is shown in Fig. 3.11. There are some evident changes noted by visual inspection alone. The flow would appear to be disordered, particularly in the lateral aspect of the sinus. In this region at this particular point in the pulse cycle, the flow is actually moving in a reverse direction. In fact, a double helix is actually formed that is propagated into the internal carotid artery for varying distances.

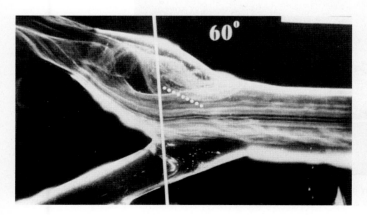

FIGURE 3.11. Flow visualization model of the normal carotid bulb in which a pulsatile system has been used. The ability to see the flow patterns is made possible by the introduction of hydrogen bubbles. This particular frame was taken right after peak systole. The flow distribution noted in the lateral aspect of the bulb is the region of flow separation. In this region, there is actual reversal of flow present. (From Ku DN, Giddens DP. Pulsatile flow in a model carotid bifurcation. *Arteriosclerosis* 1983;3:31–39, with permission.)

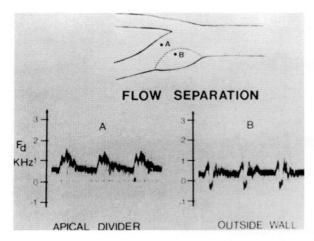

FLOW SEPARATION

FIGURE 3.12. In the example shown, when the sample volume is placed near the flow divider in this normal person, all flow is antegrade. However, when the sample volume is moved laterally in the bulb, an entirely different flow pattern is found with both forward and reverse flow components. This is the region of boundary layer separation, which is normally present.

If, based on the model studies shown, one were to predict the findings in the normal bulb, it should be possible to document both forward and reverse flow patterns during one heart cycle if the carotid bulb is free of disease. An example of such a normal study is shown in Fig. 3.12. As the sample volume is moved from the region of the flow divider to the bulb, the flow actually reverses. This is entirely consistent with the studies done in the models. This phenomenon is simple to demonstrate with the newer color systems. The fact that these flow changes can be studied with the duplex scanner is important. For example, if

boundary layer separation can be demonstrated, the bulb must be free of disease. If the posterolateral aspect of the bulb is filled with atheroma, this phenomenon cannot occur. Therefore, absence of reverse flow in the posterolateral aspect of the bulb permits recognition of the early plaque development, which is of little consequence from a clinical standpoint.

The availability of color flow has made the demonstration of the normal carotid bulb much simpler. As noted in Fig. 3.13, the flow in the area of boundary layer separation can actually reverse during each heart cycle. With color, this can be seen as an area of blue, signifying that flow has reversed. In Fig. 3.13, the picture was taken as peak systole. In Fig. 3.14 of the same subject, the frame was collected during diastole. No visible frequency shift is seen, suggesting that whatever velocity changes are taking place are below the frequency cutoff of the system. The finding of boundary layer separation signifies that the bulb is indeed free of atheroma. However, one must be aware of the fact that boundary layer separation will also occur just distal to a plaque.

What about the normal range of velocities for the carotid arteries? Müeller and associates (18) published data on the normal range of velocities in the common carotid artery as a function of age. Up to 30 years of age, the peak velocities recorded from the common carotid artery were in the range of 60 to 70 cm/sec for both men and women. However, with aging, the value decreased, so that by 70 to 80 years of age, this value had fallen to the range of 25 to 35 cm/sec for both sexes. It was of interest that the diameters of the common carotid artery progressively increased over this span of time, resulting in the volume flow's being kept in approximately the same range. This suggests that the flow to the brain was kept relatively constant, while the peak systolic velocity fell.

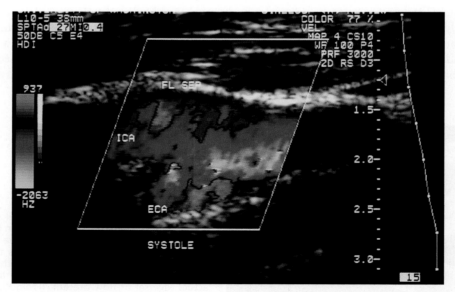

FIGURE 3.13. The boundary layer separation in the posterolateral aspect of the normal bulb is seen by the blue color signifying reverse flow at peak systole.

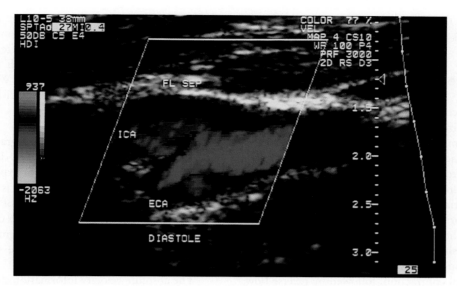

FIGURE 3.14. This photograph was taken during diastole in the normal person shown in Figure 3.13. No flow is shown in the posterolateral bulb. The velocity of the red blood cells may have been below the cutoff frequency of the system.

In our own studies of the effects of carbon dioxide on flow in the common and internal carotid arteries, the range of normal values before giving carbon dioxide was from a low value of 69 cm/sec to a high of 164 cm/sec in the common carotid artery in five presumed normal people (19). A similar range of values was found for the internal carotid artery, in which the peak systolic velocities ranged from a low of 46 cm/sec to a high of 109 cm/sec. When the volunteers breathed a mixture of 93.2% oxygen and 6.8% carbon dioxide, there was a 7% increase in the peak systolic velocity in the common carotid and a 47% increase in that recorded from the internal carotid artery (Fig. 3.15).

Because of the wide range of values noted for the absolute velocity data from the common and internal carotid arteries, it is not possible to use this type of data alone to predict the presence of a stenotic lesion and to estimate its significance. The relatively wide range of normal values at best makes this an uncertain indicator of the sta-

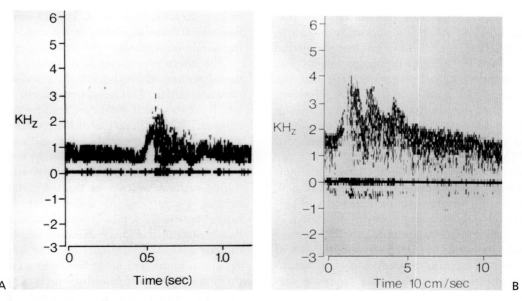

FIGURE 3.15. These velocity recordings were made from the internal carotid artery before **(A)** and after **(B)** inhaling carbon dioxide—6.8% carbon dioxide and 93.2% oxygen. (From Breslau PJ, Knox R, Fell G, et al. Effect of carbon dioxide on flow patterns in normal extracranial arteries. *J Surg Res* 1982;32:97–103, with permission.)

tus of the vessel at the site of measurement, unless some other information is available.

Peripheral Arteries

The arteries to be considered in this discussion are those large and medium-sized vessels supplying the arms and legs. Under resting circumstances, the tissues they supply have a relatively high resistance, which explains the types of velocity changes seen throughout their length. In practice, the velocity changes seen in the normal arteries of the upper limb show more variation than those from the lower limb. In about half of normal subjects, the waveforms recorded from the level of the subclavian artery to the radial and ulnar at the wrist show a triphasic velocity change (Fig. 3.16). The three components are the forward flow associated with myocardial contraction, followed by reverse flow, and then a second forward flow component in late diastole. In the latter part of the diastolic period, there is seen again a small but definite forward flow component. In people with a low level of vasomotor tone (warm hands), the reverse flow component may be absent, leaving a biphasic velocity pattern. In this circumstance, the reverse flow component is absent, and the end-diastolic flow is above zero (Fig. 3.16).

In the lower limbs, the same variability is not seen. The triphasic waveform should be seen in all normal subjects from the level of the aorta to the tibial arteries at the level of the foot (Fig. 3.17). The area beneath the systolic peak is clear, giving rise to a monotonously similar-appearing pattern throughout the entire limb.

Because the presence of reverse flow is a certain index of normality, Doppler can be used to demonstrate this phenomenon (Figs. 3.16 and 3.17). It is important to remember that the reverse flow component begins near the arterial wall during the phase of flow deceleration that follows peak systole. With color flow, a brief period of reverse flow can often be seen during each pulse cycle (Fig. 3.18). However, it must be emphasized that verification of this phenomenon can most easily be demonstrated by fast Fourier transforms (FFT) spectral analysis of the velocity patterns recorded from a pulsed Doppler.

A major advantage of color is the immediate recognition of the anatomy that it provides. This can be seen all the way from the level of the aorta to the tibial and peroneal arteries at the ankle. Examples of this are shown in Figs. 3.19 and 3.20. This saves scanning time and permits the user to make estimates of velocity at specific sites of interest. The overall scanning procedure is thus simplified, with less confusion as to the exact sampling sites being examined.

The absolute velocities recorded from the peripheral arteries of normal individuals were evaluated by Jager and colleagues [20]. The studies were done in 55 normal people (30 men, 25 women), ranging in age from 20 to 80 years old. All these subjects were free of symptoms and had normal ankle/arm indices. It was of interest that the peak aortic velocity tended to decrease with age, similar to that noted in the common carotid artery. Women were noted to have smaller arteries but with velocities that were in the same range as their male counterparts. The results are summarized in Table 3.1.

As one might expect, there is a gradual decrease in the peak systolic velocity as one proceeds down the limb. There is, however, a change that was not expected in terms of its magnitude. As you will note, there is a large drop in the peak systolic velocity from the level of the distal superficial femoral artery to the popliteal. This is certainly greater than that recorded for any other two segments in the limb or elsewhere. It is probably due to the sural arteries, which arise from this region (Fig. 3.19).

The absolute velocity information should be used only as a guide and should not be used in and of itself to indicate whether an arterial segment or one proximal to it is free of disease. This is because, in some cases with arterial narrowing, the velocities at rest may be in the normal range and can only be brought out by the stress of exercise or the injection of a vasodilating agent at the time of angiography. As will be noted in later chapters, velocity data are best used when they are compared with an arterial segment immediately proximal to the site of suspected disease.

As suggested, the true hemodynamic response of the arterial system for many of the vascular beds that fall into the intermediate-resistance category is often best characterized when the part is stimulated to increase its flow. As noted earlier, the normal peripheral arteries with a moderate stress load are able to maintain their perfusion pressure without a significant decrease. In terms of flow, the limb can increase its flow several times, depending on the workload and the resulting metabolic demands of the exercising muscle.

The effect of exercise is to reduce the resistance by vasodilatation, which converts the vascular bed into a low-resistance circuit. This has a dramatic effect on the velocity, which shows several distinctive features that are easily recognized. These include loss of the reverse flow component and an increase in the peak, mean, and end-diastolic velocities that go along with the increase in volume flow to the part. Because it is actually impossible to study these changes during exercise, patients are studied immediately after the exercise is completed when the patient has resumed the supine position. From a practical standpoint, the actual flow changes can easily be demonstrated by placing a continuous wave (CW) Doppler over the femoral artery. The velocity is monitored before and after a cuff placed on the thigh is inflated to suprasystolic pressure levels for 3 minutes. This simple experiment demonstrates the phenomenon of reactive hyperemia, transiently reducing the resistance to flow. The very short time span of this phenomenon in normal subjects is clearly seen in Fig. 3.21.

(Text continues on page 48.)

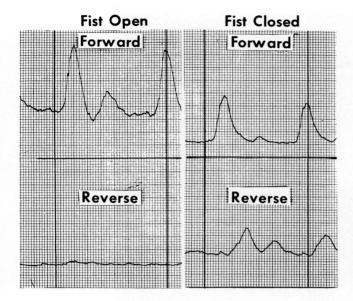

FIGURE 3.16. In the *left panel*, the recordings from the radial artery of a normal person were made with a continuous wave Doppler, displaying the changes with a zero-crossing detector. The forward and reverse flow changes are displayed on two separate channels. The waveform is biphasic, with no reverse flow component seen. However, when the person artificially increases resistance to flow by simply clenching the fist, a definite reverse flow component becomes evident, as shown in the *right panel*.

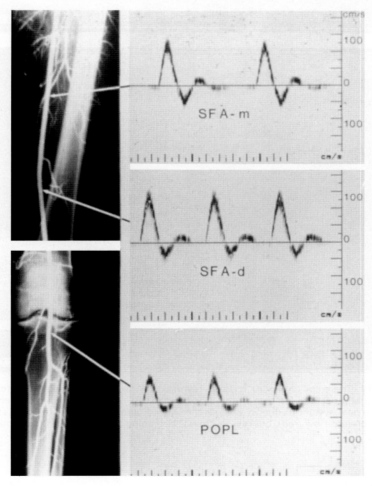

FIGURE 3.17. The velocity recordings shown were made with a duplex scanner with the sample volume placed in center stream. Note that reverse flow is seen in these normal arteries and that no spectral broadening is seen. *SFA-m*, mid-superficial femoral artery; *SFA-d*, distal superficial femoral artery; *POPL*, popliteal artery.

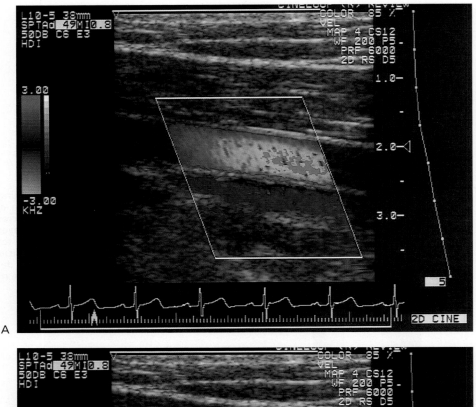

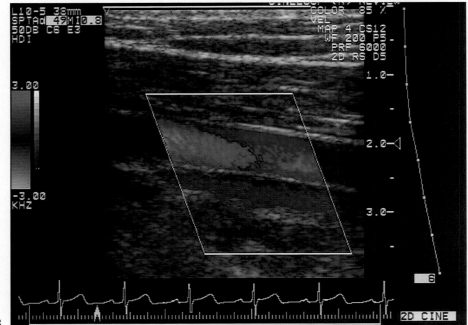

FIGURE 3.18. The color display of forward–reverse flow can be demonstrated in three phases (from a normal superficial femoral artery). **A:** After the QRS, with some aliasing in center stream shown as the peak systolic frequency exceeds the Nyquist limit. **B:** In middle to late diastole, there is ongoing forward flow *(red)*, but reverse flow is beginning to occur *(blue)*. *(Continued)*

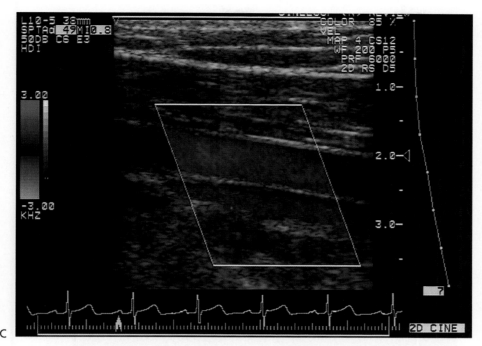

FIGURE 3.18. (*Continued*) **C:** Flow is now entirely reversed, as shown in *blue*.

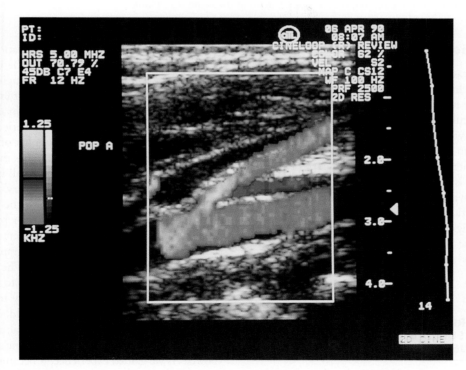

FIGURE 3.19. Color photograph of a normal popliteal artery with a large sural artery branch.

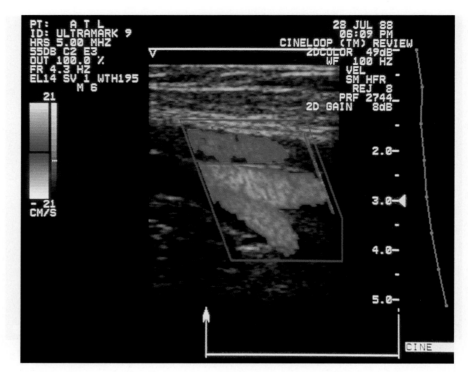

FIGURE 3.20. This image illustrates one of the advantages of color Doppler. Both the femoral artery and the deep femoral vein are shown in the same scan plane.

Visceral Arteries

From a diagnostic standpoint, major problems are seen with regard to acute and chronic mesenteric ischemia. Acute occlusions of the superior mesenteric artery are rarely called to the attention of the vascular laboratory. They usually have a dramatic presentation, with a rapid and progressive course that does not lend itself to the time required to carry out a duplex study. On the other hand, chronic mesenteric ischemia (mesenteric angina) is frequently a confusing condition, and duplex scanning provides a good method of evaluation.

The celiac, superior mesenteric, and inferior mesenteric arteries take their origin from the anterior wall of the abdominal aorta. The celiac and superior mesenteric arteries are to be found just below the diaphragm. The celiac artery gives

rise to the splenic and common hepatic arteries. These, of course, are the primary suppliers of the liver and spleen but also have important connections through potential collateral arteries with the superior mesenteric artery. These communications become extremely important in cases of chronic disease that involves the superior mesenteric artery. The superior mesenteric artery is the prime supplier of the small intestine. The inferior mesenteric artery supplies the left colon but can be important as a supplier of the small bowel when there is disease of the superior mesenteric artery.

By virtue of their location, both the celiac and superior mesenteric arteries can often be seen by B-mode imaging alone (Fig. 3.22). This can be complemented by the use of color Doppler, which permits more rapid identification of these important arteries (Fig. 3.23). The inferior mesenteric artery, by virtue of its close proximity to the mid-abdominal aorta from which it arises, is not easy to identify with certainty. Identification of this artery could, in theory, be important in cases of disease of both the celiac and superior mesenteric arteries because it would be a prime supplier of the small bowel. As we gained experience, it became clear that the inferior mesenteric artery can and should be studied in all cases in which chronic mesenteric angina is suspected.

The celiac, superior mesenteric, and inferior mesenteric arteries supply vascular beds of differing resistances. The celiac artery supplies the liver and spleen, which, like the kidney and brain, are low-resistance organs that demand a high rate of blood flow at all times. Thus, the velocity pat-

TABLE 3.1. ARTERIAL DIMENSIONS AND PEAK VELOCITIES MEASURED BY DUPLEX SCANNING IN 55 NORMAL SUBJECTS

Artery (cm/sec)	Diameter ± SD (cm)	Velocity ± SD
External iliac	0.79 ± 0.13	119.3 ± 21.7
Common femoral	0.82 ± 0.14	114.1 ± 24.9
Superficial femoral (proximal)	0.60 ± 0.12	90.8 ± 13.6
Superficial femoral (distal)	0.54 ± 0.11	93.6 ± 14.1
Popliteal	0.52 ± 0.11	68.8 ± 13.5

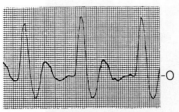

Before Reactive Hyperemia

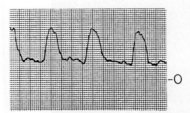

Immediately After Cuff Release

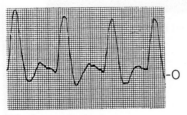

30 Seconds Later

FIGURE 3.21. Femoral artery velocity patterns. In the *upper panel*, the differential output of a direction-sensing continuous wave Doppler system is recorded using a zero-crossing detector. The triphasic velocity pattern disappears immediately with release of a cuff on the thigh inflated to suprasystolic pressure levels for 3 minutes *(middle panel)*. Within 30 seconds of releasing the pressure in the cuff, the flow velocity pattern has returned to the normal configuration *(lower panel)*.

terns seen in this vessel are similar to those seen in the internal carotid and renal arteries (Fig. 3.24).

The superior mesenteric artery and its flow patterns depend heavily on the time of day and its relationship to when the last meal was consumed. Under fasting circumstances, the flow in the superior mesenteric arteries resembles that seen in an artery supplying the lower limb. There may be reverse flow, and the end-diastolic component may return to or be close to the zero flow point (Fig. 3.24). However, after eating, there are dramatic changes in flow in the superior mesenteric but not in the celiac artery (Fig. 3.25). The flow usually reaches its maximum in 20 minutes and requires periods of time in excess of 80 minutes to return to the preprandial level (21–23).

To investigate the hemodynamics further, we studied seven healthy volunteers to examine the flow changes in the superior mesenteric artery in response to a variety of foodstuffs (23). The materials tested are shown in Table 3.2.

The baseline parameters for the celiac and superior mesenteric blood flow are shown in Table 3.3. The femoral artery flow was used as the control value for each of the times after ingestion of the materials shown in Table 3.4.

After ingesting the various foodstuffs, flow velocities and the volume flow in the superior mesenteric artery rapidly increased, reaching a peak 25 minutes after ingestion (Fig. 3.26). Because end-diastolic flow is the best indicator of the change in resistance, the values found for this parameter are shown in Fig. 3.27. As noted, there was an increase with all materials except water ($p < .05$). The maximal percentage increase for each of the tested variables is shown in Table 3.4. In making these measurements, it is important to realize that the least accurate of all is the determination of volume flow. This is because the measurement of diameter with even small errors compounds the error in the determination of flow. In addition, the assumption that the velocity vectors are parallel to the wall producing a parabolic flow profile may not be entirely correct (24,25). It is for this reason that it is prudent to use those parameters that are easily measured and at the

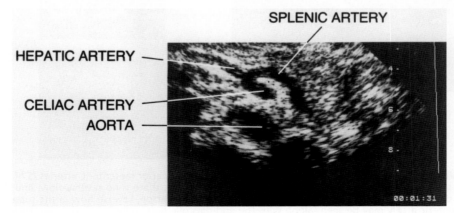

FIGURE 3.22. In this cross-sectional B-mode image of the upper abdominal region, the aorta, celiac, splenic, and common hepatic arteries are seen.

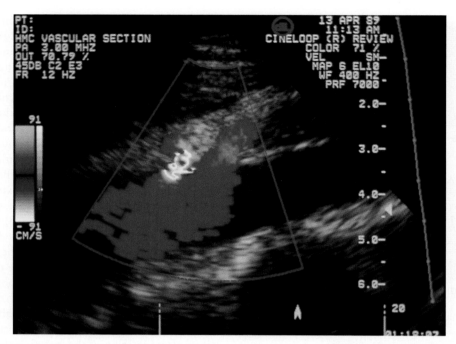

FIGURE 3.23. This color Doppler photograph shows the aorta and the first portions of the celiac and superior mesenteric arteries.

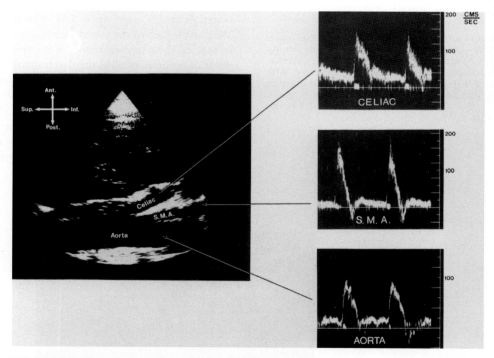

FIGURE 3.24. The velocity patterns taken from the celiac, superior mesenteric arteries *(S.M.A.)*, and the aorta in a normal fasting person. In the celiac artery, there is no reverse flow, and the end-diastolic velocity is always above normal. In the fasting person, reverse flow in the superior mesenteric artery may be seen, along with the end-diastolic flow going to zero. (From Nicholls SC, Kohler TR, Martin RL, Strandness DE Jr. Use of hemodynamic parameters in the diagnosis of mesenteric insufficiency. *J Vasc Surg* 1986;3:507–510, with permission.)

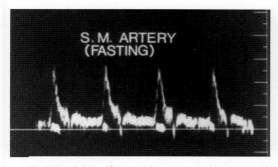 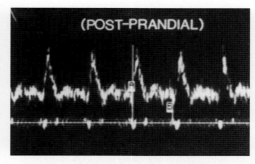

FIGURE 3.25. Changes in mesenteric artery velocities: preprandial and postprandial. Within 20 minutes of ingesting a meal, flow in the superior mesenteric *(S.M.)* artery increases. This change in terms of the velocity patterns is seen in the *right panel*. Onset of systole *(A)*. End-diastole *(B)*. There is an increase in the peak systolic velocity, the mean velocity, and the end-diastolic velocity. The reverse flow component disappears. (From Nicholls SC, Kohler TR, Martin RL, Strandness DE Jr. Use of hemodynamic parameters in the diagnosis of mesenteric insufficiency. *J Vasc Surg* 1986;3:507–510, with permission.)

TABLE 3.2. COMPOSITION OF THE MATERIAL USED TO STUDY MESENTERIC BLOOD FLOW

Mean	Volume (mL)	Calories (kcal)	Osmolarity (mOsml/L)
Mixed[a]	300	355	550
Carbohydrate[b]	300	350	550
Fat[c]	300	347	<100
Protein[d]	300	350	<100
Mannitol[e]	300	0	<550
Water	300	0	0

[a]Ensure-Plus (Ross Laboratories, Columbus, OH).
[a]Polycose (Ross Laboratories, Columbus, OH).
[c]Microlipid (Chesebrough-Ponds Inc., Greenwich, CT).
[a]Bacto-Peptone (Difco Laboratories, Detroit, MI).
[e]City Chemical, New York, NY.

TABLE 3.3. BASELINE BLOOD FLOW PARAMETERS USED IN THE STUDY OF THE EFFECTS OF VARYING FOODSTUFFS ON INTESTINAL BLOOD FLOW

	Peak systolic velocity (cm/sec)	End-diastolic velocity (cm/sec)	Mean velocity (cm/sec)	Volume flow (mL/min)
Celiac artery	101 ± 3.5	33 ± 1.4	52 ± 1.7	1083 ± 75
SMA	113 ± 3.9	15 ± 1.1	31 ± 1.4	538 ± 37
Femoral artery	83 ± 2.5	0 ± 0.2	10 ± 0.6	269 ± 22

Values expressed as the mean ± SE.
SMA, superior mesenteric artery.

TABLE 3.4. MAXIMAL PERCENTAGE INCREASE OVER FASTING FOR THE SUPERIOR MESENTERIC ARTERY[a]

	Peak systolic velocity (cm/sec)	Mean velocity (cm/sec)	Volume flow (mL/min)	End-diastolic velocity (cm/sec)
Mixed	42 ± 4	164 ± 30	164 ± 30	321 ± 100
Carbohydrate	30 ± 8	118 ± 23	118 ± 23	113 ± 20
Fat	42 ± 15	116 ± 25	117 ± 25	140 ± 47
Protein	22 ± 10	78 ± 15	78 ± 15	114 ± 21
Mannitol	33 ± 7	43 ± 10	48 ± 11	102 ± 45
Water	5 ± 7	24 ± 8	24 ± 8	34 ± 17

All values expressed as the mean ± SE.
[a]See footnote to Table 3.2 for source.

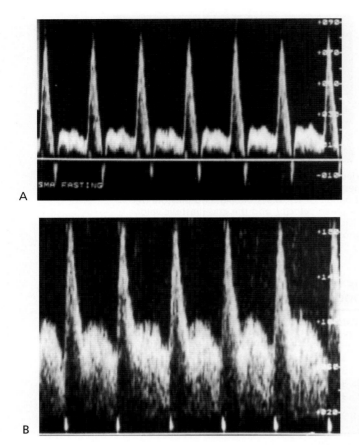

A

B

FIGURE 3.26. The fasting **(A)** and postprandial **(B)** velocity patterns from a normal superior mesenteric artery *(SMA)*. Note the dramatic increases in both the systolic and end-diastolic velocities. (From Taylor DC, Moneta GL. Duplex ultrasound scanning of the renal and mesenteric circulations. *Semin Vasc Surg* 1988;1:23–31, with permission.)

same time reflect the resistance to flow. In this regard, the end-diastolic velocity is probably the best one to use.

One of the interesting things to come out of this study was that the mixed meal produced the greatest increase in flow. This might be a useful test for those cases in which it may be desirable to determine the gut blood flow response in patients suspected of having chronic intestinal ischemia.

We now understand that flow in the inferior mesenteric artery does not normally increase with ingestion of a meal that is handled by the upper part of the small intestine and stomach. On the other hand, if one gives a substance such as lactulose, which is metabolized in the colon, flow in the inferior mesenteric artery dramatically increases when the material reaches the large bowel.

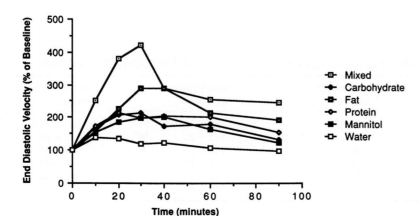

FIGURE 3.27. The end-diastolic velocity in the superior mesenteric artery after a variety of test meals. As shown, the greatest response is with a mixed meal. See text for details. (From Moneta GL, Taylor DC, Helton S, et al. Duplex ultrasound measurement of postprandial intestinal blood flow: effect of meal composition. *Gastroenterology* 1988; 95:1294–1301, with permission.)

Renal Circulation

The problem of hypertension is a major one in the United States. Gifford (26) has estimated that, of the 20 million people with hypertension, approximately 200,000 (2.6%) have it on the basis of renal arterial problems. The major problem has been and remains the identification of those patients with potentially treatable renal arterial lesions. Although intravenous urography and radionuclide studies have been proposed and used for screening purposes, they have been found to have unacceptably high false-positive rates of approximately 11% and 25%, respectively (27,28).

Intravenous digital subtraction arteriography was thought to offer promise as a screening tool, but this, too, has proved to be disappointing. Because of these facts and the improvements in duplex scanning technology, it was only natural that this method should be applied. To qualify as a reasonable screening test, it is necessary to have a very high specificity, so that large numbers of normal patients are not subjected to arteriography, which is invasive and potentially dangerous.

With the availability of lower-frequency scanheads (2.5 to 5.0 MHz), it is possible in most patients to gain access to the renal arteries throughout their length. The renal arteries are the most difficult visceral arteries to study with B-mode imaging alone. Although one can use the left renal vein as a landmark, visualization of the arteries throughout their length can be a problem. In Fig. 3.28, a B-mode image of the left renal vein and right renal artery can be seen. To be able to see the renal artery throughout its length is distinctly unusual. Color Doppler can be used to identify the origins of the renal arter-

ies, permitting the examiner the opportunity of placing the sample volume of the pulsed Doppler in its proper location (Fig. 3.29). Evaluation of the flow patterns in the renal arteries and the parenchyma of the kidney is essential in this important part of the circulation. As the initial requisite, it is necessary to review the normal flow patterns to the kidneys and to establish reasonable algorithms that could be used for screening and long-term follow-up purposes.

The kidneys are organs with high blood flow that require large volumes of blood to function properly. To accomplish this, they offer little resistance to flow, resembling very much the situations seen in the brain and the liver. Thus, the velocity patterns recorded from the renal arteries show similar characteristics with a very high end-diastolic flow rate (Fig. 3.30). Similar patterns can also be recorded from the parenchyma (Fig. 3.31).

Although it might seem feasible to generate diagnostic algorithms for the renal artery similar to those used for the carotid and peripheral arteries, this is not the case. The major problems associated with the examination relate to the depth of the arteries and the difficulty in assessing precisely the angle of the sound beam with the artery. This is made more difficult by the problem of trying to image the arteries throughout their length. This may not be possible even with the best scanners on the market.

Clearly, the best approach is to detect the sites of narrowing by a change in velocity and then to relate this to its role in activating the renin-angiotensin system. The degree of narrowing that produces a drop in the pressure beyond the stenosis, which, in theory, could be an important cause

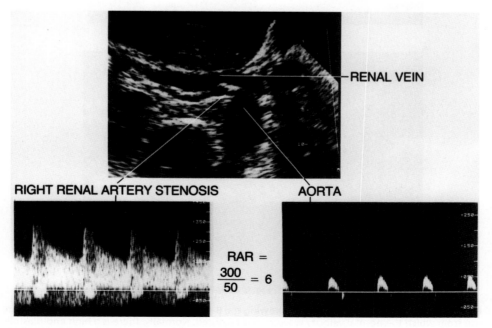

FIGURE 3.28. In this B-mode image, the abdominal aorta, the right renal artery, and the left renal vein can be seen. The velocity signal from the right renal artery is abnormal, indicating that stenosis is present. This fact would not be appreciated from the B-mode image alone.

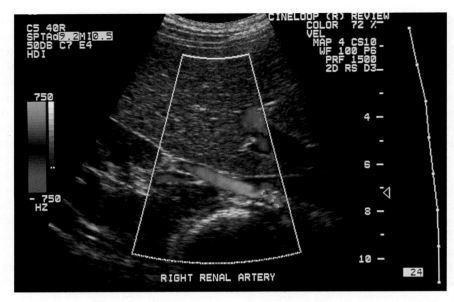

FIGURE 3.29. Color flow demonstrating the value of this modality in locating the renal arteries and their course to the kidney.

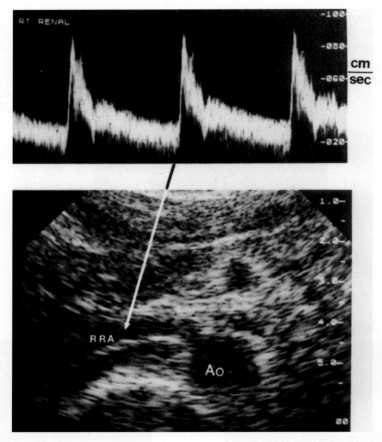

FIGURE 3.30. Renal artery duplex scan showing the B-mode image with the arrow indicating the site from which the normal velocity waveform is recorded. Normally, there is a high end-diastolic velocity without reverse flow. *Ao*, aorta; *RRA*, right renal artery. (From Taylor DC, Kettler MD, Moneta GL, et al. Duplex ultrasound scanning in the diagnosis of renal artery stenosis: a prospective evaluation. *J Vasc Surg* 1988;7:363–369, with permission.)

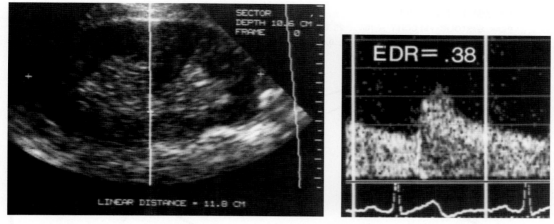

FIGURE 3.31. The velocity signal was recorded from the parenchyma of a normal kidney. Note the high end-diastolic velocity and the normal end-diastolic resistance *(EDR)*. See text for explanation.

of hypertension, appears to be a 60% diameter reduction (30). Thus, all our attempts to identify a renal artery stenosis are based on these considerations.

Because there are sites within the kidney that can lead to increased resistance and hypertension, it is also important to establish the normal range of values for this extremely important variable. Although it is possible in an animal model to measure the resistance to flow across an organ such as the kidney, this is not possible in humans. We need some measure from the velocity waveform that signifies an increase in the resistance to flow within the kidney itself (Fig. 3.31).

Fortunately, the level of resistance to flow is reflected in the velocity at end-diastole. Rittenhouse and associates (31) examined this problem and found that the ratio of peak velocity in the renal artery to the end-diastolic velocity— the end-diastolic ratio (EDR)—was a good method of estimating resistance.

As a result of all the above considerations, we elected to study a series of normal individuals to establish the normal range of values for the main renal arteries and the resistance to flow offered by the kidneys.

With regard to the main renal arteries for the detection of more than 60% stenosis, we chose to express the velocities as the ratio of the peak systolic velocity in the renal artery to that recorded from the aorta adjacent to the orifice of the renal arteries. This is referred to as the renal aortic ratio (RAR). This, combined with the measurement of the EDR, was carried out in a series of 42 normal subjects. The results of this study are shown in Fig. 3.32.

Venous System

As noted earlier, many aspects of venous function are more complex than on the arterial side of the circulation. The venous system is influenced by respiration, position, central venous pressure, arterial inflow, and muscular activity, particularly the calf muscle pump. Because duplex scanning methods are now capable of selectively sampling from major veins throughout the body, it is essential to understand the normal aspects of venous flow and how they are affected by disease. The early experience with the CW Doppler system showed quite clearly the role that respiration and body position play in venous flow in both the subclavian and femoral veins (Fig. 3.33). It should be noted from the figure that the flow dynamics for the upper extremity are quite different from the legs, which is not surprising.

The flow patterns of the lower limb veins are of particular importance, because of the frequent occurrence of acute deep venous thrombosis and the later development of the postthrombotic syndrome (32). Moneta and colleagues (33) studied 12 normal subjects to derive information on the relationship between venous dimensions and flow patterns in the common femoral vein.

The remarkable relationship between body position and femoral vein diameter was seen when the subjects were placed in positions sequentially from −10 to +30 degrees. In the −10 degrees position, the mean common femoral vein diameter corrected for body surface area was 0.47 ± 0.11 cm/m^2, as compared with 0.90 ± 0.16 cm/m^2 in the +30 degrees position, representing an increase of 92%. Conversely, as the patient was placed more upright, the mean peak flow velocity decreased. At −10 degrees, the mean peak velocity was 41 ± 10 cm/sec, as compared with 13 ± 5 cm/sec in the +30 degrees position ($p < .001$). There was a linear inverse relationship between the mean diameter of the common femoral vein and mean peak velocity: $r = -0.99$.

The relationships among body position, respiration, and events of the right heart are interesting. At −10 degrees,

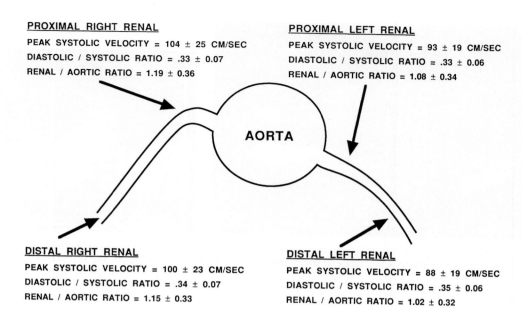

PROXIMAL RIGHT RENAL

PEAK SYSTOLIC VELOCITY = 104 ± 25 CM/SEC

DIASTOLIC / SYSTOLIC RATIO = .33 ± 0.07

RENAL / AORTIC RATIO = 1.19 ± 0.36

PROXIMAL LEFT RENAL

PEAK SYSTOLIC VELOCITY = 93 ± 19 CM/SEC

DIASTOLIC / SYSTOLIC RATIO = .33 ± 0.06

RENAL / AORTIC RATIO = 1.08 ± 0.34

AORTA

DISTAL RIGHT RENAL

PEAK SYSTOLIC VELOCITY = 100 ± 23 CM/SEC

DIASTOLIC / SYSTOLIC RATIO = .34 ± 0.07

RENAL / AORTIC RATIO = 1.15 ± 0.33

DISTAL LEFT RENAL

PEAK SYSTOLIC VELOCITY = 88 ± 19 CM/SEC

DIASTOLIC / SYSTOLIC RATIO = .35 ± 0.06

RENAL / AORTIC RATIO = 1.02 ± 0.32

N=42 (16 MALES, 26 FEMALES)

MEAN AGE = 54 MEAN BP = 129/76

FIGURE 3.32. The data were recorded from the main renal arteries of 42 normal control individuals.

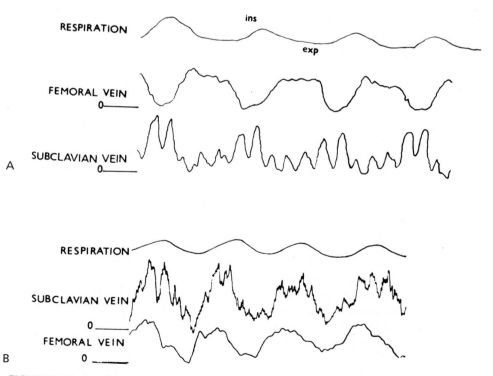

FIGURE 3.33. Simultaneous recordings of subclavian and femoral venous velocities in two positions—horizontal **(A)** and vertical **(B)**. As the position changes from the horizontal to the vertical, there is a phase shift in the femoral venous velocity. In the upright position, femoral venous velocity increases during inspiration *(ins)*, not expiration *(exp)*, as it does when the person is supine. (From Lewis J, Hobbs J, Yao J. Normal and abnormal femoral vein velocities. In: Roberts C, ed. *Blood flow measurement.* Baltimore: Williams & Wilkins, 1972:48–52,with permission.)

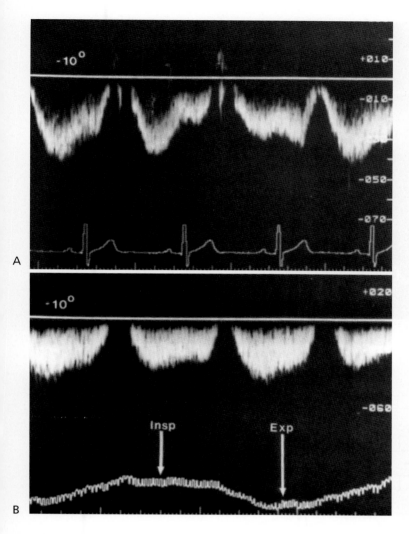

FIGURE 3.34. Femoral venous velocity patterns as related to body position. In this case, the person was at −10 degrees from the horizontal. **A:** The relationship with cardiac events. **B:** The relationship to respiratory events is shown. *Insp,* inspiration; *Exp,* expiration. (From Moneta GL, Bedford G, Beach KW, et al. Duplex ultrasound assessment of venous diameters, peak velocities, and flow patterns. *J Vasc Surg* 1988;8:286–291, with permission.)

blood flow in the femoral vein depended largely on events in the cardiac cycle. There was a marked increase during diastole, with flow decreasing or stopping shortly after the onset of systole (Fig. 3.34). When the person was placed at +30 degrees, flow in this position was more dependent on events in the respiratory cycle (Fig. 3.35).

The remarkable changes in venous diameter that can occur reflect the important capacitance function of the venous system. For example, a 100% change in diameter represents a fourfold increase in volume for that segment. Another factor concerning venous flow, which is known to all examiners who have frequently examined patients with the CW Doppler, is the role of changes in filling pressure of the right heart and the flow patterns in the veins of the leg that result. When the central venous pressure is high and the veins are distended, the effect of the cardiac events is often dramatic. This is most easily recognized by the pulsatile nature of the venous flow signal. In fact, the inexperi-

enced person listening to these velocity changes may even confuse them with arterial signals.

The most important structural elements in the venous system are the venous valves. These structures can be found from the level of the iliac veins down to the level of the foot. The greatest number of valves is found below the knee, where they provide an essential control mechanism to prevent the development of exercise-induced venous hypertension, with all of its undesirable consequences.

The venous valves close whenever there is a reversal of the transvalvular pressure gradient (34). During standing and quiet breathing, the valves remain open, permitting the necessary antegrade flow to the right heart. However, when this situation is altered by coughing, sneezing, or muscular contraction, a series of events, as displayed in Fig. 3.36, is set into play. The valves themselves are very thin and often difficult to see on B-mode imaging. Color assists in defining the location and function of venous valves, as shown in Fig. 3.37.

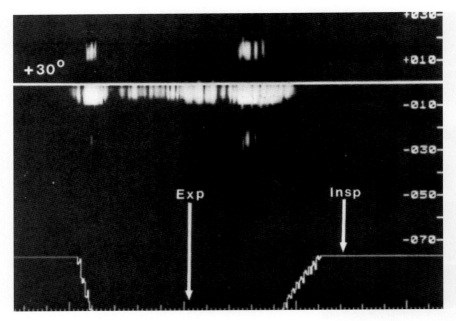

FIGURE 3.35. Femoral venous velocity patterns with the person at +30 degrees. In this position, respiration is the dominant factor affecting femoral venous flow. *Exp*, expiration; *Insp*, inspiration. (From Moneta GL, Bedford G, Beach KW, et al. Duplex ultrasound assessment of venous diameters, peak velocities, and flow patterns. *J Vasc Surg* 1988;8: 286–291, with permission.)

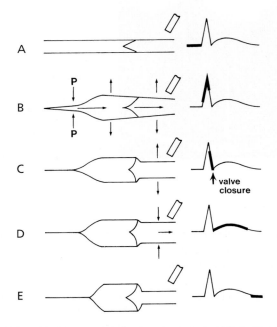

FIGURE 3.36. Sequence of valve closure when there has been a sudden increase in the transvalvular gradient. **A:** With the valve closed, there is no flow. **B:** With a sudden increase in pressure outside the vein, there is a sudden increase in venous dimensions and transient reverse flow through the valve. **C:** As the valve completely closes, flow in the distal vein will again go to zero. **D:** With elastic recoil of the vein, there will be a brief period of antegrade flow, but this is very little. **E:** While the pressure is still applied, flow in the distal vein will go to zero. (From van Bemmelen PS, Bedford G, Beach KW, Strandness DE Jr. The mechanism of venous valve closure: its relationship to the velocity of reverse flow. *Arch Surg* 1990;125:617–619, with permission.)

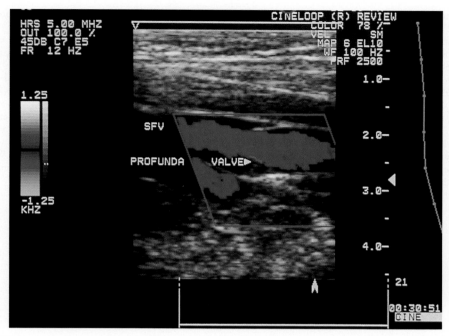

FIGURE 3.37. In this color photograph, the venous valve as seen with the B-mode image is defined more clearly by the color flow that is seen within the vein.

REFERENCES

1. Zarins CK, Giddens DP, Bharadvraj BK, et al. Carotid bifurcation atherosclerosis: quantitative correlation of plaque localization with flow velocity profiles and shear stress. *Circ Res* 1983;53: 502–514.
2. Gensler SW, Haimovici H, Hoffert P, et al. Study of vascular lesions in diabetic, non-diabetic patients. *Arch Surg* 1965;91: 617–622.
3. Strandness DE Jr, Priest RE, Gibbons GE. A combined clinical and pathological study of nondiabetic and diabetic vascular disease. *Diabetes* 1964;13: 366–372.
4. McDonald DA. *Blood flow in arteries.* Baltimore: Williams & Wilkins, 1960.
5. Kugelgen AV. Uber das verhaltnis von ringmuskulatur und innendruck in menschlichen grossen venen. *Z Zellforsch Mikrosk A Anat* 1955;43:168–183.
6. Hokanson DE, Strandness DE Jr. Stress-strain characteristics of various arterial grafts. *Surg Gynecol Obstet* 1968;127:57–60.
7. Strandness DE Jr, Sumner DS. *Hemodynamics for surgeons.* New York: Grune & Stratton, 1975:120–160.
8. Holling HE, Verel D. Circulation in the elevated forearm. *Clin Sci* 1957;16:197–213.
9. Ludbrook J. Functional aspects of the veins of the leg. *Am Heart J* 1962;64:706–713.
10. Arnoldi CC. Venous pressures in the leg of healthy human subjects at rest and during muscular exercise in the nearly erect position. *Acta Chir Scand* 1965;130:570–583.
11. Pollack AA, Wood EH. Venous pressure in the saphenous vein at the ankle in man during exercise and changes in position. *J Appl Physiol* 1949;1:649–662.
12. Langlois YE, Roederer GO, Strandness DE Jr. Ultrasonic evaluation of the carotid bifurcation. *Echocardiography* 1987;4:141–159.
13. Phillips DJ, Greene FM, Langlois Y, et al. Flow velocity patterns in the carotid bifurcations of young presumed normal subjects. *Ultrasound Med Biol* 1983;9:19–49.
14. Ku DN, Giddens DP, Phillips DJ, et al. Hemodynamics of the normal human carotid bifurcation: in vitro and in vivo studies. *Ultrasound Med Biol* 1985;11:13–26.
15. Bharadavj BK, Mabon RF, Giddens DP. Steady flow in a model of the human carotid bifurcation. I. Flow visualization. *J Biomechanics* 1982;15:349–362.
16. Bharadavj BK, Mabon RF, Giddens DP. Steady flow in a model of the human carotid bifurcation. II. Laser Doppler anemometer measurements. *J Biomechanics* 1982;15:363–378.
17. Ku DN, Giddens DP. Pulsatile flow in a model carotid bifurcation. *Arteriosclerosis* 1983;3:31–39.
18. Müeller HR, Radue EW, Buser M. Cranial blood flow measurements by means of Doppler ultrasound. In: Spencer MP, ed. *Ultrasonic diagnosis of cerebrovascular disease.* Dordrecht, Boston, Lancaster: Martinus Nijhoff, 1987:87–102.
19. Breslau PJ, Knox R, Fell G, et al. Effect of carbon dioxide on flow patterns in normal extracranial arteries. *J Surg Res* 1982;32: 97–103.
20. Jager KA, Ricketts HJ, Strandness DE Jr. Duplex scanning for evaluation of lower limb arterial disease. In: Bernstein EF, ed. *Noninvasive diagnostic techniques in vascular disease.* St. Louis: CV Mosby, 1985:619–631.
21. Nicholls SC, Kohler TR, Martin RL, Strandness DE Jr. Use of hemodynamic parameters in the diagnosis of mesenteric insufficiency. *J Vasc Surg* 1986;3:507–510.
22. Taylor DC, Moneta GL. Duplex ultrasound scanning of the renal and mesenteric circulations. *Semin Vasc Surg* 1988;1: 23–31.
23. Moneta GL, Taylor DC, Helton S, et al. Duplex ultrasound measurement of postprandial intestinal blood flow: effect of meal composition. *Gastroenterology* 1988;95:1294–1301.
24. Burns P, Taylor K, Blei AT. Doppler flowmetry and portal hypertension. *Gastroenterology* 1987;92: 824–826.

25. Gill RW. Measurement of blood flow by ultrasound: accuracy and sources of error. *Ultrasound Med Biol* 1985;11:625–641.
26. Gifford RW. Epidemiology and clinical manifestations of renovascular hypertension. In: Ernst SJ, Fry W, eds. *Renovascular hypertension.* Philadelphia: WB Saunders, 1984:77–100.
27. Treadway KK, Slater EE. Renovascular hypertension. *Annu Rev Med* 1984;35:665–691.
28. Grim CE, Luft FC, Weinberger MH. Sensitivity and specificity of screening tests for renal vascular hypertension. *Ann Intern Med* 1979;91:617–622.
29. Taylor DC, Kettler MD, Moneta GL, et al. Duplex ultrasound scanning in the diagnosis of renal artery stenosis: a prospective evaluation. *J Vasc Surg* 1988;7:363–369.
30. Haimovici H, Zinicola N. Experimental renal artery stenosis: diagnostic significance of arterial hemodynamics. *J Cardiovasc Surg* 1962;3:259–262.
31. Rittenhouse EA, Maitner W, Burr JW, et al. Directional arterial flow velocity: a sensitivity index of changes in peripheral resistance. *Surgery* 1976;79: 350–355.
32. Lewis J, Hobbs J, Yao J. Normal and abnormal femoral vein velocities. In: Roberts C, ed. *Blood flow measurement.* Baltimore: Williams & Wilkins, 1972:48–52.
33. Moneta GL, Bedford G, Beach KW, et al. Duplex ultrasound assessment of venous diameters, peak velocities, and flow patterns. *J Vasc Surg* 1988;8:286–291.
34. van Bemmelen PS, Bedford G, Beach KW, et al.. The mechanism of venous valve closure: its relationship to the velocity of reverse flow. *Arch Surg* 1990;125:617–619.

## 4

HEMODYNAMICS OF ARTERIAL STENOSIS AND OCCLUSION

The arterial system may be the site of clinical problems if one of three events occurs—if it is acutely occluded, if there is gradual arterial narrowing, or if segments become aneurysmal. The clinical presentation depends on the organ involved and the rapidity with which the process develops. Aneurysms of the abdominal aorta may rupture, with those involving the femoral and popliteal artery most commonly producing emboli or developing thrombosis. One of the remarkable aspects of the arterial system is its ability to adapt. Although this adaptation may be too slow in some cases of acute occlusion of an arterial segment, the collateral circulation is able to open and function well in most cases of chronic arterial narrowing and occlusion. This is why the patient may already have extensive disease before symptoms appear and he or she is first seen by a physician.

When the patient with arterial disease first appears, the physician needs to answer many questions that will be relevant to the subsequent workup and therapy. For aneurysmal disease, the principal question usually relates to the size and location of the lesion because it is these factors that dictate the subsequent course. The major decisions with regard to location and size can usually be determined by B-mode imaging alone and, in some cases, by computed tomography or magnetic resonance imaging. However, if there is an element of occlusive disease that may be associated with the aneurysm, examination with the duplex scanner may be of great value.

Duplex scanning is most often used in patients with chronic vascular disease; however, there are increasing numbers of patients with acute problems in whom we are being asked to evaluate the circulation. This is most commonly found in patients who have had either interventional therapy, such as transluminal angioplasty, or instrumentation with balloon pumps. Thus, it is helpful to understand the hemodynamics involved with both the acute and chronic presentations.

ACUTE ARTERIAL OCCLUSION

When an artery acutely occludes, survival of the organ without treatment is entirely dependent on the collateral circulation and its capacity to respond to the immediate need. As is well known, certain segments of the arterial circulation tolerate such an event well, whereas others tolerate it poorly. Examples of such instances include the following:

1. The abdominal aorta and common iliac arteries, when acutely occluded, lead to immediate and serious problems. The presentation is dramatic, leaving little doubt as to the cause of the event; the outcome will be poor if nothing is done to restore the circulation quickly.
2. The superficial femoral artery proximal to the superior geniculate artery to its origin can often be acutely occluded, with only transient ischemia noted.
3. In below-the-knee arteries, it is possible to occlude acutely up to two of the main arteries without significant ischemia developing. This is because the collateral communication between these vessels is extensive.
4. In the arm, isolated occlusions of the radial or ulnar artery are usually not even noticed. For the brachial artery, it depends on the site of the occlusion and its relationship to the ulnar and radial recurrent arteries. The occlusion may be recognized as only a minor and transient event, or it may be more severe.
5. For organs with high flow demands, acute occlusions are often tolerated very poorly. In some tissues, such as the brain, the time from anoxia to death of the tissues is so short that the collaterals may not have time to respond to the need. In this circumstance, the fate of the brain tissue often depends on the circle of Willis, which is known to be inadequate in about 50% of the population. The kidney is another example in which acute occlusions of the renal arteries may not be well tolerated because of the lack of large preexisting collaterals to meet the immediate needs of the tissues. The same applies to the small bowel, where acute occlusion of the superior mesenteric artery is poorly tolerated. On the other hand, if the disease develops slowly enough, the collateral supply to these areas is certainly sufficient to maintain viability and, in some cases, normal function as well.

Why should there be such striking differences from site to site when each organ has preexisting vessels that can and will serve as an alternate source of supply if the occlusion develops slowly? The survival and ultimate function of the ischemic tissue or organ depend on three elements of the collateral network: the stem vessels and the midzone and reentry arteries (1) (Fig. 4.1).

The stem arteries are those that serve as the major source of blood to the collateral arteries when the parent artery is occluded. Some common examples of the major stem artery include the profunda femoris artery, the internal iliac, and the external carotid artery. The profunda becomes the major input for all lesions, acute and chronic, that involve the superficial femoral artery. The internal iliac serves as the major stem artery when the external iliac is occluded. Both these arteries can carry large quantities of blood when called on to do so. The external carotid artery is a common collateral source to the brain via the ophthalmic artery, the small size of which limits the amount of blood that can be carried when an acute occlusion of the internal carotid artery occurs.

The midzone arteries are the most critical for most collateral circuits and are those vessels that serve as the bridging conduits between the stem and reentry vessels. Experimentally, with an acute occlusion, these arteries may be invisible by angiography immediately after the event, but with the passage of time, they become visible and greatly increase in size. Interestingly, the size of these midzone vessels correlates well with the rise in pressure that occurs in the arteries distal to the occlusion as flow improves (2).

When the collateral arteries begin to assume the transport role, flow to the regions beyond the area of occlusion will return to the main channels through the reentry arteries. For them to function as needed, the direction of flow will have to be reversed. These channels, although not as critical as those in the midzone, can also enlarge over time.

MICROEMBOLI (BLUE-TOE SYNDROME)

Microemboli are another cause of acute limb ischemia that always must be kept in mind because the etiology, recognition, and outcome are somewhat different. It is well known that atherosclerotic plaques can ulcerate, exposing the subendothelial tissue to flowing blood and permitting the accumulation of platelets and other debris from the plaque itself. If this material gets loose and embolizes, it will pass to the small arteries and arterioles of the foot, giving rise to acute ischemia.

This entity was described by Hoye and co-workers in 1959 (3), Eliot and associates in 1964 (4), and Richards and colleagues in 1965 (5). It is also important to remember that the clinical picture depends on the location of the plaque and the organs that are affected by the embolic event. For example, ulcerated plaques arising in the thoracic aorta may embolize to the renal arteries, the gut, and the lower limbs. These emboli are commonly quite small and will not occlude the large and medium-sized arteries. In some cases, cholesterol crystals will be the offending elements (Fig. 4.2).

From a clinical standpoint, the important point to remember is that these patients often have palpable foot pulses permitting the embolic material to reach the foot. When this is the case, this is not associated with total arterial occlusion. Presumably, if emboli do arise proximal to the arterial occlusion, the collateral circulation serves as a filter, delivering the bulk of the emboli to skeletal muscle. Although there is no doubt that microemboli can also pass through collaterals to the distal limb, foot, and digits, the attention is nearly always directed at the occlusions and not at looking for a source of emboli.

Duplex scanning can be of value in this setting in locating the lesion that is responsible for the embolic event.

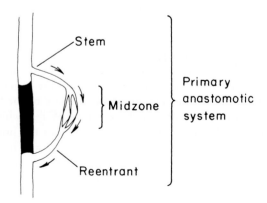

FIGURE 4.1. Schematic representation of the three major components of a collateral system that is bypassing an area of occlusion. The most critical in terms of hemodynamic performance is the midzone, where the vessels under normal circumstances may be very small. With the passage of time, these vessels increase in size, reducing their resistance to flow, which increases the distal perfusion pressure. Normally, the direction of flow in the reentrant arteries is opposite to that shown.

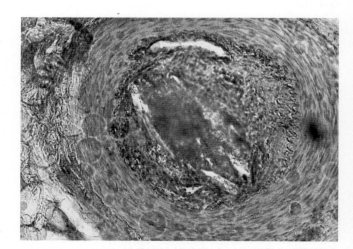

FIGURE 4.2. Photomicrograph showing occlusion of a digital artery by cholesterol crystals. (From Alksne JF. Collateral circulation. In: Strandness DE Jr, ed. *Collateral circulation in clinical surgery.* Philadelphia: WB Saunders, 1969:585–609, with permission.)

CHRONIC ARTERIAL STENOSIS AND OCCLUSION

When a patient presents with symptoms and signs of chronic arterial disease, it is certain that the offending lesions have reduced both pressure and flow to the limb. The problem in these patients is to determine the precise location and extent of the occlusive disease. This is where arteriography has traditionally played such an important role, providing a road map of the circulation. Yet, arteriography is not without its risks and should not be carried out for diagnostic purposes alone because this information can now be safely and accurately obtained by the combination of a clinical evaluation and duplex scanning.

Because each vascular bed has its own unique problems, it is not possible to generalize concerning the type of hemodynamic data that are needed and useful in evaluating a particular organ. It is common practice to address the question of "hemodynamic significance" when referring to an arterial lesion. This defines the ability of an arterial segment to provide the amounts of blood necessary for the activity demanded of it. For example, it is generally assumed that a 50% diameter-reducing lesion in a peripheral artery, by reducing the cross-sectional area of the artery by 75%, cannot support the blood flow needs of the exercising muscle. In contrast, a similar lesion in the carotid bifurcation may produce no symptoms or signs and become a problem only when the lesion becomes a source of emboli or is acutely occluded by thrombosis.

Thus, it is important when applying duplex scanning to understand the questions that need to be asked and how the information will be used. To this end, I shall review those organ systems commonly scanned and attempt to answer the pertinent questions most commonly raised.

EXTRACRANIAL ARTERIAL CIRCULATION

As is well known, atherosclerosis involving this important area of the circulation tends to localize to the origins of the arch vessels, the carotid bifurcation, and the siphon region. This is important information because it tells us where we have to look for the disease. What is the frequency of involvement at these different sites? Hass (6) studied the sites of involvement in 3,788 symptomatic patients with four-vessel cerebral arteriograms. The sites and frequency of involvement are shown in Fig. 4.3. In 75% of cases, a surgically accessible lesion was found. Forty percent were found to have intracranial lesions (Fig. 4.4). This does not mean, of course, that all observed lesions on arteriography are the source of symptoms and signs. However, when the lesions are demonstrated, it does raise the question. The clinical significance of an observed lesion depends on accumulated evidence as to its potential danger. In addition, when atherosclerotic lesions are found at one site of the

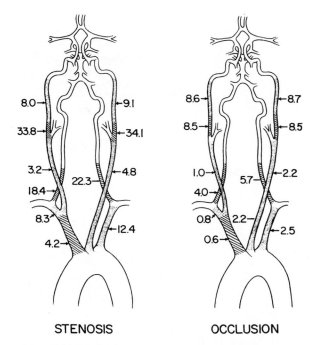

FIGURE 4.3. Distribution of extracranial arterial lesions in 3,788 patients undergoing arteriography. (From Hass WK. Joint study of extracranial arterial occlusion. II. Arteriography, techniques, sites and complications. *JAMA* 1968;203:961–968, with permission.)

extracranial circulation, they are likely to be found in other areas as well (Figs. 4.3 and 4.4). This propensity for involvement at multiple sites led Hutchinson and Yates (7) to coin the term *caroticovertebral stenosis* as a better descriptor of the process.

Because the mere presence of a lesion does not, in and of itself, predict what is likely to occur, how does it lead to problems? The early studies suggested that in the extracranial circulation, there are two major factors that might lead to and explain the occurrence of clinical events. These can be divided into the embolic and hemodynamic theories. The embolic theory states that most cerebrovascular events are secondary to the release of material from sites of ulceration—usually in the carotid bulb—to the ipsilateral hemisphere. Credit for this hypothesis must be given to Fisher (8), who reported this in 1951. It is now clear that the reason for this is loss of the integrity of the fibrous cap with either escape of the materials from within the plaque or development of a thrombus, which may fragment, releasing a portion of the thrombus into the cerebral circulation. Interestingly, this most frequently occurs in lesions that are very high grade in terms of diameter reduction and could in theory result in a fall in the flow to the ipsilateral hemisphere. This leads to the second and often hotly debated theory relating symptoms and signs to a reduction in blood flow leading to the production of symptoms. For this to occur, it presupposes that a high-grade stenosis could and

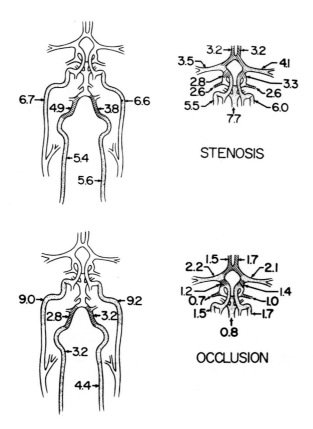

FIGURE 4.4. Distribution of intracranial arterial lesions in 3,788 symptomatic patients undergoing four-vessel arteriography. (From Hass WK. Joint study of extracranial arterial occlusion. II. Arteriography, techniques, sites and complications. *JAMA* 1968;203:961–968, with permission.)

would in many instances lead to events. The circle of Willis is so efficient in terms of providing blood flow that chronic hypoperfusion is very unlikely. On the other hand, the development of an acute thrombotic occlusion of the internal carotid artery leads to a stroke in about 25% of patients. Whether this is due to the sudden reduction of flow in the internal carotid artery or to embolization of thrombotic material is impossible to prove.

This role of high-grade lesions in the pathogenesis of stroke was obvious from the results of both the North American Symptomatic Carotid Endarterectomy Trial (NASCET) (9) and the European Carotid Surgery Trial (ECST) (10). In both of these trials, a positive relationship was found between the degree of stenosis and clinical outcome. For lesions that narrowed the diameter of carotid artery by 70% to 80% or more, there was a high incidence of stroke when these patients were treated medically. However, the end results of both of the above clinical trials did suggest that stroke events could be lowered by operation in patients with lesser degrees of stenosis (greater than 50%) but not to the same degree as with higher-grade lesions. Unfortunately, the clinical trials did not have repeat arteri-

ograms in those medically treated patients who went on to a stroke (11). In addition, neither of these trials had good ultrasound studies as a part of their protocol, which is unfortunate because we might have been provided this vital information. The higher the degree of stenosis, the more likely it was that the patient would sustain a clinical event (12).

Thiele and co-workers (13) examined the association between ischemic events and location of disease in 109 patients who underwent four-vessel angiography. In the 66 patients with ocular or hemispheric transient ischemic attacks, only 9% had no lesion found. In the 29 patients with fixed neurologic deficits, 10% were normal. The remainder of the patients in both groups had lesions in the carotid bulb. Plaque irregularity was found in 84% of the patients in the study. This study lends some credence to the role of both the carotid bifurcation and the embolic theory. Ulceration is often described by arteriography, but it is much safer to refer to the lesions as *smooth* or *irregular*. An irregular lesion is consistent with one that has lost in part the integrity of the fibrous cap.

Thus, it is quite clear that both the embolic and hemodynamic theories relative to the etiology of cerebral ischemia are correct as long as one defines the circumstances under which they are of relevance. Which of these is operative at the time of an event depends entirely on the circumstances and the nature of the changes at the bifurcation. However, it is very clear that it is the high-grade lesions that are most commonly associated with the development of a stroke.

The inability of the indirect noninvasive tests to characterize the lesions responsible for symptoms has been a problem. Periorbital Doppler and oculopneumoplethysmography were designed to test only the hemodynamic significance of lesions in the carotid artery. They did not become positive until either the collateral circulation was called into play or there was a pressure drop across the involved segment (14, 15). Although they were relatively simple to perform, the amount of information provided about the carotid artery was very limited. These tests are rarely used today because of these limitations. In addition, they cannot distinguish between a high-grade stenosis and a total occlusion. This distinction is extremely important clinically.

If the hemodynamic theory relating ischemic events to an acute reduction in flow does not answer the questions, as seen in patients who present to the noninvasive laboratory, what should be looked for? There are two aspects of this problem that can be addressed by duplex scanning. The first relates to the lesion itself and its propensity for causing problems. It is clear that there are changes within a plaque that can explain the clinical events that occur. The most obvious is the pathologic changes in the lesion itself and its propensity for leading to embolism and/or thrombosis. The ideal approach would be to identify these by imaging. From a hemodynamic standpoint, a considerable amount of time has been spent trying to measure accurately the degree of narrowing present in the carotid bulb. Why was this done? The reasons are as follows: (a) there may be a relationship between the degree of stenosis and outcome, (b) there may be a relationship between the morphologic changes in the plaque and the degree of stenosis, and (c) there must be some objective criteria that can be used for follow-up studies to monitor the progression of the disease. In this regard, the changes in velocity in a stenosis might be the most sensitive and accurate as a predictor of the degree of narrowing.

In the course of our ultrasonic studies, we soon became aware of some unique patterns of flow in the normal carotid bulb that needed to be recognized. The carotid bifurcation is the only site in the arterial system where there is a widening of the flow channel at a bifurcation. The common carotid artery divides into its two major branches with the changes that are seen in normals. These flow changes in the bulb must be understood for two major reasons. First, the localization of the atheroma in the lateral sinus region corresponds closely to the region of boundary layer separation that is normally present. Second, because the flow patterns in the normal bulb are complex, they can be a source of confusion unless understood. The finding of boundary layer separation is an important consideration when documenting the status of the carotid bulb.

As the atheroma begins to fill the bulb, it tends to convert the bifurcation into a straight and circular tube. This then eliminates the possibility of boundary layer separation. The changes in the flow patterns that might be expected when this occurs are shown in Fig. 4.5. As might be expected, if the lateral aspect of the bulb itself were completely filled with atheroma, there would be no impingement to flow in the internal carotid artery. It is also important to realize that if one uses the distal internal carotid artery as the norm, obliteration of the normal bulb configuration would not be counted as any degree of diameter reduction. This is the manner in which most arteriographers grade the degree of stenosis. On the other hand, when one uses the outer limit of the bulb as the normal reference value, it would constitute a 50% diameter reduction. If the surface of the plaque occupying the bulb were irregular, one might begin to see some flow disturbances secondary to those changes. When the plaque begins to impinge on the flow stream (i.e., exceed the limits of the bulb), a velocity increase would be expected to occur. The flow patterns immediately distal to the bulb and the stenosis would then begin to show the disturbances expected when the flow stream moved into a segment of the internal carotid artery larger than that at the site of narrowing. The flow would no longer be laminar in this region, and "poststenotic turbulence" would be expected. At what point would an actual pressure drop be expected to occur? Would it be the same as with a 50% diameter-reducing stenosis in a peripheral artery?

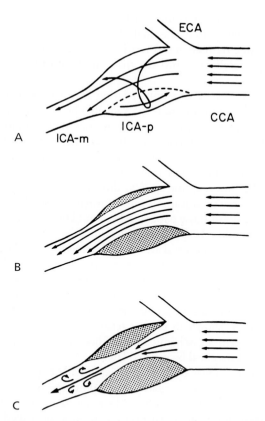

FIGURE 4.5. Schematic representation of the flow patterns seen in the carotid bulb of normal subjects **(A)**, patients with disease confined to the bulb alone **(B)**, and patients in whom the plaque has progressed beyond the confines of the bulb to impinge on the region close to the flow divider **(C)**. In **panel A**, the *dotted lines* illustrate the region in which there is normally flow reversal, referred to as the area of boundary layer separation. There can also be seen the fact that helical-type flow may occur through this region of the bulb. When the bulb is filled with an atheroma, the boundary layer separation shown in **panel A** no longer occurs. In this situation, there will be no increase in the peak systolic velocity within the region. As the plaque enlarges further, there will be an increase in the peak velocity and also some development of flow disturbances distal to the site of narrowing. This is often referred to as the zone of poststenotic turbulence.

Sillesen and Schroeder (16) examined the flow patterns in the internal carotid artery distal to a stenosis to determine whether there were findings that would be predictive of a pressure drop. By using a reduction of 20% in the mean internal carotid artery pressure, they could predict this with an accuracy of 90% to 95% by using the pulsatility index (PI), pulse rise time (RT), and systolic width (SW). As might be expected, the PI would decrease, the RT increase, and the SW also increase. For a PI of 0.71 or less, 8 of 10 arteries had an abnormal pressure gradient. When the RT exceeded 0.16 second, 8 of 9 patients had an abnormal gradient. When the SW exceeded 0.30 second, 9 of 12 patients had an abnormal gradient. The SW data were calculated as the width of the systolic waveform at the frequency that was half the sum of the peak and end-diastolic frequencies. A fast Fourier transforms system (FFT) was used to record the maximum, minimum, and mean frequencies.

There are several questions relating to such an analysis. The use of mean pressure is questionable because, for most purposes, the systolic pressure is the most accurate method of documenting hemodynamic significance. Across such a short segment, there should be no measurable systolic gradient. The mean pressure is not nearly as sensitive an indicator as the systolic pressure, and a 20% drop in mean pressure is likely to be very significant. Is this information useful? Might it be predictive of those patients who would be likely to have an event? Could it be used to predict outcome with an occlusion of the internal carotid artery? Unfortunately, one cannot give a final answer to any of these questions. Periorbital Doppler and oculopneumoplethysmography will become positive only when there is a significant drop in pressure across a stenosis and/or an occlusion, and neither of these tests has been shown to predict reliably which patients are likely to sustain an ischemic event. There are many reasons for this, and they will be covered later.

One of the most difficult problems with regard to the circulation to the brain relates to the potential importance of the circle of Willis as a collateral source, along with those extracranial-intracranial pathways that may be called on when there is a need. The circle of Willis would appear to be the ideal network connecting the right and left hemispheres with both internal carotid arteries and the basilar artery (17). It is rare for an individual component of the circle to be absent, but it is common for portions to be functionally incomplete (18). It turns out that the most common anomaly is hypoplasia of the posterior communicating artery, which can be bilateral and occur in combination with other anomalies (Fig. 4.6).

Is there proof that the circle of Willis is important in the prevention of ischemic events? The answer to this question would appear to be yes, but one must define the circumstances in which it may prevent such an occurrence (Fig. 4.7). What is most impressive is the amount of vascular disease one can possess and still remain asymptomatic. We have seen several patients with occlusions of both internal carotid arteries who are doing quite well. However, in each case, they presented with an ischemic event from which they survived and improved.

With the availability of transcranial Doppler, we may be able to answer some of these questions. We now have the capability of studying the entire circle, but relating the findings to the clinical presentations has been very difficult. Although arteriography does provide some information about the circle of Willis, I am not convinced that it helps with specific patient problems with regard to patient management or that it can be used to predict long-term outcome.

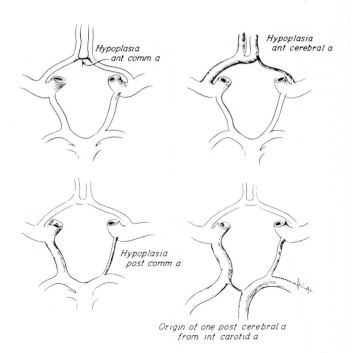

FIGURE 4.6. Most common variations seen in the circle of Willis. (From Alksne JF. Collateral circulation. In: Strandness DE Jr, ed. *Collateral circulation in clinical surgery.* Philadelphia: WB Saunders, 1969:585–609, with permission.)

In the course of validating the results of duplex scanning for classification of carotid artery disease, we had the opportunity of carrying out extensive arteriographic studies that also provided excellent views of the intracranial vessels and the circle of Willis. To study the anatomy of the collaterals, we reviewed 178 consecutive patients who had undergone selective injections of the carotid arteries and arch injections for the vertebral arteries. Towne and lateral projections were used to study the intracerebral arteries.

The patient population was divided into three groups: group I had patent carotid arteries on both sides; group II had unilateral occlusion of the internal carotid artery; and group III had occlusion of both internal carotid arteries. The presenting symptoms were divided into two groups—those with focal symptoms of a transient or fixed nature, and those who presented with nonfocal symptoms such as vertigo, ataxia, or dizziness. The anatomic details of the vessels visualized along with the direction of flow were compared in the three groups. Abnormalities of the circle of Willis were defined as nonfilling of a vessel, hypoplasia, or the presence of an atherosclerotic lesion within the vessel.

The breakdown of the groups is listed in Table 4.1. The type of symptoms found in each of the groups is shown in Table 4.2.

It was of interest that we were unable to relate the appearance of collaterals with the degree of stenosis of the internal carotid artery. In the 242 sides in group I, there were 119 (49%) with a less than 50% diameter-reducing

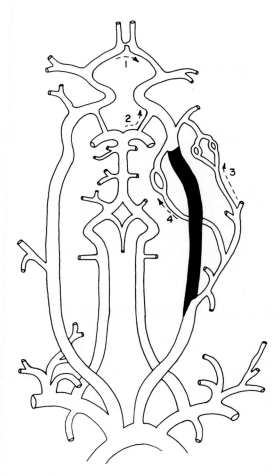

FIGURE 4.7. When the internal carotid artery becomes occluded, there are a variety of collateral pathways for blood to reach the ipsilateral cortex. As noted, two of these involve the circle of Willis. The pathways illustrated are: (*1*) from the opposite internal carotid artery through the anterior cerebral arteries; (*2*) by the basilar through the posterior communicating artery; (*3*) from the ophthalmic artery; and (*4*) the caroticotympanic artery. (Redrawn from Riggs HE, Rupp C. Variation in the form of circle of Willis: the relation of the variations to collateral circulation. Anatomic analysis. *Arch Neurol* 1963;8:8–14, with permission.)

lesion. Visible extracranial-intracranial vessels were seen in 16 sides (13%). In the 123 sides with a greater than 50% diameter-reducing stenosis, collateral pathways were seen in 18 sides (15%). With regard to the other two groups, visible collaterals were seen in five of the six patients in group

TABLE 4.1. PATIENT POPULATION AND THE DEVELOPMENT OF EXTRA- TO INTRACRANIAL PATHWAYS

	Number	Percentage
Group	(No. with visible collaterals)	
I Patent internal carotid arteries	127	13.4 (17)
II Unilateral occlusion	45	55.6 (25)
III Bilateral occlusion	6	100 (6)

TABLE 4.2. TYPE OF SYMPTOMS AT PRESENTATION

Group	Percentage with focal symptoms	Percentage with nonfocal symptoms	Asymptomatic
I (n = 127)	63 (80)	20 (25)	17 (22)
II (n = 45)	58 (26)	0 (33)	42 (19)
III (n = 6)	83 (5)	0 (33)	16.6 (1)

Numbers in parentheses, number of cases.

II on both sides. In the remaining patient, it was noted on one side. In group II, 25 (56%) of the patients had demonstrable collaterals that developed on the side of the occlusion in each case.

Most important, what was the relationship between the presenting symptoms and the appearance of visible collaterals? Because focal symptoms are the most important, we examined this relationship. The results are summarized in Table 4.3.

Although there appeared to be a trend in the patients in group I, these differences were not significant. It is interesting that one third of the patients in group II were symptomatic despite collaterals being seen.

There were 178 circles of Willis visualized that were available for analysis. The results of this aspect of the study are summarized in Table 4.4. The circle was complete in one third of patients in group III, in 18.1% in group I, and in 5.2% in group II. The highest incidence of anomalies was seen with the posterior communicating artery. This was abnormal in 63% of patients in group I and in 86% of those in group II. It is of interest that only one patient (17%) in group III had an abnormality of this vessel. The anterior communicating artery was absent in 18% of those in group I, 5% of those in group II, and 33% of those in group III. Absence of all three communicating vessels was

TABLE 4.3. RELATIONSHIP BETWEEN THE OCCURRENCE OF FOCAL SYMPTOMS AND VISIBLE COLLATERALS

Group	Collaterals	Symptomatic (%)	Asymptomatic (%)
I Patent (n = 121)	With	12.4 (15)	1.6 (2)
	Without	69.4 (84)	22.2 (10)
II Unilateral occlusion (n = 45)	With	33.3 (15)	22.2 (10)
	Without	24.4 (11)	20 (9)
III Bilateral occlusion (n = 6)	With	83.3 (5)	16.6 (1)
	Without	0	0

The patent group excludes the six with occluded or narrowed subclavian arteries because their collaterals developed in response to the disease in these vessels.
Numbers in parentheses, number of cases.

TABLE 4.4. COLLATERAL ROUTES SEEN ON ANGIOGRAPHY

Vessel derived from:	Collaterals	Vessel supplied	(%)
External carotid	Int. maxillary ophthalmic	Middle cerebral	58
External carotid	Middle meningeal	Middle cerebral	12
External carotid	Int. maxillary ophthalmic	Anterior cerebral	4
External carotid	Post. occipital	Vertebral	18
Posterior cerebral	Small superficial branches	Anterior and middle cerebral	5
Posterior cerebral	Small superficial branches	Anterior cerebral and pericallosal	4

Int, internal; Post, posterior.

seen in 10% of those in group I and in 3% of those in group II. Missing or hypoplastic forms of the anterior cerebral stem vessels were seen in 9% of group I and 2% of group II patients. There were no associations noted between the development of symptoms and the type of anomalies seen in the circle of Willis.

There were several surprising elements to this study that are worthy of comment and pertinent to the field of diagnostic methods. The fact that the degree of narrowing did not seem to correlate with the appearance of visible collaterals was most surprising. In fact, the only circumstance in which collaterals were regularly seen was with total occlusions. Perhaps the ability of the brain to autoregulate its flow even with lower levels of pressure may be a factor that is not so apparent in the peripheral circulation, where collaterals do seem to respond much earlier.

From the standpoint of duplex scanning, it is of interest that the most frequently visualized collateral route was the external carotid artery. The frequencies of the visualized collateral pathways are summarized in Table 4.4.

The findings have important implications from both a diagnostic and therapeutic standpoint. The appearance or lack of visible collaterals bore little relationship to the clinical presentation. The circle of Willis would be put to the test when both internal carotid arteries are occluded. Fields and associates (19) reported that, in such cases, an initial occlusion of one carotid artery can be well tolerated until followed by an occlusion on the opposite side. Six of 16 cases had minimal permanent deficits with an "adequate" collateral circulation. In five of our cases, well-developed collaterals were seen, but two had permanent deficits despite this. It may be, of course, that most patients with bilateral occlusions of the internal carotid artery never survive, and that those who do survive to be studied are those with an intact circle of Willis.

The collateral circulation remains critically important in most individuals even though it may fail in its role in some patients (20).

Although there is no doubt that some unilateral internal carotid occlusions are totally benign, this is certainly not always the case. Nicholls and colleagues (11) were able to follow 24 patients serially with repeat duplex scanning to assess outcome when the lesion progressed to a total occlusion. In this group, there were six strokes (25%), four tran-

sient ischemic attacks (16%), and one patient with non-hemispheric symptoms. The remaining 13 patients were asymptomatic. There is no direct evidence as to the etiology of the stroke or transient ischemic events in these patients; however, one possible theory is the abrupt fall in cerebral perfusion that accompanies the occlusion.

PERIPHERAL ARTERIAL CIRCULATION

As noted in Chapter 3, the peripheral arteries are remarkably adapted to provide flow to the limbs under widely varying conditions of demand. With normal myocardial function, large volume-flow increases can be accomplished with little energy loss. Surprisingly, this accommodation remains until there is extensive arterial involvement when the pressure losses across areas of disease are such that normal perfusion of the tissues is no longer possible. When does this occur?

A great deal of attention has been paid to the concept of the "critical stenosis." This is roughly defined as that degree of reduction in arterial cross-sectional area that is sufficient to produce a fall in pressure and flow beyond the sites of involvement under resting flow conditions. A *critical stenosis* has been defined as a 50% reduction in diameter, which corresponds to a 75% reduction in cross-sectional area (21). However, it is now recognized that much less severe degrees of stenosis can become hemodynamically significant when there is a dramatic increase in flow, such as might occur with exercise. As Schultz and colleagues (22) showed, significant pressure falls can occur across stenoses of less than 50% when the flow velocity through the narrowed segment is increased.

These considerations have important clinical implications. With a true critical stenosis, there will be a measurable pressure drop across the area of involvement with the patient at rest. This is why the measurement of ankle systolic blood pressure is such an important method of documenting the presence of occlusive disease. Systolic pressure is used for two reasons: (a) it is the most sensitive parameter for the assessment of hemodynamic significance because it is the first to fall (mean and diastolic pressures do not fall until the disease becomes much more advanced); and (b) it is easy to measure with any indirect method, such as continuous wave Doppler.

There is a subset of patients with normal resting pressures who suffer from intermittent claudication. These patients have normal peripheral pulses at rest that disappear after exercise (23). These patients usually have aortoiliac disease and a stenosis that becomes hemodynamically significant only with the stress of exercise and the increase in flow through the stenotic segment. These patients are easily recognized by measuring the ankle systolic pressure at the ankle level before and after walking on the treadmill (24,25).

As mentioned in Chapter 3, a normal person can accommodate the flow requirements of even stressful exercise without sustaining a large drop in the ankle systolic blood pressure (26). However, when there is sufficient arterial narrowing and/or occlusion to produce symptoms, the existing pressure gradient (if any) will be accentuated by the stress of exercise. It is important to understand that true vascular claudication does not and cannot occur without a drop in ankle blood pressure, the extent of which is commensurate with the degree of disability. For patients with severe, lifestyle-limiting claudication, the pressure falls after exercise to very low levels (often unrecordable), with recovery times that often exceed 30 minutes.

It must be noted that, in recording such pressure changes after exercise, it is unnecessary and misleading to record the postexercise ankle/arm ratio, which is done by many laboratories. Studies done in our laboratory have shown that the arm blood pressure increases after exercise in an almost linear fashion that is related to the workload (26). It is important to record only the fall and recovery time of the ankle systolic pressure.

In terms of the pressures seen distal to areas of stenosis or occlusions, it is important to realize that the magnitude of the pressure fall will depend on the resistance offered by the collateral circulation. In general terms, with a single-segment arterial occlusion of an iliac or superficial femoral artery, the systolic pressure at the ankle will be more than half that recorded from the arm, giving an ankle/arm index of greater than 0.50. However, when another segment becomes occluded, the resistances offered by the second series of collaterals are additive. Thus, with multisegment disease, the ankle systolic pressures are less than half that recorded from the arm, giving an ankle/arm index of less than 0.50.

It is also apparent that the most severely disabled patients are those with multisegment disease. The more disease that is present, the greater is the reduction in perfusion pressure to the foot and muscle groups. Thus, the systolic pressures at the ankle should provide clues to the severity of the problems that might be encountered clinically and also should provide some useful data on the type of duplex examination that might be necessary in evaluating the level and extent of arterial disease.

In addition to the evaluation of limb pressures, the changes that occur in the velocity patterns should also be noted. With progressive involvement, characteristic changes that occur are now well recognized. As the degree of narrowing becomes more severe, the peak systolic and end-diastolic velocities within the narrowed segment increase (Fig. 4.8). They appear to rise in an almost linear fashion, making them a potentially suitable index of the degree of stenosis. There are other changes that appear to be useful in making this distinction. For clarity, these changes should be subdivided into those cases in which the artery is totally occluded and those in which the artery is only narrowed.

Total Arterial Occlusion

Because flow is now diverted through the collateral arteries, there is a progressive fall in the peak systolic velocity with loss of the reverse-flow component. The contour of such waveforms has been described as monophasic and represents a "damped" version of the normal velocity patterns. The end-diastolic velocity remains above zero, which is a reflection of the compensatory decrease in resistance offered by the peripheral arterioles. This is the mechanism by which the limb can maintain blood flow levels to the tissue within a normal range under resting conditions. As noted earlier, this compensatory response works well, even with extensive arterial disease, but is not effective in meeting the demands placed on the circulation by the stress of exercise.

Arterial Stenosis

From a diagnostic standpoint, it is important to attempt to separate those lesions that are of clinical relevance from those that are not responsible for problems. As noted earlier, it is important to be able to detect and quantify the critical stenosis, defined as that sufficient to produce a pressure drop and a reduction in blood flow. Because duplex scanning permits an evaluation of the segments preceding and distal to the area of involvement, it is important to consider each in addition to the velocity changes within the narrowed segment itself (27).

Less than 50% Diameter Reduction

In this setting, the velocity patterns proximal to the stenosis are often entirely normal. There is an increase in the peak systolic velocity within the narrowed segment that is in the range of 30% to 100% of that from the adjacent arterial segment. There is marked spectral broadening, but the reverse-flow component is preserved. The waveform distal to the stenosis is normal.

Greater than 50% Diameter Reduction

With this critical narrowing, there may be some damping of the proximal velocity waveform due to the marked area reduction in the stenosis, although this cannot be used, in and of itself, as a measure of the degree of narrowing. Within the narrowed segment, the peak velocity increases by more than 100%, with loss of the reverse flow compo-

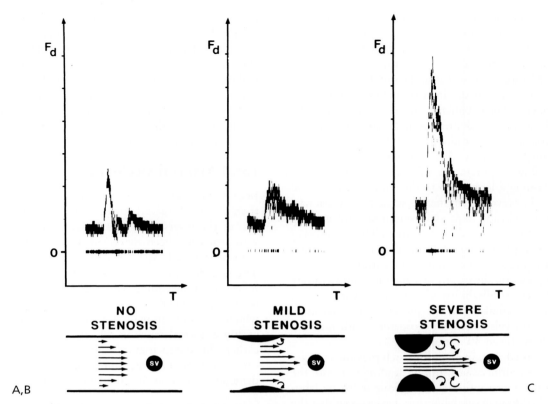

FIGURE 4.8. Some of the velocity changes that occur in a normal artery and the progressive involvement from a mild to a severe stenosis. In the illustration, the sample volume *(SV)* has been placed in the center of the artery. **A:** The waveform is very oscillatory, with a clear window beneath the systolic peak. **B:** With a mild stenosis that involves changes at the level of the wall, there is no increase in the peak systolic velocity, but there is some spectral broadening during deceleration. **C:** The degree of narrowing is such that there is an increase in both the peak and end-diastolic velocities along with spectral broadening. *Fd*, frequency shift; *T*, time. (From Roederer GO, Langlois YE, Strandness DE Jr. Comprehensive noninvasive evaluation of extracranial cerebrovascular disease. In: Hershey FB, Barnes RB, Sumner DS, eds. *Noninvasive diagnosis of vascular disease.* Pasadena: Appleton Davies, 1984:177–216, with permission.)

nent. There is marked spectral broadening with marked poststenotic turbulence. It has been noted that, with the loss of reverse flow, the pressure drop across such an area is greater than 15 mm Hg. Although unusual, we have noted that in some patients, distal to a tight stenosis, there may be a return in the reverse-flow component (28).

UPPER EXTREMITY ARTERIES

Chronic arterial occlusions of the upper extremity arteries are much less common except for the subclavian artery at its origin, which is the usual site for atherosclerotic occlusions to occur. It is extremely uncommon for atherosclerosis to involve the arteries distal to the subclavian. In fact, in my entire career, I have seen only two patients with *bona fide* lesions that resulted in clinical problems, and both of these involved the upper brachial artery. The one possible exception to this rule is in patients with chronic renal failure who have been on dialysis for long periods of time. In some of

these patients, there may be involvement of the distal arteries, palmar arch, and digital arteries, but even this is uncommon as a cause of hand ischemia except in cases where arteriovenous (A-V) shunts are placed for dialysis.

The hemodynamic changes that occur in the subclavian and innominate artery are easy to detect and evaluate by both conventional testing and duplex scanning. The simplest method is by measuring the arm blood pressures and noting the difference between the two arms. Normally, these pressures should be equal. If a difference of more than 15 mm Hg in systolic pressure is noted between the two arms, the origin of the subclavian artery might be narrowed or occluded. The velocity waveforms taken from the subclavian artery are normally triphasic, as is seen in the lower limbs. However, those recorded from the brachial, radial, and ulnar arteries may not show the typical triphasic patterns in half of normal subjects. This is probably because the arm is a lower-resistance circuit in some people, giving rise to a velocity pattern that is biphasic but still oscillatory in terms of its components.

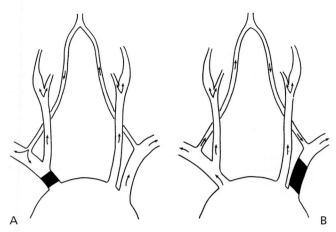

FIGURE 4.9. The collateral pathways that are invoked with occlusions of the innominate **(A)** and subclavian **(B)** arteries are shown. With a lesion of the innominate, the vertebral artery on that side can become a source of blood not only to the ipsilateral arm but also to the region supplied by the carotid artery. In rare cases with concomitant disease of the right vertebral artery, flow can be reversed in the right carotid artery as it becomes the major collateral source for the right arm. (From Roederer GO, Langlois YE, Strandness DE Jr. Cerebral arterial flow and cerebral vascular insufficiency. In: Condon RE, DeCosse J, eds. *Surgical Care II.* Philadelphia: Lea & Febiger, 1985:199–234, with permission.)

A unique feature of lesions of the subclavian and innominate artery is that the vertebral arteries can serve as an important collateral source for the arm (Fig. 4.9). This is recognized by the reversal of flow in the vertebral artery on the side of the stenosis or occlusion. The clinical significance of such a finding will be dealt with later. The velocity changes seen distal to the lesions will, as in the case of the lower limb, be monophasic, with the end-diastolic velocity above zero (29).

VISCERAL ARTERIES

Because duplex scanning can provide access to these important vessels, it becomes important to understand the pathologic changes secondary to atherosclerosis that may lead to problems. Like many other organs in the body, the symptoms and signs that develop depend on the metabolic activity of the part, the available collateral, and the types of problems that can develop. In general, the visceral arteries supply organs of both high and low resistance. The liver and the kidneys are low-resistance organs that demand high volumes of blood flow to function properly. Thus, the velocity patterns are similar to those seen in the internal carotid artery, with a high end-diastolic velocity and no reverse-flow component. The small bowel, on the other hand, demands high flow only after a meal; therefore, it is important to know the time of day during which flow information is being obtained.

The syndrome of chronic mesenteric ischemia is not common but can result in a confusing clinical picture. In short, the classic syndrome presents with postprandial abdominal cramping pain associated with explosive diarrhea and weight loss. In this form, it is not difficult to suspect but may not be easy to prove. The traditional method of providing the necessary confirming information is to do a lateral aortogram, which provides optimal visualization of the celiac, superior mesenteric, and inferior mesenteric arteries (Fig. 4.10). It is generally accepted that involvement of at least two of the three major inputs to the bowel must occur. Only recently have we been able regularly to interrogate the inferior mesenteric artery by duplex scanning. The celiac and superior mesenteric arteries are relatively easy to study because of their location in the upper abdomen, a region that is usually free of bowel gas, which interferes with sound transmission. It has been our experience that patients who truly have this syndrome *must* have high-grade stenoses of both the celiac and superior mesenteric arteries. We have not yet encountered a patient with involvement of one alone that has had the syndrome. This is because of the excellent collateral potential that exists between these two important stem vessels.

The renal arteries provide a useful and challenging area for those interested in diagnostic studies. It is well known that renal artery stenoses can produce hypertension that may be curable by either angioplasty or direct arterial surgery. For practical purposes, there are two major diseases that may involve these vessels: atherosclerosis and fibromuscular hyperplasia. The former is primarily an orificial lesion or, at best, one that involves the proximal centimeter

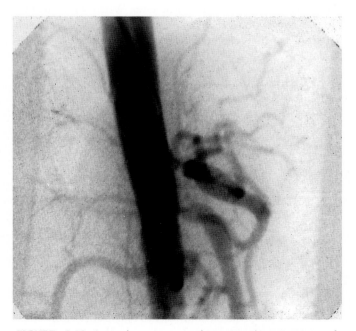

FIGURE 4.10. Lateral aortogram demonstrating stenoses of both the celiac and superior mesenteric arteries in a patient with chronic mesenteric ischemia. The inferior mesenteric artery had been sacrificed at an earlier time when an aortobifemoral graft had been placed.

of the artery. The fibromuscular lesion tends to involve the middle to distal renal arteries. It is more common in women, occurring at an earlier age than atherosclerosis.

The lesions that activate the renin-angiotensin system are generally considered to be greater than 60% diameter-reducing stenoses. Although there have been different methods proposed for screening purposes, none of these has been sensitive or specific enough to warrant its continued application. The methods have included intravenous pyelography and radionuclide studies. These methods have proved inadequate because they provide only an 80% true-positive rate with unacceptably high false-positive rates of 11% and 25%, respectively (30,31).

The types of changes seen in the renal arteries are much the same as those noted in other peripheral arteries that are narrowed. The flow in these vessels is quasi-steady, with the end-diastolic levels always above zero. As will be noted later, the major difficulties in studying the renal arteries are their position, their short length, and the problems of always knowing the exact angle of the incident sound beam with the long axis of the vessel. There is little doubt that, as this circular artery narrows, the velocity in the stenotic segment will reflect the degree of narrowing. Because of the difficulties involved, we have directed our attention to those variables that can be used to detect the lesion most prone to produce hypertension.

It has been noted by Kohler and associates (32) that aortic velocity tends to decrease as a function of age. Because of this, the velocities in the main renal artery have been related to that observed in the aorta adjacent to the renal arteries. This has been expressed as the renal/aortic ratio. When it exceeds that in the aorta by more than 3.5, it is likely to be associated with a stenosis of more than 60% diameter reduction.

REFERENCES

1. Longland CJ. The collateral circulation to the limb. *Ann R Coll Surg Eng* 1953;13:161–176.
2. Winblad JN, Reemstma K, Vernhet JL. Etiologic factors in the development of collateral circulation. *Surgery* 1959;45:105–116.
3. Hoye SJ, Teitelbaum S, Gore I, et al. Atheromatous embolism: a factor in peripheral gangrene. *N Engl J Med* 1959;261:128–131.
4. Eliot RS, Kanjuh VL, Edwards JE. Atheromatous embolism. *Circulation* 1964;30:611–617.
5. Richards AM, Eliot RS, Kanjuh VI, et al. Cholesterol embolism. *Am J Cardiol* 1951;2:696–707.
6. Hass WK. Joint study of extracranial arterial occlusion. II. Arteriography, techniques, sites and complications. *JAMA* 1968;203:961–968.
7. Hutchinson EC, Yates PO. Carotico-vertebral stenosis. *Lancet* 1957;1:2–8.
8. Fisher CM. Occlusion of the internal carotid artery. *Arch Neurol Psychiatry* 1951;65:346–377.
9. Barnett HJ, Taylor DW, Eliasziw M, et al.. Benefit of carotid endarterectomy in patients with symptomatic moderate or severe stenosis. North American Symptomatic Carotid Endarterectomy

10. Farrell B, Fraser A, Sandercock P, et al., for the European Carotid Surgery Trial Collaborative Group. Randomised trial of endarterectomy for recently symptomatic carotid stenosis: final results of the MRC European carotid surgery trial (ECST). *Lancet* 1998;351:1379–1387.
11. Nicholls SC, Bergelin RO, Strandness DE Jr. Neurological sequelae of unilateral carotid artery occlusion: immediate and late. *J Vasc Surg* 1989;10:542–548.
12. Moneta GL, Taylor DC, Nicholls SC, et al. Operative vs. nonoperative management of asymptomatic high-grade carotid stenosis: improved results with endarterectomy. *Stroke* 1987;18:1005–1010.
13. Thiele BL, Young JV, Chikos PM, et al. Correlation of arteriographic findings with symptoms in patients with cerebrovascular disease. *Neurology* 1980;30:1041–1046.
14. Barnes RW, Russell HE, Bone GE, et al. The Doppler cerebrovascular examination: improved results with refinements in technique. *Stroke* 1977;8:468–471.
15. Gee W, Mehigan JT, Wylie EJ. Measurement of collateral hemispheric blood pressure by ocular pneumoplethysmography. *Am J Surg* 1975;130:121–127.
16. Sillesen HJJ, Schroeder T. Changes in Doppler waveforms can predict pressure reduction across internal carotid artery stenoses. *Ultrasound Med Biol* 1988;8:649–655.
17. Alksne JF. Collateral circulation. In: Strandness DE Jr, ed. *Collateral circulation in clinical surgery.* Philadelphia: WB Saunders, 1969:585–609.
18. Riggs HE, Rupp C. Variation in the form of circle of Willis: the relation of the variations to collateral circulation. Anatomic analysis. *Arch Neurol* 1963;8:8–14.
19. Fields WS, Ratinov G, Weibel J, et al. Bilateral carotid artery thrombosis. *Arch Neurol* 1961;15:453–471.
20. Fields WS, Bruetman ME, Weibel J. Collateral circulation of the brain. *Monogr Surg Sci* 1965;2:183–259.
21. May AG, Van de Berg L, DeWeese JA, et al. Critical arterial stenosis. *Surgery* 1963;54:250–259.
22. Schultz RD, Hokanson DE, Strandness DE Jr. Pressure-flow and stress strain measurements of normal and diseased aortoiliac segments. *Surg Gynecol Obstet* 1967;124:1267–1276.
23. DeWeese JA. Pedal pulses disappearing with exercise: a test for intermittent claudication. *N Engl J Med* 1960;262:1214–1217.
24. Carter SA. Response of ankle systolic pressure to leg exercise in mild or questionable arterial disease. *N Engl J Med* 1972;287:578–582.
25. Strandness DE Jr. Abnormal exercise response after successful reconstructive arterial surgery. *Surgery* 1966;59:325–333.
26. Stahler C, Strandness DE Jr. Ankle blood pressure response to graded treadmill exercise. *Angiology* 1967;18:237–241.
27. Jager KA, Phillips DJ, Martin RL, et al. Noninvasive mapping of lower limb arterial lesions. *Ultrasound Med Biol* 1985;11:515–521.
28. Kohler TR, Nance DR, Cramer MM, et al. Duplex scanning for diagnosis of aortoiliac and femoropopliteal disease: a prospective study. *Circulation* 1987;76:1074–1080.
29. Roederer GO, Langlois YE, Strandness DE Jr. Cerebral arterial flow and cerebral vascular insufficiency. In: Condon RE, DeCosse J, eds. *Surgical Care II.* Philadelphia: Lea & Febiger, 1985:199–234.
30. Grim CE, Luft FC, Weinberger MH. Sensitivity and specificity of screening tests for renal vascular hypertension. *Ann Intern Med* 1979;91:617–622.
31. Treadway KK, Slater EE. Renovascular hypertension. *Annu Rev Med* 1984;35:665–691.
32. Kohler TR, Zierler RE, Martin RL, et al. Noninvasive diagnosis of renal artery stenosis by ultrasonic duplex scanning. *J Vasc Surg* 1986;4:450–456.

Trial Collaborators [see Comments]. *N Engl J Med* 1998;339:1415–1425.

5

HEMODYNAMICS OF VENOUS OCCLUSION AND VALVULAR INCOMPETENCE

The venous system in both health and disease is much more complicated and difficult to study than its arterial counterpart. The veins not only are collapsible but also contain valves that are an integral part of their structure and are essential for their performance. The venous system has not been studied in the same depth, because of both technical difficulties and the fact that there has not been the same interest in the medical community. Although pulmonary embolism remains the major source of interest and study in the Western world, there has been relatively little interest in the function of the deep venous system. This is surprising because deep venous disease is a very common cause of long-term morbidity. The postthrombotic syndrome, which consists of limb swelling, pain, hyperpigmentation, and ulceration, is a major medical problem for which there is no readily available solution. To understand the pathophysiology of the postthrombotic syndrome, it is necessary to understand the physiology and hemodynamics of both the normal and abnormal venous system.

With acute venous occlusion, transient venous hypertension may occur in the limb distal to the site of involvement. This will persist until the venous collaterals have become sufficiently developed to restore venous outflow to a normal level. Although little is known about the venous collaterals, clinical experience and more recent physiologic studies suggest that they are even more efficient in most cases than those that develop on the arterial side of the circulation.

The material in this chapter is devoted to the understanding of the changes that are seen in chronic venous disease. It is in this area that there is increasing interest and that more effort is currently being applied. It is now possible to describe in hemodynamic terms the basis for many of the changes that are observed in patients seen with these problems.

PRIMARY VARICOSE VEINS

One of the most common disorders seen in vascular clinics is varicose veins. These not only are a source of cosmetic problems but also may lead to the development of symptoms that may be of concern to the patient. The term *primary* is applied because the problem is confined to the superficial venous system. It spares both the perforating and deep veins. It is important to make this distinction because it will help in sorting out the nature of the patient's complaints and the proposed therapy.

The most striking feature of this problem is the positive family history usually obtained. Gundersen and Gauge (1) extensively studied patients presenting to the vascular clinic in Malmo, Sweden with this problem. It was noted that varicose veins were more common in women, but there also appeared to be a higher incidence of the problem in the relatives of male patients who presented with the disorder. It appeared that the inherited factors were polygenetic, but acquired factors could also be important. Another interesting factor is that the disorder appears to affect primarily the white races, with a very low incidence in black and Asian populations.

Although the genetic factors are of obvious importance in our understanding of the etiology of primary varicose veins, they do not clarify the physical factors that lead to the valvular incompetence of the superficial venous system. It is also clear that most physicians' concepts concerning the disease itself are probably incorrect. It is well known that the greater saphenous vein is the most common segment involved; however, it has not been clear to what extent. This is because until the availability of duplex scanning, there was no way of examining both the superficial and deep venous systems in their entirety.

Van Ramshorst (2) studied 31 patients with primary varicose veins by duplex scanning to determine the location and level of valvular incompetence. Saphenofemoral incompetence was found in 27 patients and saphenopopliteal incompetence in 8 patients. This is not unexpected. However, isolated valvular incompetence in the greater saphenous at the knee and calf level was found in 4 patients. Primary varicose veins that appeared to be associated with perforator incompetence were found in three limbs.

Important observations made by Folse (3), van Bemmelen and colleagues (4), and van Ramshorst (2) included the association of saphenofemoral incompetence with the presence of valvular insufficiency of the common femoral vein. Van Bemmelen and colleagues (4) found common femoral incompetence in five of seven limbs with primary varicose veins. Van Ramshorst (2), using similar methods of detecting reflux, found that pathologic levels of valve closure times were found more frequently in patients with primary varicose veins. In 10 of 27 patients with saphenofemoral incompetence, the valve closure time exceeded 2 seconds, which is the 95% value for these patients. In normal subjects, the 95% value for valve closure time in the common femoral vein is 0.88 second. These differences were significant at the $p < .01$ level. Although the association is not a perfect one, it is conceivable that incompetence of the common femoral vein, combined with loss of competence in the first valve in the greater saphenous close to its termination, might set the stage for the subsequent progressive development of valvular incompetence of most, if not all, of the greater saphenous vein.

What is peculiar about primary varicose veins is their sparing of the deep veins and their valves. Although the greater and lesser saphenous veins are, by strict definition, perforating veins, it is uncommon for the perforating veins in the lower leg to be incompetent as well. This is of more than passing interest because it may well explain the rarity of finding the typical pigmentation changes and ulceration commonly associated with the postthrombotic syndrome. It should be noted, however, that Dodd and Cockett (5) include in their classification a condition of idiopathic perforator incompetence. This is, in my experience, very unusual. In fact, I have seen only one patient who appeared to present with isolated perforator incompetence as a cause of problems in the lower leg. As noted previously, van Ramshorst (2) found primary varicose veins in conjunction with perforator disease in only three limbs of the 31 patients who presented with primary varicose veins. This would appear to emphasize the relatively uncommon association between the two.

HEMODYNAMICS OF PRIMARY VARICOSE VEINS

Because the primary defect in this disorder is incompetence of the valves, the major alteration in function will be the changes in the normal direction of flow with changes in position, coughing, sneezing, and exercise. Bjordal (6), in 1970, studied the flow changes in varicose veins using electromagnetic flow probes and pressure transducers to evaluate the hemodynamics of the problem.

In the upright position with the patient quietly standing, there was virtually no flow in the greater saphenous vein. With elevation of the foot from the ground, there was reflux

of blood down the saphenous vein, with its return to the deep venous system through the perforating veins. This set up a cyclic and circular motion of the blood, with little, if any, moving in a central direction through the saphenous vein. This pattern of flow could be immediately reversed to a normal response by manual compression of the vein at the saphenofemoral junction, showing that incompetence at this level was the primary abnormality.

A common method of studying the hemodynamics of venous problems has been to measure the venous pressure at the level of the foot in response to exercise. This procedure has permitted a separation of the normal response from those observed with both superficial and deep venous involvement (7).

In the quiet standing position, the pressure recorded at the level of the foot will reflect the height of the column of blood from the level of the right atrium. It is only with exercise that the abnormalities become evident. The changes observed are summarized in Table 5.1.

Because the measurement of venous pressure requires a venipuncture on the dorsum of the foot, it is not easily adapted for routine clinical use. The other method that has been popular is the photoplethysmograph. This method senses the amount of blood in the dermis of the skin. If it is applied to the gaitre area of the lower leg, dermal blood volume changes can be studied after five consecutive forceful dorsal and plantar flexions of the foot. The results are similar in direction and time course to the venous pressure. In normal subjects, there is a dramatic fall in dermal blood volume, which takes up to 20 seconds to return to the baseline level.

The technique can be used with and without the application of tourniquets to occlude the superficial venous system. In theory, one should be able to separate valvular reflux in the deep veins from that isolated to the superficial venous system. However, van Bemmelen and associates (8) were unable to show that this method was useful in making this separation. In their study of 151 limbs with swelling, aching, and suspected venous insufficiency, they used duplex scanning to determine the level and extent of the

TABLE 5.1. THE FALL IN VENOUS PRESSURE WITH EXERCISE

Status	Maximum fall in pressure	Recovery time
Normals	59 ± 11 mm Hg	17 ± 6 sec
Primary varicose veins Competent perforating veins	45 ± 12 mm Hg	14 ± 6 sec
Primary varicose veins Incompetent calf perforating veins	21 ± 11 mm Hg	5 ± 3 sec

From Kreissmann A. Ambulatory venous measurements. In: Nicolaides AN, Yao JST, eds. *Investigation of vascular disorders.* Edinburgh: Churchill Livingstone, 1981:461–477, with permission.

valvular incompetence. If one accepts the duplex studies of reflux as the gold standard, the photoplethysmographic method did not do well. For example, the kappa statistic for agreement between the results classified as normal, deep valvular incompetence, or superficial incompetence was only 0.12 ± 0.06, which is little better than might occur by chance.

However, one area in which the photoplethysmographic measurement of venous refill time showed some correlation was between the level of valvular incompetence and the presence of abnormal skin in the gaitre area. The results are shown in Figs. 5.1 and 5.2. Incompetent levels are defined by the number of venous segments that are in continuity and have lost valve function. The results with the photoplethysmographic method showed quite clearly that the test is of little predictive value until at least four levels of valvular incompetence are found.

It is evident that the measurement of venous pressure and the photoplethysmographic methods are of use, but they have serious limitations that must be considered by the user. It is clear that they are not the best methods for studying patients with primary varicose veins. They cannot precisely determine where the venous problem is and how extensive it might be. The finding of a normal deep venous system establishes the diagnosis of primary varicose veins with near certainty. However, with regard to the postthrombotic syndrome, the problem is much more complex. Before dealing with the chronic changes that occur and their relationships to the initiating event, it is necessary to review some of our current knowledge concerning the changes that follow the development of acute venous thrombosis and how these may affect long-term venous function. More details on the use of photoplethysmography will be covered shortly.

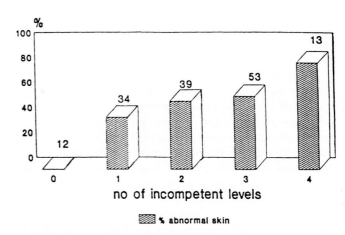

FIGURE 5.2. The percentage of patients with abnormal skin in the gaitre area of the lower leg as related to levels of valvular incompetence. (From Kreissmann A. Ambulatory venous pressure measurements. In: Nicolaides AN, Yao JST, eds. *Investigation of vascular disorders*. Edinburgh: Churchill Livingstone, 1981: 461–477, with permission.)

PATHOPHYSIOLOGY OF ACUTE VENOUS THROMBOSIS

An assumption that is nearly always made is that the sequelae we now define as the postthrombotic syndrome are the consequences of the changes that occur when the deep veins become occluded. Is this, in fact, the case? Unfortunately, until recently, we had only retrospective studies to answer this question. For example, Cockett and Jones (9) found that only 27 of 80 cases with venous ulcers could clearly be related to a previous episode of deep venous thrombosis (DVT). Browse and co-workers (10), in a retrospective review of 67 patients with DVT documented by venography, attempted to relate the extent of the initial involvement with late outcome. There was no correlation to be found. In fact, 32% of the uninvolved legs at the time the venograms were performed were noted to have symptoms at the time of follow-up 5 to 10 years after the event. In addition, one third of the limbs in which severe venous thrombosis was documented were free of symptoms at the time of the reevaluation.

The studies of Cockett and Jones (9) and Browse and associates (10) point out some of the difficulties in attempting to assess clinical outcome based on the location and extent of the venous thrombosis at the time it initially developed. It is clear that changes in the venous system occur that are not predictable. It is interesting that Browse and associates (10) found that 32% of patients with phlebographically proven deep vein thrombosis (DVT) *did not* develop the symptoms and signs of the postthrombotic syndrome after intervals of 5 to 10 years. This figure is close to that found by Strandness and colleagues (11) in their long-term study: 60% of patients with DVT developed long-

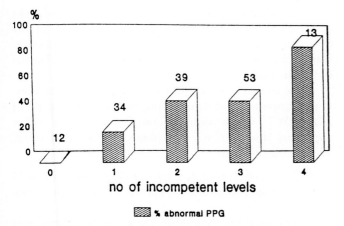

FIGURE 5.1. The percentage of patients with abnormal photoplethysmographic results as related to increasing levels of valvular incompetence. (From Kreissmann A. Ambulatory venous pressure measurements. In: Nicolaides AN, Yao JST, eds. *Investigation of vascular disorders*. Edinburgh: Churchill Livingstone, 1981: 461–477, with permission.)

term symptoms and signs, whereas the remaining 40% did not. The basis for outcome after an episode of DVT is now becoming clearer since we have had the opportunity to follow patients with sequential duplex scanning.

Based on our studies and those of van Ramshorst (2), there are two major changes in the venous system after an episode of DVT that explain many of the mysteries associated with this common disease. These are chronic deep venous obstruction and the occurrence of valvular incompetence. If one were to document the role that each of these plays, it would be necessary to follow patients from the time of the initial event for a period long enough to document the long-term outcome.

We embarked on our initial studies in 1978 (11). To be included in the long-term studies, the time of onset and the location of the venous thrombosis had to be known, either by contrast or isotope venography. There were 61 patients accepted in the study, with a mean follow-up of 39 months. All patients were seen every 6 months, at which time the clinical status of their limbs was assessed along with continuous wave (CW) Doppler studies to estimate the patency and competence of their valves in both the superficial and deep venous systems. In addition, in 39 of these limbs in 32 of the patients, venous hemodynamics were studied using photoplethysmography and venous outflow using a mercury-in-Silastic strain gauge.

During follow-up, pain and swelling developed in 67% of patients. Pigmentation developed in 15 limbs (23%), with ulcers appearing in three patients (5%). These figures are close to those reported by Browse and associates (10) in their retrospective study. The results of the hemodynamic studies will be considered in the next section.

It is clear that the fate of the patients with DVT depends on its location and its changes over time. If, in theory, the thrombus were to lyse rapidly enough, two favorable benefits might ensue, which are preservation of patency of the deep system and preservation of valve function. To evaluate the fate of the thrombus, we carried out a prospective study of 21 patients who were studied sequentially at 7, 30, 90, 180, and 270 days after the event (12). An ultrasonic duplex scanner was used to evaluate the following eight deep venous segments: the common iliac, external iliac, common femoral, superficial femoral (three locations), popliteal, and posterior tibial veins. The examination studied these segments to assess patency and the presence of valvular reflux.

With regard to the recanalization that occurred, the patients could be divided into three groups:

Group I. Recanalization in all segments by 90 days. This occurred in 11 (53%).

Group II. Extension of the thrombus at 7 days. This occurred in three (14%).

Group III. Extension of the thrombus at 30 to 180 days. This occurred in four (19%).

There were three patients (14%) who had an incomplete follow-up. The relationship of recanalization to the number of venous segments occluded is summarized in Fig. 5.3.

Valvular incompetence developed in 13 of 21 patients (62%) during the study period. Evidence for this was noted as early as 7 days in 2 patients. By 30 days, 25% of patent veins contained incompetent valves. By 180 days, 25% of patent segments contained incompetent valves, with no further changes after that period of time (Fig. 5.4). In the 8 patients who did not develop valve problems, it is conceivable that, with longer follow-up, this might occur. However, the follow-up periods were not short in 5 of the 8 patients. In 1 patient, the follow-up extended to 90 days; 2 of these patients were followed to 180 days and 2 to 270 days after the venous thrombosis. Four of these 5 patients had complete recanalization of the occluded segments by 30 days. In subsequent studies extending our follow-up in 113 patients, we noted that the median lysis time for segments developing reflux was 2.3 to 7.3 times longer than for segments not developing reflux (13). The only exception to this was found with the posterior tibial veins, where the median lysis time between the two groups was identical.

Van Ramshorst (2) carried out a similar study in 20 limbs of 18 patients. These patients had repeat duplex scans at 1, 3, 6, 12, and 26 weeks after the detection of their DVT. There were 80 venous segments that were evaluated in the long term (49 of these segments had thrombi detected). The popliteal vein had the highest prevalence of thrombosis, followed by the superficial femoral, profunda femoris, and common femoral vein. Thrombus regression (lysis?) was significant in all segments and proceeded at an exponential rate for the veins of the thigh. The extent to which this phenomenon, along with recanalization, occurred was dependent on the thrombus load and not the sites of occlusion. Recanalization was found in 23 of 31 initially occluded segments and took place within 6 weeks of presentation in 20 of 23 segments. Extension of the thrombosis occurred in 15 vein segments despite anticoagulation and did not appear to be related to the initial thrombus load.

These studies raise several issues that could be of paramount importance in determining the long-term effects of acute DVT, which would never be discovered unless sequential studies of the type done here are performed. These are as follows:

1. Early and often complete lysis of deep venous thrombi can and does occur after an episode of venous thrombosis (Fig. 5.5).
2. Extension of the thrombosis can occur quickly or even later, even though the patient is being treated with anticoagulants (Figs. 5.6 and 5.7).
3. It appears that up to 40% of the patients will never develop valve incompetence, even though major seg-

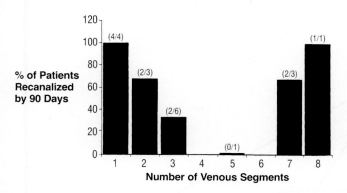

% of Patients
Recanalized
by 90 Days

FIGURE 5.3. Percentage of patients demonstrating recanalization in all the originally involved segments at 90 days. The numbers in parentheses are the numbers of patients with recanalization as compared with the total, with each number of segments originally occluded. (From Strandness DE Jr, Langlois Y, Cramer M, et al. Long-term sequelae of acute venous thrombosis. *JAMA* 1983;250: 1289–1292, with permission.)

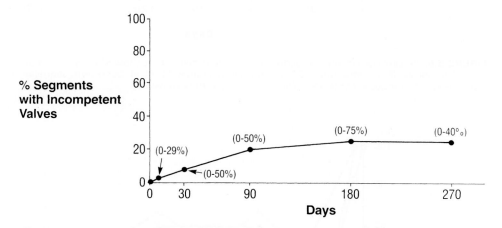

% Segments
with Incompetent
Valves

FIGURE 5.4. Mean percentage of patent segments containing incompetent valves at each time. Numbers in parentheses are the ranges for individual cases. The *arrows* indicate the percentages at days 7 and 30. (From Strandness DE Jr, Langlois Y, Cramer M, et al. Long-term sequelae of acute venous thrombosis. *JAMA* 1983;250:1289–1292, with permission.)

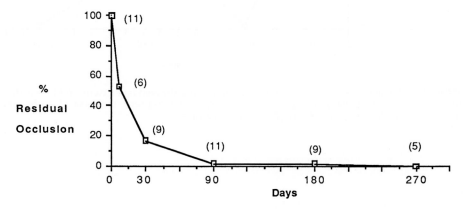

%
Residual
Occlusion

FIGURE 5.5. Mean percentage of residual occlusion for group showing early recanalization (group I). Numbers in parentheses are the number of cases studied at that time. (From Strandness DE Jr, Langlois Y, Cramer M, et al. Long-term sequelae of acute venous thrombosis. *JAMA* 1983;250:1289–1292, with permission.)

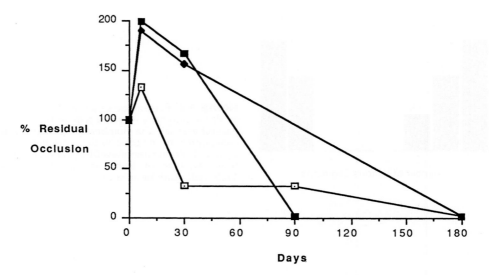

FIGURE 5.6. Percentage of residual occlusion in three patients that showed early extension of their thrombosis. (From Strandness DE Jr, Langlois Y, Cramer M, et al. Long-term sequelae of acute venous thrombosis. *JAMA* 1983;250:1289–1292, with permission.)

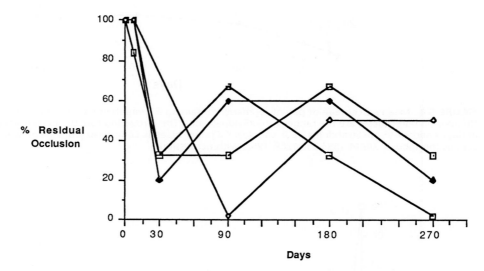

FIGURE 5.7. Percentage of occlusion in four patients who showed late extension of their thrombosis. (From Strandness DE Jr, Langlois Y, Cramer M, et al. Long-term sequelae of acute venous thrombosis. *JAMA* 1983;250:1289–1292, with permission.)

ments of the venous system have been occluded by thrombi.

4. Early lysis may be protective of valve function.
5. Johnson and colleagues (14) followed 78 patients (41 male, 37 female) with acute DVT for a median period of 3 years. A total of 41% of the patients had a feature of the postthrombotic syndrome, but only 13% developed skin complications. Limbs with the postthrombotic syndrome were three times as likely to have a combination of reflux plus obstruction.

POSTTHROMBOTIC SYNDROME

The most serious of all venous disorders occurs when the deep venous system is obstructed and the valvular mechanisms are destroyed or rendered incompetent. This is thought to occur when there has been an episode of DVT that leads to two problems: obstruction of the deep veins and subsequent destruction of the venous valves. When venous obstruction occurs, the venous blood is forced to follow alternate pathways to reach the heart. This appears to occur by two major mechanisms. The first is by the opening of alternate pathways, much as is seen on the arterial side of the circulation. These have not been well defined anatomically, but it is certain that they develop in a similar manner and fashion. The other route is to take advantage of the superficial venous system by reversing the flow in the communicating veins so that the normal direction of flow is now reversed, becoming deep to superficial rather than the opposite direction. This decompresses the deep veins but creates a whole new set of problems that have been referred to as the *high-pressure leak phenomenon*.

The location of the perforating veins corresponds well to the sites where pigmentation and ulceration develop. To clarify their role, it is necessary to summarize what is currently known about them from an anatomic standpoint. Their features are as follows:

1. They are the link between the superficial and deep veins.
2. They contain valves that normally permit flow only from the superficial to the deep veins.
3. They vary in number from 90 to 200.
4. They are to be found primarily below the knee.
5. Most are quite small and inconstant in location.
6. They are of two types: direct, which pass directly from the superficial system to link with a deep vein; and indirect, which interrupt their course by way of muscular venous channels before terminating in the deep veins.
7. The most important and most constant perforating veins link the posterior arch vein with the posterior tibial vein in the lower leg (15). These are thought to be the ones implicated in the development of the pigmentation that occurs with the postthrombotic syndrome. It is commonly believed that the perforating veins communicate with the greater saphenous vein in the lower leg,

but that is not the case. The potential role for subfascial endoscopic perforator ligation has renewed our interest in the role of the perforating veins (16,17). To what extent the procedure will become the standard remains to be seen.

Recent studies done by van Bemmelen and colleagues (4) have shed new light on and provided important information relative to the findings in patients with DVT who are seen long intervals after the initial event. In their study, 22 patients had a definite history of DVT. In this group, 12 patients developed an ulcer, whereas the remaining 10 did not. The striking difference between these two groups of patients can be seen in Fig. 5.8. Seven of 12 patients with ulceration had incompetence of the greater saphenous vein, and 8 of 12 had incompetence of the lesser saphenous vein. In the 10 patients without ulceration, none of the greater saphenous or lesser saphenous veins developed valvular incompetence. This is important because, as far as we knew, the greater and lesser saphenous veins were theoretically not involved at the time the DVT developed. This means that something transpired after the event that led to the development of valvular incompetence in these major superficial veins. It must be presumed that when this occurs, the perforating veins are also incompetent. In Fig. 5.8, it can be

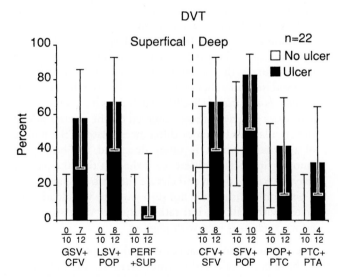

FIGURE 5.8. Percentage of venous segments found to be incompetent in patients with a previous history of deep venous thrombosis. Of the 22 patients, 12 developed an ulcer. The notable difference was the association of incompetence in the greater and lesser saphenous with ulceration. None of the patients without ulceration had incompetence of the greater and lesser saphenous veins. There was also a higher prevalence of incompetence of the popliteal and posterior tibial veins in patients with ulceration. Bars indicate the standard deviation. *GSV*, greater saphenous vein; *CFV*, common femoral vein; *LSV*, lesser saphenous vein; *POP*, popliteal vein; *PERF*, perforator veins; *SUP*, superficial veins; *SFV*, superficial femoral vein; *PTC*, posterior tibial veins in upper calf; *PTA*, posterior tibial veins at the ankle level.

seen that 5 of 12 of the posterior tibial veins in the calf and 4 of 12 in the lower leg were incompetent in the ulcer group, as compared with only 2 of the patients who did not develop an ulcer. If the study had been conducted with a more careful examination of the perforating veins, the relationships might have been even clearer.

HEMODYNAMICS OF THE POSTTHROMBOTIC SYNDROME

Before considering the hemodynamics of chronic venous obstruction and valvular incompetence, it is necessary to review briefly the clinical presentation that can occur because this will have a direct bearing on the hemodynamic abnormality that is present. This common syndrome can be characterized by the following clinical presentation:

1. Pain and swelling of the lower leg, which are most bothersome at the end of the day. The swelling is related to the upright posture and is at its minimum in the morning.
2. The pain is described as being dull and is always relieved by elevation of the limb above heart level.
3. There is hyperpigmentation of the lower limb, most commonly in the medial aspect. The pigment appears to be hemosiderin and is often accompanied by atrophy of the skin. This is also the site at which ulcers most commonly occur. The pigmentation may also involve the lateral aspect of the lower leg, but this is distinctly less common and is rarely found in isolation.
4. In some cases, the patient may complain of pain in the limb—usually the calf and thigh—which is brought on by exercise and relieved by rest. This is referred to as *venous claudication* (18–20), which does have some characteristics similar to those observed on the arterial side of the circulation. Its major differences relate to the nature of the pain, which is often described as "bursting." Another important difference is the fact that the patient may have to lie down and elevate the limb for pain relief. This problem is usually not seen with the workload associated with walking, but rather requires more strenuous effort, such as is seen with jogging.

The hemodynamic changes seen in the postthrombotic phase have been evaluated by three methods, each of which can be used to define particular aspects of venous performance: (a) photoplethysmography to define the response of the limb to simulated exercise (20) (it has been shown that the responses obtained with this method are similar to those seen with venous pressure measurements); (b) CW directional Doppler for assessment of segmental valvular competence (21,22); and (c) venous outflow plethysmography to measure the rate at which a limb can empty trapped blood after deflation of a thigh cuff inflated to 50 mm Hg (22,23).

PHOTOPLETHYSMOGRAPHY STUDIES

As might be expected, a limb that has damaged deep veins and perforating veins will have abnormalities that reflect the extent of damage to the valvular mechanisms. The photoplethysmograph uses an infrared sensor to monitor changes in the volume of blood within the dermis. These changes have been shown to mimic quite closely the venous pressure changes noted at the level of the dorsum of the foot. The test is done by placing the infrared sensor over the medial lower leg just superior to the medial malleolus. To simulate exercise, a cuff is placed on the calf, with the patient in the sitting position. The cuff is rapidly and automatically inflated to 60 mm Hg six times. This is used instead of actual exercise to avoid the motion artifacts that are associated with the voluntary motion of the limb (24).

The method employs the measurement of the venous recovery time (VRT). This is the time from the completion of the last cuff inflation until the skin blood volume returns to the prebaseline level. The values appear to be similar to those obtained when venous pressures are measured. For this study, there were 32 limbs that had a documented episode of DVT and had been followed sequentially to document the clinical outcome. The results of this study are shown in Table 5.2.

The results are interesting and show that the response appears to be different, depending on presenting symptoms. For example, if a patient had an episode of DVT but was asymptomatic, the VRT values were similar to those seen in the unaffected limb as well as to those seen in normal subjects. This means that some patients may not develop valvular incompetence after such an episode and remain free of symptoms. It also appears that the more advanced symptoms and signs are associated with very abnormal results of the type seen with extensive valvular incompetence.

Although the results of these studies may appear to be at variance with the results of van Bemmelen and colleagues

TABLE 5.2. VENOUS REFILLING TIME (VRT) IN UNAFFECTED AND AFFECTED LIMBS AFTER AN EPISODE OF DVT

Group	VRT (sec)
Unaffected limbs	24 (12)
Affected limbs	
No symptoms	21.8 (15.3)
Pain	14.6 (10.2)
Edema	9.2 (2.7)
Hyperpigmentation	8.9 (4.3)
Ulceration	9.0

Values are means ± 1 SD.
DVT, deep venous thrombosis.
From Sumner DS. Doppler evaluation of the venous circulation using the ultrasonic Doppler velocity detector. In: Rutherford RB, ed. *Vascular surgery.* Philadelphia: WB Saunders, 1977:179–200, with permission.

(8) previously discussed in this chapter, I do not believe this is true. Patients who develop the postthrombotic syndrome must have multiple levels of venous incompetence both in the deep and superficial veins. As noted previously, this appears to be the case and explains why plethysmographic studies might be of value in separating those with the syndrome from those who never develop the problem.

CONTINUOUS WAVE DOPPLER STUDIES

We conducted a long-term study of 61 patients who had an episode of DVT documented by either contrast or isotope phlebography (11). These patients were followed for a mean of 41 months. As a part of this study, we evaluated the patency and competency of the deep venous system by directional Doppler studies. If the distal veins—those below the knee—were found to be patent and competent, only 8% developed any evidence of pigmentation. This was in contrast to 40% of those in whom the distal veins were incompetent.

It was also of interest to note the relationship between the distal veins with regard to symptoms. In those 26 patients with normal distal veins, 15 were symptom free. In contrast, of the 39 patients with abnormal distal veins, only 9 did not have symptoms. These differences were statistically significant ($p < .005$). The relationship in time between the development of valvular incompetence and symptoms is shown in Fig. 5.9.

This study highlighted the importance of the venous valves for preservation of a limb that not only is free of symptoms but also is much less likely to develop the physical manifestations of the postthrombotic syndrome.

An important fact to emerge from this study was the location of the veins where valve competence seemed to be most important: the veins below the knee. This makes sense if one examines the pathophysiology of postthrombotic syndrome and the location of the stasis dermatitis that occurs. It is obvious that the great number of valves below the knee is the key in protecting the limb against the potentially damaging effects of the calf muscle pump. With activation of the calf muscle pump, muscle contraction tends to force blood in any direction not protected by valves. Normally, this is in the antegrade direction alone. When the valves in the deep veins and their communications with the superficial veins become incompetent, blood not only proceeds toward the heart but also tends to move distally and out through the perforating veins. This produces ambulatory venous hypertension as well as the high-pressure leaks through the perforating veins. This results in the ideal situation for the development of the sequelae of postthrombotic syndrome.

VENOUS OUTFLOW PLETHYSMOGRAPHY

One of the unknown aspects of chronic venous disease is the role of residual venous obstruction in the long-term outcome and its relationship to symptoms that might appear. Intuitively, it would seem that restriction of venous return—if, in fact, it exists—should be a factor in the production of symptoms.

As a part of our long-term study mentioned previously, we were able to perform venous outflow studies in 32 patients (24). We employed strain gauge plethysmography to assess the rate of venous emptying after deflation of a cuff placed around the thigh (25). The inflation pressure used was 50 mm Hg. In this procedure, the sensor used was a mercury-in-Silastic strain gauge placed around the calf. After cuff deflation, the venous outflow (VO) from 0.5 to 2.0 seconds was measured. The results of this study are summarized in Table 5.3.

It was of interest that, whereas the differences noted in the VO studies between the unaffected and affected limbs were significant ($p < .01$), the procedure was not a good

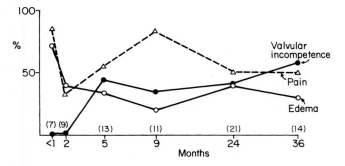

FIGURE 5.9. The relationship between the development of valvular incompetence and symptoms of pain and edema is shown. In the very early phases of the illness, the development of pain and swelling is related to the acute event itself. The valves of the deep system seem to become incompetent sometime between the second and fifth month after the episode of deep venous thrombosis. The numbers at the bottom of the graph (*in parentheses*) indicate those patients studied with the continuous wave Doppler at those intervals.

TABLE 5.3. VENOUS OUTFLOW IN UNAFFECTED AND AFFECTED LIMBS WITH AND WITHOUT SYMPTOMS

Group	Venous outflow 0–2.5 sec (mL/100 cc tissue/min)
Unaffected limbs	37.6 (10.2)
Affected limbs	28 (9.4)
No symptoms	26.5 (9.3)
Pain	28.0 (7.7)
Edema	28.3 (5.5)
Hyperpigmentation	27.7 (9.6)
Ulceration	21.0

Data expressed as the mean ± 1 SD.

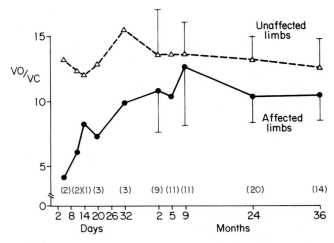

FIGURE 5.10. The relationship between venous outflow (*VO*) in the limb affected with deep venous thrombosis and the unaffected limb is shown. To normalize the values obtained for each patient, the data are expressed as the ratio of the VO in cc per 100 cc tissue per minute, to the venous capacitance (*VC*) in cc per 100 cc tissue after 2 minutes of cuff inflation.

marker for patients who were likely to develop the post-thrombotic syndrome (Fig. 5.10). As noted earlier, there is a small subset of patients with chronic venous insufficiency who will develop pain in the limb with exercise. This is referred to as venous claudication and has been reported only rarely in the literature. Cockett and co-workers (26) first described this entity in patients who developed calf pain within 5 minutes of a stepping test. It was noted to occur only in patients with iliofemoral obstruction. Hobbs (18) reported a case in which femoral vein pressures were shown to be high and to increase even further with exercise.

We have studied seven patients with this problem (19). In six cases, the left iliofemoral segment was occluded, with the remaining patient having complete occlusion of the entire deep system on the right side. These patients had VO studies done before and after exercise on the treadmill. It should be noted that these were patients who had a previous pattern of vigorous exercise, which they attempted to continue after their DVT. In fact, the exercise load required to bring out the problem was quite high, ranging from 8 minutes at 3 mph on a 15% grade to 34.5 minutes at 3 mph on a 19% grade.

The resting VO was 27.9 ± 11 mL per 100 cc tissue per minute in the affected limb and 40.8 ± 9.8 mL per 100 cc tissue per minute in the normal limb ($p < .05$). With exercise, the striking change that occurred was a decrease in the venous capacitance in the unaffected limb from 2.36 ± 0.64 mL per 100 cc tissue to 1.75 ± 0.63 mL per 100 cc tissue ($p < .05$). In the unaffected limb, there was no change. How does this explain the problem in these patients?

If the venous collaterals are not adequate to empty the leg with the increased flow during exercise, the venous vol-

ume will increase during the period of exercise but will be unable to increase any further with thigh cuff inflation. It is likely that the pain is secondary to the volume increase that occurs with venous distention.

Appreciation of the facts relating to the hemodynamics of chronic venous insufficiency is helpful in planning the type and nature of the noninvasive tests to carry out. Clearly, for most patients, it will be necessary to establish the level and extent of the valvular incompetence. The VO studies are most helpful in that small subset of patients who present with symptoms suggestive of venous claudication.

REFERENCES

1. Gundersen J, Gauge M. Hereditary factors in venous insufficiency. *Angiology* 1969;20:346–355.
2. van Ramshorst B. *Duplex scanning in the diagnosis and follow-up of deep vein thrombosis.* Thesis from Universiteit Utrecht, the Netherlands, 1992:81–94.
3. Folse R. The influence of femoral vein dynamics on the development of varicose veins. *Surgery* 1970; 68:974–979.
4. van Bemmelen PS, Bedford B, Beach K, et al. Status of the valves in the superficial and deep venous system in chronic venous disease. *Surgery* 1991;106:730–734.
5. Dodd H, Cockett FB. Primary familial varicose veins. In: Dodd H, Cockett FB, eds. *The pathology and surgery of veins of the lower limb.* London: Churchill Livingstone, 1976:61–73.
6. Bjordal RI. Simultaneous pressure and flow recordings in varicose veins of the lower extremity. *Acta Chir Scand* 1970;136:309–317.
7. Kreissmann A. Ambulatory venous pressure measurements. In: Nicolaides AN, Yao JST, eds. *Investigation of vascular disorders.* Edinburgh: Churchill Livingstone, 1981:461–477.
8. van Bemmelen PS, van Ramshorst B, Eikelboom BC. Photoplethysmography reexamined: lack of correlation with duplex scanning. In: van Ramshorst B, ed. *Duplex scanning in the diagnosis of deep vein thrombosis.* Thesis from Universiteit Utrecht, the Netherlands, 1992.
9. Cockett FB, Jones DFE. The ankle blow-out syndrome: a new approach to the varicose ulcer problem. *Lancet* 1953;1:17–23.
10. Browse NL, Clemenson G, Thomas ML. Is the postphlebitic leg always postphlebitic? *Br Med J* 1981;281:1167–1170.
11. Strandness DE Jr, Langlois Y, Cramer M, et al. Long-term sequelae of acute venous thrombosis. *JAMA* 1983;250:1289–1292.
12. Killewich LA, Bedford GR, Beach KW, et al. Spontaneous lysis of deep-venous thrombi: rate and outcome. *J Vasc Surg* 1989;9:89–97.
13. Meissner MH, Manzo R, Bergelin RO, et al. Deep venous insufficiency: the relationship between lysis and subsequent reflux. *J Vasc Surg* 1993;22:358–336.
14. Johnson BF, Manzo R, Bergelin R, et al. Flow characteristics in the deep veins of the leg during quiet respiration and with compression of the plantar veins. *J Vasc Interv Radiol* 1997;3:80–86.
15. Haeger K. The anatomy of the veins of the leg. In: Hobbs JT, ed. *The treatment of venous disorders.* Philadelphia: JB Lippincott, 1977:18–33.
16. Gloviczki P, Bergan JJ, Menawat SS, et al. Safety, feasibility, and early efficacy of subfascial endoscopic perforator surgery: a preliminary report from the North American registry. *J Vasc Surg* 1997;25:94–105.
17. Gloviczki P, Bergan JJ, Rhodes JM, et al. Mid-term results of endoscopic perforator vein interruption for chronic venous insuf-

ficiency: Lessons learned from the North American Subfascial Endoscopic Perforator Surgery registry. *J Vasc Surg* 1999;29: 489–499.

18. Hobbs JT. The postthrombotic syndrome. In: Hobbs JT, ed. *The treatment of venous disorders.* Philadelphia: JB Lippincott, 1977: 253–271.

19. Killewich LA, Martin R, Cramer M, et al. Pathophysiology of venous claudication. *J Vasc Surg* 1984;1:507–511.

20. Abramowitz HB, Queral LA, Flinn WR, et al. The use of photo-plethysmography in the assessment of venous insufficiency: a comparison to venous pressure measurements. *Surgery* 1979;86: 434–440.

21. Sumner DS. Doppler evaluation of the venous circulation using the ultrasonic Doppler velocity detector. In: Rutherford RB, ed. *Vascular surgery.* Philadelphia: WB Saunders, 1977;17:179–200.

22. Barnes RW, Collicott PE, Mozersky DJ, et al. Noninvasive quantitation of maximum venous outflow in acute thrombophlebitis. *Surgery* 1972;72:971–979.

23. Tripolitis AJ, Blackshear WM, Bodily KC, et al. The influence of limb elevation, examination technique and outflow design on venous plethysmography. *Angiology* 1980;31:154–163.

24. Killewich LA, Martin R, Cramer M, et al. An objective assessment of the physiologic changes in the postthrombotic syndrome. *Arch Surg* 1985;120: 424–426.

25. Cramer M, Langlois Y, Beach KW. Standardization of venous flow measurements by strain gauge plethysmography: the definition of normal. *Bruit* 1983;7:33–39.

26. Cockett FB, Thomas ML, Negus D. Iliac vein compression: its relation to ileofemoral thrombosis and the postthrombotic syndrome. *Br Med J* 1967;2:14–19.

6

EXTRACRANIAL ARTERIAL DISEASE

Duplex scanning was first applied to the study of the carotid artery in the neck. This unusual bifurcation, with the dilatation at the level of the proximal internal carotid artery, is a common site for the development of atherosclerosis. The disease tends to localize in the bulb region and can be a cause of transient ischemic attacks and strokes. In addition, it is now recognized that involvement at this site is a marker for atherosclerosis elsewhere, particularly in the coronary arteries. Referrals to the vascular laboratory generally fall into the following categories: (a) the asymptomatic patient with a carotid bruit, (b) the asymptomatic patient with a history of atherosclerosis elsewhere who is undergoing major vascular or cardiac surgery, (c) the patient with localizing transient ischemic attacks or a stroke, (d) the patient with nonlateralizing symptoms or signs, (e) patients suspected of having the subclavian steal syndrome, (f) patients who are part of a long-term follow-up program to assess the stability of their disease, and (g) patients who have undergone carotid endarterectomy or some other procedure to bypass lesions of the aortic arch or subclavian artery.

Since publication of the second edition of this book, several developments have occurred that greatly influence the role of the vascular diagnostic service relative to the use of duplex scanning in patients suspected of having extracranial arterial disease. Although surgeons have maintained that carotid endarterectomy was a good operation for the prevention of stroke in selected symptomatic and asymptomatic patients, this practice was subjected to considerable scrutiny by the neurologic community. The numbers of these procedures being done rapidly escalated until the mid-1980s, placing them second only to coronary artery bypass grafting in terms of numbers. In 1985, 107,000 procedures were performed in hospitals in the United States other than the Veterans Administration system (1). A report by Easton and Sherman in 1977 initially sparked the concern over the worth of carotid endarterectomy. This study showed that in Springfield, Illinois, the combined mortality and morbidity from carotid endarterectomy was 20% (2)! As a result of this study and others, several reports appeared in the literature further raising concerns about the procedure, its indications, and its results (3,4). If the operation

were to be effective, the perioperative morbidity and mortality rates would have to be lower than the projected rates of stroke and death when the patients were treated medically. For example, it had been projected that in patients presenting with transient ischemic attacks, the annual stroke rate would be 5% per year for the first 3 years, dropping to 3% per year thereafter. Although there were differences in the reported surgical results, many series showed that the operation could be performed with a combined morbidity and mortality rate of less than 5%, with many rates even better than this (5).

Even though surgical series appeared to be positive for the operation, there were neurologists who demanded that randomized clinical trials be mounted to end the debate and either prove or disprove the worth of the procedure. Two major trials in symptomatic patients have now been completed and reported their final results. These are the North American Symptomatic Carotid Endarterectomy Trial (NASCET) (6) and the European Carotid Surgery Trial (ECST) (7). To qualify for entry into these trials, patients had to present with either transient ischemic events or stroke with substantial recovery. All patients underwent arteriography to define the status of the carotid bifurcation. There were important differences in these trials as to how the degree of narrowing of the carotid artery was assessed by arteriography. This is an important issue that not enough people are aware of or have paid attention to. In the ECST trial, the method of measurement is as depicted in Fig 6.1. In the NASCET trial, the method was as shown in Fig. 6.2. Although both were primarily interested in the degree of narrowing or diameter reduction, the results of the two trials are not directly transferable, even though they both used similar numeric endpoints for the degree of stenosis. This is an important issue when the results of the trials are considered, particularly the methods used by the vascular laboratory to assess the degree of stenosis by duplex scanning. This matter will be dealt with in more detail later in this chapter.

The initial results of these trials concluded that for patients with a greater than 70% diameter reduction, carotid endarterectomy was far superior to medical therapy in the prevention of stroke. The differences in outcome

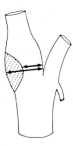

$$\% \text{ stenosis} = 100 \times \left(1 - \frac{\text{residual diameter}}{\text{normal diameter}} \right)$$

FIGURE 6.1. To estimate the degree of stenosis, the measurements were made at the level of the bulb. The outer dimension of the bulb was estimated from unsubtracted lateral views of the bulb, looking for calcium in the wall of the artery.

were evident as early as 2 years. The absolute risk reduction for stroke was 17% in the NASCET study. In the ECST study, the risk for ipsilateral stroke at 3 years was 12.3% in the surgical group, as compared with 21.9% in the medically treated group. In both studies, the results were very significant statistically. The final results of these two trials are now available. Interestingly, even the symptomatic

Residual Arterial Diameter

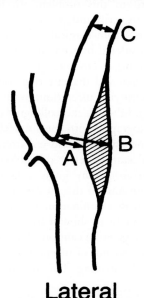

Lateral

FIGURE 6.2. The more common method of estimating the degree of stenosis. The dimension measured at *A* is compared with *C*—the internal carotid artery— rather than with *B*, which denotes the diameter of the carotid bulb. A 50% stenosis measured by this method would be equivalent to an 80% stenosis as measured by the method shown in Fig. 6.1.

patients with a 50% to 70% stenosis benefited from carotid endarterectomy (6). However, as might be predicted, the higher the degree of stenosis, the greater the risk for stroke and benefit from operation.

It should be obvious that the importance of duplex scanning will increase even further given the results of these two large clinical trials. Now that there is no question about the benefit of endarterectomy, duplex scanning becomes even more important for both screening and follow-up. Unfortunately, the NASCET investigators concluded that ultrasound was unreliable as a screening test. This was because of the lack of control over the studies and the variety of systems used, some of which were out of date at the time of the study. The methods for screening and its interpretation will be covered in detail.

STANDARD DIAGNOSTIC APPROACHES

For all patients suspected of having extracranial arterial disease, the historic method of establishing its presence or absence and its extent has been arteriography. This method has been time-tested and found to be satisfactory for clinical purposes; however, there are serious limitations and problems that limit its use except for specific indications. The most worrisome aspect of the procedure is its invasive nature and the potential for serious and, on rare occasions, irreversible complications. In fact, the asymptomatic carotid study showed that the risk for arteriography in terms of producing a stroke was nearly the same as with operation (8). This kind of evidence further supports the use of duplex scanning as the sole study done before operation.

Until duplex scanning was available and shown to be sufficiently accurate to evaluate the extracranial circulation, most tests in use were indirect. They examined the circulation at points removed from the site of disease (the bulb) and inferred from these changes the status of the arterial inflow to the hemisphere. The earliest of these tests was periorbital Doppler, which examined directional flow changes in the supraorbital and medial frontal arteries with compression of the temporal artery. Normally, flow is in an antegrade direction from the ophthalmic to the medial frontal and supraorbital arteries to supply the ipsilateral forehead (9).

When the internal carotid artery is narrowed to the point at which pressure and flow are reduced, the flow in the medial frontal and supraorbital arteries is reversed. Although this is a reasonably accurate test in experienced hands, it has major limitations that include its inability to distinguish between a high-grade stenosis and occlusion. Furthermore, it does not precisely localize the site of disease. In addition, once the test is positive, it is not possible to monitor any further changes that might take place because of the disease progression. Even though the test may be useful on occasion, it should no longer be considered a standard test for this area.

Gee and co-workers (10,11) devised the pneumoplethysmographic system, which permits an actual measurement of intraocular pressure that can, in turn, be related to the pressure in the ophthalmic artery. This method was well tested and compared against arteriography. For a diameter-reducing lesion of 60% or greater, the test has been shown to have a sensitivity of 90%. Its major problems are similar to the periorbital Doppler method, in that it cannot distinguish the site of involvement or differentiate between a high-grade stenosis and a total occlusion. In addition, it is not possible to monitor the progress of disease once the test is positive. Although this might theoretically be possible, there have been no reports documenting its use for this purpose.

Although no longer in use, the pneumoplethysmographic system was one of the screening tests used in the asymptomatic carotid surgery trial. Because the test became positive if the degree of diameter reduction exceeded 60%, this was used as the cutoff point for inclusion into the trial. This fact is not well known. A problem facing the clinician who is attempting to obtain accurate visualization by arteriographic methods has been the change in the approach used by the radiologist. The first major change was the introduction of intravenous digital subtraction arteriography (12). By administering the dye intravenously, it was possible to obtain images of the carotid bulb that, it was hoped, would be of diagnostic quality. In theory, this would be an ideal method because it would avoid all the problems associated with arterial puncture and the potential complications that can occur with injection of the contrast material. However, for the carotid artery, it proved to be disappointing, because of the lack of diagnostic quality in up to 20% of the studies. Although this method may still be used in some centers, it is not a satisfactory procedure for studying the carotid artery.

Because the digital techniques can also be used with the intraarterial injections, this method has become more popular and will, in all likelihood, become the standard method for the foreseeable future. It is possible to use smaller catheters and smaller volumes of contrast material to obtain good images that are of diagnostic quality.

Because ongoing quality control is critical for every noninvasive laboratory studying the extracranial arterial circulation, it is important to understand the accuracy of arteriography and the amount of variability that occurs in attempting to measure the degree of diameter reduction by this method. When there are disagreements, it is important to know which test may be right in resolving some of the concerns that would inevitably result.

In the course of initially evaluating the accuracy of duplex scanning for the carotid artery, we elected also to look at the intraobserver and interobserver variability of arteriography in assessing the degree of stenosis and occlu-

sion of the common, internal, and external carotid arteries (13). For this study, we used standard contrast arteriography with selective injections of the carotid artery with anteroposterior, lateral, and oblique films of the carotid bifurcation. There were 64 cases that had all views of the cervical portion of the carotid artery. All measurements of the sites of involvement were made with calipers attempting to measure the diameter in increments of 5%. There were three readers who read the films independently of one another. Unsubtracted films were used to look for calcium in the wall of the carotid bulb to define the outer limits of the artery wall to make the measurements (Fig. 6.1).

Most investigators use the dimensions of the internal carotid artery beyond the bulb as the normal reference artery. This tends to underestimate the actual degree of narrowing in the bulb itself (6) (Fig. 6.2).

Several aspects of the variability in measurement were evaluated and included the following: (a) the view of the bulb that appeared most appropriate for detecting irregularity and ulceration; (b) the variability in estimating the degree of stenosis in increments of 5%; (c) the variability in reclassifying the disease for five categories of stenosis-0%, 1% to 9%, 10% to 49%, 50% to 99%, and occlusion; and (d) the variability in reclassifying into six categories of stenosis-0%, 1% to 24%, 25% to 49%, 50% to 74%, 75% to 99%, and occlusion.

With regard to the issue of the surface of the lesion, an attempt was made to classify it into three categories—smooth, irregular, and ulcerated. For this determination, it was noted that the oblique views provided the best information with regard to this problem. In this study, no attempt was made to verify independently the presence or absence of ulceration from surgical specimens. Ulceration of the plaque is considered by some investigators to be the critical factor in leading to embolic episodes (14,15).

It is commonly believed that arteriography is an excellent method for identifying ulceration, but it is known that it can be misleading. Edwards and colleagues (16) compared the results of arteriography with the surgical specimens in 50 patients who underwent carotid endarterectomy. In 20 patients who had ulceration detected histologically, 12 were demonstrated on arteriography, giving a false-negative rate of 40%. Most important, of the 30 carotid arteries found free of ulceration with examination of the specimen, 17 (34%) had been thought to show it by arteriography. This study should encourage more caution in attempting to predict the presence or absence of ulceration by arteriography as well as by B-mode imaging. This will be considered in more detail later.

When the radiologists involved in the variability study attempted to resolve the diameter reduction by 5% increments, the measurements fell within this range in only 30% of the internal carotid arteries (13). For the five categories of disease, the carotid artery fell in the same group 75% of the time. For the six categories of stenosis, it fell to 59%.

What does this mean? It simply means that one must be cautious in attempting to resolve and classify accurately the degree of narrowing of the carotid artery for small degrees of change in the lesion. The absolute difference in percentage stenosis between readers for the internal carotid artery was 8.64 ± 9.5% (1 SD).

It must be emphasized that this study of variability in reading arteriograms was done with selective injections and multiple views of the carotid bulb. It is unusual today to obtain these types of views, unless they are specifically requested. In comparing the results of duplex scanning with the results of arteriography, it is important to realize that *both methods* will have variability in documenting both the nature of the plaque and the degree of stenosis that is present.

As noted in the introduction to this chapter, it is now apparent that the classification of the degree of stenosis is of more than academic interest. Given the results of the NASCET and ECST randomized clinical trials, patients who present with transient ischemic attacks and stroke will have their subsequent therapy determined in large part by the degree of diameter reduction in the carotid bulb (6,7). This can be assessed by duplex scanning, arteriography, or both. Because many patients now go directly to surgery on the basis of duplex scanning alone, it is very important to perform the procedure well.

THE PATIENT POPULATION

The types of patients referred to the vascular laboratory will determine the nature of the study to be done. It is important for the technologist who does the study to be familiar with the clinical problems that are under consideration. This will be helpful in optimizing the study to provide the physician with the most useful information. We classify our patient population into the following categories when they appear for study in our laboratory: (a) asymptomatic patients, (b) patients with transient ischemic attacks or strokes, (c) patients with nonlateralizing symptoms or signs, (d) patients about to undergo major cardiac or vascular surgery who are considered to be at high risk for neurologic complications, (e) patients being restudied for possible progression of disease, and (f) postoperative patients.

Asymptomatic Patients

Most patients who fit into this category have a bruit discovered on examination by their physician. Because the bruit itself does not accurately indicate the exact location and extent of the disease producing the finding, it is only natural that a suitable noninvasive test be done as the initial screen to determine the further management of the patient. What type of information is needed and useful in this setting? The major concern is whether the carotid artery is the source of the bruit, and, if so, to what degree is the artery narrowed.

In a 12-month period from January 1980 to December 1980, there were 81 asymptomatic patients with cervical bruits referred for study (17). In this very early study, 46 had unilateral bruits, and 35 had them present on both sides. The findings with regard to their carotid bifurcation were as follows: (a) normal, 4 of 116 (3%); (b) less than 50% diameter-reducing lesions, 79 of 116 (68%); (c) more than 50% diameter reduction, 31 of 116 (27%); and (d) total occlusion, 2 of 116 (2%). On the side free of a bruit, 8 (17%) had a stenosis greater than 50%, and there were no occlusions in this group of patients. Based on these early data, it was already clear that arteriography could be eliminated in a high percentage of patients screened. It is also clear based on the clinical trial data which patients should be selected as candidates for operation.

Patients with Transient Ischemic Attacks or Stroke

In this situation, it has often been stated that these patients should proceed directly to arteriography without first being studied by duplex scanning. This is clearly not the case because there are compelling reasons for suggesting that the duplex scan be done first. Some of these reasons are as follows: (a) a lesion may be found that will not warrant arteriography; (b) the internal carotid artery and, in some cases, the common carotid artery may be found to be totally occluded; (c) the carotid artery may be found to be completely normal; and (d) the test will serve as the baseline for follow-up studies.

Given the results of the NASCET and ECST studies, it is now clear which of the symptomatic patients should be considered candidates for endarterectomy (6,7). At the present time, this includes all patients with a greater than 50% diameter reduction of the carotid bulb. For patients with less than 50% stenosis, operation does not appear to offer the same amount of benefit. Given these results, it is clear how important the role of duplex scanning is in selecting which patients should proceed with operation. We will have to develop and validate criteria that will permit us to make the separation of patients into various categories of narrowing.

If the common carotid and/or internal carotid artery are occluded, these patients will not be candidates for operation. From a diagnostic standpoint, the occlusions of the common carotid and internal carotid artery should be considered separately. It is rare to miss a common carotid artery occlusion. The results of the duplex studies in this circumstance can be useful. For example, if the internal carotid artery is patent, it is possible to document this by the direction of flow in the external carotid artery. If flow in the external carotid artery is reversed, it is a collateral source to the internal carotid artery. In some cases, these patients are candidates for bypass grafting from the subclavian artery to restore normal flow to the internal carotid artery. When the common carotid artery is patent, documentation of the status of the internal carotid artery is of paramount importance.

As will be noted, we pay close attention to this question because it is such an important issue from a therapeutic standpoint. Very tight carotid bulb stenoses can be difficult to distinguish from total occlusions of the artery.

Patients with Nonlateralizing Symptoms or Signs

This group of patients consists of a confusing subset to evaluate. Their symptoms are nonspecific and suggest an overall reduction of cerebral blood flow either due to extensive extracranial arterial disease or because of disease of the vertebrobasilar blood supply. In this setting, the duplex studies can be helpful, particularly when either no disease is found or the lesions do not reduce pressure or flow. It has been thought that some patients with nonlateralizing symptoms might benefit from carotid endarterectomy when high-grade stenoses at the level of the bulb are found. This is difficult to prove because it is well known that the symptoms patients experience tend to wax and wane and may disappear entirely without any therapy at all. Vertebrobasilar symptoms are most commonly due to disease of the subclavian artery, with reversal of flow in the vertebral artery. This pattern of disease is easily ruled in or out on the basis of the duplex studies.

Patients Undergoing Cardiac or Vascular Surgery

Because atherosclerosis rarely confines itself to one arterial bed, it is only natural that there will be occasions in which disease in one location should raise some concerns about involvement elsewhere. It is a well-known fact that the finding of a bruit in the neck is an excellent "marker" for coronary artery disease (18). Conversely, if a patient has coronary and/or peripheral arterial disease, the chance of having carotid disease would appear to be high. This concern has been heightened by the observation that patients who undergo major cardiac and vascular surgery may have stroke as one of their complications. In fact, it appears that the stroke rate in patients undergoing coronary bypass grafting is in the range of 2% to 5% (19,20). The concern has focused on patients with high-grade carotid artery stenoses who, when placed on cardiopulmonary bypass, may have a drop in pressure and flow distal to a high-grade lesion, giving rise to an ischemic event. Referrals to the vascular laboratory are common for patients about to undergo major cardiac or vascular procedures (21).

The referrals generally fall into two groups: patients who are asymptomatic but are found to have a bruit, and

patients with a history of a recent or remote neurologic event. If a patient with coronary artery disease has a bruit, there is about a 50% chance that a stenosis of greater than 50% will be found by duplex scanning. There is little compelling evidence that concomitant carotid endarterectomy should be done in the asymptomatic patient at the time the patient undergoes cardiopulmonary bypass (22). If the lesion falls into the 50% to 79% stenosis category, we would simply follow the patient at 6-month intervals to evaluate the rate of change in the lesion. If a greater than 80% stenosis is found, a carotid endarterectomy would be warranted, with the timing determined by the severity of the heart disease (23,24). We prefer doing the operation as a separate procedure but realize that in some cases, the procedures are best done concurrently.

Patients Suspected of Having Vertebrobasilar Insufficiency

In 1961, Reivich and associates (25) described a syndrome in which occlusions of the proximal subclavian or innominate artery led to reversal of blood flow in the vertebral artery that was associated with events involving the posterior circulation. As reported, these patients would often develop symptoms when exercise of the arm on the side of the occlusion led to an increase in the "steal" of blood to the arm, producing the ischemia.

The mechanism for the hemodynamic changes is quite simple in that a pressure- and flow-reducing lesion in the artery proximal to the origin of the vertebral artery permits this vessel now to become an important reentry collateral to supply the arm. Although this would appear to be an ideal arrangement for the development of vertebrobasilar symptoms, it now appears clear that most patients will remain asymptomatic, even with arm exercise (26). In our laboratory, we identified 43 patients with reversal of flow in the vertebral artery. Only 7% of this group had symptoms that could be classified as classic for the subclavian steal syndrome. As will be noted later, there were some patients with *pre-steal*, defined as oscillating flow in the vertebral artery with both forward and reverse components. This represents an intermediate stage, probably reflecting a pressure gradient that is not sufficient to produce continuous reverse flow throughout the entire pulse cycle.

Involvement of the innominate artery is more likely to produce symptoms because an occlusion at this level not only will result in flow reversal in the vertebral artery but also will limit flow to the common carotid artery that could be an important source of collateral blood flow to the posterior circulation. Grosveld and colleagues (27) evaluated this in a series of 20 patients who had been investigated by both duplex scanning and arteriography. The patients were divided into two groups based on the degree of narrowing of the innominate artery. In group I, with a 40% to 80% stenosis (12 patients), only 1 patient showed symptoms with exercise of the right arm. In group II, with a greater than 80% stenosis, total occlusion, or both (8 patients), compensation through the innominate artery failed, with 6 patients developing symptoms with arm exercise. It was also shown that duplex scanning before and after exercise not only would be useful in documenting the hemodynamic response associated with exercise but also would verify that it occurred in conjunction with the development of symptoms.

The accuracy of duplex scanning for the detection of lesions involving the subclavian, innominate, and vertebral arteries is sufficiently good to recommend its use in this area. Ackerstaff and co-workers (28) evaluated the accuracy of duplex scanning for the detection of vertebral artery disease involving the prevertebral segment. There were 211 patients who underwent arteriography to verify the results obtained by duplex scanning. For the detection of a greater than 50% diameter-reducing stenosis, the sensitivity was 80%, the specificity 92%, the positive predictive value 73%, and the negative predictive value 94%. Of the occluded vertebral arteries, 87% were correctly identified.

EXAMINATION TECHNIQUE

The system must have the following elements for optimal application of the method: (a) a good high-resolution image; (b) a small sample volume, in the range of 3 mm³ at an operating range of approximately 25 mm, to permit selective sampling of at least four sites across the vessel; (c) real-time spectral analysis that permits a display of all the information in the Doppler spectrum from a range of −3 kHz to +7 kHz; (d) a hard copy output of both the image and the velocity patterns; and (e) automatic displays of the angle of incidence of the sound beam with the long axis of the vessel. Most systems available today will also permit the conversion of the frequency of the backscattered Doppler-shifted signal to velocity (angle-adjusted velocity).

There is often a great deal of confusion whether one should use frequency or velocity in reporting the results with these studies. In all our early work, the data were expressed in frequency (kHz). This was because the systems in use at the time did not permit the immediate calculation of velocity. It is important to remember that it makes no difference which approach is used for diagnostic purposes as long as one understands the rationale for the problems that can be involved—particularly for the carotid bulb—in attempting to determine an absolute velocity. This is because the flow velocity vectors in these vessels, in particular the carotid bulb, are not parallel to the long axis of the vessel either in normal subjects or in patients with stenotic lesions. We have also found that it is *very important* to attempt to make velocity recordings using a constant angle of the sound beam with the artery. Wherever possible, we try to work *as close to 60 degrees* as possible to the long axis of the vessel. This provides consistency from one study to the next, which is important (29).

Color and power Doppler have made the initial screening procedure faster and possibly more precise in terms of proper identification of the extracranial arterial blood supply. They are truly "pathfinders," particularly for depicting the anatomy. Most of the anatomic variants that are noted relate to the presence of coils and kinks, which can be confusing for even the experienced examiner. Some examples of these are shown in Figs. 6.3 and 6.4. In addition, when a stenosis is detected, it is possible to assess the direction of the jet in the narrowed segment, which is useful for accurate placement of the pulsed Doppler sample volume (Fig. 6.5). It is important to rely on the velocity data (peak systolic and end-diastolic) using the fast Fourier transforms (FFT) spectral analysis. This is because the velocities recorded from the color display alone are lower than they should be. This is due to the sampling rate required for the color and the method of analysis by the autocorrelation approach, which is used in some systems.

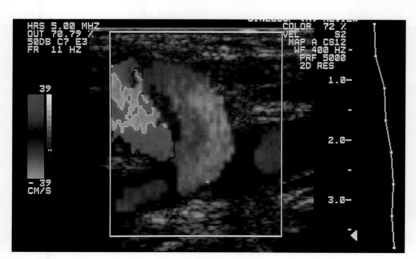

FIGURE 6.3. Color display demonstrating a kink in the internal carotid artery. This is quickly discerned by the color display's providing the technologist with the exact course of the internal carotid artery.

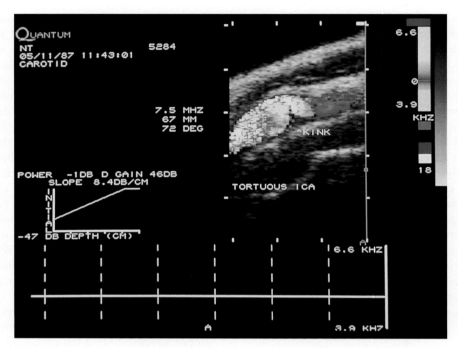

FIGURE 6.4. Another example in which color is of benefit in demonstrating the course of the extracranial arteries. Patterns of this type are not uncommon in the neck, making color very useful for this purpose.

The small sample volume becomes important when spectral broadening is used as one of the diagnostic parameters. This is illustrated in Fig. 6.6. When the carotid artery is being studied, a small sample volume is desirable (approximately 3 mm³ in our original scanner), so that spectral broadening can be used as a diagnostic parameter.

As reviewed in Chapter 3, a large sampling volume that incorporates the entire artery will pick up the steep velocity gradients near the wall. This could be interpreted as the spectral broadening that occurs in the presence of disturbed blood flow seen with a moderate to severe degree of narrowing (30–32).

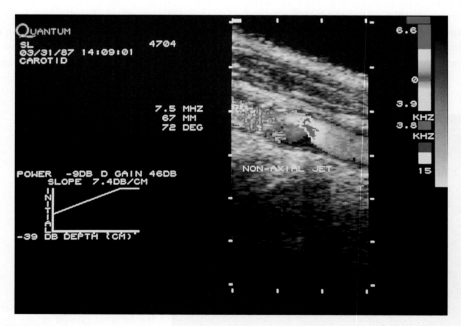

FIGURE 6.5. The direction of the jet in a stenosis may not be parallel to the walls. As noted in this figure, the jet was nonaxial.

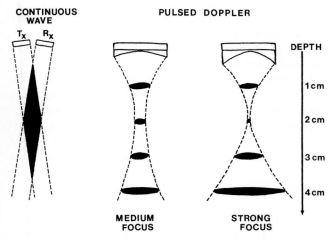

FIGURE 6.6. The more common concepts of the sample volume and its size with regard to areas that are encompassed in the vessel being studied. On the *left*, the beam of a continuous wave system with the transmitted beam (*Tx*) and the received beam (*Rx*). The *shaded areas* indicate the sites from which a velocity shift would be detected. When a pulsed Doppler is used, the effect of focusing is evident on both the width and length of the sample volume. (From Langlois YE, Roederer GO, Strandness DE Jr. Ultrasonic evaluation of the carotid bifurcation. *Echocardiography* 1987;4:141–159, with permission.)

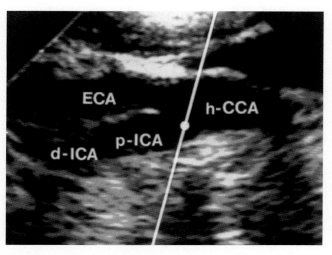

FIGURE 6.7. This longitudinal view of the carotid bifurcation shows the position of the sample volume in the middle of the artery at the junction of the high common carotid artery (*h-CCA*). The proximal (*p-ICA*) and distal (*d-ICA*) internal carotid arteries are also visualized. The origin and first few centimeters of the external carotid artery (*ECA*) are also seen. (From Roederer GO, Langlois YE, Jager K, et al.. The natural history of carotid arterial disease in asymptomatic patients with cervical bruits. *Stroke* 1984;15:605–613, with permission.)

In the course of the examination, it is important to follow the same sequence of events to avoid missing important lesions. The procedure should start by examining the low common carotid artery, paying particular attention to the velocity patterns as close to the aortic arch as possible. This will assist in the detection of stenotic lesions at that level. The B-mode image and/or the color flow display is always used as a guide for the placement of the sample volume in the center of the artery (Fig. 6.7). Complicated plaques are uncommon in the common carotid artery, but fibrous plaques are frequently observed but do not appear to be the source of problems in most patients.

The velocity patterns in the common carotid artery are a reflection of the low resistance offered by the brain and the higher resistance of the face as supplied by the external carotid artery. Normally, 70% to 80% of the blood flow in the common carotid artery is directed to the brain. A typical waveform from the common carotid artery is shown in Fig. 6.8.

The position of the flow divider is noted as the transducer is moved up the neck. This is, of course, the site at which the external carotid artery takes its origin and the bulb is located. The bulb may have several configurations; however, in most patients, the bulb is seen as the dilated segment. This is the only place in the arterial system where this configuration is found. The normal velocity patterns in the external carotid artery are characteristic enough so that the experienced technologist can recognize them by their audible character (Fig. 6.8).

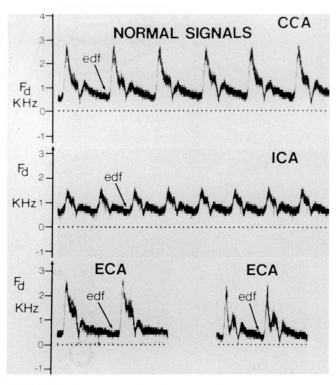

FIGURE 6.8. Normal velocity patterns from the common carotid artery (*CCA*), internal carotid artery (*ICA*), and external carotid artery (*ECA*). In the CCA and ICA, the end-diastolic velocity (*EDF*) is above the zero flow line. The flow during diastole in the ECA often goes to zero or actually reverses for a brief period of time. F_d, frequency shift.

Several flow patterns are observed in the normal carotid bulb, depending on the site of sampling and the time in the cardiac cycle. Near the flow divider, flow will be antegrade and above zero at all times in the pulse cycle. However, as the sample volume is placed in the posterolateral aspect of the carotid bulb, some complex velocity patterns are observed in the region where flow separation occurs. As noted in Fig. 6.9, flow will actually reverse at times during the pulse cycle, which is important because, when found, it means that the bulb is largely free of disease. Since we have come to recognize boundary layer separation as a normal

finding, it has become an important part of the examination sequence. As the bulb fills with atheroma, boundary layer separation cannot occur (see Fig. 4.5 in Chapter 4). Further, as has been noted by Nicholls and associates (33), the demonstration of flow separation in the bulb in patients with symptoms essentially rules out the bifurcation as a cause of the patient's problems. These authors noted that, in this circumstance, other causes and sites must be sought.

As the atheroma comes to occupy more than just the lateral aspect of the bulb, it will begin to impinge on the region near the flow divider, resulting in an increase in the

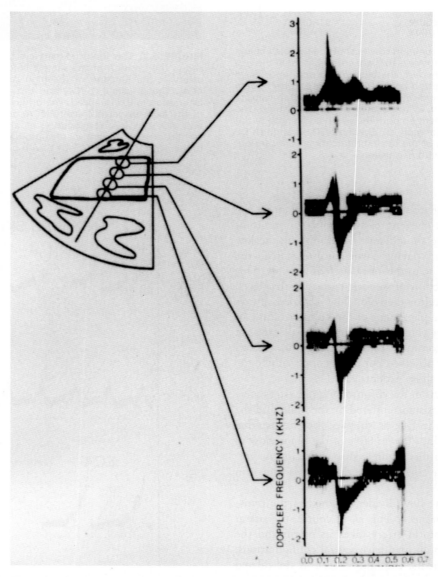

FIGURE 6.9. In this example, the sample volume was moved sequentially from a position close to the flow divider (*top*) to the posterior aspect of the carotid bulb (*bottom*). Near the flow divider, all flow is antegrade; whereas in the bulb, it reverses. This is the region of boundary layer separation. (From Phillips DJ, Greene FM Jr, Langlois YE, et al. Flow velocity patterns in the carotid bifurcation of young, presumed normal subjects. *Ultrasound Med Biol* 1983;9:33–49, with permission.)

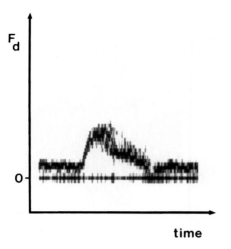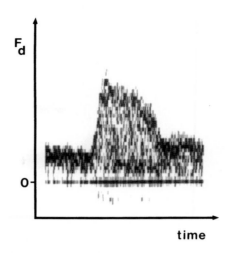

FIGURE 6.10. The velocity spectra on the *left* are from the common carotid artery. Those on the *right* are from the internal carotid artery and of the type noted with a 16% to 49% stenosis. The peak frequency (F_d) is below 4 kHz (125 cm/sec). The major diagnostic criterion used is marked spectral broadening, which obliterates the systolic window. (From Roederer GO, Langlois YE, Jager K, et al.. The natural history of carotid arterial disease in asymptomatic patients with cervical bruits. *Stroke* 1984;15:605–613, with permission.)

velocity through this area. When this is noted, it is important to pay attention to four factors: (a) the peak systolic velocity, (b) the end-diastolic velocity, (c) the amount of spectral broadening, and (d) the nature of the flow patterns distal to the region of stenosis.

The categories of disease that can be recognized by duplex scanning are as follows:

1. Normal
2. 1% to 15% stenosis
3. 16% to 49% stenosis
4. 50% to 79% stenosis
5. 80% to 99% stenosis
6. Total occlusion

The category for minimal disease (1% to 15%) has been a source of confusion. During the early validation studies of duplex scanning, some of the patients were noted on their arteriograms to have intimal irregularity that was not sufficient to produce any narrowing of the artery. It appeared that, in such patients, the only change in the velocity pattern was some spectral broadening, which occurred primarily in diastole. This turned out to be imprecise and difficult to separate from the normal velocity patterns recorded. At the present time, we make this categorization *only* if there is no flow reversal in the bulb and no increase in the peak systolic velocity at the site of disease involvement.

For the 16% to 49% diameter-reducing stenosis, the changes noted include no increase in peak systolic velocity but a marked spectral broadening that obliterates the systolic window (Fig. 6.10). It is important for the technologist to be sure that the sample volume is in the center stream of the internal carotid artery and not near the wall, where steep velocity gradients are known to be present (see Fig. 3.9 in Chapter 3).

When the atheroma begins to impinge on the region of the flow divider, the criteria used begins to depend on the levels of the peak systolic and end-diastolic velocities recorded from the site where the greatest velocity is detected. We have shown that, once the peak frequency exceeds 4 kHz (125 cm/sec), the degree of narrowing has now exceeded 50%. The end-diastolic velocity in this case is below 4.5 kHz (140 cm/sec). If one is using frequency units, these values would correspond to those obtained using a 5-MHz transmitting frequency at an angle of insonation of 60%. For lesions of this type, there is spectral broadening as well, even though this is not one of the diagnostic criteria that are used (Fig. 6.11).

In our early development of the algorithms for the separation of the various stenosis categories, we used only one category for the greater than 50% diameter-reducing stenoses. Because of the feeling that a further division of this rather large category could be of clinical importance, we developed an algorithm that permitted the separation into a 50% to 79% and an 80% to 99% grouping. Roederer and colleagues (34) noted that the use of the end-diastolic frequency would appear to be a suitable cutoff point to make this separation. It appeared that an end-diastolic frequency of 4.5 kHz (140 cm/sec) was a good and sensitive endpoint to make this distinction (Figs. 6.12 and 6.13). It is important to realize that the stenosis may be so tight that it can easily be missed if the technologist does not diligently search for the high-velocity jet in the narrowed segment. An example of the velocity changes recorded in a patient who progressed to this degree of stenosis is shown in Fig. 6.14.

The detection of occlusions is of obvious importance because it will essentially rule out the patient's need for surgery to improve blood flow to the hemisphere. We have

(Text continues on page 97.)

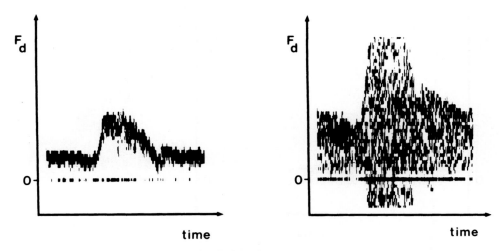

FIGURE 6.11. The velocity spectra on the *left* were from the common carotid artery. Those on the *right* were from a 50% to 79% stenosis of the internal carotid artery. The peak systolic frequency (F_d) exceeds 4 kHz (125 cm/sec). (From Roederer GO, Langlois YE, Jager K, et al. The natural history of carotid arterial disease in asymptomatic patients with cervical bruits. *Stroke* 1984;15:605–613, with permission.)

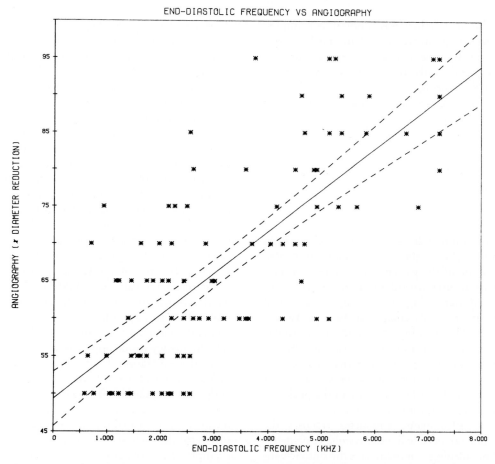

FIGURE 6.12. This figure illustrates the relationship between the degree of stenosis as estimated by arteriography and the end-diastolic frequency at the site of stenosis. The *solid line* represents the regression line, and the *dashed lines* represent the 95% confidence limits. The data were from 98 sides. (From Roederer GO, Langlois YE, Jager KA, et al. A simple spectral parameter for accurate classification of severe carotid artery disease. *Bruit* 1989;3:174–178, with permission.)

END-DIASTOLIC FREQUENCY

	<4.5 KHZ	≥4.5 KHZ	
<80% DIAMETER REDUCTION	64	9	73
≥80% DIAMETER REDUCTION	4	21	25
	68	30	98

ANGIOGRAPHY

FIGURE 6.13. The relationship between end-diastolic frequency and the diameter reduction of a stenosis of the internal carotid artery.

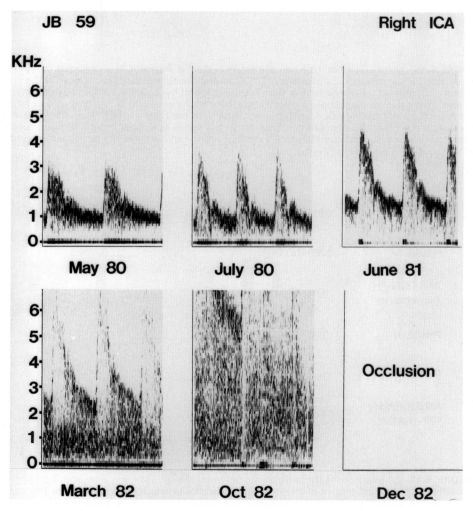

FIGURE 6.14. The spectral display from the right internal carotid artery (*ICA*) in May 1980 was consistent with a 16% to 49% stenosis. In June 1981, the peak frequency exceeded the 4-kHz level, placing the patient in the 50% to 79% diameter-reduction group. By October 1982, the end-diastolic frequency was 5.5 kHz and of the type seen with an 80% to 99% stenosis. The ICA occluded in December 1982, and the patient sustained a stroke. (From Roederer GO, Langlois YE, Jager K, et al.. The natural history of carotid arterial disease in asymptomatic patients with cervical bruits. *Stroke* 1984;15:605–613, with permission.)

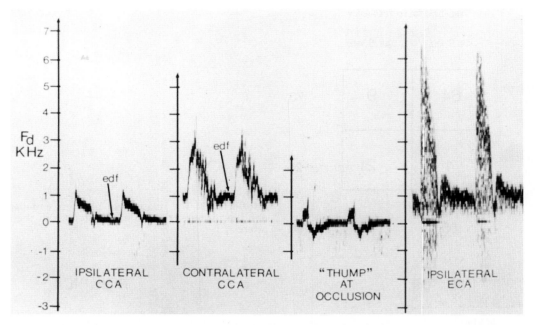

FIGURE 6.15. The major findings when the internal carotid artery (ICA) is occluded. In the *left panel*, flow in the common carotid artery (*CCA*) at end-diastole goes to zero. Flow in the contralateral carotid artery will be higher than is usually found because it now supplies both hemispheres. When the sample volume is placed at the base of the occlusion, a "thump" may be heard that reflects no net forward flow at that point. Finally, in the *right panel*, flow in the ipsilateral external carotid artery (*ECA*) might be increased; it now serves as a major collateral source for the brain. However, caution is urged because a stenotic lesion can also give rise to the same velocity pattern. *EDF*, end-diastolic frequency.

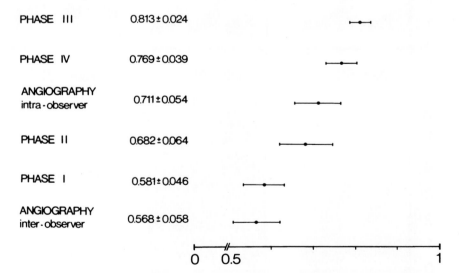

FIGURE 6.16. Comparison of the agreement between duplex scanning and arteriography for the different validation phases of the studies done at the University of Washington. The kappa values for the intraobserver and interobserver arteriographic studies are also shown (see text).

found four rules that must be followed to make this distinction accurately (Fig. 6.15):

1. Flow in the common carotid artery on the side of an occlusion will go to zero at end-diastole. In 36 cases with documented total occlusion, flow went to zero in 34 instances.
2. Look for the low-velocity "thump" at the point of the occlusion. This simply means that there is no net forward flow through the carotid artery at this point.
3. The region of the bulb must be diligently searched for the high-velocity jet that might be missed with very high-grade stenoses.
4. The internal carotid artery beyond the bulb must be examined for any evidence of flow. If flow is found, the internal carotid artery must be considered to be open. Because the internal carotid artery has no branches in the neck, there would be no detectable flow in the internal carotid when there is a total occlusion of the bulb or proximal internal carotid artery.

To evaluate the comparative accuracy of duplex scanning against arteriography, we have computed the kappa statistic for each phase of our validation studies (30). These are summarized in Fig. 6.16. The kappa statistic is a measure of the agreement between two methods corrected for chance. A kappa value of 1.0 represents complete agreement between two methods. A kappa value of zero indicates that the observed results occurred by chance. The validation of duplex scanning went through the following phases:

Phase 1. These were the results obtained with the prototype of the ultrasonic duplex scanner developed at the University of Washington. There were 270 sides in which comparison with arteriography was possible.

Phase 2. These results were obtained with the first commercially available duplex scanners that had a medium-focus scanhead; 169 sides were available for comparison.

Phase 3. In this phase, the scanhead was replaced with a short-focus transducer; 77 sides were available for comparison with arteriography.

Phase 4. The data accumulated for this phase were with the computer-based pattern recognition program; 170 sides were available for comparison (35,36).

For phases 1 through 4, the category for high-grade lesions included only the 50% to 99% category, rather than the current breakdown into 50% to 79% and 80% to 99% categories. As will be noted, for each phase of the validation trials, the concordance between duplex scanning and arteriography improved. This was due to the following facts:

- Awareness that boundary layer separation was a normal finding in the carotid bulb. The specificity of the test improved from a level of 37% to 84%
- Recognition of the factors previously reviewed in documenting the presence of a total occlusion of the internal carotid artery
- Realization that the size of the sample volume be kept small for screening the carotid bifurcation

It should be noted that the kappa value for duplex scanning and arteriography is nearly the same as that for one arteriographer rereading the same film, but better than one radiologist's readings compared with another.

The most recent validation data are shown in Table 6.1. Will this improve further? This is probably doubtful, given the inherent variability for tests of this type. The procedure does, however, satisfy the requirements for a satisfactory screening test of populations with both a high and low prevalence of the disease (37). It should be noted that those normal subjects classified as having disease were all in the 1% to 15% category and not for higher grades of involvement that could, in some cases, lead to having an arteriogram performed.

During the past few years, there have been published reports showing that the criteria for classifying the extent of narrowing in a carotid artery, which is contralateral to a total occlusion of the internal carotid artery, may have to be modified. In theory, when one internal carotid artery is totally occluded, flow to the hemisphere on the side of the obstruction will have to be supplied by collateral sources

TABLE 6.1. CONCORDANCE DUPLEX SCANNING VERSUS ANGIOGRAPHY

Angiography	Duplex results (% diameter reduction)[a]					
	Normal	1–15%	16–49%	50–79%	80–99%	Occlusion
Normal	47	9				
1–15%	4	49	8			
16–49%		14	62	4		
50–79%		1	7	56	8	
80–99%				5	22	1
Occlusion					1	38

[a]There were 336 sides studied, and they form the comparison for these two methods of evaluating the carotid bulb.
Duplex scanning has a sensitivity of 99% and a specificity of 84% for this study.

(37). The most obvious source would be the contralateral common and internal carotid arteries that could supply both hemispheres if the anterior communicating artery is patent. Thus, in this situation, the flow through the common carotid artery could be double that found when both internal carotid arteries are patent. It has been suggested by Cato and co-workers (38) and Fujitani and colleagues (39) that when this occurs, the standard spectral criteria tend to overcall the degree of stenosis. This is an important consideration that should be considered in some detail.

Fujitani and colleagues (39) carried out a retrospective review of 154 patients with arteriographically confirmed total occlusion of one internal carotid artery. Each of the patent contralateral carotid arteries was categorized from the arteriographic studies for the categories shown in Table 6.1. The peak systolic velocities were commonly exaggerated in the presence of a contralateral occlusion. For lesions that were not hemodynamically significant (less than 50% diameter reduction), the standard velocity criteria developed at the University of Washington overestimated the degree of stenosis in 43 of 89 lesions (48.3%), giving a sensitivity of 57% and a specificity of 97%. Conversely, the prediction of a greater than 50% stenosis with the standard spectral criteria gave a sensitivity of 97% with a specificity of 57%. By using receiver operating curves, it was possible to readjust the cutoff points for deciding the cutoff frequencies that were most likely to classify the degree of narrowing correctly. The criteria suggested by Fujitani and colleagues (39) are shown in Table 6.2.

By using these modified criteria, the sensitivity and specificity for the prediction of a greater than 50% or less than 50% diameter-reducing stenosis were improved. To compare the results using the standard criteria with the modified values, Fujitani and colleagues (39) calculated the kappa statistic for these two comparisons. Using the standard criteria, the kappa was 0.577 ± 0.113, as compared with 0.872 ± 0.060 (p less than 0.001). These criteria do make sense and should be employed when a patient with an internal carotid artery occlusion is found.

Every study also includes the evaluation of the subclavian and vertebral arteries because they may contribute to the clinical picture, and involvement of these arteries may become important in planning therapy. It is our routine to measure the blood pressure in both arms at the time of the examination because this will provide clues to the status of the subclavian artery. If there is a difference of greater than 15 mm Hg in the level of systolic blood pressure, the examiner should be aware that the artery on the side of the lower pressure may have either a high-grade stenosis or a total occlusion present.

The velocity signal recorded from the normal subclavian artery is usually triphasic, as it is in peripheral arteries of the lower limb. With a stenosis, the patterns observed will reflect the high velocity in the jet with loss of reverse flow and the presence of poststenotic turbulence.

The vertebral arteries are the first major branch of the subclavian artery. They have the characteristic velocity waveforms for an artery supplying a low-resistance circuit, such as the brain. They may be confused with the thyrocervical trunk, but it has branches at that level, and the demonstration of these makes its identification certain. If there is any confusion concerning the nature of the vessel being imaged, it is possible, by tapping the distal vertebral artery at the level of the mastoid process, to see these oscillations in the velocity recordings made at the base of the neck. This provides certainty that the vessel of interest is, indeed, the vertebral artery.

The types of waveforms seen in the vertebral artery depend on the nature of the process being studied. If there is a stenosis, it will demonstrate the high-velocity jets associated with stenoses wherever they might occur. If there is a significant pressure drop across the subclavian artery, flow in the vertebral artery will be reversed, as it now becomes an important collateral source for the arm (Fig. 6.17). There is a subset of patients who will have a to-and-fro pattern in the vertebral artery that will totally reverse when reactive hyperemia of the arm on the side of the lesion is produced. This has been characterized as pre-steal. Although its significance has not been fully elucidated, it may be associated with symptoms compatible with vertebrobasilar insufficiency.

TABLE 6.2. MODIFIED SPECTRAL CRITERIA FOR THE CLASSIFICATION OF CAROTID ARTERIES CONTRALATERAL TO AN OCCLUSION OF THE INTERNAL CAROTID ARTERY

Arteriographic lesion	Modified criteria
A (normal)	Peak systolic frequency <4 kHz (<125 cm/sec); minimal to no spectral broadening in deceleration phase of systole
B 1–15%	Peak systolic frequency <4 kHz (<140 cm/sec); minimal spectral broadening in deceleration phase of systole
C 16–49%	Peak systolic frequency >4 kHz, (>125 cm/sec); end-diastolic frequency <5.0 kHz, (<155 cm/sec), minimal spectral broadening (open window)
D 50–79%	Peak systolic frequency, >4.5 kHz, (>140 cm/sec); end-diastolic frequency <5.0 kHz, (<155 cm/sec), marked spectral broadening
D+ 80–99%	Peak systolic frequency >4.5 kHz, (>140 cm/sec); end-diastolic frequency >5.0 kHz, (>155 cm/sec), marked spectral broadening

The end-diastolic frequency and velocity values are used for the classification criteria for the 80%–99% stenoses. The frequency values are based on a 5-MHz pulsed Doppler carrier frequency with a 60° angle of insonation.

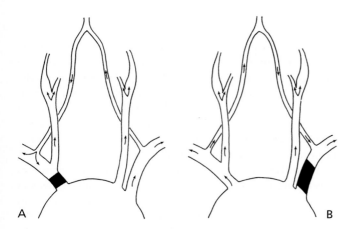

FIGURE 6.17. The types of situations in which reverse flow in the vertebral artery are shown. **A:** With occlusion of the innominate, flow to the common carotid artery is reduced, with the vertebral artery supplying not only the arm but also the right side of the brain. **B:** Occlusion of the subclavian artery with flow reversal in the left vertebral artery. (From Roederer GO, Langlois YE, Strandness DE Jr. Cerebral arterial flow and cerebral vascular insufficiency. In: Condon RE, DeCosse J, eds. *Surgical care II.* Philadelphia: Lea & Febiger, 1985:199–234, with permission.)

OTHER ALGORITHMS

During the formulation of the study procedures and the methods of classifying the degree of stenosis, we evaluated other algorithms that might be helpful for the further stratification of lesions in the 50% to 99% category. There were two approaches that we investigated for this separation. Because the peak systolic velocity in the narrowed portion of the internal carotid artery should increase with increasing degrees of narrowing, we investigated the ratio of the

peak systolic velocity in the internal carotid artery to that recorded from the common carotid artery (VICA systole/VCCA systole) (40,41). As noted in Fig. 6.18, the ratio was below 0.8 in all normal subjects and above 1.5 in all vessels with a diameter-reducing stenosis greater than 50%. It appeared that, although the method could not be used for gradation of lesions that narrowed the artery by less than 60%, it could be used for the classification of lesions that exceeded the 60% diameter-reducing range.

If one chose to examine the relationship between the peak systolic velocity in the stenosis and the end-diastolic velocity in the common carotid artery (VICA-systolic velocity/VCCA-diastolic velocity), it appeared feasible to subdivide further the degree of narrowing above the 60% diameter-reducing range. When 86 arteries with carotid artery disease were evaluated in this fashion, the following accuracy could be obtained:

- 60% to 99% stenosis (42 sides); ratio, 7.5; accuracy 95%
- 65% to 99% stenosis (36 sides); ratio, 11.0; accuracy 97%
- 90% to 99% stenosis (10 sides); ratio, 18.0; accuracy 100%

As noted previously, we no longer use this ratio because use of the end-diastolic velocity alone is adequate for the diagnosis of a greater than 80% diameter-reducing stenosis. However, this method may be useful for the long-term follow-up of patients, for whom the results of one examination will need to be compared with the previous study.

Because the interim results of the NASCET and ECST studies showed that greater than 70% diameter-reducing stenosis in the carotid artery was best treated by endarterectomy, there was a need to modify, to some extent, the velocity criteria that are commonly used (6,7). The criteria that we

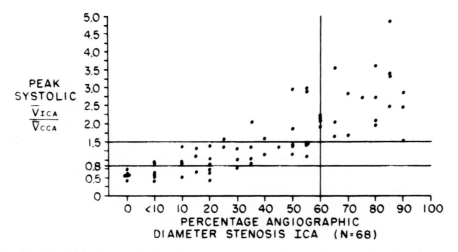

FIGURE 6.18. Relationship between the peak systolic velocity in the stenoses to that recorded from the common carotid artery. (From Blackshear WM Jr, Phillips DJ, Chikos PM, et al. Carotid artery velocity patterns in normal and stenotic vessels. *Stroke* 1980;11:67–71, with permission.)

developed separate the 50% to 79% and 80% to 99% categories with sufficient sensitivity and specificity. If a symptomatic patient were found to have a greater than 80% stenosis, there would be no question as to therapy. However, what about a symptomatic patient whose lesion falls into the 50% to 79% group? Can we develop additional duplex criteria to identify the 70% and over degree of narrowing?

Moneta and co-workers (42,43) examined this problem and came up with some suggestions that will be useful. They conducted a retrospective review of 100 carotid arteriograms that were read using the NASCET criteria. In this group, 58 (32%) carotid arteries fell into the 70% to 99% category. By using the velocity values from the common carotid artery and the site of stenosis, it was possible to construct receiver operator curves to determine which values provided the best cutoff for the 70% to 99% degree of stenosis. These authors concluded that the use of the ratio of the internal carotid artery peak systolic to common carotid artery peak systolic value provided the best single measure for this distinction. A value of 4.0 provided a sensitivity of 91%, a specificity of 87%, positive predictive value of 76%, and negative predictive value of 96%. The overall accuracy was 88%.

A similar analysis was done to arrive at a ratio for the greater than 60% stenosis as noted in the asymptomatic carotid surgery trial. The ratio that we use for this cutoff is 3.0 (44). These changes for reporting were made to accommodate those physicians who wanted to follow the recommended guidelines of the randomized clinical trials. These ratios are now calculated and become a regular part of our reporting back to the referring physician.

Another aspect of importance in duplex scanning is the relationship between the findings and clinical events. As noted earlier, the results of the NASCET and ECST studies showed quite clearly that risk in symptomatic patients could best be related to the degree of narrowing. The tighter the degree of stenosis, the more likely it was for the patient to have an ischemic event. The risk for a subsequent stroke increased for each 10% increment of narrowing above the cutoff level of 70%. Are there ultrasonic criteria that may also be used to provide an estimate of risk for this subset of patients? Moneta and co-workers (43) examined this issue with particular emphasis on the very high-grade lesions (greater than 80%) that we have found to be so dangerous. These authors examined the end-diastolic velocities at the site of maximal narrowing in the internal carotid artery in an attempt to relate these findings to clinical outcome. There were 73 patients with a greater than 80% diameter-reducing stenosis who were followed but not treated surgically. In this group, there was a relationship between the level of the end-diastolic velocity noted at the site of narrowing and clinical events. If the end-diastolic velocity was between 140 and 200 cm/sec, 30% had an event within the next 2 years. When the end-diastolic velocity exceeded 200 cm/sec, 68% had an event within the same time period.

The final report of the ECST also confirmed that the greatest risk was in patients with a greater than 80% stenosis (7).

It also appears that total occlusion of the internal carotid is not an unusual event that occurs when patients with high-grade carotid lesions are being followed. When the internal carotid artery becomes occluded, the stroke rate is in the range of 25%, with another 10% to 15% sustaining a precipitating episode of amaurosis fugax. It is also known that the risk for thrombosis is greatest during the early months after the lesion is first discovered.

It is also important to remember that the chance of developing a second ischemic event is essentially equivalent to the perioperative morbidity and mortality that one might expect from carotid endarterectomy. In NASCET, the stroke rate during the first 32 days in the medical arm of the trial after randomization was nearly the same as that occurring secondary to operation (6). This again emphasizes the danger of the high-grade lesions in terms of precipitating a clinical event.

LIMITATIONS OF DUPLEX SCANNING

One of the most glaring shortcomings of the method is that it can be used only for those vessels in the neck that are accessible to this form of energy. Early in our experience, we were concerned we might miss lesions of the great vessels of the aortic arch, which might be the cause of symptoms. With better scanheads and our ability to "look" down toward the origin of the major vessels, we have not missed any hemodynamically significant lesions at the level of the aortic arch. Nonetheless, the technologist must always be aware of this and diligently search for such stenotic lesions at the time of every examination.

Other "silent" areas are the carotid siphon and inside the skull (Fig. 6.19). With regard to the siphon, we investigated its potential as a cause for symptoms as well as the outcome after carotid endarterectomy (45). The prevalence of disease in this region was reviewed in 141 patients who had undergone 149 endarterectomies. We reviewed the arteriograms of these patients and classified the degree of narrowing into the following categories: (a) 20% to 49% diameter reduction, found in 42% of sides; (b) 50% to 99% diameter reduction, found in 9% of sides; and (c) occlusions found in 10% of sides. Most (65%) were smooth. We could find no relationship between the severity of the siphon lesions and those found in the carotid bulb. In addition, there was no relationship between the severity of the siphon stenosis and symptoms. Furthermore, the degree of siphon involvement bore no relation to the outcome after carotid endarterectomy. It is this author's belief that most of the lesions in this region are rarely the cause of problems.

The one area that cannot be examined by duplex scanning is inside the skull. To investigate this problem from an arteriographic standpoint, we reviewed the studies of 109 patients with symptomatic cerebrovascular disease not only to evalu-

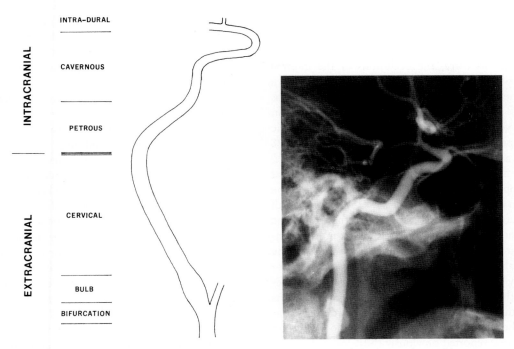

FIGURE 6.19. The anatomic extracranial and intracranial course of the internal carotid artery.

ate the nature of the findings in the bulb but also to examine both the siphon and the arteries inside the skull (46).

In this study, the major factors examined were the status of the bulb, the siphon, and the presence or absence of communicating arteries inside the head. In the 29 patients with fixed neurologic deficits, 26 (90%) had intracerebral abnormalities of either the siphon or the communicating arteries. This is in contrast to those patients who presented with transient ischemic attacks where only 29% had an abnormality of the intracranial vessels and the communicating arteries.

In theory, transcranial Doppler (TCD) should be able to perform two major roles that could be critically important for the evaluation of patients who present with symptoms of either the anterior or posterior circulation. The first would be to identify sites of stenosis and occlusion of vessels, such as the middle cerebral artery (47–50).

Because the intracranial collateral potential depends so heavily on the role of the circle of Willis, TCD may come to play an important role here. Because all elements of the circle can be outlined, at least in terms of their patency and direction of flow, this may provide the best method available to understand better its role in the pathogenesis of permanent deficits that occur in patients with both extracranial and intracranial arterial disease. This requires an enormous amount of work to ferret out all the details and the innumerable permutations and combinations that are possible. Perhaps it can also begin to shed some light on the perplexing disorders of the posterior circulation that are so hard to

understand at the present time. However, TCD has not been able to help ferret these patients out who are most likely to sustain a permanent deficit when carotid stenosis is the major problem. However, there is no doubt that TCD can detect narrowing of the middle cerebral artery, which can be a cause of a neurologic deficit.

STUDIES AFTER ENDARTERECTOMY

Although carotid endarterectomy has been shown to be better for the prevention of stroke than conventional medical therapy, in symptomatic patients with greater than 50% diameter-reducing stenosis, there is more information of value that can be obtained by duplex scanning. The questions that are of great importance include the following:

1. Does the bifurcation remain free of disease after operation and for how long?
2. How often does the internal carotid artery occlude during and after operation?
3. Are the events that occur after operation related to residual disease in the bulb, or do they occur from other causes?

Healy and associates (51) carried out a prospective study of 200 consecutive patients who had undergone carotid endarterectomy between 1980 and 1987. All of these patients were followed at regular intervals with a mean follow-up time of 31 months. At each visit, repeat duplex scans were performed to assess the status of the operated artery and the contralateral side. There were five occlusions of the internal carotid artery—one occurring during operation and four during follow-up. In three, the occlusions of the internal carotid artery were accompanied by the development of a stroke. A restenosis secondary to myointimal hyperplasia was found in 19.7%. The mean stroke incidence after operation was 2.8% per year for the patients with transient ischemic attacks, 6.2% per year for patients with stroke, and 0.65% per year in the asymptomatic patient group.

Although it is possible to use duplex scanning in the first few days after operation, we do not recommend it, unless the simple question of patency of the internal carotid artery is all that is of concern. Unless one is experienced, there are some unusual flow patterns seen during this time that may be confusing. There are changes during the healing process in the bulb that may alter the flow patterns and make it difficult to assess accurately the status of the area. For this reason, we recommend that the first study be done 6 weeks to 3 months after the procedure has been carried out. If it is done at that time or later, the results, as compared with angiography, are as accurate as those reported previously (52).

A point that must be emphasized for the studies done after endarterectomy is to know whether the artery had been patched. If a patch is used, the bulb may no longer have a normal configuration, and the flow patterns may be confusing to the observer. Although even the prosthetic patches are sonolucent after they are placed, the type of material used is also of interest. What effect this will have on the subsequent course of the patient and the ultrasonic studies will have to await further, more detailed, evaluation.

An important question relates to the frequency of study required after operation and its relevance to outcome. Can we justify the routine surveillance of the carotid artery after plaque removal? Given the very low incidence of clinical events even in the face of a 10% to 20% restenosis rate, it is difficult to justify follow-up studies unless there are specific indications (53).

One important aspect of the carotid endarterectomy procedure is the relatively high incidence of myointimal hyperplasia and the low incidence of problems associated with its development at this site. Although a stenosis in the 50% to 79% range rarely leads to the development of symptoms when it develops in the carotid bulb, this is clearly not the case when it occurs in other arterial beds. For example, a similar degree of stenosis in a vein graft placed either in the leg or the heart would make the patient symptomatic and require repair. This is not true in the carotid artery, thus making it an ideal place both to monitor and perhaps modify this interesting arterial wall response to injury.

Other changes have taken place with regard to duplex scanning that are of great importance in monitoring the process of myointimal hyperplasia. The most important is the dramatic improvement in B-mode image and color and power Doppler quality that is now available. We now have the opportunity of monitoring the healing changes in the endarterectomized segment from the early postoperative period up to the point of maximal development and stability of the lesion. We have embarked upon a program to investigate the postoperative changes. We have been able to do the following, which may be of value to those interested in monitoring the changes that take place after operation:

1. The sutures placed in the bulb can be used as fiducial markers, permitting an examination of the same site at each examination (Figs. 6.20 and 6.21).

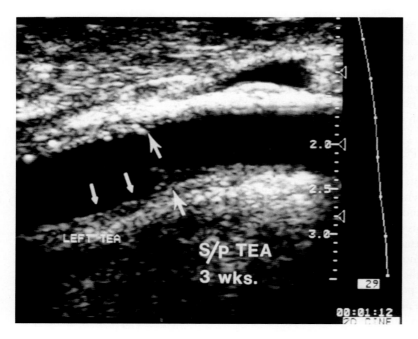

FIGURE 6.20. In this B-mode image taken 3 weeks after carotid endarterectomy, one of the sutures (*large arrow anterior wall*) can be seen. The prominent shelf on the posterior wall can also be easily seen. This is the site of transection of the plaque (*large arrow*). The *smaller arrows* point out the residual posterior wall segment from which the plaque was removed.

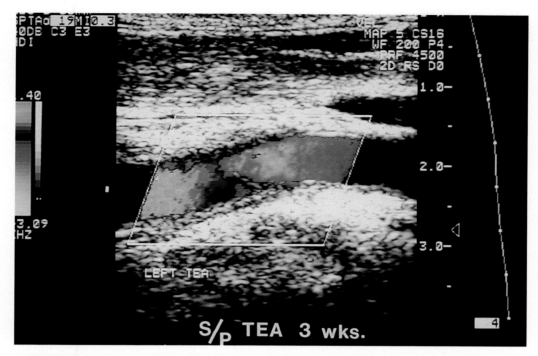

FIGURE 6.21. The same view as noted in Fig. 6.20 is now depicted with the addition of color. The sudden transition from red to blue is due to the change in the angle of the sound beam to the velocity vectors and does not represent a dramatic change in flow direction.

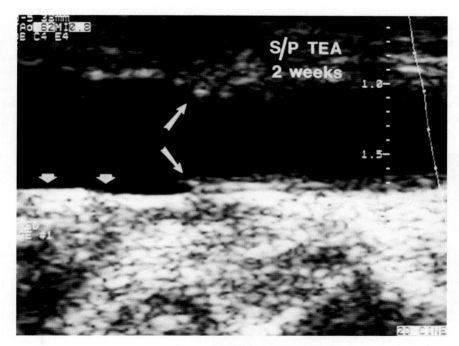

FIGURE 6.22. This picture was taken 2 weeks after carotid endarterectomy. The *large arrows* point to a suture on the anterior wall and the transected shelf on the posterior wall. The *shorter arrows* indicate the site of plaque removal.

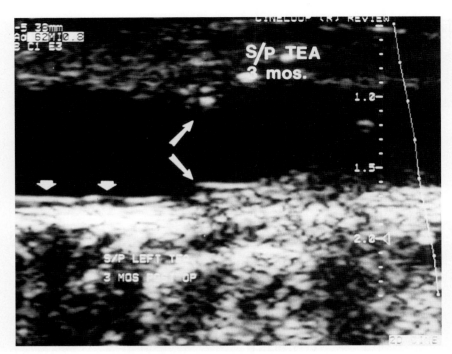

FIGURE 6.23. After 3 months, the segment of carotid artery shown in Fig. 6.22 now appears to have a *double line*, which suggests that the healing process is now complete. This image is similar to what one would observe from a normal carotid artery. The *double line* is thought to represent the total thickness of the intima and media.

2. It is also possible to use the proximal "shelf" at the point of plaque transection along with the sutures as sites to monitor the healing response. As shown in Figs. 6.22 and 6.23, in the interval of 2 weeks to 3 months, a "normal" double line has developed.

3. It is also possible to document the development and progression to myointimal hyperplasia as shown in Fig. 6.24. In this patient, the lesion was stable.

4. As is known, the myointimal hyperplastic response develops early (weeks to months) and is nearly always complete within the first 2 years (Figs. 6.25–6.27).

5. After 2 years, any changes that take place in the bulb can usually be ascribed to atherosclerosis (53). When this does occur, the clinical approach that one employs will depend entirely on the presenting complaints of the patient and the degree of narrowing (Fig. 6.28).

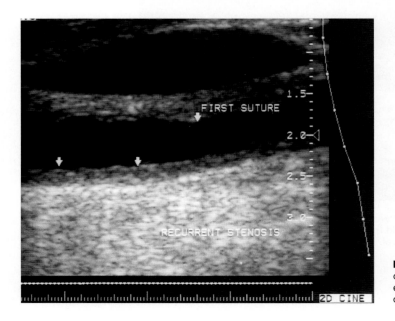

FIGURE 6.24. This figure illustrates a fully developed area of myointimal hyperplasia. The uniform pattern of the thickened area on the posterior wall (*small arrows*) should be contrasted to that shown in Fig. 6.23.

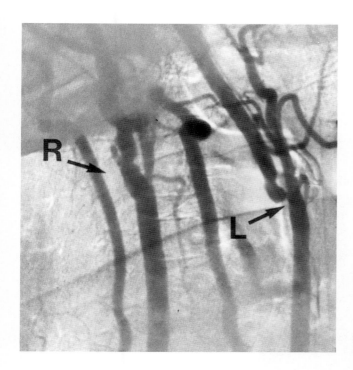

FIGURE 6.25. This patient with bilateral carotid bifurcation disease underwent staged endarterectomies.

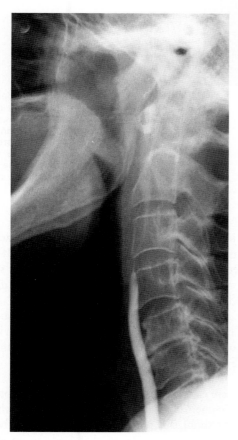

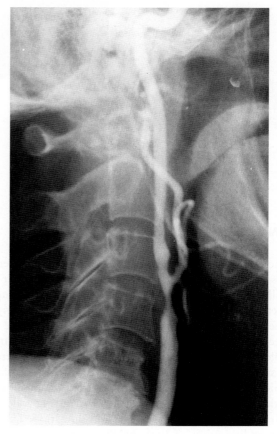

FIGURE 6.26. Six weeks after the left carotid endarterectomy was performed on the patient shown in Fig. 6.25, a recurrent, nearly total occlusion developed. The patient was asymptomatic.

FIGURE 6.27. On the right side, a recurrent stenosis developed within 6 weeks after endarterectomy. The preoperative view is shown in Fig. 6.25.

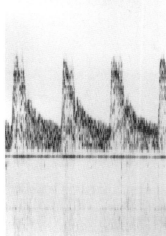

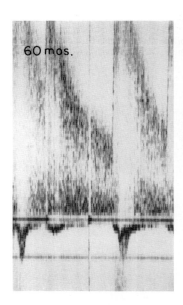

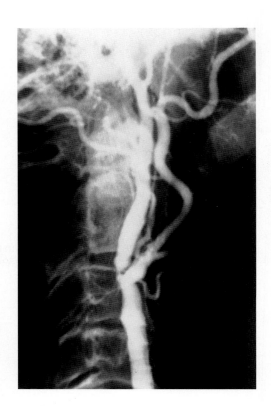

FIGURE 6.28. The spectra recorded at 48 months after endarterectomy were compatible with a borderline 50% stenosis of the internal carotid artery. By 60 months, the changes in the velocity patterns are of the type seen with a more than 80% stenosis. The arteriogram done at that time demonstrates recurrent atherosclerosis, which is found in its usual location.

LONG-TERM STUDIES

Although a major role for duplex scanning is screening patients with suspected extracranial arterial disease, it also fulfills an important role for the long-term follow-up of patients with the problem. A major deficit in nearly all aspects of arterial disease is the lack of quantitative and objective data on the fate of the lesions. For most clinical studies, the endpoints chosen are clinical, such as stroke, transient ischemic attacks, and death. In this type of epidemiologic study, there is no information obtained on the relationship between events that occur during follow-up and the status of the diseased carotid bifurcation. This was a major limitation of both NASCET and ECST (6,7). Duplex scanning should be used more frequently for studies such as following the rate of progression of the diseased

bifurcation. It will provide information on the fate of the lesion itself and its rate of change over time. If we are interested in the role of therapy, be it medical or surgical, this is a critically important question that must be answered.

How then can duplex scanning be used for such purposes? There are several questions for which we can begin to derive some answers that are unobtainable by any other means. Some of these are as follows:

1. Are there elements in the lesion itself that are predictive of outcome? It is obvious to all workers who have thought about this problem that there has to be something unique in the plaque that leads to an event. It might be the presence of ulceration, intraplaque hemorrhage, or the degree of stenosis (54–58).

2. Does the "activity" of a plaque in terms of its morphologic changes and the rate at which these occur bear any relevance to outcome? For example, if we can demonstrate progression of a lesion, does this mean that a poor outcome can be expected? One might guess that this is the case, but we do not have much in the way of hard evidence except for the case where the progression proceeds to a greater than 80% diameter-reducing stenosis. When this occurs, the risk for an ischemic event is very high (59).

3. Is it possible to document the role of various methods of intervention and their effects on disease progression, and, ultimately, on the outcome of the therapy, be it medical or surgical? I think this might be one of the best research applications for duplex scanning. For example, in the NASCET and ECST studies, the information on natural history of the plaques themselves is totally lacking because of the failure to use a comprehensive ultrasound program during the follow-up phases of the studies.

4. Is it possible to work out the optimal surveillance scheme that should be used for monitoring changes in the status of the disease and its effect on the production of clinical events? In 1995, we reported our long-term follow-up of 232 patients who were asymptomatic and with lesions that narrowed the carotid artery by less than 80% (60). Progression of disease was found in 23%, with nearly half progressing to a greater than 80% lesion. The cumulative stroke risk for patients with a less than 50% stenosis was 6%, and the risk for stroke was 11.8% in patients with a lesion in the 50% to 79% category. The follow-up extended to 10 years, with each patient being studied every 6 months.

Based on these studies, the following guidelines are suggested:

1. For a less than 50% stenosis, I don't believe that follow-up intervals of less than 1 year can be justified. The chance of an ischemic event is very low—approximately 3% per year.

2. For lesions that are in the range of 50% to 79%, I suggest a follow-up interval of 6 months. If progression is noted and the degree of stenosis reaches the 80% level, I recommend operation because these are dangerous lesions. The issue of carotid endarterectomy for the 60% stenosis remains controversial in spite of the clinical trial results.

If progression appears to be ongoing but not to the 80% level, I believe that repeat studies at 3-month intervals should be suggested.

THE ATHEROSCLEROTIC PLAQUE

As noted earlier, it is the morphology of the lesion itself that will ultimately determine its biologic behavior. In this regard, it is important to review the role of atherosclerotic lesions in the arteries supplying the brain, as contrasted with those supplying other organs in the body. Although it is clear that a diameter-reducing lesion sufficient to reduce pressure and flow is sufficient to produce symptoms in the legs, this is not true in the carotid and vertebral arteries. Indeed, it is common to find high-grade lesions in these vessels and yet have the patient remain entirely asymptomatic. How can this occur? Two major factors are at work. The first is the ability of the brain to autoregulate flow down to very low levels of perfusion pressure. Normally, this is in the range of a mean pressure of 50 mm Hg. Second, the ever-present circle of Willis may be able to compensate for a marked reduction of flow in one vessel and quickly accommodate by providing flow from another source through its communicating arteries.

What, then, are the mechanisms by which the brain gets into trouble with lesions of the extracranial arteries? First and most commonly accepted is the embolic theory, which states that, as a lesion loses its surface covering, platelets and other debris may accumulate in the denuded area to become embolic at some later time. The other and less recognized problem that can occur is the development of thrombosis in the region of the lesion. This has not been fully appreciated because of the infrequent study of patients over time to document the frequency of this occurrence and its relationship to the development of ischemic events. This is a common mechanism for the development of myocardial infarction and may be the most common mechanism for the development of occlusion of arteries in the leg at sites where atherosclerotic plaques develop.

Given this as a background, it is only natural that we should attempt to document the nature of the atherosclerotic plaque and attempt to classify it in terms of its ultrasonic characteristics. The role of ultrasound has been dictated, in large part, by the findings in the lesions themselves that appear to correlate with clinical events. The most obvious factor that has been associated with the development of embolic events is ulceration. What is an ulcerated area? Strictly speaking, it is an area with loss of the usual surface covering that exposes the underlying collagen and other materials, leaving a site for the accumulation of material such as platelets to form a "thrombus." The classic method of demonstrating this is arteriography, but, even here, the track record is not particularly impressive if the surgical specimen is considered to be the gold standard. As noted earlier, Edwards and colleagues (16) examined the accuracy of the arteriogram in predicting the presence of ulceration and found it to be correct about half the time. When ultrasound has been compared with arteriography and the surgical specimen, similar and disappointing results have been obtained. It is not accurate enough to state with any certainty that ulceration is either present or absent (54). It is our own view that imaging with both ultrasound and arteriography has such serious problems in this regard that they should be used only to describe the surface of the lesion as smooth or irregular.

Another factor that has been implicated in the course of events that may explain why patients suddenly become symptomatic is the presence of intraplaque hemorrhage. The theory is that the plaque will suddenly increase in size, which, in some cases, may actually lead to an intimal disruption, in turn leading to activation of the coagulation cascade with thrombosis (55,56)

How would intraplaque hemorrhage be seen ultrasonically, and what would its morphologic characteristics be? Before dealing with the specifics, it is important to define the types of lesions seen regularly when scanning is carried out. These lesions are basically of two types—the homogeneous and the heterogeneous. The former is, by definition, uniform in its echo character and has a smooth covering. This would be classified by a pathologist as the fibrous plaque and, although not known for certain, it appears to be the precursor of the complicated lesion responsible for most patients' symptoms. The heterogeneous lesion consists of different echo patterns within the lesion, the presence of calcium, and the loss of the smooth covering. This would be most consistent with the plaque described by pathologists as the complicated lesion (57).

Is this distinction important clinically? Several authors have used this approach and compared the scanning results not only with the specimen but with the clinical events as well. Reilly and associates (57) showed that the heterogeneous lesions accounted for 91% of the intraplaque hemorrhages and 100% of the ulcerated lesions. In 41 of 50 specimens (82%), ultrasound correctly identified the presence or absence of intraplaque hemorrhage. The false-positive studies occurred when there were large amounts of lipid or cholesterol in the lesion. Similar results were found by Bluth and colleagues (58) in their study of 50 patients who had the lesions examined. A rather surprising finding in this study was the poor correlation between the symptoms that occurred and the nature of the lesion. In the patients with heterogeneous plaques, 65% were symptomatic, as compared with 52% in the homogeneous group. Thus, it would not appear that such findings can be directly associated with the symptomatic status of the patient. Conversely, it would appear that, at present, ultrasound findings should not be used to predict the type of clinical events likely to occur.

We have struggled with this problem for the past several years. Although there is no doubt that we can demonstrate ultrasonic changes in a lesion, we cannot be sure of what these mean clinically. For example, in Fig. 6.29, a "hole" is clearly seen in a lesion. This patient had two episodes of amaurosis fugax. When this plaque was examined after removal, there was clearly an area of hemorrhage within the plaque that explained this hypolucent area. Unfortunately, other changes in the complex lesions can give rise to similar ultrasonic features. Areas of necrosis can give a similar pattern. Does it have similar clinical connotations? We do not have this answer at the present time.

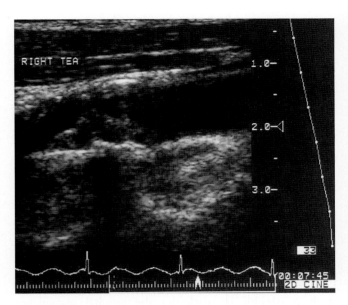

FIGURE 6.29. The B-mode image of this plaque clearly demonstrated a "hole" in the middle of the lesion. When this was examined histologically, it was found to be an area of hemorrhage.

PLAQUE MORPHOLOGY AND OUTCOME

The findings of the NASCET and ECST studies once again emphasize that some carotid bifurcation plaques are dangerous, whereas others appear to be rather benign (6,7). In the NASCET study, 23% of the symptomatic patients developed a completed stroke within the first 24 months of follow-up. However, it must be remembered that the remaining 77% of the patients with similar degrees of narrowing did *not* develop an ischemic event. This suggests that there was something other than the degree of narrowing alone that led to an event. This suggests that most of the plaques within this time frame remained stable, whereas those lesions that produced an event must have undergone some change that precipitated the stroke.

There have been many suggestions as to what these changes might be. They include the sudden development of intraplaque hemorrhage, with a resulting sudden increase in the size of the lesion (55–58). Another plausible reason is the loss of the protective fibrous cap, which would expose the underlying collagen and other materials to the flowing blood. An important question relates to whether ultrasound can detect these changes and thus provide a method of detecting the plaques that are the most dangerous.

In my laboratory, we have had a skeptical interest in such an idea. This was due largely to our belief that the reported studies were not rigorous enough to prove the point. In addition, a major flaw of such an approach is that to prove such findings, one would have to follow patients with such changes in a prospective fashion to assess outcome and its relationship to the observed changes in the plaques. This has not been done, and it is unlikely to be done given the current criteria for operation.

Nonetheless, we have embarked on a long-term study of plaque morphology that is based on extensive histologic studies to assess plaque content, volume, and distribution of materials within the lesion. By using modern imaging methods, it is possible to do a three-dimensional reconstruction from the histology done on plaques removed at the time of carotid endarterectomy. Once the plaque has been reconstructed, it would be possible to relate the changes seen on ultrasound to those observed within the plaque (60–62).

The results can be summarized as follows:

1. Ultrasonically, it is impossible at present to distinguish between hemorrhage or necrosis and lipid.
2. There was no relationship between the volume of lipid, necrosis or hemorrhage, or fibrous tissue and clinical status.
3. It is not possible using ultrasound to characterize the integrity of the fibrous cap.
4. Magnetic resonance imaging may be more likely to help confirm the status of the fibrous cap.

There is general agreement that it is the fibrous cap that holds the key to the development of ischemic events.

RESULTS OF FOLLOW-UP STUDIES

One of the major advantages of duplex scanning is its potential for providing natural history data on the results of therapy, be they medical or surgical. One of the major defects of all the clinical trials to examine the clinical outcome of atherosclerosis is that they have examined outcome only, without regard to the changes in the lesions that may have led to the event. For example, if one were to enter a trial, be it medical or surgical, and the only endpoints chosen were transient ischemic attacks and strokes, one would never know whether the lesion responsible had remained stable, had undergone degeneration, or had progressed to total occlusion. With the availability of duplex scanning, many of these questions can now be answered.

What information is available and with what confidence can we trust it? The most certain information at the moment is the degree of stenosis and its change over time. We know from the validation studies reported previously that the positive predictive value, particularly for lesions that exceed a 50% diameter reduction, is 90% or greater. In addition, for follow-up studies for which repeat information is available, we have confidence in the findings from one visit to another and whether an apparent change persists with additional studies.

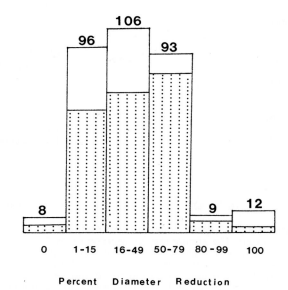

FIGURE 6.30. Distribution of disease in the asymptomatic patients with cervical bruits at the time they entered the follow-up study. (From Roederer GO, Langlois YE, Jager KA, et al. The natural history of carotid arterial disease in asymptomatic patients with cervical bruits. *Stroke* 1984;15:605–613, with permission.)

Our own natural history studies were first initiated in the asymptomatic patients with cervical bruits. Because these patients' risk for ischemic events was unknown, it was legitimate to ask the question as to which lesions were potentially dangerous and which ones would be safe to follow. A prospective study was initiated in 1980, which included 167 patients (63).

In this group, the distribution of the disease at the time of entering the study is shown in Fig. 6.30. As is noted, there were 93 sides with a 50% to 79% stenosis, 9 with an 80% to 99% stenosis, and 12 with total occlusion. The remaining sides were less than 50% in terms of diameter reduction. The annual event rate for the entire group was only 4% per year (transient ischemic attacks and strokes). The rate of progression from a less than 50% to a greater than 50% stenosis was 8% per year. More than 60% of the sides showed some evidence of progression (Fig. 6.31).

The striking finding in this study was the relationships among the degree of narrowing, progression of disease, and outcome. As noted in Table 6.3, the most important finding was the relationship between the presence of an 80% to 99% stenosis and progression to this level. As noted, only 4 of the 262 sides with a less than 80% stenosis had an event, as compared with 12 of the 25 sides with a greater than 80% stenosis ($p < 0.00001$).

The patterns of progression were of interest and bear some relevance to the type of follow-up schedule one might use for sequential studies in such patients. Two examples are indicative of the rate at which it can occur and the uncertainty that one is faced with in dealing with this disease. Figure 6.32 shows the findings from a patient who under-

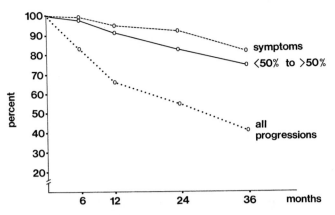

FIGURE 6.31. Life-table analysis of asymptomatic patients with cervical bruits. The annual rate of symptoms was 4%. For progression to a more than 50% stenosis, it was 8% per year. During the 3-year follow-up, 60% of the patients showed some progression. (From Roederer GO, Langlois YE, Jager KA, et al. The natural history of carotid arterial disease in asymptomatic patients with cervical bruits. *Stroke* 1984;15:605–613, with permission.)

TABLE 6.3. RELATIONSHIP BETWEEN PROGRESSION BEYOND THE 80% STENOSIS RANGE AND OUTCOME

Clinical state	Stenosis category on follow-up	
	<80%	>80%
No complication	258	13
TIA[a] only	1	4
TIA with occlusion	0	1
TIA followed by stroke and occlusion	0	1
Stroke with occlusion	0	3
Asymptomatic occlusion	3	3
Total complications	4	12

[a]TIA, transient ischemic attack.

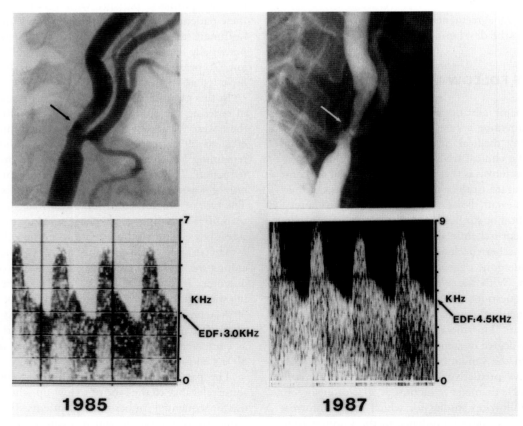

FIGURE 6.32. At the time of the original study in 1985, the end-diastolic frequency *(EDF)* was 3.5 kHz. Within the next 2 years, it increased to 4.5 kHz. The repeat arteriogram demonstrated the progression of the lesion associated with the change.

went a carotid endarterectomy on the right in 1985. During follow-up, the contralateral carotid artery remained stable for 1 year but then progressed rather rapidly to approach the 80% stenosis range. No apparent cause for this change was evident in any factors we could elucidate.

In some cases, the disease may remain stable for years but then suddenly change for no apparent reason. This is illustrated in Figs. 6.33 and 6.34, of a patient whose follow-up spanned a 10-year period. This gentleman remained stable for 10 years and then suddenly progressed on both sides to a greater than 80% stenosis. The arteriograms taken at the time of entry into the study and at the time of progression are shown.

Because the greater than 80% stenoses appeared to be related to subsequent ischemic events, we began to treat these lesions more aggressively and offer operations to those patients who appeared fit enough to have the procedure. During a 4-year period, we were able to identify 129 asymptomatic high-grade lesions in 115 patients. In this group, there were 56 sides that underwent operation, with 73 lesions treated nonoperatively (63). The results of this study confirmed the potentially dangerous nature of these lesions when not removed. The results can be summarized as follows.

To document the natural history of the entire gamut of asymptomatic patients with carotid disease, we studied a total of 232 patients who were found to have carotid disease by duplex scanning but had no previous surgery (63). These patients (136 men and 96 women) were seen at 6 months, at 1 year, and yearly thereafter. The total follow-up time was 10 years with enough follow-up data for a 7-year life table analysis. To qualify, the patients had to have mild (less than 50% stenosis) or moderate degrees of narrowing (50% to 79% stenosis). Progression to a higher degree of stenosis was seen in 23% of patients, with nearly half of these progressing to either a greater than 80% lesion or total occlusion. The risk for progression to the high-grade stenosis or occlusion was greatest in those with the moderate degree of narrowing at the time of entry. The cumulative stroke risk with mild stenosis was 6% increasing to 11% with those in the moderate category. In this group, carotid endarterectomy was performed in 27 patients. In 13 patients, the indication was an ischemic event ipsilateral to the stenosis, and in 14 patients, it was an asymptomatic progression to a high-grade (greater than 80%) stenosis.

In the patients who had endarterectomy, the perioperative stroke rate was 1.8%, and there were no in-hospital deaths. There were no immediate or long-term occlusions. In the nonoperated patients, nine strokes and 14 transient ischemic events occurred, with most developing within 6 months of discovery of the lesion. There were five internal carotid arteries that became occluded in the nine patients who developed a stroke. In the 14 patients who developed transient events, 3 of these events were associated with the occurrence of a total occlusion. Although this study was not

randomized, it clearly highlights the value of duplex scanning as a method of sequential follow-up to document outcome as related to the lesion of interest. There are no other methods that can do this.

Another area where serial duplex scanning has had an impact is in our understanding of the long-term outcome after carotid endarterectomy and the problems that may occur. We have examined this problem from two standpoints—first, with regard to the rate of occlusion of the internal carotid artery; second, with regard to the issue of myointimal hyperplasia, which is a common cause of early restenosis. In 200 patients whom we had the opportunity of monitoring for a mean follow-up period of 30 months, the occlusion rate was 2.5%. There was only one perioperative occlusion, with the others being detected months to years after the procedure (51).

The problems with regard to restenosis after operation became evident only with the availability of duplex scanning. Although it was known that symptomatic recurrences were in the range of 5% or less, the actual rate of restenosis and its time frame and outcome were not known (53).

We have investigated this problem in phases. Our initial report on the subject showed that early restenosis was not uncommon and occurred in 19% of sides. These were defined as lesions that reduced the artery diameter by greater than 50%. In some cases, the lesion appeared to regress. In a later study with longer follow-up, we were again able to document the benign nature of the lesion. For reasons that are not well understood, the lesion remained smooth and rarely progressed to a total occlusion. For this reason, we feel it is important simply to follow these lesions and not be aggressive in their management (52,53).

An example of the myointimal hyperplasia and the rapidity with which it can occur is shown in Figs. 6.25–6.27.

Carotid Endarterectomy without Arteriography

Given what appears to be the accuracy of well-performed duplex scanning, why not consider this as the only testing procedure that needs to be done before operation (64–67)? Before this can even be considered, we must satisfy ourselves that the following questions have been satisfactorily answered:

1. Is the accuracy of our testing comparable to that obtained by arteriography? The only way to determine this is to compare the two modalities in a blinded fashion. Not all laboratories can or should try this until they have a quality control program in place that monitors their performance against arteriography before considering this approach.
2. Can carotid endarterectomy and its associated costs and risks be eliminated without losing vital clinical information? As noted earlier, we don't believe that lesions of the carotid siphon play an important role in the etiology of ischemic events; therefore, our inability to study these by

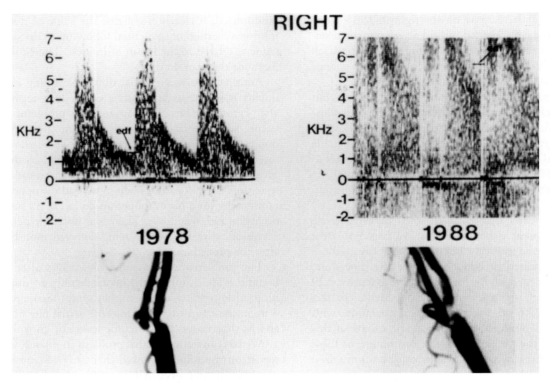

FIGURE 6.33. This illustrates the change in the velocity pattern from the right internal carotid artery. This patient had remained stable for 10 years before progressing to more than 80% stenosis.

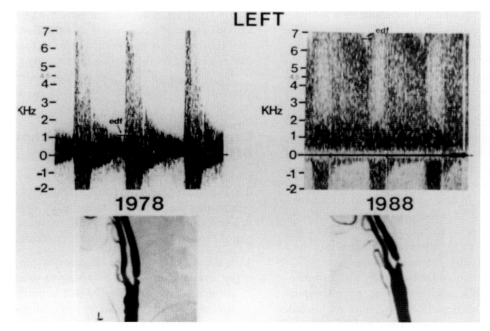

FIGURE 6.34. These are the spectral and arteriographic changes in the left internal carotid artery from the patient shown in Fig. 6.33. This side also remained stable for 10 years before suddenly progressing to more than 80% stenosis.

duplex scanning would not appear to be a serious problem (45). On the other hand, the availability of TCD may give us this information.

If we assume that 150,000 carotid arteriograms are done annually, the following outcomes might be expected (68,69):

1. About 7,500 transient neurological events would take place.
2. About 1,500 permanent neurologic deficits would result.
3. There might be 100 deaths, most of which would be stroke related.
4. If $3,000 is taken as the average cost for arteriography, the total cost of arteriography alone would be $750 million dollars. This does not take into account the cost of the complications and deaths listed in 1, 2, and 3.
5. If the patients had duplex alone, the total cost would be in the range of $37.5 million.

To investigate the feasibility of such an approach, we prospectively asked members of the vascular section to record their management plan after reviewing the results of a duplex scan. Of the 111 consecutive patients, the therapeutic plan was recorded before arteriography being performed. In these 111 patients, the duplex scan was diagnostic in 88 (95%). In those cases with discrepancies, the following was noted:

1. The disease was not limited to the distal common carotid artery or bifurcation in four patients.
2. It was not possible to obtain satisfactory Doppler signals to estimate the degree of stenosis in one patient.
3. An internal carotid occlusion could not be distinguished from a high-grade stenosis in two patients.

When a technically adequate duplex scan was obtained, arteriography contributed information that might have affected management in only one case. This patient had a middle cerebral artery occlusion distal to a high-grade carotid bifurcation stenosis. However, even in this case, it is likely that carotid endarterectomy would have been done even if that information had been available before the operation. Based on these data, we perform endarterectomy in more than 90% of our cases without the need for arteriography. We are satisfied with this approach and see no need to change (70).

INTERNAL CAROTID ARTERY DISSECTION

Dissections of the internal carotid artery can occur secondary to trauma or be entirely spontaneous. Although the arterial pathology with a tear in the intima may be similar in the two varieties, the clinical outcome is often very different. A stroke related to the dissection is much more common in the traumatic type. The spontaneous dissections appear to be more common in young to middle-aged women and may in many cases be related to underlying fibromuscular disease. Classically, when the dissection develops, the patient will have a severe unilateral headache, which may be accompanied by the appearance of Horner's syndrome. The dissection nearly always involves the middle to distal internal carotid artery. In some cases, the artery may become totally occluded, but it will in most cases reopen as the blood in the dissected channel is resorbed. By B-mode imaging, it is possible to identify the two channels and note the absence of flow or very low flow in the false channel. In most cases, this improves over time, so that ultrasound can be used to follow the progress of the process.

Therapy is conservative, using warfarin sodium (Coumadin) until it becomes clear that the lesion has stabilized or improved. However, in a few cases, there may be repeated dissections that become a serious problem. To illustrate this, we saw a 48-year-old woman with a 25-year history of hypertension. She experienced her first carotid dissection in 1991, at which time it was also noted that she had fibromuscular dysplasia of her renal arteries. Her carotid dissections continued to occur, and she developed a false aneurysm at the base of the skull. With each dissection, the patient developed severe headache and transient neurologic events, which cleared. Because of the ongoing dissections and the presence of the false aneurysm, it was elected to have this bypassed by an extracranial to intracranial bypass graft, which was done in 1993. She recovered from this procedure and has been studied in our laboratory since to document the status of the bypass graft and to monitor the fibromuscular dysplasia (FMD) involvement of one renal artery. At the time of her last follow-up study done in April 1999, the bypass graft remained patent with normal middle cerebral artery velocities on that side. The patient does have a moderate stenosis at the origin of the bypass, but that remains stable, and she is free of symptoms.

THE FUTURE

Given that duplex scanning is the preferred method of screening for carotid artery disease, how long will this be the case, and are there any serious competitors that might change this picture? At the moment, the only possible alternative as a totally noninvasive test is magnetic resonance arteriography (MRA). This modality has the potential of providing diagnostic information from the level of the aortic arch to the intracranial circulation and at no risk (71). This could be the only test that is required. It may also have the potential for providing data on flow parameters such as velocity and volume flow. However, there are serious drawbacks that may not be resolved over the next several years. These are as follows:

1. The technology is expensive and even after purchase requires sophisticated maintenance.
2. There will only be a limited number of systems available, even in first-rate facilities. This means that the sys-

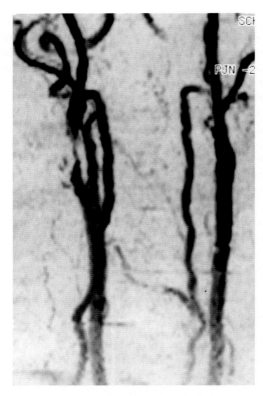

FIGURE 6.35. This magnetic resonance arteriogram clearly demonstrates a tight stenosis of the internal carotid artery.

tems will have to be used for other purposes as well. This will limit their availability for vascular studies.

3. This is not a test that is ideal for follow-up because of facts listed previously.
4. Because of the nature of the test, many patients cannot be studied, including not only patients with metal in their bodies but also patients who are claustrophobic.
5. Problems remain with regard to resolution that will need to be addressed and worked out before this method can be accepted as the only test needed for therapeutic decision making.

Although I agree that the technology continues to evolve, it is my view that MRA at present has too many problems to put it in the same category as contrast arteriography.

1. In some cases, the MRA studies are good enough to demonstrate clearly an area of stenosis (Fig. 6.35).
2. In other cases, the resolution in the presence of turbulence may lead to signal dropout, which can mimic total

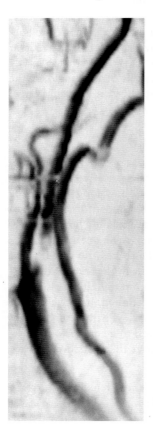

FIGURE 6.36. In this magnetic resonance arteriogram, there is signal dropout, which occurred secondary to turbulence. In some cases, this could suggest that a total occlusion is present and pose a serious problem.

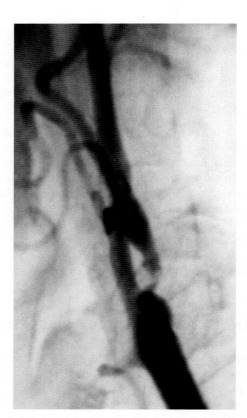

FIGURE 6.37. This is the contrast arteriogram that corresponds to the lesion seen by magnetic resonance imaging and shown in Fig. 6.36.

occlusion (Fig. 6.36). The corresponding contrast arteriogram is shown in Fig. 6.37.

If MRA reaches the level of contrast studies, it will be able to complement but not replace duplex studies for the evaluation of carotid artery disease.

INTRAOPERATIVE STUDIES

It has become increasingly clear that some of the studies done before operation can also be brought to the operating room to assist the surgeon in performing the operation and confirming the results. The technique, along with our findings, will be covered later, but in brief these are some of the problems and perhaps indication of the solution.

Transcranial Doppler

There are two problems in the operating room that have always been a source of debate and considerable confusion. The first is whether or not to use a shunt during the procedure to provide cerebral protection. The surgical community is sharply divided on this issue, with very little evidence that one practice is better than the other in terms of stroke prevention. There appears to be an element of truth on both sides—in other words, some patients will benefit from a shunt, whereas others will not. The question has always been, how do we identify those patients who need to be shunted? There have been two ways to do this. The first is to measure the stump pressure, and the second is electroencephalogram monitoring. There is no information available that will concretely tell the surgeon which to use and how. In fact, all of this debate boils down to surgeon's preference.

Transcranial Doppler has brought a new dimension to the field because we now can monitor flow in the middle cerebral artery and document the presence of emboli during the procedure. The value of this procedure has been documented by Ackerstaff and colleagues (72–74). It is clear based on their excellent studies that the development of emboli during and after the operation can adversely affect outcome. It is on the basis of these studies that we have instituted this practice at the University of Washington.

Evaluation of the Carotid Artery at the Time of Operation

If a carotid endarterectomy is well done without problems, the bulb area should be clean of any debris, and the distal endpoint should be free of a stenosis. With the duplex scan done in the operating room, these questions can be answered. The method of doing this is covered in some detail in Chapter 14 along with examples of how useful it appears to be.

REFERENCES

1. Pokras R, Dyken ML. Dramatic changes in the performance of endarterectomy for diseases of the extracranial arteries of the head. *Stroke* 1988;10:1289–1290.
2. Easton JR, Sherman DG. Stroke and mortality in carotid endarterectomy: 228 consecutive operations. *Stroke* 1977;8: 565–568.
3. Barnett HJM, Plum F, Walton JN. Carotid endarterectomy: an expression of concern. *Stroke* 1984;15:941–943.
4. Chambers BR, Norris JW. The case against surgery for asymptomatic carotid stenosis. *Stroke* 1984;15:964–967.
5. Matchar DB, Goldstein LP, McCrory DC, et al. *Carotid endarterectomy: A literature review and ratings of appropriateness and necessity.* Rand Corp., ISBN:0-8330-1246-0, 1992.
6. Barnett HJ, Taylor DW, Eliasziw M, et al. Benefit of carotid endarterectomy in patients with symptomatic moderate or severe stenosis. North American Symptomatic Carotid Endarterectomy Trial Collaborators [see Comments]. *N Engl J Med* 1998;339: 1415–1425.
7. Farrell B, Fraser A, Sandercock P, et al. Randomised trial of endarterectomy for recently symptomatic carotid stenosis: final results of the MRC European Surgery Trial (ECST) *Lancet* 1998; 35:1379–1381.
8. Executive Committee of the Asymptomatic Carotid Atherosclerosis Study. Endarterectomy for asymptomatic carotid artery stenosis. *JAMA* 1995;273:1421–1428.
9. Barnes RW, Russell HE, Bone GE, et al. Doppler cerebrovascular examination: improved results with refinements of technique. *Stroke* 1977;8:468–471.
10. Gee W, Mehigan JT, Wylie EJ. Measurement of collateral cerebral hemispheric blood pressure by ocular pneumoplethysmography. *Am J Surg* 1975;130:121–127.
11. Gee WG. Ocular pneumoplethysmography: diagnostic and surgical techniques. *Surv Ophthalmol* 1985;29:276–292.
12. Mistretta CA, Crummy AB. Diagnosis of cardiovascular disease by digital subtraction angiography. *Science* 1981;214:761–765.
13. Chikos PM, Fisher LD, Hirsch JH, et al. Observer variability in evaluating extra-cranial carotid artery stenosis. *Stroke* 1983;14: 885–892.
14. Houser OW, Thorale M, Sundt T, et al. Atheromatous disease of the carotid artery: correlation of angiographic, clinical and surgical findings. *J Neurosurg* 1974;41:321–331.
15. Moore WS, Hall AD. Ulcerated atheroma of the carotid artery: a cause of transient cerebral ischemia. *Am J Surg* 1968;116: 237–242.
16. Edwards JH, Krichell II, Riles T, Imparato A. Angiographically undetected ulceration of the carotid bifurcation as a cause of embolic stroke. *Radiology* 1979;132:369–373.
17. Fell G, Breslau P, Knox RA, et al. Importance of noninvasive ultrasonic Doppler testing in the evaluation of patients' asymptomatic carotid bruits. *Am Heart J* 1981;102:221–226.
18. Chambers BR, Norris JW. Outcome in patients with asymptomatic neck bruits. *N Engl J Med* 1986;315: 860–865.
19. Reul GH, Morris GC, Howell JF, et al. Current concepts in coronary artery surgery. *Ann Thorac Surg* 1972;14:243–259.
20. Hertzer NR, Loop FD, Taylor PC, et al. Staged and combined surgical approach to simultaneous carotid and coronary vascular disease. *Surgery* 1978;84:803–811.
21. Breslau PJ, Fell G, Ivey TD, et al. Carotid arterial disease in patients undergoing coronary artery bypass operations. *J Thorac Cardiovasc Surg* 1981;82:765–767.
22. Ivey TD, Strandness DE Jr, Williams DB, et al. Management of patients with carotid bruit undergoing cardiopulmonary bypass. *J Thorac Cardiovasc Surg* 1984;87:183–189.

23. Barnes RW, Marszalek PB, Rittgers SE. Asymptomatic carotid disease in preoperative patients. *Stroke* 1980;2:1361(abst).

24. Turnipseed WD, Berkoff MA, Belzer FO. Postoperative stroke in cardiac and peripheral vascular disease. *Ann Surg* 1980;192: 365–368.

25. Reivich M, Hollins HE, Roberts B, et al. Reversal of blood flow through the vertebral artery and its effects on cerebral circulation. *N Engl J Med* 1961;265:878–885.

26. Bornstein NM, Norris JW. Subclavian steal: a harmless hemodynamic phenomenon. *Lancet* 1986;2:303–305.

27. Grosveld WJHM, Lawson JA, Eikelboom BC, et al. Clinical and hemodynamic significance of innominate artery lesions evaluated by ultrasonography and digital angiography. *Stroke* 1988;19: 958–962.

28. Ackerstaff RGA, Grosveld WJHM, Eikelboom BC, et al. Ultrasonic duplex scanning of prevertebral segment of the vertebral artery in patients with cerebral atherosclerosis. *Eur J Vasc Surg* 1988;2:387–393.

29. Phillips DJ, Beach KW, Primozich J, et al. Should results of ultrasound Doppler studies be reported in units of frequency or velocity? *Ultrasound Med Biol* 1989;15:205–212.

30. Langlois YE, Roederer GO, Strandness DE Jr. Ultrasonic evaluation of the carotid bifurcation. *Echocardiography* 1987;4: 141–159.

31. Roederer GO, Langlois YE, Jager K, et al. The natural history of carotid arterial disease in asymptomatic patients with cervical bruits. *Stroke* 1984;15:605–613.

32. Phillips DJ, Greene FM Jr, Langlois YE, et al. Flow velocity patterns in the carotid bifurcation of young, presumed normal subjects. *Ultrasound Med Biol* 1983;9:33–49.

33. Nicholls SC, Phillips DJ, Primozich J, et al. Diagnostic significance of flow separation in the carotid bulb. *Stroke* 1989;20: 175–182.

34. Roederer GO, Langlois YE, Jager KA, et al. A simple spectral parameter for accurate classification of severe carotid artery disease. *Bruit* 1989;3:174–178.

35. Knox RA, Greene FM, Beach KW, et al. Computer-based classification of carotid arterial disease: a prospective assessment. *Stroke* 1982;13:589–594.

36. Langlois YE, Greene F, Roederer GO, et al. Computer-based pattern recognition of carotid artery Doppler signals for disease classification: a prospective validation. *Ultrasound Med Biol* 1984;10: 581–595.

37. Roederer GO, Langlois YE, Strandness DE Jr. Cerebral arterial flow and cerebral vascular insufficiency. In: Condon RE, DeCosse J, eds. *Surgical care II.* Philadelphia: Lea & Febiger, 1985:199–234.

38. Cato FR, Bandyk DL, Livigni D, et al. Carotid collateral circulation decreases the accuracy of duplex scanning. *Bruit* 1986;10: 68–73.

39. Fujitani RM, Mills JL, Wang LM, et al. The effect of unilateral internal carotid artery occlusion upon contralateral duplex study criteria for accurate interpretation. *J Vasc Surg* 1992;16:459–468.

40. Blackshear WM Jr, Phillips DJ, Chikos PM, et al. Carotid artery velocity patterns in normal and stenotic vessels. *Stroke* 1980;11:67–71.

41. Knox RA, Breslau PJ, Strandness DE Jr. A simple parameter for the detection of severe carotid disease. *Br J Surg* 1982;69: 230–233.

42. Moneta GL, Edwards JM, Chitwood RW, et al. Correlation of North American Symptomatic Carotid Endarterectomy Trial (NASCET) angiographic definition of 70%–99% internal carotid stenosis with duplex scanning. *J Vasc Surg* 1992;17: 152–160.

43. Moneta GL, Taylor DC, Zierler RE, et al. Asymptomatic high-grade internal cartoid artery stenosis: is stratification according to

44. Moneta GL, Edwards JM, Papanicolaou G, et al. Screening for asymptomatic internal carotid artery stenosis: duplex criteria for discriminating 60–90% stenosis. *J Vasc Surg* 1995;21: 989–994.

45. Roederer GO, Langlois YE, Chan ARW, et al. Is siphon disease important in predicting outcome after carotid endarterectomy? *Arch Surg* 1983;118:1177–1181.

46. Thiele BL, Young JV, Chikos PM, et al. Correlation of arteriographic findings and symptoms in cerebrovascular disease. *Neurology* 1980;30:1041–1046.

47. Spencer MP. Intracranial carotid artery diagnosis with transorbital pulsed wave (PW) and continuous wave (CW) Doppler ultrasound. *J Ultrasound Med* 1983;2(10 Suppl 2):61(abst #912).

48. Niederkorn K, Neumayer K. Transcranial Doppler sonography: a new approach in the non-invasive diagnosis of intracranial brain artery disease. *Eur Neurol* 1987;26:65–68.

49. Kirkham FJ, Neville BGR, Levin SD. Bedside diagnosis of stenosis of the middle cerebral artery [Letter]. *Lancet* 1986;1:797–798.

50. Hennerici M, Rautenberg W, Schwartz A. Transcranial ultrasound for the assessment of intracranial arterial flow velocity. II. *Surg Neurol* 1987;27:523–532.

51. Healy DA, Clowes AW, Zierler RE, et al. Immediate and long-term results of carotid endarterectomy. *Stroke* 1989;20: 1138–1142.

52. Roederer GO, Langlois YE, Chan ATW, et al. Post-endarterectomy carotid ultrasonic duplex scanning. *Ultrasonic Med Biol* 1983;9:73–78.

53. Nicholls SC, Phillips DJ, Bergelin RO, et al. Carotid endarterectomy: relationship of outcome to early restenosis. *J Vasc Surg* 1985;2:375–381.

54. Katz ML, Johnson M, Pomajzl MJ. The sensitivity of real-time B-mode carotid imaging in the detection of ulcerated plaques. *Bruit* 1983;8:13–16.

55. Imparato A, Riles T, Mintzer R, et al. The importance of hemorrhage in the relationship between gross morphologic characteristics and cerebral symptoms in 376 carotid plaques. *Ann Surg* 1983;197:195–203.

56. Lusby R, Ferrell L, Ehrenfeld W, et al. Carotid plaque hemorrhage: its role in production of cerebral ischemia. *Arch Surg* 1982;117:1479–1488.

57. Reilly LM, Lusby RJ, Hughes L, et al. Carotid plaque histology using real-time ultrasonography. *Am J Surg* 1983;146:188–193.

58. Bluth EI, Kay D, Merritt CRB, et al. Sonographic characterization of carotid plaque: detection of hemorrhage. *Am J Roentgenol* 1986;146:1061–1065.

59. Moneta GL, Taylor DC, Nicholls SC, et al. Operative versus nonoperative management of asymptomatic high-grade internal carotid artery stenosis: improved results with endarterectomy. *Stroke* 1987;18:1005–1010.

60. Hatsukami TS, Ferguson MS, Beach KW, et al. Carotid plaque morphology and clinical events. *Stroke* 1997;28:95–100.

61. Hatsukami TS, Thackray BD, Primozich JF, et al. Echolucent regions in carotid plaque: preliminary analysis comparing three-dimensional histologic reconstructions to sonographic findings. *Ultrasound Med Biol* 1994;20:743–749.

62. Roederer GO, Langlois YE, Jager KA, et al. The natural history of carotid arterial disease in asymptomatic patients with cervical bruits. *Stroke* 1984;15:605–613.

63. Johnson BF, Verlato F, Bergelin RO, et al. Clinical outcome in patients with mild and moderate carotid stenosis. *J Vasc Surg* 1995;21:120–126.

64. Dawson DL, Zierler RE, Kohler TR. Role of arteriography in the prospective evaluation of carotid artery disease. *Am J Surg* 1991;161:619–624.

65. Flanigan DP, Schuler JJ, Vogel M, et al. The role of duplex scanning in surgical decision making. *J Vasc Surg* 1985;1:15–25.
66. Moore WS, Ziomek S, Quininones-Baldrich WJ, et al. Can clinical evaluation and noninvasive testing substitute for arteriography in the evaluation of carotid artery disease. *Ann Surg* 1988; 208:91–94.
67. Ricotta JJ, Holen J, Schenk E, et al. Is routine arteriography necessary prior to carotid endarterectomy? *J Vasc Surg* 1984;1:96: 96–102.
68. Mani RL, Eisenberg RL, McDonald EJ Jr, et al. Complications of catheter cerebral arteriography: analysis of 5,000 procedures. I. Criteria and incidence. *Am J Roentgenol* 1978;131: 861–865.
69. Earnest F, Forbes G, Sandok BA. Complications of cerebral arteriography: prospective assessment of risk. *Am J Roentgenol* 1984; 142:247–253.
70. Dawson DL, Zierler RE, Strandness DE Jr, et al. The role of duplex scanning and arteriography before endarterectomy: a prospective study. *J Vasc Surg* 1993;18:673–683.
71. Riles TS, Eidelman EM, Litt AW. Comparison of magnetic resonance arteriography, conventional arteriography and duplex scanning. *Stroke* 1992;23:341–346.
72. Ackerstaff RGA, Jansen C, Moll FL. Carotid endarterectomy and intraoperative emboli detection: correlation of clinical, transcranial Doppler, and magnetic resonance findings. *Echocardiogr J Cardiovasc Ultrasound Allied Tech* 1996;13:543–550.
73. Ackerstaff RGA, Jansen C, Moll FL, et al. Regarding "The significance of microemboli detection by means of transcranial Doppler ultrasonography monitoring in carotid endarterectomy" [Reply]. *J Vasc Surg* 1996;23:735–736.
74. Ackerstaff RGA, Jansen C, Moll FC, et al. The significance of microemboli detection by means of transcranial Doppler ultrasonography monitoring in carotid endarterectomy. *J Vasc Surg* 1995;21:963–969.

7

PERIPHERAL ARTERIAL SYSTEM

As reviewed in Chapter 2, patients with either acute or chronic arterial occlusion should have been evaluated by a complete history, physical examination, and measurement of the ankle/brachial index before they are considered candidates for duplex scanning (1). It is neither reasonable nor feasible to scan all patients with arterial occlusive disease *unless* some form of direct intervention is being planned. At the present time, we consider the indications for duplex scanning to be essentially the same as for arteriography. When an increase in blood flow is needed, the types of intervention that can be carried out include transluminal angioplasty and direct arterial surgery.

Although the field continues to evolve, transluminal angioplasty has been most successful in the treatment of stenotic lesions in the aortoiliac segment. There is no doubt that total occlusion involving these arteries can also be treated by balloon angioplasty; however, it has been our practice to confine this procedure primarily to stenotic lesions alone. With the recent addition of newer methods of endovascular therapy, there has been interest in extending the indications to occlusions in the femoropopliteal segment and the arteries below the knee. The results in this area, except for very short lesions of less than 3 cm, have been very disappointing. Whether this effort will be successful in extending the procedure to a larger group of patients remains to be determined.

Direct arterial surgery can be used to revascularize the limb from the level of the aorta to the small arteries at the level of the ankle. Thus, in evaluating patients for these operations, we must supply all the data necessary to plan the appropriate procedures. This will require information that is essentially equivalent or superior to that obtained by arteriography in order to be useful.

As noted in Chapter 2, patients with acute arterial occlusions should not, in general, be considered candidates for duplex scanning unless the limb is clearly viable and time is not of importance in preserving limb viability. Any delays in revascularizing a limb can have disastrous consequences when its blood supply is not sufficient to perfuse the tissues of the distal limb. However, in a hospital setting where an acute arterial occlusion might occur secondary to place-

ment of a balloon pump, bedside duplex scanning can be of great help.

IMPORTANT INFORMATION BEFORE SCANNING

For patients with chronic limb ischemia, it is important to separate the clinical presentation into the following categories at the time the patients are first seen:

1. Patients with intermittent claudication constitute the largest number with atherosclerosis of the limb arteries. It is important to determine whether the problem limits the lifestyle of the patient or is simply a nuisance. For the latter group, it is not necessary to proceed beyond the standard workup because interventional therapy is rarely indicated. These patients should simply be followed, with repeat measurement of the ankle/brachial index to document the status of their disease (2). For patients with severe claudication, the initial evaluation is helpful in defining the level and extent of the arterial occlusive disease. The following information is helpful:

   a. If the patient has an ankle/arm index of more than 0.50, it is likely that he or she has single-segment disease either at the aortoiliac or femoropopliteal level. If the femoral pulse is absent, it is likely to signify that proximal disease is present. If a pulse is palpable, but there is a bruit heard over the iliac artery, then the possibility of a stenotic lesion must be entertained. A normal femoral pulse without bruits being heard at that level, in combination with an absent popliteal pulse, is suggestive of femoropopliteal disease.

   b. When the ankle/arm index is less than 0.50, the likelihood of multisegment disease must be considered. When all pulses in the limb are absent, it is likely that the patient has both aortoiliac and superficial femoral artery involvement. This is a common combination.

2. Most patients with limb-threatening ischemia have multisegment disease and an ankle/arm index of less than 0.50. The one exception to this is patients who present with

the sudden onset of rest pain in the digits and forefoot but who have normal peripheral pulses and an ankle/arm index that may even be in the normal range. Here, it is likely that the patient has microemboli to the foot from an ulcerated plaque in the arterial supply at some point proximal to the foot level.

With an increase in our aging population, there is an increase not only in the prevalence of arterial disease but also in other conditions that might lead to exercise-induced leg pain. These generally center on the common patient who has neurospinal disease secondary to degenerative joint problems. This can lead to pain with ambulation that might be confused with true intermittent claudication. With these patients, the walk-pain-rest cycle is not constant from day to day. In addition, these patients may need to sit down or lie down for relief of their pain. The other, much less common problem is seen in patients who have venous claudication. This can develop when the patient has an episode of deep venous thrombosis and is left with chronic venous obstruction, which is usually in the iliofemoral venous segment. When these patients exercise vigorously, they develop a bursting pain in the thigh that can be relieved only by cessation of exercise and elevation of the limb.

When the cause of the leg pain is in question on the basis of the history, physical examination, and preliminary measurement of the ankle/arm index, it is important to carry out an exercise test to establish whether the leg complaints are in fact secondary to arterial disease. If the patient is truly suffering from intermittent claudication, the postexercise ankle blood pressure must fall. If there is no fall in this parameter, the patient does not have arterial disease as a cause of the leg pain.

Once this information has been obtained, it is possible to obtain a reasonable assessment of the patient's status and the form of therapy that may be required. It cannot be emphasized too strongly that the need for therapeutic intervention is based on the clinical status and limitations of the patient. If a decision is made not to proceed with direct therapy (surgical or endovascular), there is no need to proceed with duplex scanning.

However, if the patient is a candidate for further consideration of therapy, it is appropriate to proceed with duplex scanning. The type of preliminary information obtained is also of great value to the technologist, who can focus on those areas of greatest interest.

DUPLEX SCANNING

If an arteriogram is to be done anyway, why should this be preceded by duplex scanning? There are several reasons that make it not only justifiable but also worthwhile. Even at present, duplex scanning is accurate enough to plan the definitive procedure that will follow. This is important preliminary information for the patient and the physician, who can then plan the procedure and also counsel the patient on the likelihood of success. For example, it is now possible to determine which patients will be candidates for angioplasty. In fact, when segmental hemodynamically significant stenoses are found in the aortoiliac segment, the patient is scheduled for the procedure (Figs. 7.1 and 7.2). It is also helpful for the radiologist to have this information because it pinpoints the arterial segments involved. In addition, it permits the discovery of lesions that may pose problems and compromise the outcome. An example of this is the finding of disease in the profunda femoris artery, which may require special attention.

Another major advantage of this approach is that it provides a baseline for future studies. If, for example, an angioplasty is done, it is possible to reexamine the same segment to determine to what extent the narrowing has been corrected (Fig. 7.3). This is the most direct method of determining the success or failure of the angioplasty.

Duplex scanning complements the arteriographic findings and can compensate for their limitations in defining the hemodynamic significance of areas of involvement. Bruins Slot and associates (3) were among the first to point out the inadequacy of single-plane arteriograms. These problems are evident when it is remembered that atherosclerotic lesions do not narrow the vessel in an axisymmetric fashion. In fact, the most common site of involvement is on the posterior wall of the involved arterial segments. Visualization of this region of the artery may, to some extent, be overcome by biplanar views, but these are not always obtainable (Fig. 7.4). Although these biplanar views are, in theory, more helpful, there is little evidence that they have increased the accuracy of interpretation.

Clinical evidence to support the inadequacy of aortography alone predicting the hemodynamic significance of lesions, particularly in the aortoiliac region, was provided by the report of Sumner and Strandness (4). This study noted that up to 30% of patients who had combined aortoiliac and femoropopliteal disease did not show hemodynamic improvement after a proximal reconstruction alone. This confirmed the inadequacy of arteriogram alone in predicting the need for a proximal arterial reconstruction such as an aortobifemoral graft.

Because of these problems with arteriography, there have been several methods tested that are designed to identify the hemodynamic significance of stenoses in the iliac arteries. Most of this work has been done using parameters derived from common femoral artery velocity patterns to estimate the status of the iliac arteries. These include pulsatility index, Laplace transform damping factor, and principal component analysis (5–7). Although these methods have had some success, they have not been widely applied for the solution of the problem.

A conclusion reached by most investigators, including us, was that any attempt to predict hemodynamic signifi-

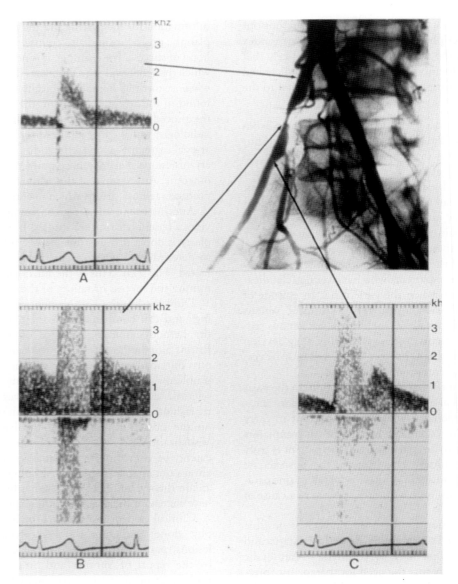

FIGURE 7.1. This patient presented with severe claudication involving the right leg. A duplex scan revealed a tight right common iliac artery stenosis. The arteriogram and the corresponding velocity proximal to, in, and distal to the stenosis are shown. *A*, common iliac artery; *B*, site of narrowing; *C*, proximal external iliac artery.

cance of stenosis in the aortoiliac segment must be verified by direct intraarterial pressure measurements made at the time of arteriography (8). Normally, the change in systolic pressure from the abdominal aorta to the femoral artery should be so small that it would be difficult to measure. It must be remembered that there is a less than 10-mm Hg mean pressure drop from the level of the aorta to the small unnamed arteries of the lower limb and foot.

In practice, it is generally accepted that a systolic pressure gradient from the aorta to the common femoral artery is normally taken to be less than 10 mm Hg. If a gradient of less than 10 mm Hg is noted, intraarterial papaverine is given. This will lead to a transient vasodilatation and increase in flow. This is designed to mimic the flow increase seen with exercise. If a systolic pressure gradient of more than 20 mm Hg develops, this is considered to be hemodynamically significant (9).

When intraarterial pressure gradient criteria were used to test the hemodynamic status of the aortoiliac segment, it was possible to test the visual reading of arteriograms against a realistic hemodynamic gold standard. Thiele and Strandness (10) reported on a comparison of arteriographic readings with intraarterial pressures in 73 aortoiliac segments. In 39 segments, significant pressure drops were

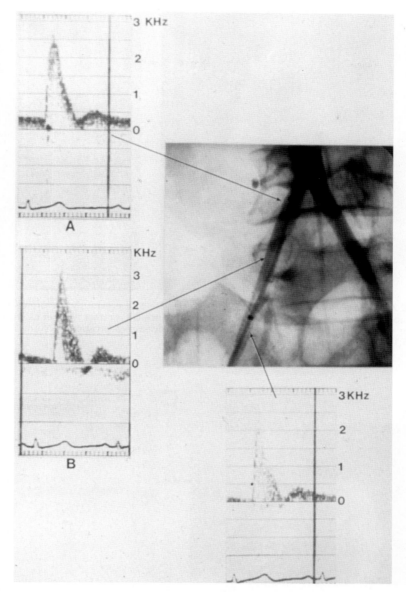

FIGURE 7.2. A balloon angioplasty was performed on the patient shown in Fig. 7.1. After the dilatation, the stenosis is no longer seen. The velocity ranges proximal to, in, and distal to the dilated segment are now nearly normal. *A*, common iliac artery; *B*, site of narrowing that has been dilated; *C*, external iliac artery.

found at the time of arteriography. Two vascular surgeons reviewed the arteriograms without prior knowledge of the pressure gradient results. The results of the comparisons were as follows:

1. Reader 1 identified 34 visualized arterial segments as being hemodynamically significant. In 24 cases, this was true.
2. Reader 2 identified 37 arteries he considered significant. In 27 of these segments, this was verified by the intraarterial pressure measurements.

3. For those 34 aortoiliac segments that did not have an abnormal pressure gradient, reader 1 correctly identified 27, with reader 2 identifying 24.

There is little doubt that intraarterial pressure measured at the time of arteriography should be considered the gold standard for documenting the hemodynamic status of the aortoiliac segment. In fact, these measurements must be done when stenotic lesions are found and angioplasty is being contemplated (8). Furthermore, the pressure gradient should be measured again after the completion of the

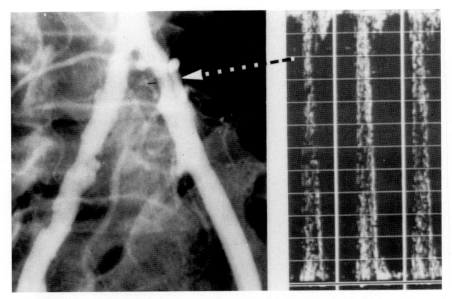

FIGURE 7.3. The patient's velocity recorded from the site of a previously perfomed translumi-nal angioplasty is again abnormal. (From Kohler RR, Nance DR, Cramer MM, et al. Duplex scan-ning for diagnosis of aortoiliac and femoropopliteal disease: a prospective study. *Circulation* 1987;76:1074–1080, with permission.)

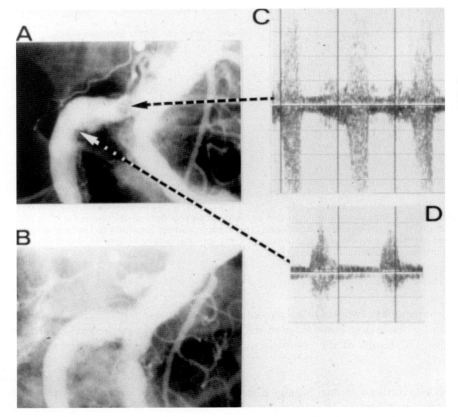

FIGURE 7.4. The stenosis in the iliac artery was not well seen *(A)*. However, the increased veloc-ity in this area was clearly seen *(C)* and was reduced distal to the lesion *(D)*. After angioplasty, the small filling defect is no longer seen *(B)*.

dilatation to document the immediate result. Having prearteriographic duplex scanning data relevant to this arterial segment can be helpful for the radiologist.

The preparation of the patient before the duplex scan is important, since a key area that needs to be examined is the aortoiliac segment. The major obstacle to the use of ultrasound in the abdomen is the presence of bowel gas. Because of this, we prefer to study the patient after a 12-hr fast and, if at all possible, the first thing in the morning. The procedure is much easier to do, with a greater likelihood of one's being able to do a complete study.

Many of our early attempts to use duplex scanning to examine the abdominal and limb vessels were frustrated by our inability to reach these vessels because of the lack of low-transmitting frequency scanheads with a focal point at the appropriate depths. The early systems were designed for studying only the carotid arteries and were not intended for examining arteries or veins in other areas of the body. In addition, it did not appear clear that it would be worthwhile to spend the necessary time investigating the entire length of the arterial supply to the lower limbs. It seemed impractical but, as we have subsequently learned, a great

deal of useful information may be obtained (11). In addition, because we know where the atherosclerotic lesions commonly tend to occur, we know where to focus the attention of the study.

The use of duplex scanning for peripheral arteries is based on the assumption that the velocity increase found in the area of narrowing can be related to the degree of diameter reduction. In contrast to the carotid artery, where hemodynamically significant lesions may not produce ischemic problems, this is not true for the arteries supplying the lower extremities. In these arteries, when the diameter reduction exceeds 50%, there is a drop in pressure and flow that will lead to the development of intermittent claudication (12). This, then, is the type of lesion and its location that we are trying to detect. To recognize such areas of narrowing, it is necessary to monitor the velocity changes along the entire course of the arterial supply. From this type of survey, it became feasible to develop criteria that could be used to estimate the degree of stenosis. Stenoses that under resting levels of flow do not have an abnormal gradient may develop one with the stress of when the flow is dramatically increased (13).

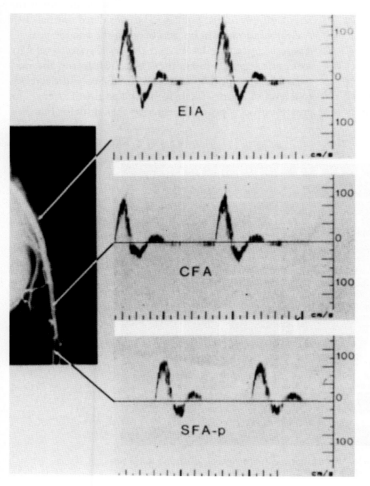

FIGURE 7.5. The normal velocity waveforms in the iliac, common femoral, and proximal superficial femoral are triphasic. *EIA,* external iliac artery; *CFA,* common femoral artery; *SFA-p,* proximal superficial femoral artery.

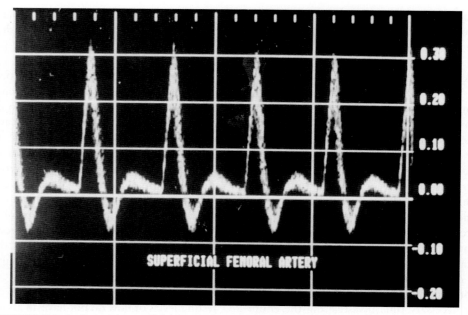

FIGURE 7.6. In the mid-superficial femoral artery, the triphasic waveform is normally present.

Although the normal findings in the arterial system have been discussed in Chapter 3, it will be helpful to review the critical factors in such an evaluation. The normal findings include the following:

1. A triphasic velocity waveform is normally found in the arteries from the level of the abdominal aorta and iliac arteries to the tibial arteries at the ankle (Figs. 7.5 to 7.7). The reverse flow component must be present if the arterial supply to that point is to be considered normal (14). A clear window must be seen beneath the systolic peak.

2. There is a gradual decrease in the peak systolic velocity from one segment to another (Fig. 7.8). In the abdominal aorta, it is in the range of 100 cm/sec and decreases to a level of about 70 cm/sec in the popliteal artery. The greatest drop appears to be across the adductor hiatus.

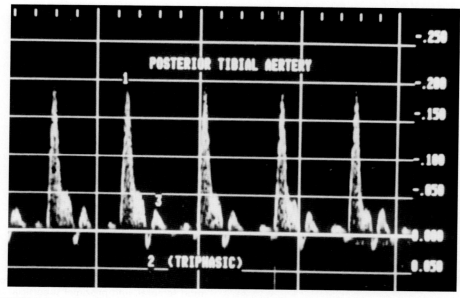

FIGURE 7.7. In the tibial arteries at the ankle, the triphasic waveform would normally be present. *l*, Peak-systolic; *2*, reverse flow; *3*, secondary forward flow.

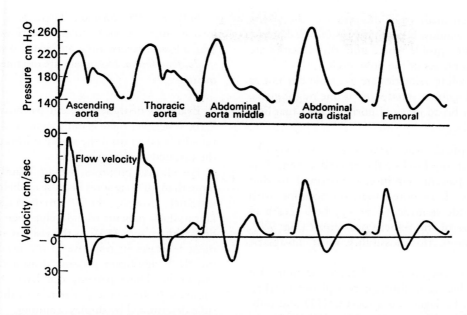

FIGURE 7.8. Changes in the intraarterial blood pressure and velocity of flow from the level of the ascending aorta to the femoral artery. The peak systolic pressure increases. The peak velocities recorded from similar sites show a gradual decrease. (Adapted from McDonald DA. *Blood flow in arteries.* Baltimore: Williams & Wilkins, 1960:271, with permission.)

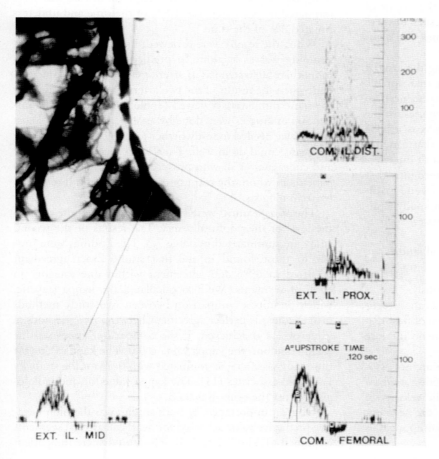

FIGURE 7.9. Normalization of arterial waveforms. In this patient, there was a tight iliac artery stenosis with the corresponding increase in peak systolic velocity. Distal to the stenosis, the waveform regained its reverse flow component. *COM IL DIST,* distal common iliac artery; *EXT IL PROX,* proximal external iliac artery; *COM FEMORAL,* common femoral artery; *EXT IL MID,* mid-external iliac artery.

3. Recordings, when made from the center of the artery, will have a clear window beneath the systolic peak, characteristic of a flow profile where uniform velocities are found during all phases of the pulse cycle.
4. Data on the absolute velocities are available but not as useful from a diagnostic standpoint as one might guess. There is a rather broad range of normal values that limits their usefulness.

Whenever a triphasic waveform with a clear systolic window is found at any level of the arterial system, it is unlikely that the patient has disease proximal to that point. However, we have noted that, on occasion with distal to a high-grade stenosis, there may be a return in the triphasic nature of the velocity waveform (Fig. 7.9). Although uncommon, this possibility must always be kept in mind.

Our evaluation of the accuracy of duplex scanning for peripheral arteries has gone through two phases (11,15). The first was done by Jager and associates (11) and published in 1985. In this trial, there were 330 arterial segments in 30 patients (54 limbs) that were evaluated by both duplex scanning and arteriography. For the arteriographic measurements, calipers were used to make the estimations of diameter reduction. Two arteriographers were involved, so that we could also determine the amount of interobserver variability present in attempting to measure the extent of diameter reduction by the arteriogram. The results of these studies led to the formulation of the guidelines and algorithms we currently use.

The classification scheme used for scanning the arterial supply to the lower limbs is slightly different than for the carotid arteries. In peripheral arteries, there is no need to subdivide the degree of stenosis into more categories for the 50% to 99% group because once a lesion exceeds a 50% reduction in diameter, it is a critical stenosis that can and will, in most patients, lead to the development of intermittent claudication. However, it is important to recognize that some stenotic lesions that do not produce a pressure gradient and flow reduction at rest can become hemodynamically significant when the flow velocity increases, such as occurs with exercise (13).

The categories that resulted from our initial studies are as follows:

Normal. These criteria were outlined previously.

Wall irregularities (1% to 19%). In this case, the irregular nature of the wall may lead to the generation of flow disturbances that lead to spectral broadening but no increase in peak systolic velocity.

20% to 49% Stenosis. These types of lesions are not associated with a pressure gradient at rest. The criterion used for this category is an increase in the peak systolic velocity of more than 30% but less than 100% from the segment immediately preceding it. The reverse flow component is preserved.

50% to 99% Stenosis. There is a more than 100% increase in the peak systolic velocity within the narrowed area, a loss of reverse flow, and marked spectral broadening.

Total occlusion. No signals are obtained from imaged segment.

Examples of these different patterns are shown in Fig. 7.10. Whenever there is multisegment disease, the reference velocity is taken from the segment immediately proximal to the diseased area in question.

For clinical purposes, we are mainly interested in the more than 50% stenoses because of their hemodynamic significance. However, the 20% to 49% lesions can be important in those patients who develop their abnormal gradients only with exercise (13). As the velocity in the narrowed segment increases in response to the needs of the exercising muscle, a significant pressure drop and reduction in flow can occur. These patients can have their arterial disease "unmasked" by an exercise test, with the exact sites responsible determined by duplex scanning.

In the initial studies done by Jager and associates (11), there were 30 patients (15 male and 15 female). The mean ankle/arm index was 0.61 on the right and 0.62 on the left. The segments and the results are summarized in Table 7.1. The overall agreement for the segments was 76% (258 of 338). By the duplex criteria, the degree of disease was overestimated by two categories 1.5% of the time and underestimated 3% of the time.

When the results were reviewed, it appeared that duplex scanning was as accurate in predicting the presence of a more than 50% stenosis as arteriography. This became evident when the results of the two arteriographers' readings of the same films were reviewed (Table 7.2). Because the initial duplex studies were done by an experienced angiologist (Jager), we needed to test whether technologists performing the scans could do as well. This led to the study by Kohler and colleagues (15), who prospectively studied another 20 patients in whom the scans both were done and interpreted by technologists.

The areas scanned were similar and included the aorta to the level of the popliteal artery. The results of the second study are summarized in Table 7.3. The findings were similar to those found in the first study. Exact agreement occurred in 69% and agreement within one category in 87% of segments. We also calculated the kappa statistic, which permits a comparison between two study methods (16). If there is perfect agreement between two methods, a value of 1.0 is achieved. If the comparison appears to be totally random, the kappa value is 0.0. The kappa value for this study was 0.55, as compared with 0.69 for the study by Jager and associates (11). The kappa value for one radiologist against the other was 0.63.

Of great importance for both studies was the high negative predictive value achieved for nearly all arterial segments examined (Tables 7.1 to 7.3). This could spare the patient

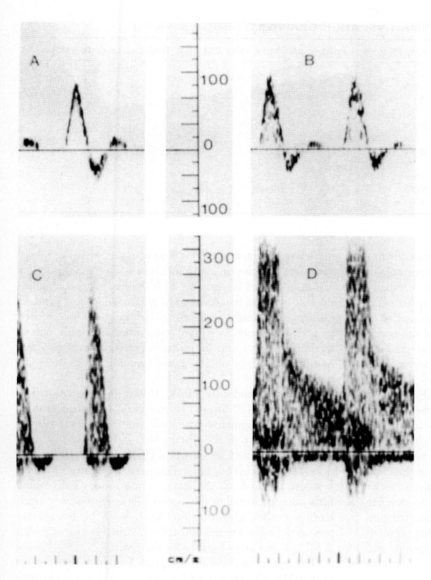

FIGURE 7.10. Examples of the velocity changes noted for the various categories of disease: *A,* normal; *B,* 1% to 19% stenosis; *C,* 20% to 49% stenosis; *D,* 50% to 99% stenosis. See text for explanation. (From Jager KA, Phillips DJ, Martin RL, et al. Noninvasive mapping of lower limb arterial lesions. *Ultrasound Med Biol* 1985;11:515–521, with permission.)

TABLE 7.1. COMPARISON OF DUPLEX SCANNING AND ARTERIOGRAPHY (<50% VS. >50%)

Arterial segment	Sensitivity (%)	Specificity (%)	Positive predictive value (%)	Negative predictive value (%)
Iliac	81	100	100	92
Common femoral	56	96	71	91
Profunda	86	100	100	98
Superficial femoral				
Proximal	71	100	100	88
Superficial femoral				
Mid	80	100	100	87
Superficial femoral				
Distal	77	90	77	90
Popliteal	80	100	100	93
All segments	77	98	94	92

TABLE 7.2. COMPARISON OF ANGIOGRAPHER 1 VS. ANGIOGRAPHER 2 (<50% VS. >50%)

Arterial segment	Sensitivity (%)	Specificity (%)	Positive predictive value (%)	Negative predictive value (%)
Iliac	94	96	94	96
Common femoral	66	100	100	91
Profunda	33	91	40	88
Superficial femoral Proximal	95	100	100	93
Superficial femoral Mid	100	84	82	100
Superficial femoral Distal	91	85	78	94
Popliteal	91	100	100	95
All segments	87	94	88	93

from having a potentially dangerous operative procedure on an arterial segment that might appear to be important on the arteriogram. For the iliac arteries, the negative predictive value was 96%, which is extremely high for an area that has always been difficult to examine. With a sensitivity of 89%, it is then possible to direct the attention of the arteriographer to this area so that intraarterial pressure gradient measurements can be made at the time of arteriography to arrive at a final decision.

Another interesting finding in the study by Kohler and colleagues (15) was the relationship between the findings and actual pressure gradient measurements done at the time of arteriography. There were eight patients who had gradients measured. Gradients exceeding 15 mm Hg were noted in seven segments. In six cases, they were placed in the more than 50% category by duplex scanning and in five cases by arteriography. In the four cases with a less than 15-mm Hg gradient, both methods classified two as less than 50% and one as a more than 50% stenosis. The remaining segment was classified as less than 50% stenosis by arteriography and more than 50% by duplex scanning.

ROLE OF COLOR

All of the validation studies done with duplex scanning have been completed with standard "black-and-white"

duplex scanning; however, it is only natural that the role of color either alone or in conjunction with standard duplex scanning should be considered. It is important to establish the role of color, where it can be applied, and how it might influence the results of scanning. This has been investigated by several authors. As with all modalities, it is important to establish how it works in normal subjects, the type of information that can be obtained, and how this might be modified by disease.

Hatsukami and co-workers (17) studied the color flow patterns from 420 arterial segments in 10 normal volunteers. These segments extended from the level of the abdominal aorta to the distal tibial and peroneal arteries. The sites examined are shown in Fig. 7.11. All studies were done with a QUAD-1 Angiodynograph (Quantum Medical Systems, Issaquah, WA). This system was not ideally suited for studies proximal to the inguinal ligament but was excellent for studies below the groin level. A 3-MHz linear array was used for the arteries above the inguinal ligament with a 5-MHz linear array used below the groin.

The quality of the scans was graded as good, poor, or not obtainable. The areas in which some difficulty was encountered most frequently were above the inguinal ligament, where 10% to 15% of the arteries could not be examined at all with this system. Below the knee, the arterial segment most difficult to examine included the proximal and distal peroneal, where no information was obtained in 15% to

TABLE 7.3. DUPLEX SCANNING VS. ANGIOGRAPHY (STUDY 2) (<50% VS. >50%)

Arterial segment	Sensitivity (%)	Specificity (%)	Positive predictive value (%)	Negative predictive value (%)
Aorta	100	100	100	100
Iliac	90	90	75	96
Common femoral	67	98	80	96
Superficial femoral	84	93	90	88
Profunda	67	81	53	88
Popliteal	75	97	86	93
All segments	82	92	80	93

None of the aortic segments had a >50% stenosis.

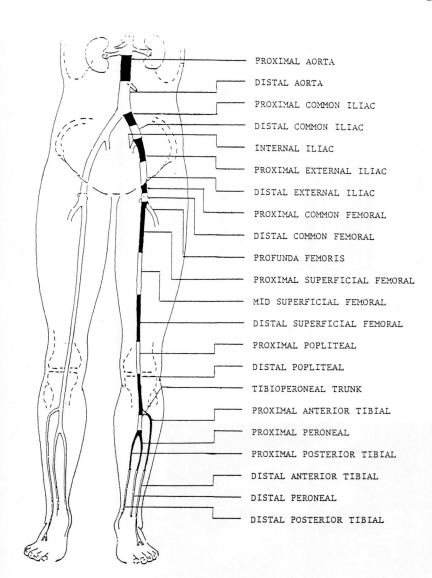

PROXIMAL AORTA

DISTAL AORTA

PROXIMAL COMMON ILIAC

DISTAL COMMON ILIAC

INTERNAL ILIAC

PROXIMAL EXTERNAL ILIAC

DISTAL EXTERNAL ILIAC

PROXIMAL COMMON FEMORAL

DISTAL COMMON FEMORAL

PROFUNDA FEMORIS

PROXIMAL SUPERFICIAL FEMORAL

MID SUPERFICIAL FEMORAL

DISTAL SUPERFICIAL FEMORAL

PROXIMAL POPLITEAL

DISTAL POPLITEAL

TIBIOPERONEAL TRUNK

PROXIMAL ANTERIOR TIBIAL

PROXIMAL PERONEAL

PROXIMAL POSTERIOR TIBIAL

DISTAL ANTERIOR TIBIAL

DISTAL PERONEAL

DISTAL POSTERIOR TIBIAL

FIGURE 7.11. Sites examined with color Doppler system. (From Hatsukami TS, Primozich J, Zierler RE, et al. Color Doppler characteristics in normal lower extremity arteries. *Ultrasound Med Biol* 1992;18:167–171, with permission.)

20% of normal subjects. For all other areas, good studies were possible in more than 90% of the normal subjects.

The peak systolic velocities obtained at each level of the circulation are shown in Fig. 7.12. As noted, there is an apparent decrease in the peak systolic velocities between the proximal and distal common femoral artery and across the adductor canal to the popliteal artery. This is apparently secondary to the large branches that arise from these segments. These quantitative velocity data can be quite useful in clinical scanning, but as noted earlier, it is more reliable to examine the velocity changes from one segment to another.

The color in and of itself is not used for the estimation of absolute velocities. This is because the color alone does not provide an accurate reflection of the true velocities. It tends to underestimate the true velocities (see Appendix). On the other hand, the color is a good pathfinder, permitting the identification of the target vessels to allow accurate placement of the sample volume of the pulsed Doppler. The

addition of power Doppler provides another useful technique for detailing the anatomy of suggested sites of disease.

In normal subjects, the major factor that distinguishes the velocity patterns from those seen in patients with arterial disease is the presence or absence of reverse flow. This can most reliably be seen with the spectral displays as shown in Figs. 7.5 and 7.6. To test the role of color alone, Hatsukami and co-workers (17) examined this in the 10 normal subjects they studied. The agreement between spectral waveform detection and its observance with color alone was greater than 94%, except for the internal iliac, profunda femoris, and peroneal arteries. An example of reverse flow seen in early diastole with color alone is shown in Fig. 7.13.

Based on this preliminary experience with color Doppler, Hatsukami and co-workers (17) concluded the following:

- Color greatly aids in the identification of arteries and veins at all levels of the lower extremities.

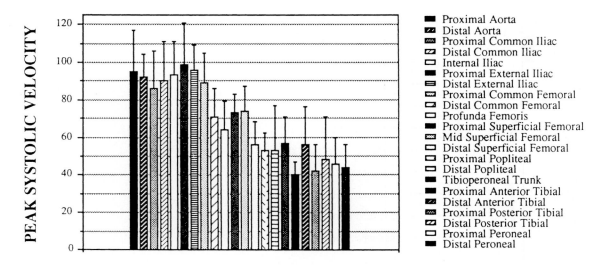

ARTERIAL SEGMENT

FIGURE 7.12. The peak systolic velocities recorded from the target arteries using the color Doppler system. The color was used for vessel identification with the single-sample pulsed Doppler for estimation of velocity. (From Hatsukami TS, Primozich J, Zierler RE, et al. Color Doppler characteristics in normal lower extremity arteries. *Ultrasound Med Biol* 1992;18:167–171, with permission.)

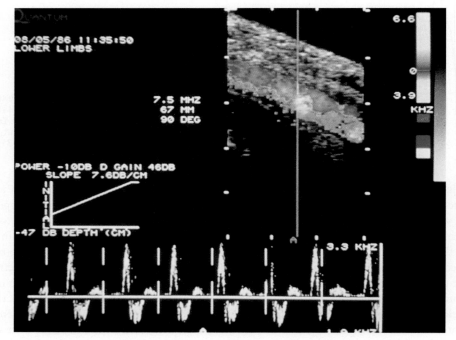

FIGURE 7.13. With color, the reverse flow component is seen along one or both walls in early diastole. This corresponds to that observed when a spectral display of the velocity patterns is obtained.

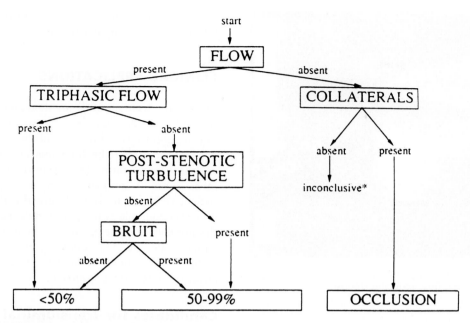

FIGURE 7.14. The algorithm used for documenting the status of the arteries from the level of the abdominal aorta to the ankle. (From Hatsukami TS, Primozich JP, Zierler RE, et al. Color Doppler imaging of lower extremity arterial disease: a prospective validation study. *J Vasc Surg* 1992;16:527–533, with permission.)

■ It is possible with color alone to recognize the triphasic flow pattern seen in normal peripheral arteries.

■ Color is particularly helpful in vessel identification below the knee.

■ Color alone should not be used to replace the fast Fourier transforms (FFT) analyzed velocity waveforms on a hard-copy printout.

With the experience using color flow in normal subjects, it became possible to explore its application in patients with arterial disease.

To investigate the role of color in a blinded fashion, Hatsukami and associates (18) studied 29 men before arteriography using the QUAD-1 color Doppler system. All patients were studied from the level of the infrarenal aorta to the tibial and peroneal arteries at the ankle. As in the studies of normal subjects, a 3-MHz linear array was used above the inguinal ligament with a 5-MHz probe distal to the groin. In this study, only color alone was used for the determination of the degree of stenosis. The algorithm used for the study is shown in Fig. 7.14. The criteria were, briefly, as follows:

■ If triphasic flow was seen, the segment was considered to be normal (Fig. 7.13).

■ If flow was absent and collaterals were seen, the artery was considered to be occluded (Fig. 7.15).

■ If poststenotic turbulence was seen with a bruit in the surrounding tissue, the artery was classified as having a more than 50% stenosis (Fig. 7.16).

■ When a bruit was absent, the artery was not considered to harbor a more than 50% stenosis (Fig. 7.17).

There were 910 arterial segments studied by color Doppler. Less than 66% of those from the infrarenal aorta to the external iliac artery were well visualized. This low figure was due in part to the QUAD-1, which does not perform as well above the inguinal ligament as other, later ver-

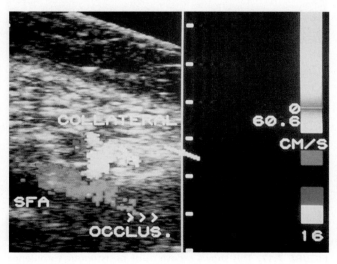

FIGURE 7.15. An example of total arterial occlusion with apparent collaterals.

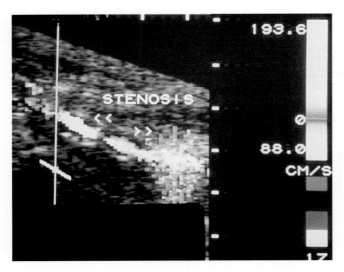

FIGURE 7.16. The mixing of colors outside the artery is consistent with a pressure- and flow-reducing stenosis.

sions or other systems currently available. However, distal to the inguinal ligament, more than 90% of the arteries could be satisfactorily seen. By using the criteria listed previously, at less than 50% or more than 50% stenosis, the specificity and negative predictive value were more than 90%, except for the tibial and peroneal arteries (88%) and the posterior tibial artery (84%). The sensitivity ranged from 50% to 100%. Larger numbers would be required to determine the value of color alone in terms of its sensitivity. It needs to be emphasized that the quality of the data collected is highly operator dependent, which is a major disadvantage. For this reason, we strongly recommend that color never be used alone but rather be combined with the FFT estimate of velocity change from one segment of the

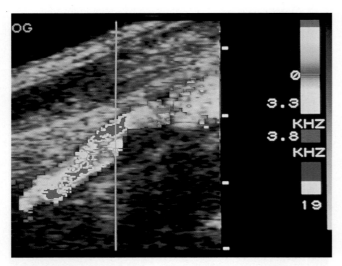

FIGURE 7.17. This shows a pattern of poststenotic turbulence without an associated bruit seen in the adjacent soft tissue. In this setting, a stenosis of less than 50% was suspected.

arterial system to another. This will provide the maximum information and the best results.

CLINICAL APPLICATIONS

Because the accuracy of the method approaches that of arteriography, under what circumstances can it provide useful information for the clinician and the patient? There is little need for the study to be done unless there are adequate indications for some form of intervention to be carried out. The most common complaint seen in a vascular clinic is the patient with claudication. As noted earlier, the indications for either angioplasty or operation depend on the severity of the problem and the extent to which it interferes with the patient's lifestyle. The following are offered as guidelines, along with examples of how the results of the study can affect the subsequent approach.

Candidates for Transluminal Angioplasty

Although there are differences in opinion and these are continually evolving, the guidelines used here are as follows:

1. Iliac lesions are the most successful and have the best long-term results.
2. There is no doubt that occlusions can be dealt with; however, we generally reserve angioplasty for patients with stenotic lesions.
3. Femoropopliteal stenoses can be dilated, but the results are not as good as those in the iliac artery. The one subset of patients in whom this may not be the case includes those with short lesions (3 cm or less). In this setting, we might recommend this approach.

The clinical presentation is helpful in suggesting the course most likely to be pursued. The most straightforward clinical presentation is the patient with calf and thigh claudication who has a palpable femoral pulse with a loud bruit heard over the iliac artery and transmitted to the groin. In this case, there may be pulses palpable at the level of the popliteal and foot as well; it is likely that the patient has a stenosis of the iliac artery.

The more common situation is that of an absent femoral pulse with or without a bruit. The examiner in this case is not sure of two things: (a) Is the iliac lesion a stenosis, occlusion, or both? (b) Are there additional lesions in either the common femoral, profunda femoris, or superficial femoral artery? Under these circumstances, the level of suspicion will be high, but it is important to have this verified, preferably by duplex scanning if at all possible.

An example of a patient with an iliac stenosis diagnosed by duplex scanning and scheduled for the procedure is shown in Figs. 7.1 and 7.2. As noted, the changes that occurred with the angioplasty could be verified by repeat duplex scanning and provided immediate hemodynamic assessment of the result.

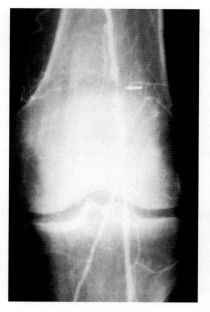
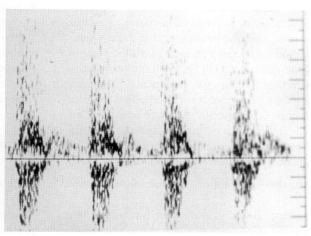

FIGURE 7.18. Popliteal artery velocities before angioplasty. This patient presented with mild ischemic rest pain and a nonhealing ulcer of one digit. The ankle systolic pressure was 40 mm Hg. The duplex scan identified the high-grade popliteal stenosis.

The patient illustrated in Fig. 7.18 shows the utility of scanning in a patient with mild ischemic rest pain and an open ulcer on one of her digits who was not a candidate for direct arterial surgery because of severe myocardial problems. Her ankle systolic pressure was 40 mm Hg on that side. The duplex scan showed a focal popliteal stenosis that was ideal for angioplasty. There was an immediate increase in her ankle pressure to normal levels, and her ulcer healed. The immediate velocity change confirmed the good anatomic result (Fig. 7.19). During follow-up, her ankle

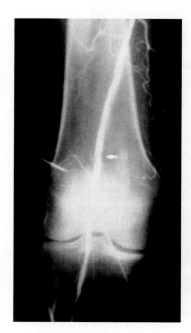
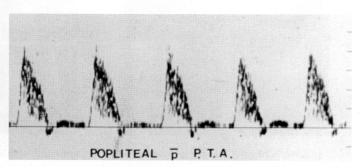

FIGURE 7.19. Popliteal artery velocities after angioplasty. The postdilatation duplex scan verified the return in the velocity signal to normal.

pressure began to fall and the stenosis recurred, yet she remained free of pain. Her lack of pain with the recurrence of the stenotic lesion was because her ulcer, the site of her discomfort, remained healed. Her ankle pressure also decreased to the predilatation level.

Although it is instructive to present illustrative cases, it is necessary to test rigorously the hypothesis that duplex scanning can be a method for selecting patients for balloon angioplasty. Edwards and colleagues (19) reviewed our prospective experience in selecting patients for angioplasty by duplex scanning. There were 110 arteriograms preceded by a duplex scan. From this group, 50 cases (45%) were scheduled for angioplasty based on the results of duplex scanning. The procedure was performed on 47 of these cases (94%). In the three cases not dilated, the reasons were as follows:

- In one patient, the lesion appeared to be too dangerous to dilate.
- In another patient, although the lesion was seen, there was not a measurable pressure gradient across the lesion.
- In the final patient, an occlusion distal to a high-grade stenosis was missed, hence the patient was not treated.

It must be remembered that the criteria we use for selecting patients for angioplasty are simple. We dilate lesions that are short, discrete, and for the most part not total occlusions. In this series of 47 patients with angioplasty, only two occlusions were treated in this fashion. There are several advantages of this method of study that we consider to be important. These are as follows:

- The patients are fully informed of the likely course of therapy before arteriography.
- The radiologist can plan the site of catheter placement without prior angiographic verification.
- It is not necessary to do a "diagnostic" arteriogram and then review the study to determine whether an angioplasty is warranted. Although I do not have proof that this is a common practice, it is my impression that it is more common than one might expect. Clearly, a second arteriographic study should not be necessary for this purpose.

Documentation of the Source of Emboli

There is a subset of patients who present with what appears to be microemboli to the foot and, on occasion, both feet. This syndrome is suspected by the distribution of the ischemia, which nearly always involves all the digits, with a prominent pattern of livido reticularis of the forefoot. Pulses are often palpable, and the problem usually involves locating the site from which such emboli may arise. A case in point is shown in Fig. 7.20. This elderly gentleman was without symptoms until he suddenly noted the appearance of mild ischemic rest pain in his toes along with a decrease in skin temperature and profound color changes. He had palpable pulses, so it was clear that his major arteries to the level of the foot were, in all likelihood, patent. A duplex scan revealed the tight popliteal stenosis, shown in Fig.

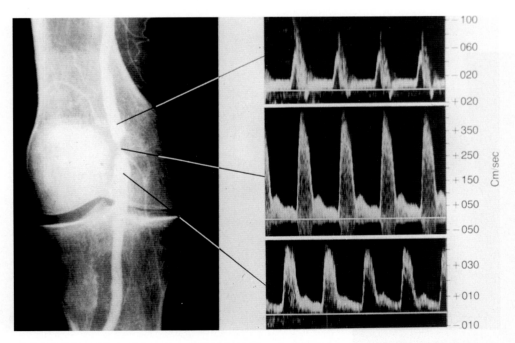

FIGURE 7.20. This patient presented with microemboli to the toes and forefoot. The site from which the emboli arose was demonstrated by the velocity changes shown and verified by arteriography. A vein bypass graft was placed with ligation of the artery to prevent further embolization.

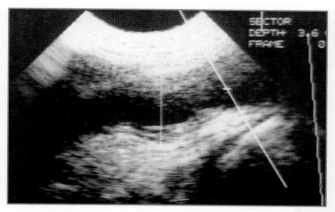

FIGURE 7.21. This longitudinal scan of the popliteal artery revealed aneurysmal dilatation with a mural thrombus. No flow was detected immediately distal to the mycotic aneurysm.

7.20. A reversed saphenous vein graft was placed, and the site of the stenosis was excluded with a good result.

Unusual Cases of Claudication

The most common cause of intermittent claudication is atherosclerosis; however, there are, on occasion, other

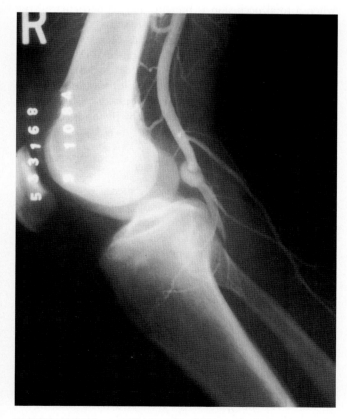

FIGURE 7.22. The arteriogram from the patient shown in Fig. 7.21 revealed the aneurysm and the arterial occlusion.

causes that can be elucidated by duplex scanning. The patient shown in Figs. 7.21 and 7.22 is a case in point. He was hospitalized for the treatment of subacute bacterial endocarditis. While in the hospital, he noted some mild cramping pain in the calf with walking. His foot pulses were absent, and his ankle pressure was below normal. The ultrasonic duplex scan revealed a popliteal aneurysm with an occlusion of the artery just distal to the lesion. This was a mycotic aneurysm that was treated by excision and performance of an *in situ* vein graft.

The duplex scan was helpful in making the diagnosis and suggesting the form of therapy that might be needed, even before the arteriogram was carried out. In addition, as will be discussed shortly, the same method will be useful in following the course of vein grafts to document problems that can be corrected and thus preserve long-term patency.

False Aneurysms

One of the most useful applications of duplex scanning is for the detection and now treatment of false aneurysms that occur secondary to catheter injury. With the increasing use of diagnostic cardiac methods and indwelling devices such as balloon pumps, the chance of injury to the arterial wall with leakage and of generation of a false aneurysm is heightened. It is recognized by the swelling, which is pulsatile and varies considerably in size. When the patient is first seen with this problem, the following several questions are often asked:

1. What is the relationship of the aneurysm to the site of the needle or catheter placement?
2. What is the size of the aneurysm?
3. Is the aneurysm occluded, and if not, how much of the lumen is occluded by thrombus?
4. Can the aneurysm be compressed, and will the flow stop within the sac?

Cox and colleagues (20) described their experience in 47 patients (50 pseudoaneurysms) with graded compression using a duplex scanner to promote thrombosis. The overall success of this approach was 90%. It is of interest that success was also achieved with those that had been present for longer than 30 days. The average time required for success for the early lesions was 30 minutes, increasing to 75 minutes for those that had been present for longer than 30 days. There were two recurrences: one at 24 hours, the other at 16 days. These were successfully treated by repeat compression. The aneurysms ranged in size from 0.7 to 5.2 cm (average, 2.4 cm).

Cox and colleagues (20) also examined the results in patients who were on anticoagulants at the time of detection and therapy. The success rate was lower in those on anticoagulants, being 67%. This is not unexpected given the fact that the success is dependent on thrombosis within the sac of the aneurysm.

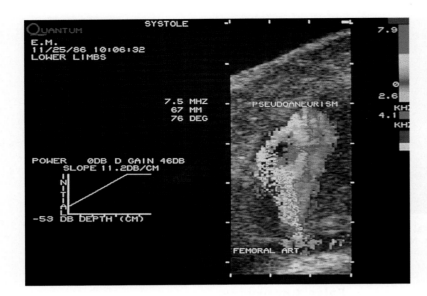

FIGURE 7.23. Color Doppler findings with a large false aneurysm of the femoral artery.

There is no doubt that many of these lesions can be compressed and thus cured by the simple application of pressure with the ultrasound probe. However, it is important to remember that many of these false aneurysms will spontaneously close and do not require a direct form of intervention for a cure. However, even if one is conservative about the management of these lesions, duplex scanning is the ideal method for follow-up. An example of the types of studies that can be obtained with color duplex is shown in Fig. 7.23. Recently, there has been evidence presented that the injection of thrombin under ultrasound guidance can greatly assist in the thrombosis of these aneurysms. This newer approach will be covered in detail.

Evaluating the Results of Fibrinolysis

In some cases of acute or subacute arterial occlusion, it may be possible to use a fibrinolytic agent to clear the occlusion. The initial workup does not always clarify the underlying cause of the thrombosis. The two major causes of acute occlusion are thrombosis in the vicinity of a high-grade atherosclerotic plaque and embolism from a proximal site, such as the heart. Duplex scanning can serve two purposes here. The first is to identify the extent of the involvement, and the second is to evaluate the previously occluded segment to determine whether there might be a lesion that could explain the event. An example is shown in Fig. 7.24. After the thrombolysis, the scan revealed that there were no areas of stenosis that could have been implicated as a cause of the occlusion (Fig. 7.25). The patient was placed on long-term anticoagulant therapy. Another advantage of the method is that it is feasible to monitor the pattern and rapidity with which lysis is occurring. This

can be important in determining how long the fibrinolysis should be continued.

It must be remembered that a preliminary duplex scan in patients with acute or subacute arterial occlusion may not indicate what the underlying cause may be. This is true when a total occlusion is present. This is particularly true when a previously patent graft is found to be occluded. Because the event that led to the occlusion may be "hidden" by the thrombus, it is only with clearance of the thrombus that the cause may be found. In most cases, this is noted by the follow-up arteriogram and not duplex scanning. Yet, the results of the intervention, be it angioplasty or direct arterial surgery, can readily be monitored by methods to be considered in later sections.

Intraoperative Monitoring

One of the key elements in the early success of any vascular operation is to ensure at the time of the procedure that the intended goal has been accomplished. The procedures that I have followed over the past several years are the use of the continuous wave Doppler and more recently duplex scanning. The manner in which this is accomplished is as follows:

1. For peripheral reconstructions, be they bypass grafts or endarterectomy, the criterion of success is restoration of flow to normal or near-normal levels. To assess this, it is possible simply to examine all components of the reconstruction, which are the inflow, the reconstruction, the artery at the site of graft insertion, and the contribution to the distal arteries. The advantage of duplex scanning is that it can be run along the entire reconstruction, listening for the telltale signs of a stenosis by noting a sudden increase in the velocity. Finding this should prompt the performance of

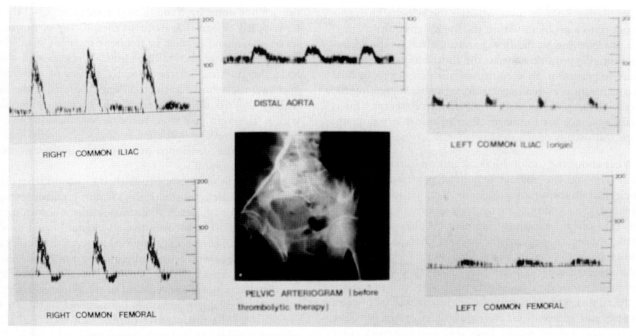

FIGURE 7.24. This patient presented with a sudden change in temperature of the left foot. A duplex scan demonstrated an occlusion in the iliac artery system that was later verified by arteriography.

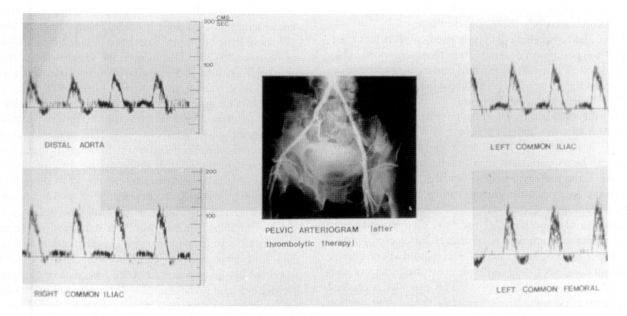

FIGURE 7.25. Blood flow velocities after thrombolytic therapy for acute iliac occlusion. After intraarterial thrombolysis, the artery is now cleared of the thrombus. The velocity recordings are now nearly normal.

an arteriogram to determine whether the velocity change is secondary to a problem within the bypass conduit.

2. By listening to the flow patterns distal to the reconstruction, it is possible to assess the contribution of the procedure to perfusion. By compressing the graft, one can note the contribution in qualitative terms, further suggesting the success of the procedure. If there are any concerns, this is certain evidence for the need of an operative arteriogram, which will usually reveal the cause.

What about the use of duplex scanning in the operating room? This has the obvious benefit of providing not only velocity data but also a high-quality B-mode image. Color will aid in the rapidity of the scan by identifying suspicious areas that can be selectively sampled by placement of the sample volume to examine the velocity changes across discrete areas.

Although there is no doubt that this method will work, it does require moving the equipment to the operating room for the completion studies. However, it may well be possible to justify this approach for arterial reconstructions in which an operative failure would have dire consequences. One example of this is the renal artery, in which correction of areas of stenosis may be by endarterectomy or bypass grafts. If an operative problem is not discovered, the outcome could be truly catastrophic. Failure might lead to loss of the kidney, which could not be reversed even if reoperation were to take place within a relatively short period of time.

Hallet and co-workers (21) have used color duplex scanning for the evaluation of renal artery reconstructions. They reported on 35 patients who were undergoing reconstructions on 64 renal arteries. Technical problems were found in 10.9%. These included two occlusions, three intimal defects, one extrinsic band, and one anastomotic stenosis. Correction of these defects resulted in a satisfactory outcome. It is in this type of reconstruction that immediate results can be so important for the long-term function and outcome of the patient. I believe that this type of operation monitoring easily justifies the additional time and expense of the screening procedure.

Bandyk and associates (22) reviewed their experience in the intraoperative studies of carotid endarterectomy (N = 210), lower limb bypass grafts (N = 210), and visceral artery reconstructions (N = 23). Duplex detected defects that required repair in 37 cases (10%). This provided a method for preventing postoperative complications and graft failures.

Monitoring Grafts

One of the major contributions made in the vein bypass grafting procedures is the realization that long-term patency may be accomplished by careful monitoring of the graft after it has been placed. This has become most evident in

the studies done by Bandyk and associates (22–24), who have clearly shown that frequent monitoring of *in situ* and reversed saphenous veins at frequent intervals may permit early detection of the "failing" graft. These careful studies have also pointed out the potential causes of graft failure and how they can be corrected. Venous grafts in the lower leg, be they *in situ* or reversed, fail because of problems within the vein itself, at the sites of anastomosis, and because of outflow problems. Although grafts can fail because of the development of inflow problems, this is much less common.

An example of a case in which the preoperative duplex studies of a patient scheduled for a femoropopliteal vein graft were ignored with nearly disastrous results is shown in Figs. 7.26 and 7.27. The preoperative arteriogram failed to reveal any stenoses in the popliteal artery. However, the duplex scan revealed an area with a markedly increased peak systolic and end-diastolic velocity (Fig. 7.26). At the time of operation, the distal anastomosis was placed in the popliteal artery. An operative arteriogram revealed a tight stenosis at the site documented by the preoperative duplex scan (Fig. 7.27). This was corrected by an endarterectomy and a vein patch.

Although it is also possible to use repetitive measurements of ankle pressure, this does not appear to be as sensitive as the data derived from velocity indices in the graft itself. Because the grafts are in a relatively superficial position within the limb, it is a simple matter to scan their entire length and to do it quickly. The parameters used for the surveillance of grafts have been detailed by Bandyk and associates (26–28). The most important variables include the peak systolic and end-diastolic velocities. The values used in these studies are shown in Table 7.4.

The major findings of this study showed that the peak systolic velocity decreased from the intraoperative value for the femoropopliteal grafts ($p < .05$). The peak systolic velocity of the femorotibial grafts was lower than that obtained from the femoropopliteal grafts at the time of operation. The end-diastolic velocities by 30 days for all grafts were significantly lower than they were for the measurements done at operation. This is as it should be because, at the time of graft placement, there is a reduction in peripheral resistance secondary to reactive hyperemia that will gradually subside over time. The return in vasomotor tone is reflected by the appearance of the reverse flow component.

Bandyk and associates (23–25) were able to classify the postoperative grafts into three categories based on their hemodynamic performance. These are as follows:

Category 1. Low graft peak systolic velocity, less than 40 cm/sec (N = 13).
Category 2. Normal graft peak systolic velocity, more than 40 cm/sec; end-diastolic velocity more than zero with an increase in the ankle/arm index of more than 0.3 to a normal or stable value (N = 96).

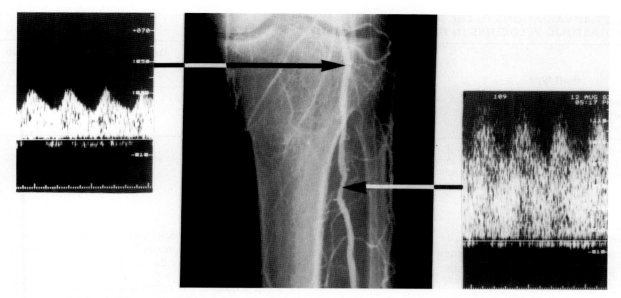

FIGURE 7.26. The duplex scan revealed a short segment with markedly increased systolic and end-diastolic velocities. Although this was suggestive of a stenosis, this was not seen on the arteriogram (see text).

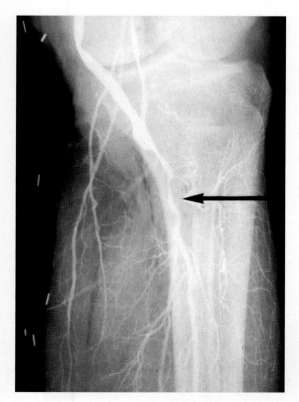

FIGURE 7.27. The operative arteriogram from the patient shown in Fig. 7.26 demonstrated a high-grade stenosis. This was the site at which the high-velocity signal was detected on the preoperative duplex scan. This was corrected by endarterectomy and vein patch (see text). The *arrow* identifies the site of stenosis.

TABLE 7.4. VARIATIONS IN THE PEAK SYSTOLIC AND END-DIASTOLIC VELOCITIES IN IN SITU VEIN GRAFTS

Graft type	No.	Intraoperative		Day 1		Day 30	
		V – p	V – d	V – p	V – d	V – p	V – d
Femoropopliteal	48	81 ± 18	19 ± 11	77 ± 18	16 ± 11	72 ± 12	2 ± 4
Femorotibial	71	74 ± 21	18 ± 11	79 ± 23	22 ± 12	74 ± 16	5 ± 5
Femoropopliteal (Isolated segment)	5	62 ± 17	14 ± 5	63 ± 12	14 ± 8	68 ± 18	7 ± 6

V – p, peak systolic velocity (cm/sec); V – d, end-diastolic velocity (cm/sec).
Adapted from Bandyk DF, Kaebrick HW, Bergamini TM, et al. Hemodynamics of in situ saphenous vein arterial bypass.
Arch Surg 1988;123:477–482, with permission.

Category 3. High graft velocity with a progressive increase in the ankle/arm index; these are small veins that may gradually increase in size in the postoperative period (N = 28).

For those grafts in category 1, there is a problem that will need correction. In the 13 grafts so identified by Bandyk and associates (22–24), 8 were found to be caused by problems that were revised at the time of operation. A sequential graft was applied to three cases, with an improvement in their velocity parameters. There were three in which no problem was identified, and all failed early.

For grafts in category 2, there were 96 with normal graft hemodynamics. One graft failure was caused by heparin-induced thrombocytopenia. Three other grafts had to be revised within 1 month of operation.

For the flow-restrictive grafts in category 3 (N = 28), the problem resolved itself by the end of the first month, due, in most cases, to a small-diameter vein segment. Interestingly, none of the 28 grafts in this category required early revision.

Since the first edition of this book, we have begun an intensive research study of vein grafts to develop better methods of monitoring the changes that occur, their site, and most importantly their natural history (26). Our data support the data of Bandyk in nearly every respect. We studied 61 grafts at intervals of 1, 2, 3, 4, 6, 9, and 12 months, then annually. The secondary graft patency at 3 years was 93.2%. In addition, owing to the improvements in B-mode imaging, we have been able to locate the valves in the reversed saphenous veins and categorize them (27). Although some valves become frozen in the mid-position, producing a stenosis, this was uncommon. In our practice, we have adopted a ratio of more than 3.5, a drop in the ankle/arm index and return of symptoms as an indication for intervention.

The following case illustrates several of the problems that can be encountered, how they can be detected, and how they should be treated.

Case: This 73-year-old white man first underwent a left femoral-popliteal (AK) vein graft 1.5 years before. During fol-

low-up, the patient developed problems at several sites within the vein and in the proximal popliteal artery immediately distal to the insertion of the vein graft.

The lesions at the upper anastomosis (Fig. 7.28) and at the apparent site of a valve cusp (Fig. 7.29) in the distal vein graft were detected by follow-up duplex scanning. Another lesion was detected just distal to the insertion of the vein graft (Fig. 7.29).

The proximal vein graft lesion was repaired with a vein patch, with the distal one handled by sleeve resection and

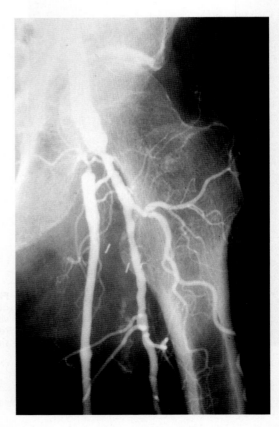

FIGURE 7.28. This illustrates the very tight stenosis that developed at the proximal anastomosis of this saphenous vein graft.

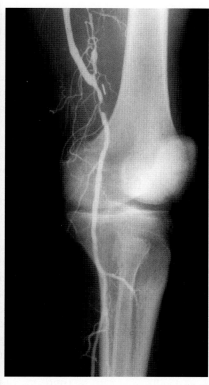

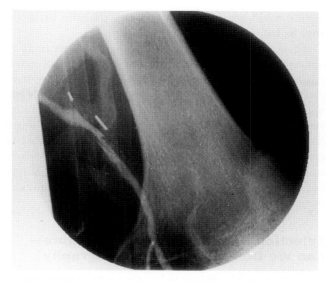

FIGURE 7.30. Immediate results with intraoperative angioplasty.

FIGURE 7.29. The very tight stenosis that occurred at the site of a valve cusp in the distal vein is shown. The stenosis in the proximal part of the popliteal artery is also shown. This was corrected by balloon angioplasty at the time of operation.

an end-to-end repair. The lesion in the popliteal artery was treated intraoperatively by balloon dilatation with an immediate good result (Fig. 7.30).

The above therapeutic measures were effective in restoring the limb hemodynamics to normal. However, by the end of the second month of surveillance, it was clear that new problems were developing in the popliteal artery beyond the anastomosis. The arteriogram depicting the changes that occurred in the artery is shown in Fig. 7.31.

This patient illustrates several aspects of vein graft function and failure that are worthy of comment. First, the problem that developed at the site of the proximal anastomosis was a myointimal lesion typical of that which occurs at all sites of vascular injury. The valve lesion, although appearing much the same as that seen at the proximal anastomosis, was discrete and may have been an old injury. The popliteal artery lesion may represent a recurrent atherosclerotic lesion or another myointimal lesion.

The striking finding was the rapidity with which these lesions can develop and the extent to which they can involve the graft or artery. For example, the extensive popliteal artery involvement shown in Fig. 7.31 developed in less than 3 months. This undoubtedly was the result of

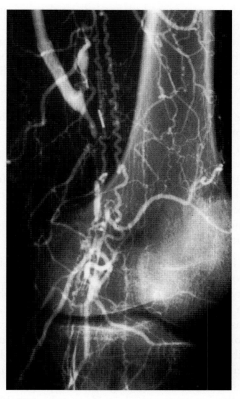

FIGURE 7.31. The extent of the stenoses involving the popliteal artery is shown. This artery had been the site of a balloon angioplasty less than 3 months before this arteriogram.

the intimal injury that took place at the time the intraoperative balloon angioplasty was performed.

These studies of graft performance are important to understand because, for the first time, we can use objective guidelines to monitor grafts and increase their long-term patency. The practice of performing a vein bypass graft and not regularly monitoring its performance at frequent intervals during the first year is no longer acceptable. Although the time frame for follow-up may vary, it is my view that an early postoperative scan (within 1 month), followed by a study every 3 months, should be done. If a lesion is found, the follow-up interval may have to be shortened to document the stability of the lesion.

Selection of the Operative Procedure— Can We Do Away with Arteriography?

If duplex scanning appears to be as accurate as angiography, why can't it be used to select the operative procedure and bypass the invasive studies altogether? It is already apparent to me that it is possible to select those patients who will be candidates for angioplasty, which is a major step forward in planning the therapy for a segment of our population. The problem with selecting the operative procedure, however, is much more complex and will require careful study for the following reasons:

- The choice of a procedure depends on the accurate identification of disease at many levels.
- It is necessary not only to be able to predict the extent of the involvement but also to be able to evaluate both the inflow and, most important, the outflow in the limb.
- There is a need to predict the sites at which the anastomosis can be placed.
- There is a wide variation in surgeon preference for various procedures that may be based on personal bias as much as on the findings.
- There is an impression that the arteriogram not only is essential but also provides the surgeon with a "feel" for the disease he or she is approaching. This is one of those subjective factors that may be the most difficult to surmount. Can we ever convince a surgeon to operate based on data that are heavily functionally oriented?

This is not as novel an idea as it might appear because some groups, including our own, are already doing carotid endarterectomy without the benefit of arteriography. The problem with the carotid artery is not as complex as with the limbs. In the case of the carotid artery, all we have to be certain of is whether the disease seen by duplex scanning is compatible with the clinical picture that is present. Because most cerebral ischemic events occur secondary to high-grade carotid stenoses, carrying out the operation without the benefit of arteriography is unlikely to be a problem.

To test the hypothesis that duplex scanning can be used to predict the proper form of therapy to be employed, we enlisted the assistance of six well-known vascular surgeons (28). These surgeons were asked to choose a treatment plan consisting of eight possible categories from which they could select their preference. The categories of decisions allowed were (a) no intervention, (b) percutaneous angioplasty, (c) operative endarterectomy, (d) aortobifemoral bypass, (e) femorofemoral bypass, (f) femoropopliteal bypass, (g) combined aortofemoral and femoropopliteal bypass, and (h) other. The duplex scans and arteriograms from 29 patients were selected as the target group. The data from both the duplex scan and the arteriograms were transferred to an anatomic diagram and submitted in a random fashion in two batches. They were presented with a brief clinical history along with the ankle/arm indices and, where appropriate, the results of an exercise test.

The intraobserver agreement between different surgeons was good (mean kappa statistic of 0.70 with exact agreement in 76% of the cases). Interobserver agreement was not as good, with a mean kappa statistic of 0.56. It was of interest that there was significant disagreement in 43% of the cases in which the data available on the duplex scan and arteriogram were identical. This discrepancy suggests that the major differences were in the decision-making process and not based on the data per se.

Legemate and colleagues (29) in 1989 also addressed the potential for arteriography to be replaced by duplex scanning. This study included 40 patients with 620 arterial segments that had been studied by both duplex scanning and arteriography. The criteria they employed were slightly different than those developed by us. They used a more than 150% increase in peak systolic velocity from one segment to another as indicative of a more than 50% diameter-reducing lesion. For the aortoiliac area, these criteria gave a sensitivity of 92% with a specificity of 98%. For the femoropopliteal segment, the sensitivity and specificity were 90% and 100%, respectively. For the detection of occlusions in the aortoiliac segments, the sensitivity and specificity were each 100%. Based on the excellent studies done here and in Holland, we believe it is time to avoid the preoperative arteriogram in selected cases (29).

What does this mean? It perhaps indicates that, with further study, we may be able to define those circumstances in which it will be adequate to proceed with the operation without resorting to angiography as an essential step.

REFERENCES

1. Marinelli MR, Beach KW, Glass MJ, et al. Noninvasive testing versus clinical evaluation: a prospective study. *JAMA* 1979;241: 2031–2034.
2. Beach KW, Bedford GB, Bergelin RO, et al. Progression of lower extremity arterial occlusive disease in type II diabetes mellitus. *Diabetes Care* 1988;11:464–472.
3. Bruins Slot HCK, Strijbosch L, Greep JM. Interobserver variability in single plane arteriography. *Surgery* 1981;90:497–503.
4. Sumner DS, Strandness DE Jr. Aortoiliac reconstruction in

patients with combined iliac and superficial femoral occlusion. *Surgery* 1977;28:348–355.

5. Gosling RG, Dunbar G, King DH, et al. The quantitative analysis of occlusive arterial disease by a noninvasive ultrasonic technique. *Angiology* 1971;22:52–55.

6. Skidmore R, Woodcock JP. Physiological interpretation of Doppler-shift waveforms: theoretical considerations. *Ultrasound Med Biol* 1980;6:7–10.

7. Sheriff SB, Barber DC, Martin TRP, et al. Mathematical feature extraction applied to the Doppler shifted signal obtained from the common carotid artery. In: Taylor D, Stevens AL, eds. *Blood flow: theory and practice,* 14th ed. London: Academic Press, 1983: 235–259.

8. Strandness DE Jr. Transluminal angioplasty: a surgeon's viewpoint. *Am J Roentgenol* 1980;135:998–1000.

9. Thiele BL, Bandyk DF, Zierler RE. A systematic approach to the assessment of aortoiliac disease. *Arch Surg* 1983;18:477–485.

10. Thiele BL, Strandness DE Jr. Accuracy of angiographic quantification of peripheral atherosclerosis. *Progr Cardiovasc Dis* 1983; 26:223–236.

11. Jager KA, Phillips DJ, Martin RL, et al. Noninvasive mapping of lower limb arterial lesions. *Ultrasound Med Biol* 1985;11:515–521.

12. May AG, DeWeese JA, Rob CG. Hemodynamic effect of arterial stenosis. *Surgery* 1963;53:513–524.

13. Carter SA. Response of ankle systolic pressure to leg exercise in mild or questionable arterial disease. *N Engl J Med* 1972;287:578–582.

14. McDonald DA. *Blood flow in arteries.* Baltimore: Williams & Wilkins, 1960:271.

15. Kohler RR, Nance DR, Cramer MM, et al. Duplex scanning for diagnosis of aortoiliac and femoropopliteal disease: a prospective study. *Circulation* 1987;76:1074–1080.

16. Cohen J. A coefficient of agreement for nominal scales. *Educational and psychological measurement* 1960;20:37–46.

17. Hatsukami TS, Primozich J, Zierler RE, et al. Color Doppler characteristics in normal lower extremity arteries. *Ultrasound Med Biol* 1992;18:167–171.

18. Hatsukami TS, Primozich JP, Zierler RE, et al. Color Doppler imaging of lower extremity arterial disease: a prospective validation study. *J Vasc Surg* 1992;16:527–533.

19. Edwards JM, Coldwell DM, Goldman ML, et al.. The role of duplex scanning in the selection of patients for transluminal angioplasty. *J Vasc Surg* 1991;13:69–74.

20. Cox GS, Young JR, Gray BH, et al. *Ultrasound guided compression of traumatic pseudoaneurysms.* Midwestern Vascular Surgical Society, Cincinnati, September 11, 1992 (abstr).

21. Hallet JW, Dougherty MJ, James EM, et al. Optimizing technical success of renal revascularization: does intraoperative color flow duplex ultrasonography enhance results? Midwestern Vascular Surgical Society, Cincinnati, September 11, 1992 (abstr).

22. Bandyk DF, Mills JL, Gahtan V, et al. Intraoperative duplex scanning of arterial reconstructions: fate of repaired and unrepaired defects. *J Vasc Surg* 1994;20:426–432; discussion, 432–433.

23. Bandyk DF, Cato RF, Towne JB. A low blood flow velocity predicts failure of femoropopliteal and femorotibial bypass grafts. *Surgery* 1985;98:799–809.

24. Bandyk DF, Kaebnick HW, Bergamini TM, et al. Hemodynamics of in situ saphenous vein arterial bypass. *Arch Surg* 1988;123: 477–482.

25. Bandyk DF, Schmitt DD, Seabrook GR, et al. Monitoring functional patency of in situ saphenous vein bypasses. *J Vasc Surg* 1989;9:286–296.

26. Caps MT, Cantwell-Gab K, Bergelin RO, et al. Vein graft lesions: time of onset and rate of progression. *J Vasc Surg* 1995;22:466-475.

27. Tullis MJ, Primozich J, Strandness DE Jr. Detection of "functional" valves in reversed saphenous vein bypass grafts: identification with duplex ultrasonography. *J Vasc Surg* 1997;25: 522–527.

28. Kohler TR, Andros G, Porter JM, et al. Can duplex scanning replace arteriography for lower extremity arterial disease? *Ann Vasc Surg* 1990;4:280–287.

29. Legemate DA, Teeuwen C, Hoeneveld H, et al. The potential for duplex scanning to replace aortoiliac and femoropopliteal angiography. *Eur J Vasc Surg* 1989;3:49–54.

8

THE RENAL ARTERIES

Renovascular hypertension is the most common cause of secondary hypertension (1). Its prevalence is a source of debate primarily because there has never been a suitable, simple screening test to document its presence. It is estimated that it may involve between 1% and 6% of unselected hypertensive patients. In patients older than 50 years of age, atherosclerosis is the most common cause, with more than 80% of the lesions involving the proximal renal artery. In patients younger than 40 years of age, fibromuscular dysplasia (FMD) is most common; the involvement can occur at all levels of the renal artery.

The screening procedures designed to detect these patients have been disappointing. These have included the rapid-sequence urogram, radionuclide renal scanning, and, more recently, intravenous digital subtraction arteriography (2,3). The urogram and radionuclide studies have a true positive rate of only 80%, with an unacceptably high false-positive rate of 11% and 25%, respectively.

Intravenous digital subtraction arteriography, although initially promising, has not lived up to its expectations. The method does not have sufficient resolution, nor does it provide enough views of the renal arteries to support its use either for screening or as a definitive method of documenting the areas of involvement and estimating their hemodynamic significance (4).

Standard contrast studies remain the definitive diagnostic approach for documenting the location and degree of arterial stenosis. Because of the invasive nature of these studies, they are reserved for those patients who are considered candidates for some form of intervention. Another problem that is of concern is the potential hazard of contrast-induced renal failure. This is a particular risk for patients with preexisting renal disease or disease secondary to bilateral renal artery stenosis. Although digital intraarterial studies can be done with a much lower load of contrast material, they also present some risk in the setting of renal damage, whatever the cause.

The diagnosis of renovascular hypertension requires three elements: (a) documentation of narrowing of one or both renal arteries, (b) evidence that the lesions are hemodynamically significant, and (c) evidence that the lesions are compatible with the clinical picture of a renal vascular cause of the elevation in blood pressure.

Gifford (1) has provided a picture of the magnitude of the problem, which is enormous, given the total number of patients who might be candidates for screening and follow-up if a suitable noninvasive test were available. The total population with hypertension in the United States is in the range of 20 million people. Of this group, about half have fixed hypertension. Within this fixed group of hypertensive patients, 500,000 have chronic renal disease, 400,000 have renal arterial disease, and 260,000 have true renovascular hypertension.

In practice, not all patients with hypertension are candidates for screening. Vaughan (4) has established the following guidelines for screening purposes:

- Malignant hypertension
- Young patients with hypertension
- Presence of a bruit
- Decreased serum potassium
- Azotemia.

For patients who do not fit into these categories but do have severe hypertension, Vaughan proceeds with plasma renin levels. If these are high, the workup includes differential renal vein and inferior vena cava renin level tests with captopril, followed by selective arteriography if lateralization is noted.

It would be ideal if a noninvasive test could provide the necessary data on the renal arteries and the parenchyma of the kidney when the patient is considered to be a potential candidate for treatment. It would be useful if the main renal arteries could be shown either to be free of involvement or to harbor high-grade stenoses. For a screening test to be of value, it must not result in a large number of false-positive results, in which case unnecessary arteriography might be the end result. In addition, a high false-negative rate is not desirable because patients will be missed who might well benefit from some direct form of intervention such as angioplasty or surgery.

The pharmacotherapy of hypertension has made great strides. In most patients with renovascular hypertension, control of blood pressure is not the problem. The one issue that is becoming more important and relevant to the entire field is that of renal failure secondary to bilateral renal artery stenosis. It is this subset of patients in whom there is little evidence that drugs used to control the hypertension may affect the progressive nature of the renal artery atherosclerosis and the subsequent renal failure. If we are to make any progress with this aspect of the problem, we must be able to identify patients who will be at risk for the subsequent development of renal failure. These patients must be identified before the renal parenchymal changes become irreversible and not treatable by any of the currently available direct means, be it surgery or angioplasty. As will be noted in this chapter, we have made some progress in this regard, and the use of duplex scanning will come to play an increasingly important role in the long-term evaluation of patients with renovascular hypertension.

The ability to examine the renal arteries directly has a great advantage. Because the same test could be used to follow patients to monitor the results of therapy, whether it is surgery, angioplasty, or medical treatment, this would be important particularly if the method were without risk to the patient. This is one of the major potential advantages of duplex scanning. It is the only noninvasive method that can be used for long-term repetitive studies. Assessing the natural history of renal artery stenosis will be one of the major applications of duplex scanning.

ROLE OF DUPLEX SCANNING IN THE STUDY OF THE MAIN RENAL ARTERIES

Several improvements in the technology of duplex scanners have made it feasible to study the renal arteries: (a) improvements in scanhead design, (b) the addition of real-time spectral analysis, (c) the availability of lower transmitting frequencies, (d) the addition of microprocessor-based software, and (e) better image resolution. Norris and co-workers (5) first used the method to study 120 patients who had undergone arteriography. In 10 of 12 patients with stenosis of more than 60%, an increase in the peak systolic velocity was detected in the renal artery. In eight arteries with a less than 40% diameter reduction and in four arteries with a 40% to 50% diameter reduction, there was no apparent increase in the peak systolic velocity.

Greene and colleagues (6) and Avasthi and associates (7) found that duplex scanning was 89% sensitive and 73% specific in detecting stenoses that exceeded 50% in terms of diameter reduction. In these studies, four parameters were used to make the diagnosis of renal artery disease: (a) a peak velocity more than 100 cm/sec, (b) absence of flow at end-diastole, (c) absence of flow denoting an occlusion, and (d) the finding of a broad band of frequencies due to turbulence.

When we began to examine this area and the potential for duplex scanning, there were several questions that needed to be answered in the course of evaluating the method:

1. With what regularity can the renal arteries be imaged?
2. Can reproducible velocity signals be obtained from the renal arteries?
3. Would estimates of renal size be important?
4. Are changes in the parenchyma of the kidney important?
5. Will it be possible to detect multiple renal arteries and occlusion of the main renal artery?
6. Is it possible to detect changes in renovascular resistance secondary to disease of the renal parenchyma?
7. Will it be possible to use duplex scanning to detect rejection of the transplanted kidney?

Before considering each of these questions, it is important to review the procedure used for scanning because it is critically important in achieving the best possible results. This examination is the most difficult that we carry out, and it requires the greatest amount of dedication by the technologist. This test should be done only by those who are willing to take the time to understand the procedure and to do a complete examination. The depth of the arteries, the motion imposed by respiration, and intraabdominal gas contribute to the problems in doing the study. Because of these factors, it is important that the patients be studied early in the morning if at all possible and after an overnight (12-hour) fast. This will diminish the amount of bowel gas and also ensure that the stomach is empty.

The procedure begins with the patient in the supine position and the head of the bed elevated about 30 degrees. A low-frequency scanhead (2.5 to 3.0 MHz) is used to image the abdominal aorta longitudinally from an anterior midline approach. A representative aortic velocity waveform is recorded at the level of the renal arteries. This serves as the reference signal for comparison with those recorded from the renal arteries. Although we are not sure of its significance, we have noted that the peak aortic velocity tends to decrease as a function of age (8). It may be that, with aging, there is a progressive dilatation of the large arteries, which explains this decrease. Whether this will be reflected in the renal artery velocity patterns is as yet unknown, but we have elected to use this information for the studies that will be reviewed shortly. It is possible in nearly all cases to identify the left renal vein, which serves as an important landmark in the search for the renal arteries.

To localize the renal arteries, the scanhead is rotated 90 degrees. Even though the image resolution of most systems in use has improved considerably, it is still not sufficient in many cases to see the renal arteries throughout their length. The technologists will first identify the origin of the renal arteries and then follow them by the velocity signals obtained. It is important that signals be obtained from the entire length of the vessels to avoid missing any lesions that might be present. It is also important that the technologist be aware of the possibilities of multiple renal arteries because these can also harbor lesions that are responsible for the development of renovascular hypertension.

It is important to realize that it is often difficult to know the precise relationship of the incidence of the sound beam with the long axis of the vessel. As noted in Chapter 7, in assessing the velocity changes from peripheral arteries, it is possible to use the angle of incidence more regularly, because of the regular and predictable course of the vessels. It is for this reason that we have chosen to express the results in terms of ratios relating the velocity to that recorded from the aorta.

For estimation of renal size and to assess the flow patterns from the renal medulla and the cortex of the kidney, the patient is rolled to the side, and the kidney is approached from the flank.

REGULARITY OF IMAGING THE RENAL ARTERIES

By using the 12-hour fast, it is possible to study 90% of the patients who are referred for the study. The failures are largely due to the presence of bowel gas, previous surgery, or obesity. If the problem is due to bowel gas, it is possible to reschedule the patient for another examination that may be successful the second time. The technologist is also able, in most cases, to determine the extent to which the examination has been successful. This is important because it is not acceptable to obtain spurious data or to provide results that may be wrong and place the patient in an improper category.

A great advantage of the method is the fact that, once a patient has been studied successfully, it is likely that repeat studies can be done with the certainty that additional information can be obtained. This is of great importance for follow-up studies designed to monitor the changes that might have occurred.

The diagnosis of renal artery stenosis depends entirely on the velocity changes detected along the course of the renal arteries. Imaging is of value only for locating the necessary landmarks for identification of the renal arteries. The renal arteries supply an organ that requires high flow for optimal performance. This places it in the category of a low-resistance organ, such as the brain and liver. Thus, one would expect high end-diastolic flow, with no reverse flow component at any time during the heart cycle (Fig. 8.1). Although the normal waveform usually shows a clear window beneath

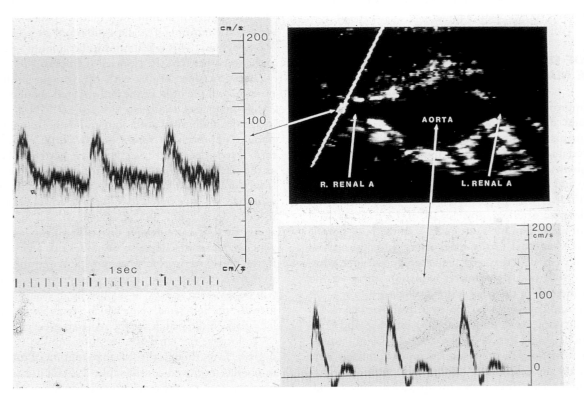

FIGURE 8.1. The normal velocity pattern recorded from the mid-portion of the right renal artery. There is a high end-diastolic velocity that is characteristic of an organ with a low peripheral resistance. (From Taylor DC, Kettler MD, Moneta GL, et al. Duplex ultrasound scanning in the diagnosis of renal artery stenosis: a prospective evaluation. *J Vasc Surg* 1988;7:363–369, with permission.)

the systolic peak, spectral broadening cannot be used reliably as an index of stenosis. This is because the sample volume size used to monitor the flow is normally increased to encompass the entire artery during the study. This prevents the sample volume from moving out of the field of interest, making the examination more difficult and time-consuming. This is an advantage because the distance between the abdominal wall and the artery changes—often a great deal with each respiration.

EFFECT OF DISEASE ON THE RENAL ARTERY VELOCITY PATTERNS

The effects of narrowing the lumen of the renal artery are similar to those in other areas of the circulation (Fig. 8.2). There is an increase in the velocity within the narrowed segment that reflects the degree of narrowing. Although it would be desirable to grade the degree of narrowing into the same categories used for peripheral arteries, this is not possible at the present time. The major goal of the study is to identify the velocity changes that are consistent with the degree of stenosis sufficient to activate the renin-angiotensin system. As noted in Chapter 3, this appears to be a diameter reduction that exceeds 60%. Of course, it is also important to be able to detect a total occlusion of the renal artery.

Because of the difficulties in separating the entire spectrum of disease of the renal artery, we explored those velocity criteria that might lend themselves to the diagnosis of a more than 60% stenosis. It soon became apparent that the best variable to use was the ratio of the peak systolic velocity in the renal artery to that obtained from the aorta (RAR). This has the benefit of using the aortic velocity as the reference in each patient and does, to some extent, get around the problem of attempting to assess the velocity in absolute terms.

To test the potential validity of the RAR as a diagnostic endpoint, we retrospectively examined its relationship to the findings in 43 renal arteries that had arteriographic confirmation. An RAR of 3.5 appeared to provide good separation in 90% (20 of 22 diseased arteries). This served as the basis for the prospective evaluation subsequently carried out and reported by Taylor and colleagues (9).

The prospective study group consisted of 250 duplex scans, with 58 renal arteries that had arteriography within 1 month of the study. The duplex studies and the arteriograms were read independently of each other. The results of this trial are summarized in Fig. 8.3 and Table 8.1.

The results of the screening procedure gave a sensitivity of 84% and a specificity of 97%, with a 93% overall agreement with arteriography Are these results satisfactory as a screening test? For a population with a low prevalence of disease such as renal vascular hypertension, it is important that the number of normal subjects who are thought to have the problem be kept as low as possible to avoid an invasive and dangerous procedure such as arteriography. If these results hold true, it appears that only 3 of every 100

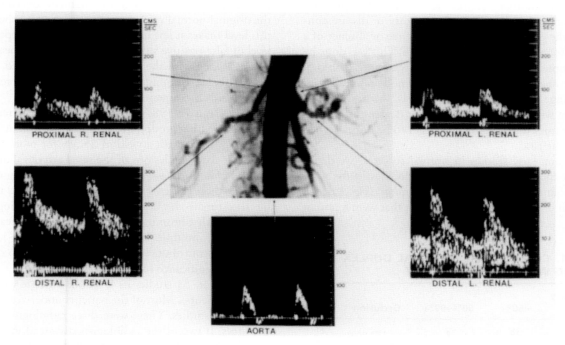

FIGURE 8.2. Bilateral renal stenosis. In this patient with bilateral fibromuscular hyperplasia, there is a large increase in the peak systolic velocities recorded from the areas of stenosis as compared with the normal levels found in the proximal right and left renal arteries.

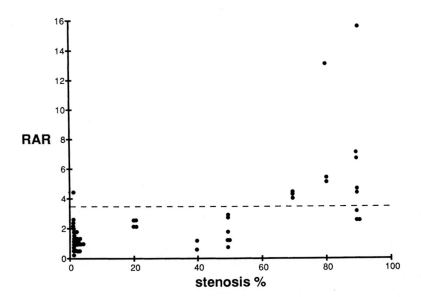

FIGURE 8.3. The renal/aorta ratio *(RAR)* plotted against the degree of renal artery stenosis as determined by arteriography. (From Taylor DC, Kettler MD, Moneta GL, et al. Duplex ultrasound scanning in the diagnosis of renal artery stenosis: a prospective evaluation. *J Vasc Surg* 1988;7:363–369, with permission.)

normal subjects screened might be subjected to the invasive procedure. The sensitivity is lower, but, here, the results are better than reported with other screening procedures.

In this study, there were five renal artery occlusions with four detected. We have come to recognize that renal size can be important in suggesting the presence of an occlusion. If the kidney length is less than 9 cm, it is important to look closely for an occluded renal artery.

In the study reported in 1991, Hoffman and associates (10) included another variable not used in the previous studies. As noted earlier, the only category of disease considered in the early studies was the presence or absence of a more than 60% diameter-reducing lesion. This was done by simply computing the RAR ratio; if it was more than 3.5, the patient was classified as having a hemodynamically significant range of narrowing. Obviously, with this ratio alone, there will be patients with lesser degrees of stenosis that will be missed and perhaps thought to be normal when that is not the case.

During our early studies in normal subjects, we determined that the normal peak systolic velocities in the renal artery were in the range of 100 ± 20 cm/sec (Fig. 8.4). In theory, then, if a velocity value exceeding that were found, it

could be associated with a renal artery stenosis. If we were able to determine accurately the angle of incidence of the sound beam with the renal artery, we would be able to estimate precisely the peak systolic velocity. However, because of the depth and course of the renal arteries, it is often difficult to determine precisely this angle and hence to measure an accurate peak systolic velocity. Because of this problem, we elected to use a peak systolic velocity of 180 cm/sec as the cutoff level for normal subjects. A velocity threshold of 180 cm/sec represents more than two standard deviations above the original normal values we obtained. Setting the cutoff at this level makes it less likely to lead to an unacceptably high level of false-positive studies. Incorporating the peak systolic velocity along with the RAR, we again evaluated the accuracy of duplex scanning for both the detection of renal artery disease and an estimation of its severity.

From January 1987 to August 1989, we screened 427 patients. In this group, we were able to obtain complete studies in 87%, with a yield of 25.3% for more than 60% diameter-reducing lesions of the renal arteries. For the purpose of this study, we investigated the accuracy of duplex for only those patients with atherosclerosis. It is not possible to estimate the degree of stenosis by arteriography in patients with fibromuscular disease. This is because there are usually multiple lesions ("string of beads"), each of which may contribute in an uncertain manner to the hemodynamic significance of the process (Fig. 8.5).

There were 51 studies in 47 patients (there were 5 studies in 3 patients). Most of the patients underwent intraarterial digital studies. There were three radiologists who read the films. If two of the radiologists disagreed in their reading, the third radiologist was involved, and his reading was considered to be the correct one.

The criteria used for the duplex study were as follows:

TABLE 8.1. COMPARISON OF RENAL DUPLEX SCANNING WITH ARTERIOGRAPHY

Arteriography duplex (%)	<60%	60%–99%	Occlusion	Total
0–59	38	3	—	41
60–99	1	11	1	13
Occlusion	—	—	4	4
Total	39	14	5	58

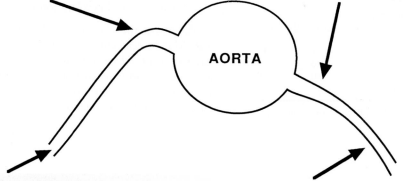

PROXIMAL RIGHT RENAL

PEAK SYSTOLIC VELOCITY = 104 ± 25 CM/SEC

DIASTOLIC / SYSTOLIC RATIO = .33 ± 0.07

RENAL / AORTIC RATIO = 1.19 ± 0.36

PROXIMAL LEFT RENAL

PEAK SYSTOLIC VELOCITY = 93 ± 19 CM/SEC

DIASTOLIC / SYSTOLIC RATIO = .33 ± 0.06

RENAL / AORTIC RATIO = 1.08 ± 0.34

AORTA

DISTAL RIGHT RENAL

PEAK SYSTOLIC VELOCITY = 100 ± 23 CM/SEC

DIASTOLIC / SYSTOLIC RATIO = .34 ± 0.07

RENAL / AORTIC RATIO = 1.15 ± 0.33

DISTAL LEFT RENAL

PEAK SYSTOLIC VELOCITY = 88 ± 19 CM/SEC

DIASTOLIC / SYSTOLIC RATIO = .35 ± 0.06

RENAL / AORTIC RATIO = 1.02 ± 0.32

N=42 (16 MALES, 26 FEMALES)
MEAN AGE = 54 MEAN BP = 129/76

FIGURE 8.4. Data on the peak systolic velocity, the diastolic/systolic velocity ratio (EDR), and renal/aortic ratio (RAR) in 42 normal subjects.

- If the peak systolic velocity was less than 180 cm/sec, the patient was considered normal.
- If the peak systolic velocity was more than 180 cm/sec, the patient was classified as having a stenosis, but no attempt was made to classify it on this basis alone.

- If the RAR was less than 3.5 with a peak systolic velocity of more than 180 cm/sec, the diagnosis of a stenosis of less than 60% was made.
- If the RAR was more than 3.5 with a peak systolic velocity of more than 180 cm/sec, the diagnosis of a more than 60% diameter-reducing lesion was made.
- If there was no detectable renal artery signal with a kidney length of less than 9 cm, the diagnosis of renal artery occlusion was made.

The results as compared with arteriography for the detection of disease based on a peak systolic velocity of 180 cm/sec are shown in Table 8.2.

FIGURE 8.5. It is impossible to estimate accurately the degree of narrowing when the "string of beads" of fibromuscular disease is found.

TABLE 8.2. RESULTS OF USING 180 CM/SEC PEAK SYSTOLIC VELOCITY AS THE CUTOFF POINT FOR THE DETECTION OF RENAL ARTERY STENOSIS

	Arteriography		
Duplex	Normal	Disease	Total
Velocity < 180 cm/sec	9	4	13
Velocity > 180 cm/sec	1	60	61
Total	10	64	74

Sensitivity, 94%; specificity, 90%; accuracy, 93%; kappa statistic, 0.74.

TABLE 8.3. COMPARISON OF DUPLEX VS. ARTERIOGRAPHY FOR DETECTION OF A >60% DIAMETER REDUCING STENOSIS

| Duplex | Arteriography | | | |
	<60% diameter reduction	>60% diameter reduction	Occluded	Total
RAR < 3.5	15	3	1	19
RAR > 3.5	11	45	0	56
Occluded	0	0	10	10
Total	26	48	11	

Sensitivity, 92%; specificity, 58%; accuracy, 81%; kappa statistic, 0.66.
RAR, renal/artery ratio.

The results of detecting a more than 60% diameter-reducing stenosis are shown in Table 8.3. It should be noted that the specificity of 58% is quite low. However, in the 11 cases with an RAR of more than 3.5 in which the arteriographic reading was less than 60%, it was not that duplex missed a stenosis but, rather, a matter of disagreement as to how tight the lesion was. It has also been our experience that, if a patient has hypertension and we find a renal artery stenosis, an arteriogram may be ordered if the clinical picture supports the diagnosis of renovascular disease and if some form of intervention may be needed.

In this early study, accessory renal arteries could not be reliably detected by duplex scanning. Seven accessory renal arteries were seen on the arteriograms, and none of these was seen on duplex study. However, in none of the cases in this series were lesions in an accessory renal artery the basis for the hypertension. With experience and the assistance of color and power Doppler, accessory renal arteries are detected more frequently.

ROLE OF HILAR DUPLEX SCANNING FOR SCREENING PURPOSES

Because of the difficulties in performing the standard renal artery duplex study outlined previously, some authors have proposed the use of hilar scanning as a much simpler method of screening. Handa and co-workers (11) and Martin and colleagues (12) have proposed this as an alternative method for detecting significant renal artery lesions. The procedure is much simpler in that one does not attempt to locate and identify the main renal arteries but rather confines one's efforts to the recording of the arterial signals from the hilum of the kidney using a translumbar approach. There are basically three elements that are used in the classification scheme for screening purposes. These are as follows:

1. Pattern of the recorded velocity as shown in Fig. 8.6. This is simply a pattern recognition method that notes the presence or absence of certain elements within the waveform.
2. Determination of the acceleration index (Fig. 8.7).
3. Measurement of acceleration time (Fig. 8.7)

Based on the criteria of Handa and co-workers (11) and Martin and colleagues (12), the changes considered indicative of a hemodynamically significant stenosis are an acceleration time of less than 100 msec and an acceleration index of more than 291 cm/sec^2. If any one of these three are found to be positive, a complete duplex scan

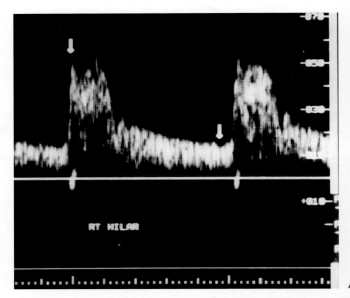

A

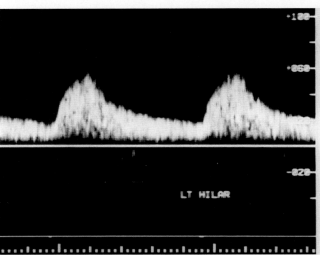

B

FIGURE 8.6. Normal **(A)** and abnormal **(B)** hilar velocity signals. The abnormal signals are observed distal to a high-grade renal artery stenosis.

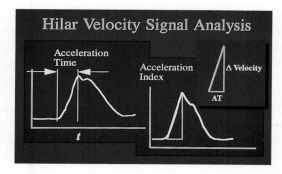

FIGURE 8.7. Hilar velocity signal analysis. This illustrates the measurement of the acceleration index and acceleration time.

ARE CHANGES IN RENAL PARENCHYMA IMPORTANT?

It is clear, as already noted, that some patients with hypertension will have the problem on the basis of parenchymal changes that may add to the resistance to flow and be a primary cause of the blood pressure elevation. It would be ideal if the renal duplex scan could, in addition to providing information on the status of the renal arteries, also provide data on the resistance to flow within the kidney. As noted earlier, the end-diastolic flow to a low-resistance organ, such as the kidney, should be well above zero. Conversely, if the resistance to flow is abnormally high, the end-diastolic velocity should be closer to zero and, in some cases, reach zero (5).

Because it is not possible for duplex scanning to give all the parameters for a quantitative evaluation of peripheral resistance, we chose to express the end-diastolic velocity in relation to the peak systolic velocity (the end-diastolic ratio, or EDR). To arrive at this figure, the end-diastolic velocity or frequency is divided by the peak systolic velocity or frequency. We evaluated this ratio in 42 normal subjects with a mean age of 54 years (16 men, 26 women). Their mean blood pressure was 129/76 mm Hg. The results for the EDR, as well as the RAR, are shown in Fig. 8.4.

To evaluate the relationship between the serum creatinine and the EDR, we studied this in 80 patients who had an RAR of less than 3.5. As the serum creatinine level increased, there was a progressive decrease in the EDR (−0.46; $p < .01$). The EDR may have two uses: first, to identify parenchymal disease as a cause of the hypertension when the renal arteries are free of involvement; second, as a predictive element in deciding which patients are apt to improve or not when a renal artery corrective procedure is carried out. Our data to the present are not complete enough to warrant definitive conclusions. However, we have encountered patients who have gone into renal failure secondary to causes other than renal artery problems in whom the EDR did reflect a marked increase in resistance to flow.

One of the major problems has been to verify the ongoing pathologic process within the kidney during the study. It is also important to show that the duplex findings can be modified or changed by the therapy being given. The ultra-

should be carried out. If this approach were satisfactory, it would make the entire screening process much simpler, easier to perform, and more readily accepted by the vascular diagnostic laboratories in the United States and abroad.

We have investigated this approach in a series of 44 patients who were screened for renal artery stenosis by two technologists. One completed the standard duplex scan, and the second completed only the hilar study. Eighty-six renal arteries were scanned in this manner. The mean examination time for the standard test was 69 minutes, as compared with 14 minutes for the hilar scan. Using the RAR as the diagnostic cutoff point for a more than 60% stenosis, the results are shown in Table 8.4. When a test is used for the study of a population with a low prevalence of disease, such as is found with renovascular hypertension, it is important to have a test with a high sensitivity. Because the prevalence of disease (here defined as a more than 60% stenosis) is low, a high specificity and negative predictive value are less meaningful. The low sensitivity of hilar scanning suggests that it is not a satisfactory method for screening patients for the presence of a high-grade renal artery stenosis. If this method had been used alone for this study, 38% of the more than 60% stenoses would have been missed. Another defect of the hilar scan is that it does not differentiate between a high-grade stenosis and a total occlusion of the renal artery.

TABLE 8.4. RESULTS OF HILAR DUPLEX SCAN AS COMPARED TO STANDARD APPROACH

Hilar indices	Specificity (%)	Sensitivity (%)	PPV (%)	NPV (%)	Accuracy (%)
Acceleration time	89	62	50	93	85
Acceleration index	79	62	35	92	76

PPV, positive predictive value; NPV, negative predictive value.

sonic studies include recordings from the main renal artery, those in the renal hilum (segmental or interlobar), and those at the junction of the medulla and the cortex of the kidney. The studies also include an estimate of renal parenchymal resistance that, in the case of our laboratory, would be the EDR. There are other indices that look at similar changes but are expressed in a different manner and referred to by another name. It has been established both clinically and experimentally that the end-diastolic velocity appears to be the most sensitive index of changes in resistance to flow. Norris and colleagues (5) and Rittenhouse and associates (13), in experimental preparations, demonstrated that, as the resistance to flow increased, the end-diastolic flow decreased.

RENAL ARTERY SCANNING AND LONG-TERM FOLLOW-UP

When a patient is scanned and found to have a high-grade stenosis, this information is important in planning the form of therapy that might be in order. The patient shown in Fig. 8.8 was a middle-aged woman with severe intractable hypertension. The scan demonstrates high lesions in the middle and distal renal arteries that were consistent with the diagnosis of FMD. The arteriographic study and the plan for angioplasty were determined from this study. She underwent a bilateral angioplasty with immediate relief of her hypertension. However, within a few weeks, it was noted that her hypertension was recurring. Repeat duplex scanning revealed that the originally detected stenoses had not been relieved. Another attempt at angioplasty produced the same results, and she went on to have bilateral vein grafts to the renal arteries with good results.

The patient illustrated in Fig. 8.9 posed a particular challenge. She was a 35-year-old woman who had lost her right kidney as a child secondary to an accident. She developed severe hypertension that was not possible to control.

The duplex scan revealed fibromuscular hyperplasia that involved the middle and distal renal artery and the branch vessels as well. Dilatation was done and was successful in controlling her blood pressure for a few days. The repeat scan showed no changes. She went on to have an *ex vivo* repair by Dr. Richard Dean.

One of the major unknowns in the field of renal vascular hypertension has been the fate of the lesions and its relationship to the clinical outcome. The traditional measure of success has been the response of the blood pressure to the therapy applied.

There have been few studies that have documented the fate of the high-grade stenoses involving the renal arteries. Schreiber and colleagues (14) studied 85 patients with repeat arteriograms over a period of 52 months. The following were found:

1. Progression of the lesions occurred in 37 patients (44%).
2. Total occlusion occurred in 14 patients, and this was most common when there was a more than 75% stenosis noted at the initial study.
3. A decline in renal function was most common in those patients who had disease progression.

We were able to follow 19 renal arteries in 15 patients who had a more than 60% stenosis and no intervention (15). All 19 arteries remained patent, but there was a significant decrease in renal size (mean difference in renal length of more than 1.0 cm, $p < .01$) during a follow-up period of 13 months. This is an intriguing finding in that the decrease in renal mass may be the first indication that renal failure may occur. This would be true, of course, only if there were bilateral involvement. As noted earlier, when the renal artery is occluded, the renal length has been below 9 cm.

There were five patients who underwent angioplasty on six arteries. There was relief of the stenosis by duplex scanning in two patients, with improvement in their hypertension. There was continued evidence of a high-grade steno-

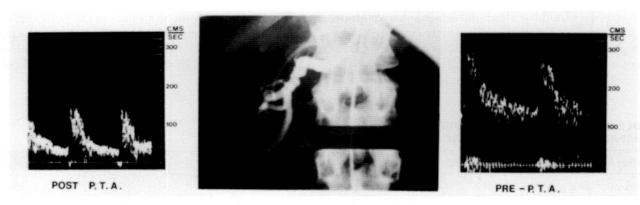

FIGURE 8.8. This patient with fibromuscular hyperplasia underwent a transluminal angioplasty with restoration of the velocity signals to normal. Within a few weeks, these lesions recurred (see text).

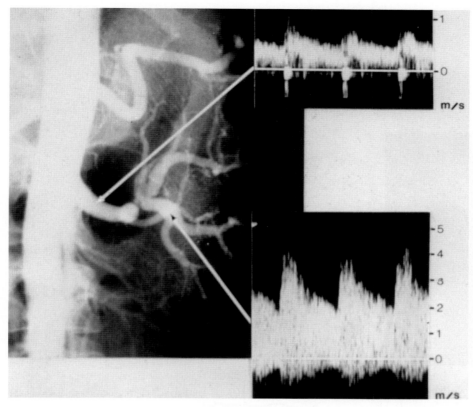

FIGURE 8.9. This 35-year-old woman with a solitary left kidney and severe hypertension was noted by duplex scanning to have a high-grade stenosis of the terminal renal artery (see text).

sis in three patients whose hypertension did not improve. There were 10 stenotic arteries in seven patients who underwent surgical bypass grafting. At a mean follow-up of 9 months, repeat studies revealed continued patency in eight arteries and occlusions in two that were unsuspected. Examples are shown in Figs. 8.10 and 8.11.

The one subset of patients with renovascular hypertension that is most favorable for transluminal angioplasty includes those with fibromuscular hyperplasia (16). These patients are discovered by the presence of lesions that usually involve the middle to distal renal artery. As noted earlier, the lesions are usually multiple, making it difficult to assess the hemodynamic significance. In our institution, when fibromuscular hyperplasia is found by duplex scanning, the patient is often referred for arteriography and transluminal angioplasty. The response to the dilatation is based on the response of the blood pressure and more recently to the changes in the RAR. Because duplex scanning was used in the first instance to detect the lesions, it is only natural that it would be repeated to document the results of therapy.

To assess the role of duplex scanning as a monitor of the endpoint after transluminal angioplasty, we have studied 18 renal arteries in nine patients that had been treated directly

(16 arteries had angioplasty, 2 had surgery for failed angioplasty) (16). The patients were classified into two groups based on their clinical response. These are as follows:

Group 1. Patients with a beneficial blood pressure response (less than 150/90 mm Hg) and no medications were considered successes. In addition, patients who were normotensive with medications or had a diastolic pressure of less than 90 mm Hg without medications were considered successes.

Group 2. Patients who did not show a blood pressure response to the treatment as listed in Group 1 were considered to be failures.

The patient treatment groups consisted of all women, with a mean age of 38.9 ± 8.6 years. Hypertension was present in 100%. The average duration of hypertension was 6.5 ± 10 years. Mean systolic and diastolic blood pressures were 172 ± 49 mm Hg and 97 ± 18 mm Hg. The treatment given averaged 1.8 antihypertensive medications per patient (range, 1 to 3).

For 14 of the 18 treated arteries, there was a satisfactory blood pressure response. In each case, there was a fall in the RAR to levels below 3.5. In two of the four patients whose blood pressure did not respond to therapy, the RAR

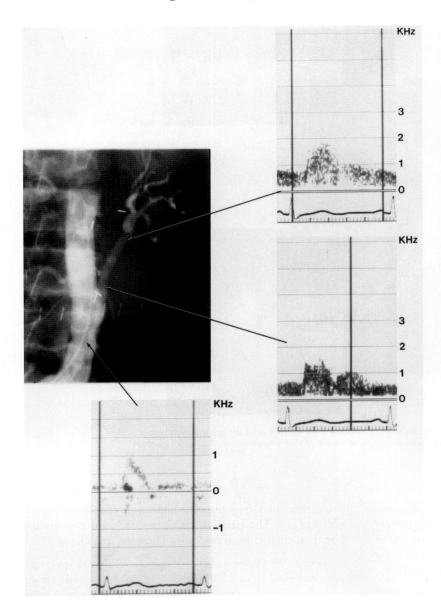

FIGURE 8.10. This postoperative study of a left aortorenal graft confirmed continuing patency and normal velocity signals.

remained high (more than 10 in each instance). In one of the other failures, the RAR fell from 9.0 to 3.5. In the final patient, the RAR went from 3.9 to 4.1. There were two patients who had single or multiple recurrences after angioplasty. In each patient, the recurrence was accompanied by an increase in both the blood pressure and the RAR. Because duplex scanning can be used for detection of renal artery stenosis, we believe it should be more widely used for monitoring the response to therapy, be it endovascular or surgery. One of the striking features of FMDs that may explain their favorable response to angioplasty is their very low parenchymal resistance.

Frauchiger and colleagues (17) examined the prognostic significance of intrarenal resistance in patients with renal artery intervention. In a group of 32 patients with 35 interventions, the EDR appeared to be predictive of outcome.

Patients in the FMD group did well and had an EDR of more than 0.3, which was in the upper range of normal for young adults. This is clearly not the case in patients with renal artery atherosclerosis.

Why should patients with atherosclerosis have evidence of parenchymal vascular disease? The classic studies of Goldblatt (18) predicted that this might occur. Our own studies (19) examining this issue tend to support the hypothesis of Goldblatt. However, this still does not explain why patients with FMD are so different in this respect.

It is clear that duplex scanning will be the only feasible method of long-term follow-up. The repeat studies are easier to do because we know the initial status of the artery and the procedure that was done to relieve the problem. Because of these facts, we have embarked on a natural history study of patients with duplex-detected renal artery disease who

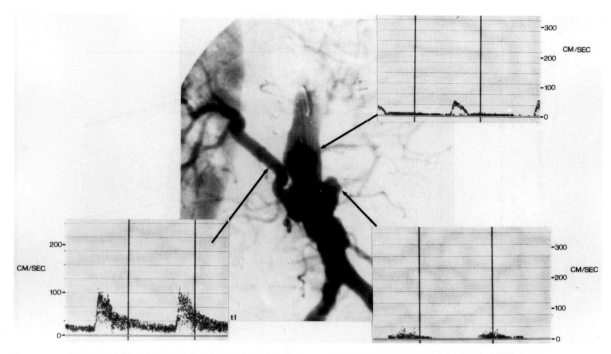

FIGURE 8.11. Velocity waveforms obtained after operation in a patient with bilateral aortorenal grafts. The occluded graft on the left was not suspected. (From Tullis MJ, Zierler RE, Glickerman DJ, et al. Results of transluminal angioplasty for atherosclerotic renal artery stenosis: a follow-up with duplex sonography. *J Vasc Surg* 1997;25:46–54, with permission.)

are being treated for hypertension (20). The purpose of this study is to document the natural history of renal artery lesions and to assess which parameters are most useful for predicting outcome both in terms of the hypertension and, most importantly, renal function.

Guzman and associates (20) reviewed the effects of having renal artery disease on several parameters, the most important of which is renal mass. A total of 54 patients (22 men, 32 women; mean age, 65.2 years) were followed for an average of 14.4 months (range, 4 to 24 months). The criteria used for detection of renal artery stenosis were as outlined previously using both the peak systolic velocity and the RAR for classification of the degree of disease in the renal artery. In this group, 101 sides were available for analysis. The patients were seen every 6 months, and at each visit, a clinical questionnaire and repeat duplex study was performed. We also performed blood urea nitrogen and creatinine tests as rough indices of renal function.

As noted previously, estimation of renal mass was an important part of this long-term follow-up study. For this measurement, the patient was placed in the lateral decubitus position, and the B-mode image was optimized to bring the maximal renal length into view. Three separate measurements were made for both the longitudinal and width dimensions from which the averages were calculated. On the basis of a variability study using a single observer and the same duplex scanner, a measurement threshold of more than 0.71 cm was regarded as a significant change in size between measurements. This represented two standard deviations above the mean in variability. For the purpose of the long-term changes, kidney length changes of more than 1 cm were considered significant. The changes in kidney length were compared with those obtained at the time of the baseline visit. The disease class at study intervals for patients who sustained a more than 1 cm decrease in renal length is shown in Table 8.5. The average rate of decrease in

TABLE 8.5. DISEASE CLASS IN KIDNEYS THAT DECREASED IN SIZE BY >1 CM IN LENGTH

	Months of follow-up				
Disease class at baseline	6	12	18	24	Total
Normal	0/5	0/2	0/10	0/8	0/24
<60% stenosis	0/13	0/5	0/7	0/7	0/32
>60% stenosis	1/9	4/7	7/24	2/10	14/50

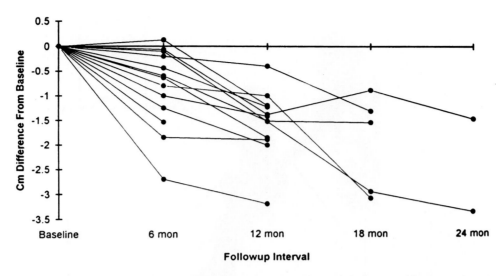

FIGURE 8.12. Time course of change in kidney length in those that decreased by more than 1 cm.

size for patients with a more than 1 cm decrease in size is 0.15 cm (range, 0.6 to 0.27) per month (Fig. 8.12).

When length changes are considered by patients, the data are as shown in Table 8.6. When the data are displayed by life-table analysis for the sides with a more than 60% stenosis, the risk for a more than 1-cm decrease in size at 12 months is 20%. The pattern with regard to those with unilateral and bilateral stenoses of more than 60% is shown in Fig. 8.13. These data strongly suggest that a high-grade renal artery stenosis is associated with a progressive loss of renal mass.

Although we have established that stenoses of more than 60% by our criteria were associated with loss of renal mass, we carried out a much larger study examining the risk factors that might be associated with this loss (21). For this study, we included 204 kidneys in 122 patients who had been followed for a mean of 33 months. It was again confirmed that renal atrophy was likely to occur when the stenosis was more than 60%. There were several baseline risk factors that were predictive of a loss of 1 cm or more of renal length. These were:

- Systolic pressure of more than 180 mm Hg. Cumulative incidence of atrophy was 35% at 2 years ($p = .01$).
- Renal artery peak systolic velocity of more than 400 cm/sec. Cumulative incidence of atrophy was 32% at 2 years ($p = .02$).
- Renal end-diastolic velocity of less than 5 cm/sec. Cumulative incidence of atrophy was 29% at 2 years ($p = .046$).

These data are graphically shown in Figs. 8.14 to 8.17. Finally, one element of the problem that needed to be examined was the rate of progression of the renal artery stenosis. For this study, we included 295 kidneys in 170 patients followed for a mean of 33 months (22). The 3-year cumulative incidences of progression were 18%, 28%, and 49% for arteries initially classified as normal, less than 60%, and more than 60% stenosis, respectively. There were nine renal artery occlusions, each of which was associated with a more than 60% stenosis at baseline. The baseline risk factors associated with progression were as follows:

- Systolic blood pressure of more than 160 mm Hg; RR = 2.1; $p = .006$

TABLE 8.6. DISEASE STATUS IN PATIENTS WITH A >1 CM DECREASE IN RENAL LENGTH

Disease class at baseline	Months follow-up				
	6	12	18	24	Total
Unilateral >60% stenosis					
Contralateral normal	0/1	0/0	1/9	1/5	2/15
Contralateral <60% stenosis	1/3	2/3	0/4	1/2	4/12
Contralateral occluded, nephrectomy	0/3	0/1	4/6	0/0	0/4
Bilateral >60% stenosis					
Contralateral	0/1	1/1	4/6	1/2	6/10

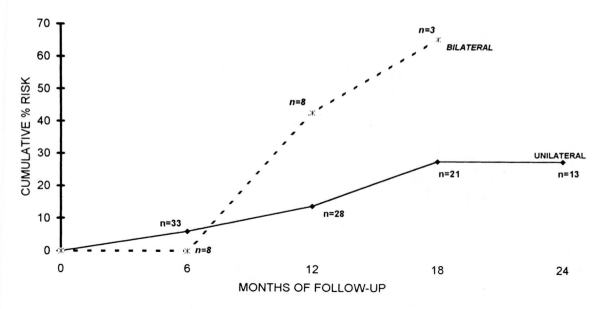

FIGURE 8.13. Cumulative risk of change in renal length (>1 cm) among patients with unilateral as compared with bilateral more than 60% stenosis.

- Diabetes mellitus; RR = 2.0; p = .009
- High-grade ipsilateral renal artery stenosis; RR =1.9; p = .004
- High-grade contralateral renal artery stenosis; RR = 1.7; p = .04

Remarkable about these data is the relationship between the variables collected at baseline and the long-term outcome.

Because renal artery stenosis is theoretically correctable by either angioplasty or surgery, there is a clear role for duplex follow-up. Caps and colleagues followed 41 patients (26 men, 16 women; mean age, 65 years) for a mean of 34 months (22). The cumulative incidences of restenosis from a normal artery to a stenosis of more than 60% were 13 % at 1 year and 19% at 2 years. The cumulative incidences of restenosis from a less than 60% stenosis to a more than 60% lesion were 44% and 55% at 2 years.

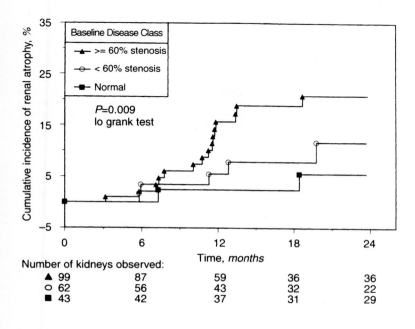

FIGURE 8.14. Cumulative incidence of renal atrophy stratified according to baseline renal artery disease classification. Standard error is less than 10% through 24 months.

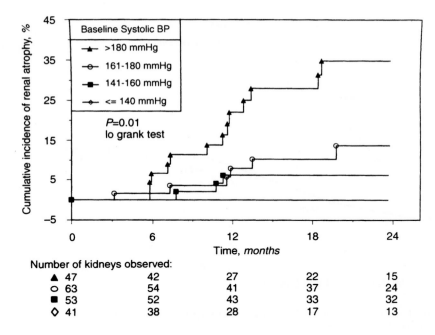

FIGURE 8.15. Cumulative incidence of renal atrophy as related to baseline systolic blood pressure. Standard error is less than 10% through the 24 months.

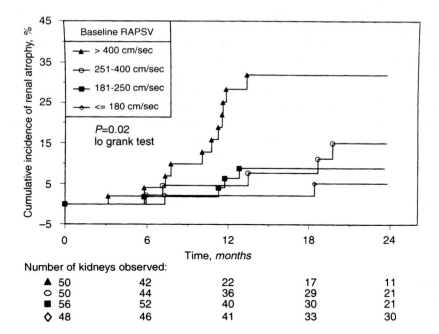

FIGURE 8.16. Cumulative incidence of renal atrophy stratified according to the baseline peak systolic velocity at the site of stenosis. Standard error is less than 10% for the 24 months.

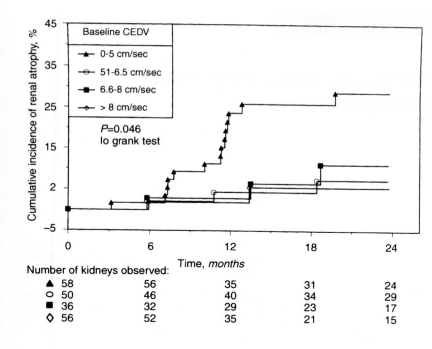

FIGURE 8.17. Cumulative incidence of atrophy as related to the baseline cortical end-diastolic velocity in cm/sec. Standard error is less than 10% for the 24 months of follow-up.

REFERENCES

1. Gifford RW. Epidemiology and clinical manifestations of renovascular hypertension. In: Stanley J, Ernst C, Fry WJ, eds. *Renovascular hypertension.* Philadelphia: WB Saunders, 1984;5:77–99.
2. Grim GE, Luft FC, Weinberger MH. Sensitivity and specificity of screening tests for renal vascular hypertension. *Ann Intern Med* 1979;91:617–622.
3. Treadway KK, Slater EE. Renovascular hypertension. *Annu Rev Med* 1984;35:665–691.
4. Vaughan ED. Renovascular hypertension. *Kidney Int* 1985;27: 811–827.
5. Norris DS, Pfeiffer JS, Rittgers SE, et al. Noninvasive evaluation of renal artery stenosis and renovascular resistance: experimental and clinical studies. *J Vasc Surg* 1984;1:192–201.
6. Greene ER, Venters MD, Avasthi PS, et al. Noninvasive characterization of renal blood flow. *Kidney Int* 1981;20:523–529.
7. Avasthi PS, Voyles WF, Greene ER. Noninvasive diagnosis of renal artery stenosis by echo-Doppler velocimetry. *Kidney Int* 1984;25:824–829.
8. Kohler TR, Zierler RE, Martin RL, et al. Noninvasive diagnosis of renal artery stenosis by ultrasonic duplex scanning. *J Vasc Surg* 1986;4:450–457.
9. Taylor DC, Kettler MD, Moneta GL, et al. Duplex ultrasound scanning in the diagnosis of renal artery stenosis: a prospective evaluation. *J Vasc Surg* 1988;7:363–369.
10. Hoffman U, Edwards JM, Carter S, et al. Role of duplex scanning for the detection of atherosclerotic renal artery disease. *Kidney Int* 1991;39:1232–1239.
11. Handa N, Fukunaga R, Etani H, et al. Efficacy of echo-Doppler examination for the evaluation of renovascular disease. *Ultrasound Med Biol* 1988;14:1–6.
12. Martin RL, Nanra RS, Wlodarczyk J, et al. Renal hilar Doppler analysis in the detection of renal artery stensosis. *J Vasc Technol* 1991;15:173–180.
13. Rittenhouse EA, Maitner W, Burr JW, et al. Directional arterial velocity: a sensitive index of changes in peripheral resistance. *Surgery* 1976;79:350–355.
14. Schreiber MJ, Pohl MA, Novick AC. The natural history of atherosclerotic and fibrous renal artery disease. *Urol Clin North Am* 1984;11:382–392.
15. Taylor DC, Moneta GL, Strandness DE Jr. Follow-up of renal artery stenosis by duplex ultrasound. *J Vasc Surg* 1989;9: 410–415.
16. Edwards JM, Zaccardi MJ, Strandness DE Jr. A preliminary study of the role of duplex scanning in defining the adequacy of treatment of patients with renal artery fibromuscular dysplasia. *J Vasc Surg* 1992;15:604–609.
17. Frauchiger B, Zierler RE, Bergelin RO, et al. Prognostic significance of intrarenal resistance indices in patients with renal artery interventions: a preliminary duplex sonographic study. *Cardiovasc Surg* 1996;4:324–330.
18. Goldblatt H. Studies on experimental hypertension. I. The production of persistent elevation of systolic blood pressure by means of renal ischemia. *J Exp Med* 1934;59:347–379.
19. Tullis MJ, Zierler RE, Glickerman DJ, et al. Results of transluminal angioplasty for atherosclerotic renal artery stenosis: a follow-up with duplex sonography. *J Vasc Surg* 1997;25:46–54.
20. Guzman RP, Zierler RE, Isaacson JA, et al. Progressive renal atrophy with renal artery stenosis: a prospective duplex evaluation. *Hypertension* 1994;23:346–350.
21. Caps MT, Zierler RE, Polissar NL, et al. Risk of atrophy in kidneys with atherosclerotic renal artery stenosis. *Kidney Int* 1998; 53:735–742.
22. Caps MT, Perissinotto C, Zierler RE, et al. Prospective study of atherosclerotic disease progression in renal artery. *Circulation* 1998;98:2866–2872.

## 9

THE MESENTERIC AND PORTAL CIRCULATION

The major clinical problems that can be addressed by duplex scanning involve the arterial supply to the small bowel and the portal circulation to the liver. In the case of the arterial supply to the intestine, it is common for atherosclerotic lesions to involve these vessels, particularly at or near their origins. In the case of the portal circulation, it is the problems associated with portal vein thrombosis or liver disease that lead to the syndromes that are often seen. With atherosclerosis involving the aortic branch vessels to the intestine, the disease adds to the resistance of the inflow vessels, as compared with a disorder such as cirrhosis, which adds to the outflow resistance of the organ. As might be expected, these produce entirely different situations from both the clinical and diagnostic standpoints.

Because the diagnostic procedures used are different, the problems associated with mesenteric ischemia and portal hypertension will be discussed separately.

ARTERIAL SUPPLY

The celiac, superior mesenteric, and inferior mesenteric arteries all originate from the anterior wall of the aorta. About 1 to 2 cm from its origin, the celiac artery divides into its three major branches—the common hepatic, splenic, and left gastric arteries (Fig. 9.1). Those that are easiest to visualize include the celiac, common hepatic, and splenic arteries. The superior mesenteric artery originates about 1 to 2 cm distal to the origin of the celiac artery (Fig. 9.2). It has connections with the celiac artery through the superior and inferior pancreaticoduodenal arteries, which can become important collateral sources to the gut when the superior mesenteric artery becomes diseased. The inferior mesenteric artery is more difficult to visualize and study, but with experience and the availability of color Doppler, it has become much easier to access. Because one of the major problems associated with the development of atherosclerosis is a gradual reduction in blood supply through the involved arteries, it is important to review, in brief, the potential collateral blood supply to the viscera

because it may play a key role determining to what extent the patient becomes symptomatic. The major available pathways are as follows:

1. The left inferior phrenic artery, through its connections with the left gastric artery, can be an alternate source of blood flow to the small intestine in cases of involvement of the superior mesenteric artery.
2. The pancreaticoduodenal arcade is a relatively constant and important connection between the celiac axis and the superior mesenteric arteries. When the lesion involves the superior mesenteric artery alone, this arcade is sufficient to provide normal blood flow to the small bowel.
3. The left colic-middle colic artery anastomosis. The left colic artery, which is normally a branch of the inferior mesenteric artery, will join with the middle colic branch of the superior mesenteric artery. With occlusive disease of the superior mesenteric artery, this artery may enlarge

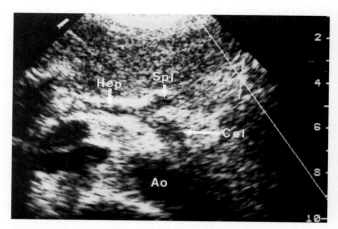

FIGURE 9.1. Ultrasonic cross-sectional image of the abdominal aorta *(Ao)* at the level of the celiac artery *(Cel)* . The hepatic *(Hep)* and splenic *(Spl)* branches of the celiac artery are shown. (From Taylor DC, Moneta GL. Duplex scanning of the renal and mesenteric circulation. In: Rutherford RB, ed. *Seminars in vascular surgery.* Philadelphia: WB Saunders, 1988:23–31, with permission.)

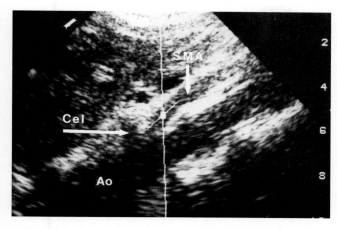

FIGURE 9.2. Longitudinal image of the abdominal aorta showing the position and relationship of the superior mesenteric artery *(SMA)* to the celiac artery *(Cel)* and the aorta *(Ao)*. The sample volume is in the SMA. (From Taylor DC, Moneta GL. Duplex scanning of the renal and mesenteric circulation. In: Rutherford RB, ed. *Seminars in vascular surgery.* Philadelphia: WB Saunders, 1988:23–31, with permission.)

enough to keep the blood supply to the small bowel in a normal range.

4. The internal iliac artery. This artery, through the middle and inferior rectal arteries, has a rich anastomosis that can become important for occlusive lesions in the inferior mesenteric artery.

These rich potential pathways explain why symptomatic chronic mesenteric angina is so rare. For this problem to develop, the atherosclerotic involvement has to be extensive and involve all the major arterial inflow arteries supplying the gut.

CLINICAL SYNDROMES

The major clinical problems seen with regard to the blood supply to the small bowel include acute mesenteric ischemia and chronic mesenteric angina. If the blood supply to the small bowel is suddenly interrupted and the collateral circulation does not have time to respond, the clinical presentation and outcome, if untreated, are quite certain. The small bowel does not tolerate the interruption in its blood supply without the development of dramatic and severe pain, which is crampy in nature and is accompanied by very active peristalsis. This entity is so dramatic that it should not be missed. With this type of clinical presentation, time is of the essence if the small bowel is to be revascularized before the onset of necrosis. The major diagnostic tool used is arteriography, which provides the surgeon with a map of the location of the occlusion and, in some cases, a clue to the etiology of the event. In this circumstance, duplex scanning is not usually done. Arteriography must be done

quickly to avoid any delay in the patient's trip to the operating room. Although confirmation of acute occlusion of the superior mesenteric artery by duplex scanning may be adequate for immediate transport to the operating room, this remains to be shown. The number of cases with acute mesenteric ischemia is not sufficiently large to permit firm conclusions to be made at this time.

Chronic mesenteric ischemia is also uncommon, even though atherosclerosis involving the major arteries supplying the bowel is not unusual (1). The reason for the rarity of the condition relates to the excellent collateral potential that exists in this region. It is well known that, for chronic mesenteric angina to occur, there must be involvement of all three major inputs to the bowel, including the celiac, superior mesenteric, and inferior mesenteric arteries (2). It is also clear, as noted earlier, that the internal iliac artery can be an important collateral pathway to the small bowel. Its contribution to the prevention of developing the syndrome is hard to appreciate but theoretically could be very important. There has been no effort to my knowledge to attempt to study this vessel or its primary branches and their supply to the gut. As will be noted later, we have not seen a case of chronic mesenteric ischemia that has not had involvement of both the celiac and superior mesenteric arteries.

Patients with chronic mesenteric angina present with the "fear of food" syndrome. Every time they eat, they develop cramping abdominal pain and diarrhea that leads to a weight loss that can be profound. They soon find that eating smaller meals more frequently may permit them to get along somewhat better, but, ultimately, the weight loss continues and they are forced to seek medical attention.

The physical findings are usually of little assistance in suggesting the underlying diagnosis. In some cases, an abdominal bruit may be noted in the epigastrium, but this is nonspecific and of little help. Short of proceeding directly to aortography with lateral views of the aorta, there are no other diagnostic tests that provide useful information. Because the diagnosis rests on the finding of high-grade stenoses or occlusions of the major arteries supplying the small bowel, it is only natural that duplex scanning should be used and proves helpful in sorting out the problems associated with making the diagnosis (3,4).

EXAMINATION TECHNIQUE

Patients should be studied in the fasting state (1). This will minimize the amount of gas in the bowel that may interfere with the study. The patient is studied in the supine position with the head of the bed elevated 10 degrees. A 3-MHz scanhead is placed slightly to the left of the midline to permit visualization of the abdominal aorta in a longitudinal plane. When the transducer is aligned in the proper plane with the aorta, the origins of

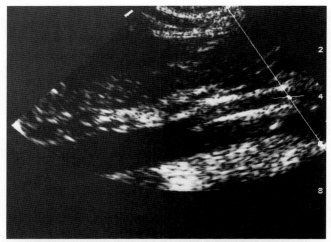

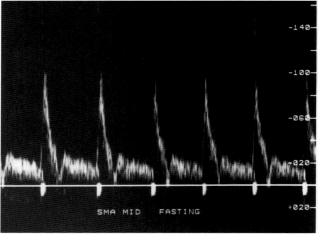

FIGURE 9.3. The waveforms taken from the superior mesenteric artery (*SMA*) in the fasting state.

the celiac and superior mesenteric arteries can be seen. Although demonstration of the arteries on the B-mode image is important, the velocity findings are the critical factors used in making the diagnosis (Fig. 9.3). The sample volume is adjusted to be slightly smaller than the diameter of the arteries. In addition, it is important for the angle cursor to be placed in such a way that the orientation of the incident sound beam with the long axis of the vessel can be recognized and recorded.

As with other examinations looking for areas of stenosis, it is important to search for the highest-velocity signal that can be found. Because atherosclerosis most frequently involves the orifice and first 1 or 2 cm, these areas are carefully examined for areas of narrowing. Although difficult, it is possible, in some patients, to identify and evaluate the inferior mesenteric artery, which may be an important collateral source to the small bowel and may be very large. This is often referred to as a "meandering" inferior mesenteric artery. When present, it is easy to visualize arteriographically.

Moneta and colleagues (3) have shown that in some cases it is possible not only to investigate the inferior mesenteric artery in cases of celiac and superior mesenteric artery occlusions but also to study its blood flow response to a meal. An example of such a case is shown in Fig. 9.4. In this patient with occlusion of the celiac and superior mesenteric arteries, the major source of blood flow to the gut was through the inferior mesenteric artery. This case also demonstrated the fact that the blood flow response to feeding could be entirely normal even though the blood supply to the intestine is through this collateral artery alone.

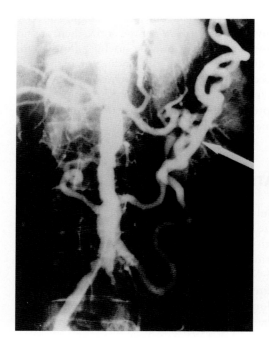

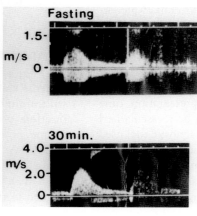

FIGURE 9.4. Illustration of a very large collateral vessel from the inferior mesenteric artery that is supplying the small bowel. There was a normal blood flow response to feeding, as noted in the velocity change. (From Moneta GL, Cummings C, Castor J, et al. Duplex ultrasound demonstration of postprandial mesenteric heperemia in splanchnic circulation collateral vessels. *J Vasc Technoln* 1991;15:37–39, with permission.)

SPLANCHNIC ARTERY WAVEFORMS

As noted in earlier chapters, each organ in the body has its own characteristic velocity patterns that are related primarily to its metabolic activity and the time of day when the examination is carried out. The liver and spleen are low-resistance organs, like the brain and kidney, so that one would expect there would be no reverse-flow component with a high end-diastolic velocity. This is the case. On the other hand, flow in the superior mesenteric artery should vary, depending on the metabolic activity of the gut. In the fasting state, the blood flow patterns reflect the relatively high resistance with the occasional reverse-flow component and the low end-diastolic velocity (Fig. 9.3). As noted in Chapter 3, with eating, this pattern dramatically changes as the resistance to flow decreases and the flow increases (Fig. 9.5).

The normal peak systolic velocity in the abdominal aorta adjacent to the origin of the celiac and superior mesenteric arteries is in the range of 100 ± 20 cm/sec. In theory, then, the normal value for the first few centimeters, which is the most common site for disease to develop, should be somewhat higher because of the change in the diameter of the two arteries. Because it has been possible to establish normal values for other areas of the arterial circulation that might be useful for screening, what about the visceral arteries supplying the gut? One of the confounding problems with the visceral circulation is that the finding of a high-grade stenosis of the celiac and superior mesenteric arteries has little meaning because of the excellent potential collateral circulation that is available.

One of the common reasons for referral to the laboratory is chronic abdominal pain that may or may not be related to eating. When the treating physicians cannot find a cause and the patient is in the age group in which chronic mesenteric angina is a possibility, a referral for study may result. This is not unreasonable because in nearly all cases, the diagnosis can be ruled out with certainty. If we understand the process as previously outlined, the syndrome cannot exist if one or both of the celiac and superior mesenteric arteries is either normal or has lesions that are not pressure and flow reducing. The criteria for normalcy require studies in both normal subjects and patients subjected to arteriography when a reasonable estimate of arterial dimensions can be obtained.

What are normal velocities for these two major inputs to the small bowel? Moneta and co-workers (4) studied patients admitted to their vascular service over an 18-month period who underwent routine mesenteric duplex scanning and, whenever possible, lateral aortography. These studies were done without regard to the presence of abdominal symptoms or signs. The lateral aortograms were graded to determine the presence or absence of a more than 70% diameter-reducing stenosis in the celiac and superior mesenteric arteries. The peak systolic velocities were recorded without any information relative to the arteriographic findings. The study was terminated when 100 patients had been accumulated. All arteries were satisfactorily visualized by arteriography, making grading of the degree of narrowing possible. In these 100 patients, the duplex studies were satisfactory in 93% of the superior mesenteric arteries and 83% of the celiac arteries.

Moneta and co-workers (4) tested the accuracy of using values of more than 200 cm/sec peak systolic velocity for the celiac artery and more than 275 cm/sec for the superior mesenteric artery in detecting a more than 70% diameter-reducing stenosis. The findings were as follows:

- For the superior mesenteric artery, the results showed a sensitivity of 92%, specificity of 96%, positive predictive value of 80%, negative predictive value of 99%, and overall accuracy of 96%.
- For the celiac artery, the results showed a sensitivity of 87%, specificity of 80%, positive predictive value of

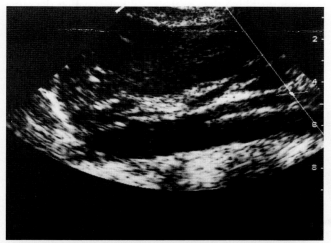
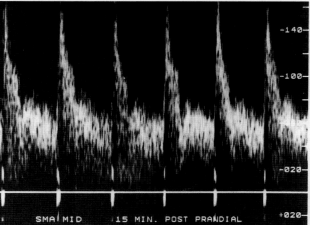

FIGURE 9.5. The dramatic increase in both the peak systolic and end-diastolic velocities is seen. Fasting levels are shown in Fig. 9.3.

63%, negative predictive value of 94%, and overall accuracy of 82%.

These studies have demonstrated the accuracy of detecting these high-grade lesions in the major inputs to the small bowel as compared with arteriography. The variability of arteriography in estimating the degree of stenosis was not tested in the study by Moneta and co-workers (4); therefore, we cannot be sure what the true range of estimations might be for these arteries. The key questions are, How should this type of information be used clinically? and What impact might it have on decision making for patients with suspected chronic mesenteric angina? Fortunately, it is rare when the actual grading of the observed lesions comes into play in making the diagnosis. In part, this may be because the symptoms that are often highly suggestive of the syndrome, when combined with the duplex findings, make the diagnosis relatively straightforward (5).

The anatomic and velocity changes that occur normally after a meal have been well characterized. The changes that occur can be described as follows:

1. There is an increase in the diameter of the superior mesenteric artery. Jäger and colleagues (6) found that the diameter of this artery was 0.60 ± 0.09 cm in the fasting state. Forty-five minutes after ingestion of a meal, the diameter was found to be 0.67 ± 0.09.

2. The velocity changes include an increase in the peak systolic velocity (120 to 190 cm/sec; mean values from 20 persons) and a threefold or greater increase in the end-diastolic velocity.
3. The reverse flow component disappeared.
4. As might be expected, there was also an increase in the time-averaged mean velocity as well as the volume flow to the small bowel. Similar findings have been reported by Nicholls and associates (7) and Moneta and co-workers (8).

In patients with chronic mesenteric angina, there have been dramatic areas of narrowing and/or occlusion of both the celiac and superior mesenteric arteries (5,7). We have not yet encountered a case in which the celiac artery was normal but the inferior mesenteric artery was either occluded or stenosed to a degree sufficient to reduce intestinal blood flow to a critical level during digestion. It has not been necessary to use a food challenge to unmask a stenosis that was not hemodynamically significant in the fasting state. This remains a theoretic possibility that must be kept in mind for the future.

One of the major advantages of this method of documenting the blood flow to the small bowel is that the same studies can be done postoperatively to document the results of therapy, be it direct arterial surgery or angioplasty. Examples of the usefulness of such studies are illustrated in Figs. 9.6 and 9.7.

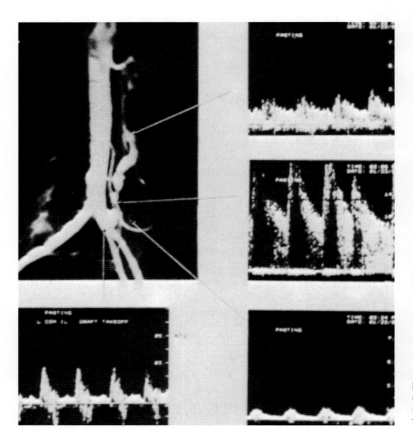

FIGURE 9.6. Nine months after placement of a vein graft from the left common iliac artery, the symptoms recurred. By duplex scanning, a stenosis was found at the proximal end of the vein graft.

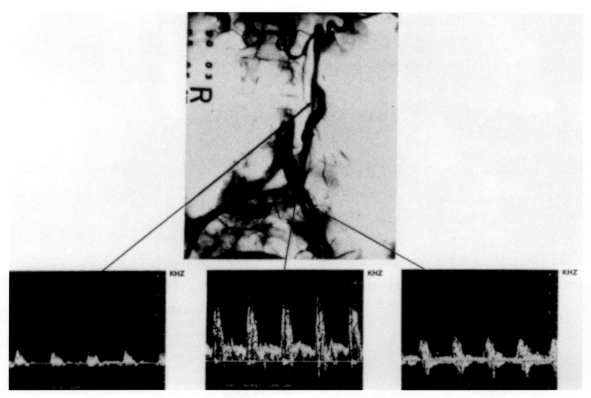

FIGURE 9.7. A transluminal angioplasty was performed on the proximal end of the vein graft shown in Fig. 9.5. There is an improvement in the velocities through the narrowed segment. *DIST SMA*, distal superior mesenteric artery; *PROX ANAST SMA GRFT*, proximal superior mesenteric artery graft; *L COM IL*, left common iliac artery.

THE PORTAL SYSTEM

The blood supply to the liver is unique because of the two inputs through the hepatic artery and the portal vein (Fig. 9.8). Although lesions involving the hepatic artery rarely, if ever, lead to ischemia of the liver, diseases of the liver commonly produce problems that not only destroy the parenchyma but also lead to progressive changes in the resistance to flow that dramatically alter the pathways that the blood in the portal system normally takes (9). In undertaking studies to investigate the portal system, it is important to keep in mind that not all disorders have their origin within the liver. Indeed, portal hypertension can occur because of changes at three sites—prehepatic, intrahepatic, and posthepatic. The most common cause of prehepatic portal hypertension is thrombosis of the portal vein or, less commonly, extrinsic compression, which may have the same effect (Fig. 9.9). In this setting, liver function is found to be normal.

Posthepatic causes of portal hypertension include thrombosis of the hepatic veins or the inferior vena cava. Thrombosis of the hepatic veins most commonly occurs in the setting of a hypercoagulable state such as polycythemia,

a myeloproliferative syndrome, or paroxysmal nocturnal hemoglobinuria. The inferior vena cava may be the site of obstruction because of extrinsic compression by tumors, such as hepatocellular or renal carcinoma.

The most common cause of the intrahepatic form of the disorder that leads to portal hypertension is alcohol, but it must be remembered that there are other etiologic factors, such as postnecrotic and postviral cirrhosis. However, regardless of the underlying cause, the portal hypertension that develops in response to the changes in the liver is the same. Ultrasound and, in particular, duplex scanning are not the primary methods for establishing the diagnosis of portal hypertension; however, they can provide useful information and responses to the following points:

1. The cause of the elevated portal pressure may be identified as being prehepatic, posthepatic, or intrahepatic.
2. It is possible, on the basis of the location and direction of flow, to establish whether the collaterals seen are portohepatic or portosystemic.
3. The direction of flow in the portosystemic collaterals may be of value in determining the potential risk for bleeding. If the direction of flow is toward the superior

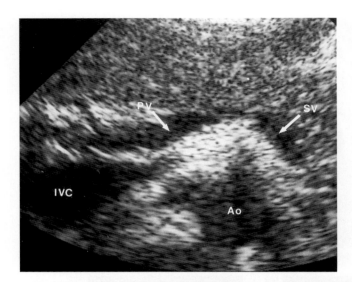

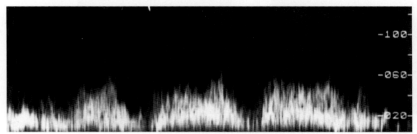

FIGURE 9.8. Top: B-mode image of the right upper quadrant showing the portal vein *(PV)*, splenic vein *(SV)*, inferior vena cava *(IVC)*, and aorta *(Ao)*. **Bottom:** The normal phasic blood flow pattern is noted in the portal vein. (From Taylor DC, Moneta GL. Duplex scanning of the renal and mesenteric circulation. In: Rutherford RB, ed. *Seminars in vascular surgery.* Philadelphia: WB Saunders, 1988:23–31, with permission.)

vena cava, there may be a subsequent risk for bleeding. If the direction is toward the inferior vena cava, there is not any danger of bleeding from esophageal varices.

4. The patency of surgical shunts can be determined, along with the direction of flow. The method is ideal for the long-term follow-up of such patients.

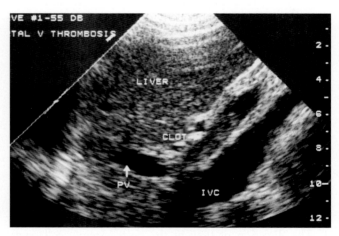

FIGURE 9.9. B-mode scan of the right upper quadrant showing the portal vein *(PV)* and a thrombus that is occluding it. The inferior vena cava *(IVC)* is also shown.

Clinical Applications

The impact of duplex scanning for this area of the circulation has expanded considerably beyond its use for the detection of atherosclerosis of the major visceral arteries discussed earlier in this chapter. To present its current uses, it will be necessary to summarize briefly those areas of greatest interest, and how duplex scanning can play an important role.

Portal Hypertension and Liver Disease

Ultrasound was used for the evaluation of portal hypertension before the availability of duplex scanning. Bolondi and colleagues in 1984 (10) reviewed the role of B-mode alone for the evaluation of portal hypertension in 150 patients. The criteria found to be of value included the following:

- Portal vein diameter of more than 13 mm
- Dilatation of the umbilical vein
- Presence of intraabdominal collaterals
- Splenomegaly with dilatation of radicles of the splenic vein with loss of the normal cyclic variations in size with respiration

All of the above can of course be documented more easily by the added use of the pulsed Doppler, which facilitates identification of the vessels and also provides information relative to the direction of flow.

Attempts have also been made to quantify portal venous flow volume using information from the B-mode image and velocity data from the pulsed Doppler. Moriyasu and associates (11,12) determined portal volume flow by multiplying the product of the mean velocity and the cross-sectional area of the portal vein. The mean velocity was calculated by multiplying the maximal velocity by a coefficient of 0.57. Similar studies were done by Ohnishi and co-workers (13) in 1985. These authors used a coefficient of 0.60 for the estimation of the mean velocity. Ackroyd and colleagues (14) and Gill (15) also studied the role of duplex scanning in the measurement of portal venous volume flow by using the mean flow velocity and venous cross-sectional area. As with estimations of volume flow from this and other areas, there is a wide range of reported normal values (462 to 900 mL/min). This range of normal values is not unexpected given the difficulties in estimating diameter alone, when very small errors give rise to very large errors in calculating the cross-sectional area.

The many problems associated with estimation of portal venous volume flow were reviewed by Burns and associates (16). An assumption that there is a constant relationship between peak velocity and the mean velocity may be incorrect. Because the mean velocity depends on the velocity profile, it is important to know what this is, if at all possible. The velocity profile is dependent on many factors, including flow rate, resistance, vessel compliance, pressure changes, and time of sampling relative to flow from the gut. In addition, as noted previously, serious errors can occur secondary to estimation of the diameter. All of these considerations make the clinical use of volume flow measurements in this area uncertain and unlikely (at least at present) to be of much value. Although portal hypertension appears to result in a decrease in portal venous flow in some patients, this is of no clinical relevance in making the separation between normal subjects and patients with chronic liver disease.

The use of duplex scanning remains important, however, particularly for the documentation of the direction of flow and the presence or absence of thrombi in the portal system. This information is of great value in the evaluation of patients and in selecting the type of shunt that may be of clinical value.

Given the fact that imaging along with Doppler interrogation can be used to document the presence or absence of flow along with its direction, it should not be surprising that Duplex scanning would find an invaluable place in the evaluation of patients after portosystemic shunt surgery. Several authors have used duplex scanning for this purpose, including Ackroyd and colleagues (14), Helton and associates (17), and Grant and co-workers (18). The shunts most easily visualized are the direct portocaval shunts. The information available includes direct visualization of the shunts, flow characteristics, and direction. The sensitivity and specificity have been reported to be nearly 100% for documentation of shunt patency.

Liver Transplantation

Because successful liver transplantation depends on patency of the portal vein, hepatic artery, hepatic veins, and inferior vena cava, duplex scanning should become a part of the routine preoperative screening process. After transplantation, duplex scanning provides the only simple and direct method of documenting patency of the hepatic artery (19–21). Segel and co-workers (21) reported a 100% sensitivity and specificity rate in the 29 patients who were evaluated for consideration of hepatic artery patency. The method can also be used to determine the patency of the inferior vena cava and portal vein.

For all these indications, the use of the Doppler component of the duplex system is absolutely essential to obtain the information. With imaging alone, most of the important information is missing.

REFERENCES

1. Taylor DC, Moneta GL. Duplex scanning of the renal and mesenteric circulation. In: Rutherford RB, ed. *Seminars in vascular surgery.* Philadelphia: WB Saunders, 1988;1:23–31.
2. Fry WJ. Arterial circulation of the small and large intestine. In: Strandness DE Jr, ed. *Collateral circulation in clinical surgery.* Philadelphia: WB Saunders, 1969;24:508–536.
3. Moneta GL, Cummings C, Castor J, et al. Duplex ultrasound demonstration of postprandial mesenteric heperemia in splanchnic circulation collateral vessels. *J Vasc Technoln* 1991;15:37–39.
4. Moneta GL, Lee RW, Caster JD, Cummings CA, et al. Mesenteric duplex scanning: a blinded prospective study. *J Vasc Surg* 1993;17:79–87.
5. Jäger KA, Fortner GS, Thiele BL, et al. Noninvasive diagnosis of intestinal angina. *J Clin Ultrasound* 1984;12:588–591.
6. Jäger KA, Bollinger A, Valli C, et al. Measurement of mesenteric blood flow by duplex scanning. *J Vasc Surg* 1986;3:462–469.
7. Nicholls SC, Kohler TR, Martin BS, et al. Use of hemodynamic parameters in the diagnosis of mesenteric insufficiency. *J Vasc Surg* 1986;3:507–510.
8. Moneta GL, Taylor DC, Helton WS, et al. Duplex ultrasound measurement of postprandial intestinal blood flow: effect of meal composition. *Gastroenterology* 1988;95:1294–1301.
9. van Leeuwen MS. Doppler ultrasound in the evaluation of portal hypertension. In: Strandness DE Jr, Taylor KW, eds. *Duplex Doppler ultrasound.* New York: Churchill Livingstone, 1989.
10. Bolondi L, Mazziotti A, Arienti V, et al. Ultrasonographic study of portal venous system in portal hypertension and after portosystemic shunt operations. *Surgery* 1984;95:261–269.
11. Moriyasu F, Ban N, Nishida O, et al. Quantitative measurement of portal blood flow in patients with chronic liver disease using an ultrasonic duplex system consisting of a pulsed Doppler flowmeter and B-mode electroscanner. *Gastroenterol Jpn* 1984; 19:529–536.
12. Moriyasu F, Ban N, Nishida O, et al. Clinical application of an ultrasonic duplex system in the quantitative measurement of portal blood flow. *J Clin Ultrasound* 1986;14:579–588.
13. Ohnishi K, Saito M, Nakayama T, et al. Portal venous hemodynamics in chronic liver disease: effects of posture change and exercise. *Radiology* 1985;155:757–761.
14. Ackroyd N, Gill R, Griffiths K, et al. Duplex scanning of the portal vein and portasystemic shunts. *Surgery* 1986;99:591–597.

15. Gill RW. Pulsed Doppler with B-mode imaging for quantitative blood flow measurement. *Ultrasound Med Biol* 1979;5:223–225.

16. Burns P, Taylor K, Blei AT. Doppler flowmetry and portal hypertension. *Gastroenterology* 1987;92: 824–826.

17. Helton WS, Montana MA, Dwyer DC, et al. Duplex sonography accurately assesses portacaval shunt patency. *J Vasc Surg* 1988;8: 657–660.

18. Grant EG, Tessler FN, Gomes AS, et al. Color Doppler imaging of portosystemic shunts. *Am J Roentgenol* 1990;154:393–397.

19. Dalen K, Day DL, Ascher NL, et al. Imaging of vascular complications after hepatic transplantation. *Am J Roentgenol* 1988; 150:1285–1290.

20. Longley DG, Skolnick ML, Zajko AB, et al. Duplex Doppler sonography in the evaluation of adult patients before and after liver transplantation. *Am J Roentgenol* 1988;151:687–696.

21. Segel MC, Zajko AB, Bowen A, et al. Hepatic artery thrombosis after liver transplantation: radiologic investigation. *Am J Roentgenol* 1986;146:137–141.

10

DEEP VENOUS THROMBOSIS AND THE POSTTHROMBOTIC SYNDROME

Deep venous thrombosis is the most common vascular disorder that affects patients in the hospital. It has been estimated that at least 800,000 cases are detected each year in the United States. It may be nothing more than a harmless interlude in some patients with minor calf vein thrombosis, but it places other patients at risk for the development of pulmonary embolism and the postthrombotic syndrome. Even though the disease has been with us since antiquity, it still remains a problem in terms of both its recognition and management. Why should this be? It appears that many members of the medical community still feel that it is possible to recognize the condition on the basis of the history and physical examination alone. Nothing could be further from the truth.

It is now clearly recognized that the bedside diagnosis is so inaccurate that an independent objective method must be used to verify the status of the patients' deep veins (1,2). Another factor that has contributed to this problem is the continued use of Homans' sign for the diagnosis, which is not a reliable physical finding and should not be employed.

Before considering the noninvasive tests that can be used to make the diagnosis of deep venous thrombosis, it is important to review the one instance in which the bedside diagnosis for deep venous thrombosis can be useful. The only entity that should not be confused with any other is acute iliofemoral thrombosis (phlegmasia cerulea dolens). This is the result of extensive thrombosis not only of the iliofemoral system but also of the lower leg veins. The clinical picture is dramatic with the sudden onset of total leg swelling, severe pain, cyanosis, and coolness of the limb.

As noted in Fig. 10.1, the entire right leg is swollen from the level of the groin to the ankle. When this is seen, the thrombi occupy not only the iliofemoral system but also those veins distal to the inguinal ligament. In its most severe form, venous gangrene can result.

Another disorder that should not be a diagnostic problem is superficial thrombophlebitis. This is an inflammatory condition with local tenderness, redness, and a palpable venous cord. There is often a rise in the body temperature as well. The process is always accompanied by thrombosis of the involved veins. Its etiology is often obscure, and in my view, it is a distinctly separate entity from deep venous thrombosis. In fact, I

do not use the term *thrombophlebitis* in referring to deep venous thrombosis because this is not an inflammatory condition. Similarly, although it is common to describe the long-term complications of deep venous thrombosis as the *postphlebitic syndrome*, this is also incorrect. The terminology used in this chapter for the long-term complications will be the *postthrombotic syndrome*.

Before reviewing the available noninvasive tests and their application, it is necessary to review the problem of deep venous thrombosis with regard to its clinical significance and the relationship between the levels of involvement and ultimate outcome. The most immediate concern when the diagnosis is suspected relates to the potential for the development of pulmonary embolism. It is well known that emboli that are most likely to be fatal originate from the iliofemoral segment. These are very large veins, and the thrombi that develop there are capable of complete occlusion of the pulmonary circuit. Those that arise from the superficial femoral and popliteal veins may or may not be a cause of death, depending on the extent of the pulmonary circuit that is obstructed and the underlying cardiac and pulmonary disease that is present. It is clearly the large proximal veins that are the most serious in terms of immediate outcome.

The one area of the venous circulation that is relatively silent in terms of both symptoms and signs is venous thrombosis developing below the knee. It is well known that thrombi arise within the soleal sinuses, but they can also arise *de novo* from the tibial and peroneal veins as well as the gastrocnemial veins. If the thrombi remain confined to the area below the knee, they are rarely the cause of significant or even detectable pulmonary emboli. Problems can occur when thrombi propagate to involve the popliteal and superficial femoral vein. This happens in up to 20% of patients if they are untreated (3).

The involvement of veins below the knee is the most confusing and controversial area of the limb with regard to deep venous thrombosis, its recognition, and treatment. As noted earlier in this chapter, the high incidence of calf vein thrombosis was recognized only because labeled fibrinogen was used for the detection of the process. In clinical practice, the instances of calf vein thrombosis confined to below

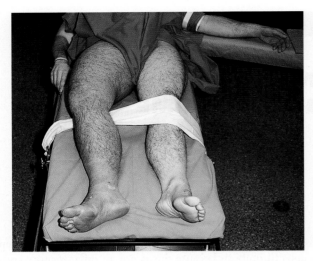

FIGURE 10.1. The entire right leg became massively swollen and was accompanied by severe pain and coolness. This is the typical presentation with iliofemoral thrombosis (extensive). This is also referred to as *phlegmasia cerulea dolens.*

the knee alone are relatively uncommon. In our study of 833 patients with suspected deep venous thrombosis, there were 209 who had a positive duplex study confirming the presence of deep venous thrombosis (4). The distribution of thrombi by leg is shown in Fig. 10.2. It should be noted that the prevalence of isolated-below-the-knee thrombi is low for both the right and left legs (less than 10%).

Because it would appear that both treatment and outcome would depend in large part on the location and extent of venous thrombosis in the lower limbs, it is important to spend some time discussing what we know and its ramifications for both diagnosis and therapy. The reader is urged to consult the appropriate references to this problem. I would like to summarize the important points from my vantage point, which are as follows:

1. Thrombi confined to a single venous segment are unusual. In this context, a single segment is defined as a vein with a proper name. Thus, the superficial femoral vein would be a single segment.
2. The left leg is more commonly involved, which is a fact that is well known. It is thought that the element of

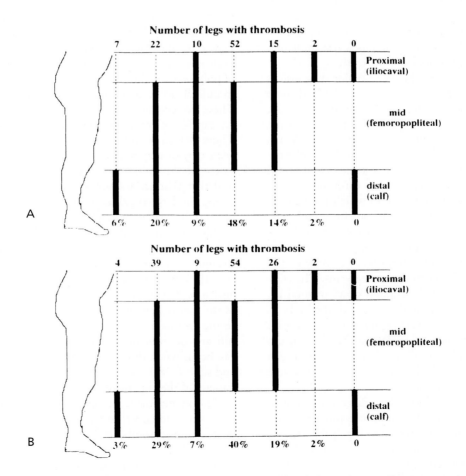

FIGURE 10.2. Distribution of thrombi in the right leg of patients with acute deep venous thrombosis **(A)**; distribution of thrombi in the left leg of patients with acute deep venous thombosis **(B)**.

chronic compression of the left common iliac vein by the right common iliac artery may play a role here.

3. Although patients most often complain of symptoms in one leg only, bilateral involvement was observed in at least 17% of the patients we have studied.

4. The veins most frequently involved in order of frequency are superficial femoral (74%), popliteal (73%), common femoral (58%), posterior tibial (40%), deep femoral (29%), greater saphenous (19%), and the inferior vena cava in only 2%. As noted in Fig. 10.2, multisegment involvement is the most common occurrence with this problem.

5. Although total occlusion of the venous segments occurred in most cases, partially occluding thrombi were not rare, being observed in 18% of patients with acute deep venous thrombosis.

6. Total leg involvement (iliocaval, femoropopliteal, and calf) occurred in 10% of patients. It is this subset of patients who may have the poorest long-term prognosis.

If the patient is treated for deep venous thrombosis, the long-term outcome depends on two major factors—the location and extent of the residual obstruction and the extent of the valvular incompetence that develops. However, it is difficult, if not impossible, to predict the long-term outcome based on the initial presentation. For example, Browse and colleagues (5) showed that it would be impossible to predict, on the basis of the location and extent of the initial involvement, what the long-term results might be. These authors reviewed the phlebograms 5 to 10 years after the event in 67 patients with deep venous thrombosis. In one third of the patients with "severe" thrombosis, there were no undesirable long-term sequelae! Even more confusing is the report by Cockett and Jones (6) that only 27 of 80 patients with venous ulcers gave a history of a previous episode of venous thrombosis.

These studies not only point out the difficulty of predicting the natural history of patients with an initial episode of deep venous thrombosis but also emphasize the need for longitudinal studies in this patient population. We conducted a study of 61 patients who had an episode of deep venous thrombosis verified by objective tests and were followed to document outcome as related to the status of their deep venous system (7). The follow-up period ranged from 1 to 144 months. Pain, swelling, or both were noted in 67% of the patients. Pigmentation occurred in 23% and ulceration in three patients. The most important factor appeared to be the status of the distal deep veins. If these veins were found to be patent and competent, the long-term outcome was good with regard to both symptoms and the development of pigmentation. Only 8% of the limbs with competent distal veins developed pigmentation, as compared with 40% of those with occlusion or incompetence of the valves.

The other long-term, but much less common, complication of deep venous thrombosis is the development of venous claudication. These patients develop severe pain, usually in the thigh, that is brought on by exercise and relieved by rest. In contrast to claudication secondary to arterial disease, the time required for relief of the pain is much greater and may even require elevation of the limb for relief (8). Venous claudication most commonly develops when there is chronic occlusion of the iliofemoral venous segment. The primary problem here is not related to valvular incompetence but to the chronic residual obstruction, which severely limits the rate at which blood can be drained from the limb during strenuous exercise.

All the above information on localization of acute venous thrombi and their relationship to outcome is important to understand when diagnostic methods are being applied. It becomes even more important when it is recognized that what is found with the initial episode may not be the case in the long term. This was highlighted by the study by Killewich and associates (9), who investigated the rates at which thrombi lyse and their relationship to outcome in 21 patients with acute venous thrombosis.

In the patients studied by Killewich and associates (9), spontaneous lysis occurred rapidly in most, even though they were receiving conventional anticoagulant therapy and not fibrinolytic agents. In 11 of the 21 patients, recanalization occurred in all segments by 90 days after the event. In four patients, extension of the thrombi occurred, even though patients appeared to be on adequate anticoagulant therapy. This study highlights the need for sequential and long-term study if any sense is to be made of the data and their predictive nature. It is clear that, if one were to take the level and extent of occlusion at the time the diagnosis was made and attempt to relate it to long-term outcome, the results would be incorrect. The dynamic nature of the changes that occur probably explains the results reported by Browse and co-workers (5) in their 1981 study.

INDIRECT NONINVASIVE TESTS
Continuous Wave Doppler

The development of deep venous thrombosis by definition results in the obstruction (partial or complete) of the involved venous segments. Because continuous wave (CW) Doppler can be used to determine patency of the superficial and deep veins, it was only natural to use this method to detect this problem (10). The great advantage of the method is its ability to study the flow patterns in many of the veins that are commonly the site of venous thrombosis.

In practice, all that is required is a pocket-sized unit that has a transmitting frequency of 5 MHz and an audible output of the velocity patterns that are detected. Because many of the flow changes detected with the pocket units are also used with the duplex scanning method, these will be reviewed now.

The venous flow patterns in the lower limbs are normally dominated by the events and pressure changes that occur with respiration. For example, in the supine position, there is an increase in the intraabdominal pressure with inspiration. The intraabdominal pressures reached are sufficient to result in a transient obstruction in venous outflow from the lower limb. This finding is most evident in the large veins that are accessible to the ultrasonic energy (external iliac, common femoral, and superficial femoral veins). At the level of the ankle, the flow pattern's response to respiration is not so evident in many people, particularly if there is any element of vasoconstriction present.

The method provides useful information if it is carried out in a systematic manner with careful attention to detail. Because the technique is "blind," in a sense, one must use the adjacent artery as the landmark for proper identification of the companion vein. This is most easily accomplished for the large veins down to the level of the popliteal vein. The problems are more difficult when the veins below the knee are examined. Here, it is not possible to be certain that the venous signal being detected is, in fact, the named vein of interest. For this reason, it is common to examine only the posterior tibial veins at the level of the medial malleolus.

If the flow in the major deep veins is phasic with respiration, this is certain evidence that the veins proximal to this point are patent. One obvious concern is with nonocclusive thrombi, which may still permit flow to occur in a normal fashion. In addition, it is not possible to determine the presence of anatomic variants, such as paired major veins, that can occur, particularly in the superficial femoral and popliteal veins. Failure to demonstrate spontaneous flow in the posterior tibial veins does not have the same significance as with the more proximal segments. Here, it is necessary to demonstrate patency by compression of the foot, which will augment the flow to a detectable level (11).

Venous thrombosis affects the flow in two major ways. In the obstructed vein, no flow will be detectable. If the vessel is proximal to the level of venous obstruction, the flow pattern will be continuous and not affected by respiration. In this situation, the flow is being diverted around the area of obstruction by the collaterals and does not appear to be influenced by the normal pressure changes associated with respiration. A key factor in a successful examination is the comparison of the flow patterns from identical sites of both limbs. This is important because there are changes in flow that can occur because of central causes. For example, any increase in venous pressure due to problems involving the right heart and/or the pulmonary circuit can lead to alterations in venous flow that might be interpreted as being secondary to acute venous occlusion.

How accurate is this method? It is not the purpose of this chapter to review in detail the results of the numerous studies that have been done. The reader should refer to the survey of results as summarized by Yao and Blackburn (12). The overall accuracy of the method, as compared with venography, ranges from 49% to 96%. It is clear that the accuracy is dependent on the experience of the technologist carrying out the examination. For the acute occlusions involving the major proximal veins (popliteal to external iliac), the diagnosis should not be missed.

The problems with the CW Doppler method that make it less than optimum for routine screening are as follows:

1. It is entirely dependent on the skill and experience of the examiner.
2. It cannot be quantitated.
3. It cannot distinguish between an occlusion and extrinsic compression.
4. It is of little value in a patient with suspected recurrent venous thrombosis.
5. It is of limited value for thrombi below the knee.
6. It is not a good method for monitoring the results of therapy.

Phlebography

The classic study of Bauer in 1940 (13) demonstrated the utility of this method for visualization of the venous system and the detection of thrombi. This procedure has been the gold standard for the detection of deep venous thrombi but even before the availability of duplex scanning was not widely applied. As mentioned earlier, its lack of widespread acceptance and use has been due to several factors. Probably the greatest factor has been the belief that the bedside diagnosis is adequate. Even Bauer himself in 1957 (14) made a statement that would be unacceptable today:

I may seem to have dwelt unduly long on a description of these symptoms but I am firmly convinced that if a combination of several of the aforementioned general and local signs are recorded, one can be reasonably certain that early thrombosis is present. It is no longer necessary to rely on phlebography to establish the diagnosis. This method was of great value as long as the whole problem was still in the course of investigation, but it is quite superfluous nowadays. The diagnosis can be made by means of routine clinical methods

Although phlebography has been the gold standard, there are serious problems associated with its use. The method itself is designed to provide complete opacification of the deep veins from the level of the calf to the inferior vena cava. There are a variety of methods in use; that described by Rabinov and Paulin (15) is one of the best. With this approach, the dye is injected into a vein on the dorsum of the foot with the patient at 40 degrees with the legs not bearing weight; thus, the muscles are completely relaxed. Even with the best possible technique, there are areas that are not routinely visualized in all patients. The deep femoral vein is visualized in only 50% of patients (16). Another concern is the lack of routine visualization of the common femoral and iliac veins, which occurs in about 18% of patients (16).

Aside from these problems, there has always been a concern that the use of the contrast media may, in and of itself, induce venous thrombosis. This is a difficult issue to prove because it would require a repeat study, which is not often done. In addition, even if the patient develops more symptoms after the study, this is often interpreted as being due to the disease itself. Athanasoulis (16), in a study of patients undergoing total hip replacement who had venograms, found that 53.2% of the patients had normal phlebograms. Clinically evident "phlebitis" developed in 10.6% of this group. When repeat studies were done on these patients, thrombi were demonstrable in 6.4%. Finally, patients find the procedure unpleasant because of the discomfort associated with the injection of the contrast media. The use of nonionic contrast material will make this less of a problem, but the other concerns will remain. Nevertheless, phlebography will remain an important diagnostic test to settle some of the questions that can arise, even with the use of duplex scanning.

Duplex Scanning

The ideal method of investigating the venous system for suspected deep venous thrombosis would be to combine the imaging component of the method with the use of the pulsed Doppler to permit an investigation of the flow patterns that are present. It is of interest that, with the availability of the imaging component, most investigators have implied that the Doppler adds little to the evaluation (17,18). In fact, most of the early studies have emphasized only two aspects of the evaluation: the presence of a visible thrombus and the inability to compress the vein being studied. The presumption is that, if the vein cannot be compressed with the probe, it must be occupied by a thrombus. Before considering whether this is, in fact, the case, there are some obvious areas where this cannot be tested. It is not possible to compress the iliac veins and the inferior vena cava (Fig 10.3). Are these veins insignificant? How can one evaluate them if flow in the visualized segment is not used?

Lensing and associates (19), who used imaging alone, acknowledged that it is impossible to compress the iliac veins but pointed out that isolated iliac vein obstruction is rare in symptomatic patients. I am not convinced that this is, in fact, true, and, even if it were rare, this is the one major venous segment where disease should not be missed because of the potentially disastrous outcome when thrombi of this size become emboli. Furthermore, if one were to take this stand with regard to imaging alone, then it would be imperative to use some other diagnostic test, such as venous outflow plethysmography, to establish the patency or occlusion of this critical venous segment.

To evaluate the role of duplex scanning in the diagnosis of deep venous thrombosis, we conducted a prospective double-blind study in 47 patients who had confirmatory phlebography. This study included one patient with bilateral deep venous thrombosis and two patients who had two duplex scans and phlebograms within the first week after presentation. Thus, there were 50 studies that were included in the analysis (20).

The study was done using a 3.5-MHz transducer for the iliac veins and vena cava and a 7.5-MHz transmitting frequency for the veins of the thigh and below the knee. For examination of the tibial veins, a 10-MHz transmitting frequency was used. All veins were examined in longitudinal sec-

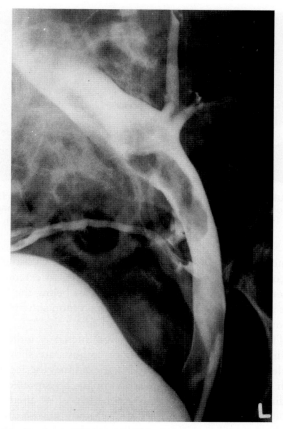

FIGURE 10.3. An example of a nonocclusive venous thrombus detected by duplex scanning in an iliac vein (see text).

tion for the presence of thrombi and the evaluation of flow at that site using the pulsed Doppler. The flow parameters that were investigated included the presence of spontaneous flow, phasicity with respiration, augmentation of flow with distal compression, and augmentation of flow with release of proximal compression or Valsalva's maneuver. In addition, reflux of flow was tested for each venous segment by either proximal limb compression or Valsalva's maneuver. To test compressibility of the venous segments, the probe was rotated 90 degrees to see the vein in cross-section. The criteria used for a positive diagnosis were as follows:

- Visualization of a thrombus (Fig. 10.4).
- Incompressibility of a venous segment. The areas that could not be compressed included the iliac veins, the inferior vena cava, and the superficial femoral vein in the adductor canal.
- Absence of venous flow and/or the lack of phasicity with respiration. The lack of spontaneous flow in the posterior tibial veins was not taken as indicative of venous thrombosis because detection of spontaneous flow is not common, even in normal subjects.

In this initial study, we did not attempt to study the soleal sinuses, peroneal vein, or gastrocnemius veins. It was difficult, with the "black-and-white" systems, to identify

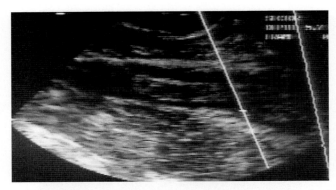

FIGURE 10.4. A nonocclusive thrombus in the superficial femoral vein of a woman in the second trimester of pregnancy. This had propagated from a thrombus in the popliteal vein.

accurately the veins below the knee. However, with the use of color and power Doppler, it is possible to extend the venous studies to include all of the veins below the knee. The anterior tibial vein is such an uncommon site for deep venous thrombosis that it is not studied.

The results of the these various parameters as indicators of the presence of deep venous thrombosis are shown in Tables 10.1 through 10.4. Table 10.1 examines the accuracy with imaging of the thrombus. As might be expected, the finding of a thrombus has a very high positive predictive value (95%). On the other hand, the failure to see a thrombus has a very low negative predictive value of 37%. This is not surprising because it is apparent that, as a thrombus ages, it tends to lose its echogenicity (21,22).

The issue of incompressibility and its importance from a diagnostic standpoint is shown in Table 10.2. Although some groups advocate compressibility alone as the only necessary diagnostic maneuver, this was clearly not the case in our study (20,23). It was our failure to be able to compress veins in some areas, such as the pelvis and the adductor region, that gave rise to these disappointing results. Although one may argue that ignoring these segments may not be a problem, we strongly disagree. If one adopts this attitude, thrombi that could be a serious problem might be missed.

TABLE 10.1. ACCURACY OF VISUALIZATION OF THE THROMBUS

Contrast venography (no. of cases)	Thrombus visualization (no. of cases)		
	Positive	Negative	Total
Positive	19	19	38
Negative	1	11	12
Total	20	30	50

Sensitivity, 19/38 = 50% (95% confidence limits = 34%–66%).
Specificity, 11/12 = 92% (95% confidence limits = 62%–98%).
Positive predictive value, 19/20 = 95% (95% confidence limits = 69%–100%).
Negative predictive value, 11/30 = 37% (95% confidence limits = 14%–59%).

TABLE 10.2. ACCURACY OF VEIN INCOMPRESSIBILITY FOR DIAGNOSIS OF VENOUS THROMBOSIS

Contrast venography (no. of cases)	Vein incompressibility (no. of cases)		
	Positive	Negative	Total
Positive	30	8	38
Negative	4	8	12
Total	34	16	50

Sensitivity, 30/38 = 79% (95% confidence limits = 66%–92%).
Specificity, 8/12 = 67% (95% confidence limits = 40%–93%).
Positive predictive value, 30/34 = 88% (95% confidence limits = 67%–95%).
Negative predictive value, 8/16 = 50% (95% confidence limits = 18%–82%).

If we examine the role of the detected velocity patterns in the diagnosis of venous thrombosis, the results are not surprising. The absence of flow from any visualized vein must mean that the vessel is occluded. There can be no other explanation, unless the flow in that vein is below the velocity threshold for the system. However, as we have learned, if spontaneous flow cannot be elicited, it is a simple matter to augment flow by compression of the limb distal to the site being examined. When this parameter was examined, in and of itself, the results were as shown in Table 10.3.

The other sensitive parameter is the phasicity of flow. As noted earlier, normal venous flow is characterized by cyclic increases and decreases in flow that occur with the respiratory cycle. Alterations in this pattern with venous thrombosis have been known, beginning with our early experience with CW Doppler. When one examines a patent vein that has lost this finding, it is suggestive of a more proximal narrowing or occlusion that has altered the flow patterns. The accuracy of this finding is shown in Table 10.4.

If we examine the combination of variables, the two that had the highest sensitivity were visualization of the throm-

TABLE 10.3. ACCURACY OF ABSENCE OF SPONTANEOUS FLOW IN THE DETECTION OF THROMBI

Contrast venography (no. of cases)	Absence of spontaneous flow (no. of cases)		
	Positive	Negative	Total
Positive	29	9	38
Negative	0	12	12
Total	29	21	50

Sensitivity, 29/38 = 76% (95% confidence limits = 63%–90%).
Specificity, 12/12 = 100% (95% confidence limits = 88%–100%).
Positive predictive value, 29/29 = 100% (95% confidence limits = 85%–100%).
Negative predictive value, 12/21 = 57% (95% confidence limits = 29%–85%).

TABLE 10.4. ACCURACY OF ABSENCE OF PHASICITY OF FLOW IN DETECTING VENOUS THROMBOSIS

Contrast venography (no. of cases)	Absence of phasicity of flow (no. of cases)		
	Positive	Negative	Total
Positive	35	3	38
Negative	1	11	12
Total	36	14	50

Sensitivity, 35/38 = 92% (95% confidence limits = 79%–97%).
Specificity, 11/12 = 92% (95% confidence limits = 62%–98%).
Positive predictive value, 35/36 = 97% (95% confidence limits = 81%–91%).
Negative predictive value, 11/14 = 79% (95% confidence limits = 41%–92%).

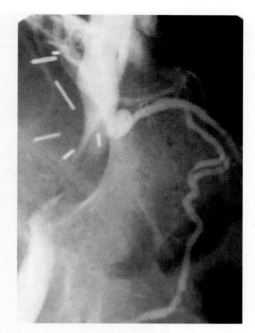

FIGURE 10.5. Acute venous obstruction by external compression of a lymphocele. After drainage of the lymphocele, the venous obstruction was relieved.

bus and the absence of phasicity of flow (95%, with 95% confidence limits of 82% to 98%). The same occurred for specificity, which was 83%, with 95% confidence limits of 52% to 95%. The key factor in the results of our study was the fact that all available information, both with regard to imaging and the Doppler findings, should be used when patients suspected of having deep venous thrombosis are studied. Unless this is done, errors will be made that can be serious. In some cases, confirmatory venography can help prevent errors from occurring (Fig. 10.5).

All of the studies done to confirm the accuracy of duplex scanning were done in black and white. Although this modality alone is satisfactory for the proximal veins (popliteal to inferior vena cava), its greatest limitations were for the venous segments below the knee. Here, the duplication of veins and their size made scanning difficult. However, with the availability of color and power Doppler, the situation has changed. Atri and co-workers used compression ultrasonography and color Doppler imaging to evaluate its accuracy in detecting calf vein thrombi (24). In the comparison with venography in 108 symptomatic limbs,

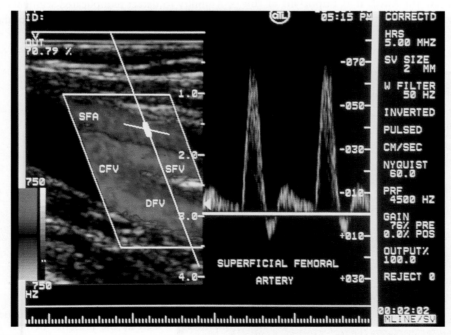

FIGURE 10.6. The use of color to demonstrate the anatomy of the confluence of the common femoral (*CFV*), superficial femoral (*SFV*), and deep femoral veins (*DFV*).

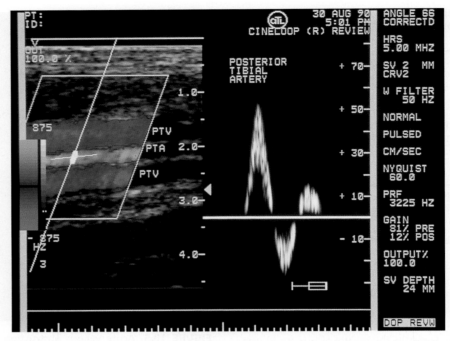

FIGURE 10.7. Anatomy of the paired posterior tibial veins (*PTV*) and the posterior tibial artery (*PTA*) at the level of the ankle.

the method had a sensitivity of 88% (kappa statistic = 0.60). The availability of color has simplified and has sped up the evaluation process. The location of the patent venous segments can immediately be appreciated, as can the adjacent artery. It is also of help in immediately recognizing the partially occluding thrombus by the presence of flow around the thrombus. Examples of the value of color can be seen in Figs. 10.6 to 10.9. Color has become essential for studying the veins below the knee. It is important at this point to note that venous flow in the below-knee segments

may be difficult to detect if the ambient temperature is quite low or if the patient is vasoconstricted. Some systems have "low-flow" transducers to permit detection of very low velocities. This can be of great help, but one must remember that artifacts caused by simple motion of the transducer may introduce disturbing bursts of color in the soft tissues, which can be annoying to the technologist.

Another advantage of both black and white and color is the ability to detect reduplicated segments of the venous system. Reduplication of the superficial femoral, popliteal, or both

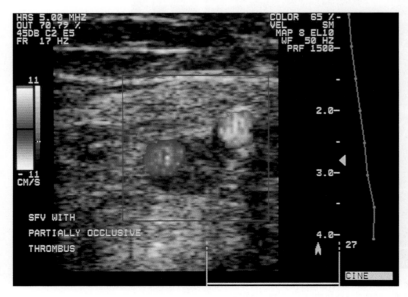

FIGURE 10.8. A partially occluding thrombus can be seen by the presence of flow around the thrombus occupying a portion of the circumference of the vein.

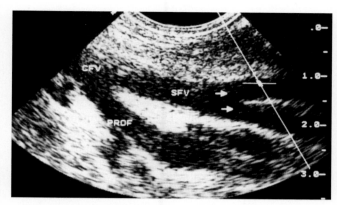

FIGURE 10.9. Reduplication of the superficial femoral vein (*SFV*).

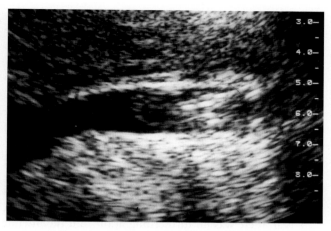

FIGURE 10.10. The filter in the inferior vena cava can be visualized by ultrasound. A thrombus is seen attached to the distal end of the filter.

veins can be seen in up to 20% of the population. This can be extremely important because thrombi may develop in one, leaving the other segment normal. Failure to recognize this could well lead to a false-negative finding and failure to treat a potentially dangerous thrombus. An example of a reduplicated superficial femoral vein is shown in Fig. 10.9.

DOCUMENTATION OF INFERIOR CAVA FILTER FUNCTION

Duplex scanning can be used for the detection of deep venous thrombosis and therefore should prove to be helpful in documenting the long-term outcome after filter placement. Because filters are permanent and are a foreign body, they have the potential for long-term complications. The filters are designed to protect the patient from serious, and on occasion fatal, pulmonary embolism by trapping emboli released from sites of thrombosis. Long-term function may also be dependent on the site of insertion. Until recently,

most filters were placed through the internal jugular vein by a cut-down procedure for exposure. With the availability of smaller catheters, it has become possible to insert these percutaneously through the common femoral vein. This makes the procedure simpler because it can be done in the radiology suite with better imaging methods available. With experience with duplex scanning, it became apparent that the inferior cava could be imaged as well as the filters placed to prevent the development of pulmonary emboli (Fig. 10.10).

Markel and colleagues (25) have reported their experience with long-term surveillance of caval filters by duplex scanning. There were 27 patients (8 men, 19 women; mean age, 60 years) who had filters placed and became a part of the long-term evaluation. The filters used were Simon Nitinol (17 patients), Bird's nest (9 patients), and Venatech (1 patient). These filters are shown in Fig. 10.11. The inser-

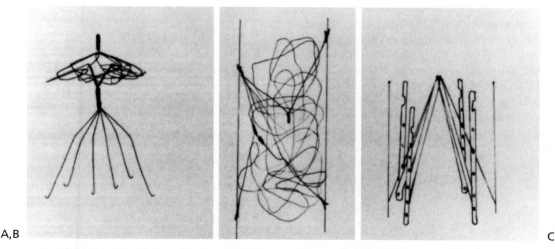

A,B

C

FIGURE 10.11. The filters used were the Nitinol **(A)**, Bird's nest **(B)**, and the Venatech **(C)**. (From Markel A, Goldman M, Coldwell DM, et al. Follow-up of percutaneous placed inferior vena cava filters by duplex scanning. *J Vasc Inv* 1992;16:74–78, with permission.)

tion site was common femoral in 24 patients and the jugular vein in the remaining 3 patients. Nineteen patients were available for follow-up at intervals of 3 months to 2 years. The follow-up studies were performed at 1 day, 1 week, 1 month, and then every 3 months during the first year and annually thereafter.

The complications of filter placement were as follows:

1. In one patient, extravasation of contrast material occurred at the time of placement with no further problems.
2. Tilting of the filter occurred in one patient, but this did not affect long-term function.
3. In one patient with a Bird's nest filter, the wires migrated to above the renal veins on the second day. However, at 1 year, there was no further migration, and the inferior cava was found to be patent.

Duplex follow-up was available in 19 patients (12 with the Nitinol filter and 7 with the Bird's nest device). During long-term follow-up, the complications relative to the filters were few. In 2 patients, it was not possible to visualize the filter. The long-term results were as follows:

1. Filter position did not change.
2. In a patient with a Nitinol filter, a partially occluding thrombus developed proximal and distal to the device at 12 months. After 6 months, there was nearly complete recanalization.
3. Pulmonary embolism developed 1 month after insertion in a patient with a Bird's nest filter. In another patient with a Nitinol filter, pulmonary embolism was suspected at 1 month. The source of the emboli was not determined in either patient. The inferior vena cava was patent and free of thrombus in both patients.

THE TRANSITION: ACUTE TO CHRONIC

Thrombus Lysis and Valve Function

As noted earlier in this chapter, intrinsic fibrinolysis not only occurs in patients treated with heparin but also can occur quickly, often leading to a totally occluded segment becoming widely patent. Our own studies of this phenomenon started with the observations of Killewich and associates (9), followed by the studies of Markel and colleagues (26) and Meissner and associates (27). These studies were performed as a part of our long-term study of the natural history of deep venous thrombosis, with particular interest in those factors that may lead to and be associated with the development of the postthrombotic syndrome. In the interval from 1986 to 1991, patients presenting at the University Hospital in Seattle with duplex-documented acute deep venous thrombosis were recruited for long-term follow-up whenever possible. The criteria for inclusion were as follows:

■ Acute deep vein thrombosis as determined by duplex scanning
■ No historical or clinical evidence of chronic venous disease

■ Ability to return for follow-up visits

The patients were seen at intervals of 1 day, 7 days, 1 month, and every 3 months for the first year. They were then asked to return annually thereafter. At the time of restudy, the patients were queried for any changes in symptoms or signs, and a complete venous duplex study of both lower limbs was carried out. The venous segments from the level of the inferior vena cava to the ankle were examined. The superficial femoral vein was divided into three segments. There were 127 patients with acute deep venous thrombosis that were examined in this time interval. A total of 113 patients presented who were followed for a sufficient interval to document complete lysis in at least one major venous segment. The presence or absence of reflux was defined by the status of the venous segment at the last follow-up visit. The occurrence of transient reflux, which later reversed, was noted but not considered to be an important contributor to long-term outcome. The study group contained 62 men (55%) and 51 women (45%). The average age was 52 years (range, 10 to 82 years). The mean follow-up time was 17.6 (SD ± 15.3) months. Only thrombosed segments undergoing complete recanalization were considered. The follow-up times differed among venous segments.

The median lysis times for all venous segments are shown in Table 10.5 and Fig. 10.12. As noted, the median lysis times were shorter for all venous segments that did not develop reflux subsequently except for the posterior tibial vein. Those segments in which the differences were significant were the superficial femoral vein in its mid-portion, the profunda femoris vein, and the popliteal vein. In addition, there was a clear trend toward significance for all other segments except the posterior tibial vein. Even given the apparent benefit of early lysis on valve function, it must be remembered that there are exceptions. Some segments with early lysis may go on to develop reflux, whereas some that recanalize late may not.

Reflux developed at varying times after the development of thrombosis for the various venous segments. With recanalization, the median time for the appearance of reflux varied considerably as follows:

■ Common femoral vein: 94 (28 to 364) days
■ Proximal superficial femoral vein: 118 (94 to 267) days. Mid-superficial femoral vein: 104 (91 to 184) days. Distal superficial femoral vein: 184 (100 to 304) days
■ Popliteal vein: 194 (35 to 274) days
■ Posterior tibial vein: 62 (38 to 234) days
■ Profunda femoris vein: 245 (184 to 577) days
■ Greater saphenous vein: 165 (103 to 191) days

Although reflux generally appeared in a similar time interval that coincided with complete recanalization of the occluded segments, there were exceptions. For example, in the mid-superficial femoral vein, reflux appeared before complete recanalization occurred.

Van Ramshorst and colleagues (28) conducted a similar study examining the development of valvular reflux after an

TABLE 10.5. LYSIS TIME AND VENOUS REFLUX

| Segment | N | Reflux | | N | No reflux | | p |
		Medium lysis time (days)	Interquartile range		Median lysis time (days)	Interquartile range	
Common femoral	10	279	104–577	14	111	37–208	0.14
Proximal SFV	15	214	95–474	18	73	30–245	0.086
Middle SFV	10	474	245–736	16	65	15–199	0.002
Distal SFV	7	268	230–433	13	118	34–371	0.15
Popliteal	10	260	187–388	20	93	29–190	0.006
Posterior tibial	8	72	49–130	38	80	28–182	0.85
Profunda	5	375	289–388	10	130	30–275	0.04
Greater saphenous	6	287	145–348	7	98	4–191	0.11

SFV, superficial femoral vein.

episode of deep venous thrombosis. They studied 27 patients by repeat duplex scanning with a follow-up interval of 18 to 51 months (mean, 34 months). Forty-five percent of the initially involved segments had developed valvular reflux at follow-up. Interestingly, only 3 of 40 segments that were not affected with thrombosis went on to develop valvular incompetence. This further substantiates the impression that valves that are in the thrombosed venous segments are the ones that most likely will later become incompetent.

These findings with regard to lysis, recanalization, and status of the venous valves in the affected veins are important in terms of the long-term outcome after an episode of acute deep venous thrombosis. The promotion of lysis with fibrinolytic agents and the preservation of valve function are the basis for the use of such therapy. There is no doubt that thrombolytic agents, such as streptokinase and urokinase, can promote lysis at a faster rate than occurs with intrinsic fibrinolysis. Goldhaber and co-workers (29), in a pooled analysis of six clinical trials, found that lysis, although often not complete, occurred 3.7 times faster with streptokinase than with conventional heparin therapy. The problem with most studies of fibrinolysis has been the small numbers of patients who have been followed to document the long-term effects. The reported long-term results have not been consistent. The studies by Kakkar and colleagues (30) demonstrated some early benefit for thrombolysis, but in later studies, Kakkar and colleagues (31) found the early benefit was lost over time. The long-term studies using foot volumetry did not demonstrate continued

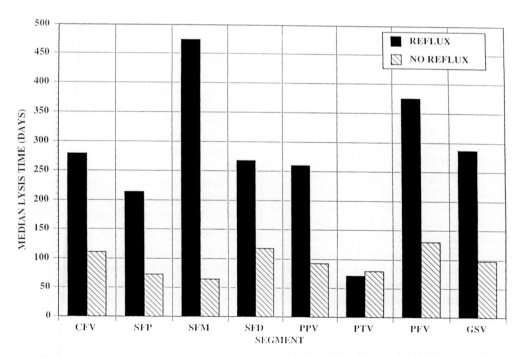

FIGURE 10.12. Median lysis time by venous segments and its relationship to the development of valvular incompetence. *CFV,* common femoral vein; *SFP,* proximal superficial femoral vein; *SFM,* mid-superficial femoral vein; *SFD,* distal superficial femoral vein; *PPV,* popliteal vein; *PTV,* posterior tibial vein; *PFV,* profunda femoris vein; *GSV,* greater saphenous vein.

efficacy for thrombolytic therapy. Albrechtsson and associates (32), in their studies, found that only 2 of 35 (6%) patients treated with streptokinase were both free of symptoms and had normal phlebographic, plethysmographic, and foot volumetry studies.

Because deep venous thrombosis is such a common disorder, it is important to determine which patients might be candidates for lytic therapy. To evaluate this, Markel and associates (33) reviewed 209 patients who had been diagnosed by duplex scanning to have deep venous thrombosis. In this group of patients, 194 (93%) of the patients were found to have contraindications to fibrinolytic therapy. The contraindications to therapy included the following:

- Recent surgery (less than 1 month)
- Recent major trauma
- Active or recent bleeding
- Brain disease (cerebrovascular accident, brain tumor, arteriovenous malformation)
- Pregnancy
- Bleeding diathesis

Two or more contraindications were present in 65 cases (31%). Recent surgery was the most frequent contraindication, being found in 71 patients. Another finding that precluded the use of lytic agents was a history of previous deep venous thrombosis in the affected leg. This was found in 45 patients. Another factor was the duration of symptoms. In this case, patients who had symptoms for more than 7 days were considered to be unsuitable for lytic therapy. The findings in this study do not mean that lytic therapy should not be considered if the patient is otherwise suitable. It would appear that patients with massive venous thrombosis, phlegmasia cerulea dolens, or concurrent pulmonary embolism should be considered as potential candidates and merit consideration for this form of therapy.

A venous registry was established to examine the outcome in patients who had received catheter-directed thrombolysis for the treatment of acute proximal deep venous thrombosis. All patients that had complete studies were followed for a period of 1 year by duplex to document the patency rates of the treated segments. Mewissen and colleagues reviewed the data on 287 patients (34). After 1 year, the primary patency rate was 60%. Several lessons were learned from this trial. If the patient had a left-sided iliofemoral thrombosis, lysis would commonly uncover the lesion in the common iliac vein that narrowed the vein leading to the thrombosis. When that was found, the primary patency was improved by the placement of a stent. These registry results suggested that in properly selected patients, thrombolytic therapy is very likely to be of benefit.

Thrombosis, Recanalization, and the Vein Wall

It is commonly accepted that an episode of deep venous thrombosis will leave the venous wall irreparably damaged, with residual changes that can be seen on duplex scanning. In fact, it is thought that these chronic changes make the use of duplex scanning suspect for the detection of new episodes of thrombosis. This is, in fact, considered to be one of the shortcomings of the method for this important subset of patients. To investigate the changes that occur after an episode of deep venous thrombosis, Meissner and colleagues (35) studied 56 patients with a duplex-documented episode of venous thrombosis. These patients were evaluated if they had been followed for more than 6 months after the event. The following studies were performed:

1. The diameters of the involved veins were measured in the standing position and compared with the uninvolved vein from the other leg. Comparisons with normal individuals were adjusted for individual variation in vein size using the ratio of ipsilateral and contralateral segments (diameter index). It was noted that in 17 normal subjects, the diameter index approached 1 for all segments.
2. To estimate venous compliance, the diameter changes that occurred with Valsalva's maneuver were also measured.

For patients with residual disease as noted on the duplex scan, the involved venous segments were 0.07 to 0.28 cm smaller than the contralateral disease-free side. This was at a significance level of $p < .05$ for the common femoral and superficial femoral veins. In contrast, for those veins with complete recanalization, the diameters of the previously occluded veins were not significantly smaller than their contralateral counterpoints.

The results with regard to compliance were also surprising. In normal subjects, the average change from baseline with Valsalva's maneuver was 20% ± 9% for the common femoral vein, 10% ± 5% for the superficial femoral vein, and 11% ± 3% for the popliteal vein. The findings in the patients with unilateral venous thrombosis are shown in Table 10.6. It is of interest that there were no significant changes regardless of the status of the vein. As noted, the compliance even in those veins with residual disease was comparable to that in veins that were completely recanalized.

These studies may have important implications for the diagnosis of acute deep venous thrombosis. Based on these observations, we would make the following observations and suggestions:

1. During the acute phase, there is evidence that the diameter of the thrombosed vein may be larger than its noninvolved counterpart. Thus, the indexed diameter may be greater than 1 at the time of detection.
2. Venous diameters with residual disease (partially recanalized) should have index diameters of less than 1.
3. Segments that have completely recanalized should have index diameters approaching 1.
4. It appears that venous thrombosis does not affect the ability of the recanalized vein to respond to a sudden increase in proximal pressure.

TABLE 10.6. UNILATERAL DVT: DISEASED SIDE VS. DISEASE-FREE SIDE DIAMETER CHANGE WITH VALSALVA

Segment	Last F/U Dx	N	Diameter change with Valsalva (mean ± SD)		Percentage diameter change with Valsalva (mean ± SD)		
			Diseased	Disease free	Diseased	Disease free	*p*[a]
CFV	Patent	14	0.23 (±0.12)	0.20 (±0.14)	23 (±14)	16 (±11)	0.25
	Residual	10	0.20 (±0.10)	0.23 (±0.09)	22 (±10)	20 (±7)	0.59
SFV	Patent	16	0.06 (±0.04)	0.06 (±0.04)	8 (±5)	8 (±5)	0.88
	Residual	15	0.07 (±0.06)	0.09 (±0.07)	17 (±18)	13 (±12)	0.69
PPV	Patent	17	0.08 (±0.06)	0.08 (±0.03)	11 (±8)	11 (±5)	0.33
	Residual	21	0.07 (±0.06)	0.09 (±0.05)	10 (±9)	11 (±7)	0.50

[a]Wilcoxon signed rank test.
DVT, deep venous thrombosis; F/U Dx, follow-up diagnosis; CFV, common femoral vein; SFV, superficial femoral vein; PPV, popliteal vein.

Although these suggestions will have to be confirmed by other prospective studies, they should serve as the basis for approaching patients with a previous history of deep venous thrombosis in a different manner. The fact that duplex scanning has rapidly become the diagnostic procedure of choice will make it possible to reexamine patients with recurrent thrombosis to determine how they should be approached.

CHRONIC VENOUS INSUFFICIENCY

Patients with chronic venous insufficiency are commonly seen in vascular clinics. They appear either because of cosmetic problems due to unsightly varicosities or because of symptoms and signs that are related to the venous system. For practical reasons that relate not only to the proper classification of the disease but also to its therapeutic implications, it is important to have a good sense of what is responsible for the clinical presentation. In general, it is sufficient to classify the patients into two categories: those with primary and secondary varicose veins. The successful separation into these groups is important and can be greatly aided by the application of indirect and direct noninvasive tests.

Before considering the entities themselves, it is important to consider those variables that are important for the understanding of venous physiology and critical for the proper classification of the disorders that can affect the venous system. From a clinical standpoint, the two elements that are the most important are valvular incompetence and chronic residual obstruction. The valves are the key to proper venous function and are found in increasing numbers as one proceeds distally from the level of the inferior vena cava to below the knee. Although valves are uncommon in the iliac veins, they are numbered in the hundreds below the knee. Here, they appear to be critical for proper venous function because of the calf muscle pump. When activated, the contracting muscle forces blood in every direction that is not protected by an intact set of valves. For example, when the valves below the knee are incompetent, blood is forced toward the heart, toward the foot, and out through the perforating veins into the superficial venous system (Fig. 10.13).

These incompetent valves lead not only to the development of ambulatory venous hypertension but also to the development of edema and, in the long-term, pigmentation in the vicinity of the medial malleolus and, less commonly, in the area of the lateral malleolus. Although there are many theories designed to explain these relationships, it is quite clear that the one factor that appears essential for this problem to develop is incompetence of the perforating veins, which are commonly located in the areas that develop the skin changes (6). The most common perforating veins are found to communicate with the posterior arch vein (Fig. 10.14) and not the greater saphenous vein, as is commonly thought by many physicians.

It is only natural that chronic obstruction of the deep venous system would be considered a key element in the pathogenesis of the postthrombotic syndrome. In fact, it has been common to relate many of the findings noted in chronic cases to the presence of residual venous occlusion. However, this has not been uniformly successful when it has been attempted. For example, as noted earlier, Browse and colleagues (5) attempted to relate the long-term outcome after deep venous thrombosis to the extent of the initial involvement. There was not a good relationship. The extent of the initial occlusion is not predictive of outcome. How can this be?

One obvious explanation is that the final extent of the occlusion may not be the same as that initially noted because of the role of the intrinsic fibrinolytic system and its activation after such an event as deep venous thrombosis occurs. Although it has been known for a long time that recanalization can occur, its rapidity and completeness have not been evaluated. Before the development of duplex scanning, the only method available for such documentation was phlebography, which was rarely repeated unless there was a specific indication to do so.

Killewich and associates (9) prospectively studied 21 patients with documented deep venous thrombosis by serial duplex scanning. As noted earlier, in 11 of 21 patients, recanalization occurred in all segments by 90 days after the event. In four patients, extension occurred despite what appeared to be adequate warfarin therapy. It was noted that

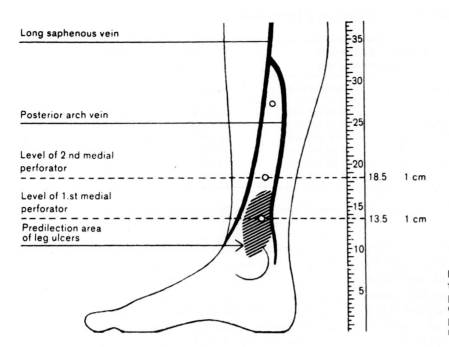

Long saphenous vein

Posterior arch vein

Level of 2 nd medial perforator

Level of 1 st medial perforator

Predilection area of leg ulcers

18.5   1 cm

13.5   1 cm

FIGURE 10.13. Diagrammatic representation of the location of the most important lower leg perforating veins. (From Markel A, Goldman M, Coldwell DM, et al. Follow-up of percutaneous placed inferior vena cava filters by duplex scanning. *J Vasc Inv* 1992;16:74–78, with permission.)

valvular incompetence developed in 13 patients, both in segments that had lysed and in venous segments that had never been involved by thrombus. This suggested that, although incompetence most commonly occurs because of injury to the valves in the occluded vein, other mechanisms must have been operating to explain the problems developing in uninvolved venous segments.

How, then, do we study patients to assess the presence and extent of valvular incompetence and residual venous obstruction? Several indirect methods have been used for this purpose. The gold standard has been the use of pressure measurements during and after exercise. In this test, the needle is placed into a vein on the dorsum of the foot, with the pressure monitored during and after cessation of exercise. Normally, as the calf muscle becomes activated, there is a steady fall in the recorded venous pressure at the level of the foot as the blood is forced in a cephalad direction and is prevented from refluxing toward the foot by the competent valves. Once the exercise stops and the patient stands quietly, the pressure slowly recovers to baseline (Fig. 10.14). As one might expect, several patterns develop that depend on the extent of both the valvular incompetence and the residual obstruction (Fig. 10.16).

Although it has been suggested that the pressure changes reflect the valvular incompetence present, pressure is also affected by the presence of obstruction and the extent to which the collateral circulation has developed (36). This is most clearly evident in patients with venous claudication, in whom there may be a marked increase in venous pressure during exercise because of the high-resistance collateral channels (37). It is also known that the changes in pressure recorded at the level of the foot do not tell the observer the

site of involvement. In addition, the loss of valve competence in the superficial veins can result in abnormal pressure changes, even though the deep venous system is normal (Fig. 10.15). Although it is true that a tourniquet placed around the calf can be used to obstruct the superficial venous system, this method is not foolproof.

Because the measurement of venous pressure requires the insertion of a needle into a vein on the dorsum of the foot, it is invasive and is not the ideal test. To this end, photoplethysmography was developed as a replacement for the direct venous pressure measurements. The method requires application of the transducer to the skin—usually in the vicinity of the medial malleolus. It can monitor changes in the skin blood volume. It has been shown to provide information similar to that obtained with the direct pressure measurements (38,39). An example of the types of recordings that are possible is shown in Fig. 10.16. Although it provides directional and time course data similar to those provided by the venous pressure measurements, it suffers from the same shortcomings. From a diagnostic and therapeutic standpoint, the important issues with regard to valvular incompetence are as follows:

- Documentation of reflux
- Localization of the valvular incompetence with regard to both the superficial and deep venous circulations
- Relationship, if any, between the demonstration of reflux and the clinical status of the patient

Outside the use of venous pressures and the photoplethysmograph, the method most widely used is CW Doppler. The principles are quite simple in that the system is used to document reverse flow in the veins during those maneuvers in

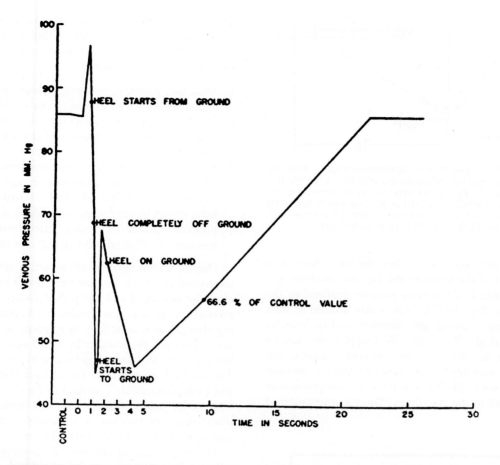

FIGURE 10.14. Changes in the venous pressure at the level of the dorsum of the foot occurring from a single step. (From Hjelmstedt A. Pressure decrease in the dorsal veins on walking in persons with and without thrombosis. *Acta Chir Scand* 1968;134:531–539, with permission.)

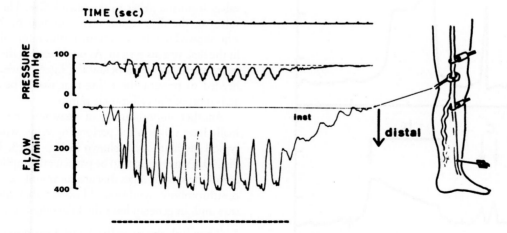

FIGURE 10.15. When there is incompetence of the greater saphenous vein, the pressures recorded from that vein do not fall with exercise *(broken line)*. As noted, there is also bidirectional flow in the greater saphenous vein. (From Hjelmstedt A. Pressure decrease in the dorsal veins on walking in persons with and without thrombosis. *Acta Chir Scand* 1968;134:531–539, with permission.)

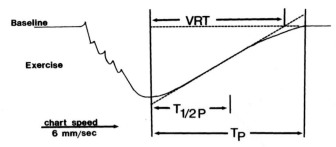

FIGURE 10.16. The types of photoplethysmographic training obtained from a normal individual during and after exercise. The most commonly used value for comparison with patients is the venous refilling time (*VRT*). $T_{1/2P}$, half peak time. (From Killewich LA, Martin R, Cramer M, et al. Pathophysiology of venous claudication. *J Vasc Surg* 1984;1:507–511, with permission.)

which it should not occur (40). When the valve closes, it is due to a reversal of the transvalvular pressure gradient secondary to a change in the venous pressure proximal to the valve in question (Fig. 10.17). This occurs because of such things as coughing, sneezing, and contraction of the muscles in the calf and thigh. With the CW Doppler, this can be tested by placing the transducer over the vein of interest and carrying out a maneuver that increases venous pressure acutely, such as with Valsalva's maneuver or compression of the limb proximal to the transducer. The documentation of

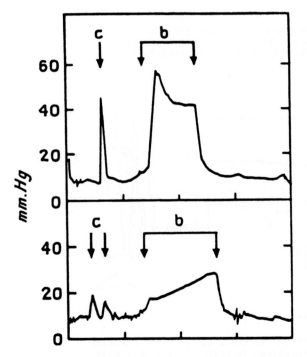

FIGURE 10.17. Effect of a cough (*c*) and Valsalva's maneuver (*b*) on the venous pressures with a competent valve in the iliofemoral regions. *Upper panel* shows pressure above the valve. *Lower panel* shows pressure below the valve. (From Ludbrook J, Beale G. Femoral venous valves in relation to varicose veins. *Lancet* 1962;1:79–81, with permission.)

reflux depends on the demonstration of reverse flow through the venous segment of interest. Although this seems simple enough, there are problems that are not commonly considered, including the following:

1. Was the pressure gradient change induced by the maneuver sufficient to result in valve closure?
2. Are there intervening valves that are competent and prevent the accurate assessment of the venous segment of interest?
3. With the CW system, it is impossible to know with certainty the vein being examined, except in areas such as the common femoral vein and external iliac vein. Even here, it may be confusing, particularly if there have been previous episodes of venous thrombosis and there are prominent collateral veins in the vicinity.

Duplex scanning offers considerable advantages for the estimation of reflux. Because the vein of interest can accurately be visualized and the pulsed Doppler can be placed precisely at the site, it is possible to examine the time-varying changes in venous flow in response to various maneuvers. However, the manner in which one verifies reflux as being present and pathologic is a more complicated matter. The methods in common use include Valsalva's maneuver and limb compression proximal to the site of interrogation. The major concern rests with the certainty that these maneuvers can produce a sufficient sudden increase in venous pressure to ensure valve closure.

Before considering the role of scanning to test valvular reflux, it is important to review the distribution of valves in the deep system because this is important in examining and interpreting the changes that occur secondary to disease. The distribution of valves in the pelvis and upper thigh is shown in Figs. 10.18 and 10.19 (41–44). The average number of valves from the pelvis to the knee is five. The distribution of valves in the iliac region was examined by Basmajian (42), who showed that it was not uncommon for valves to be absent in the iliac venous system. As noted earlier, there are hundreds of valves in the veins below the knee, where they are badly needed to prevent the reflux that would be associated with activation of the calf muscle pump.

Another important set of anastomosing veins that normally have valves is the perforating veins, which have a fairly typical distribution, as shown in Fig. 10.13. Those shown in Fig. 10.13 are thought to be particularly important in the genesis of the skin changes that are commonly associated with the postthrombotic syndrome. However, they do occur at other sites and, in general, have the following features:

1. They link the superficial and deep systems.
2. They perforate the deep fascia.
3. They generally contain valves, permitting unidirectional flow from the superficial to the deep system.
4. They vary in number from 90 to 200.
5. Most are found below the knee.
6. Most are small and inconstant in position.

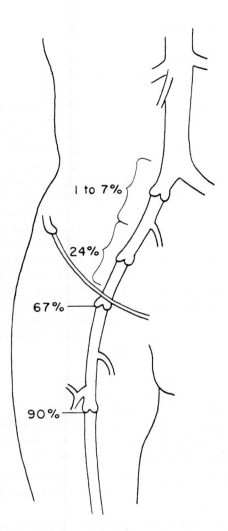

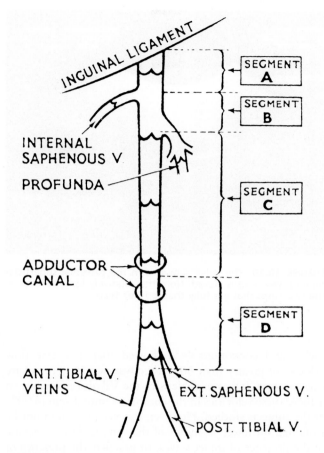

FIGURE 10.18. Frequency and location of valves in the upper thigh and pelvis. (From Basmajian JV. Distribution of valves in femoral, external iliac and common iliac veins and their relationship to varicose veins. *Surg Gynecol Obstet* 1952;85:537–542, with permission.)

FIGURE 10.19. Frequency of valves in the various segments of the thigh. *V,* vein; *ant.,* anterior; *ext.,* external; *post.,* posterior. (From Dodd H, Cockett FB. The surgical anatomy of the veins of the lower limb. In: *The pathology and surgery of the veins of the lower limb.* Edinburgh: Churchill Livingstone, 1976:18–49, with permission.)

7. There are two types. The first type communicates directly with the superficial and deep veins. The second type may interrupt their course in muscular veins before terminating in the deep veins.

It is important to realize that the two largest perforating veins in the leg are the greater and lesser saphenous veins. These veins are normally protected by a valve located close to their termination with the deep system.

The valves themselves can be seen with some regularity in some locations, such as the proximal superficial femoral vein and greater saphenous vein. They may also be seen in the popliteal vein, but it is difficult to image the valves regularly and reliably in other locations. The valves themselves are thin, and a great deal of time and effort are required to visualize them throughout their entire course of movement during opening and closing. However, when this can be

done, as shown in Fig. 10.20, something very interesting is noted. There is a great deal of redundancy in their design, as there must be to function properly when the vein changes its dimensions over the wide range of which it is capable. If this were not possible, it is clear that, with simple dilatation such as occurs when the patient assumes the upright position, the valve would not be able to close completely. It is also apparent that loss of the ability of the valve to coapt has disastrous long-term effects in the venous function and the integrity of the skin subserved particularly by the perforating veins, which ultimately become the Achilles heel in the progression to the fully developed postthrombotic syndrome.

Given these considerations, what is the role of the various maneuvers designed to test competence of the valvular mechanism? If we first consider the proximal venous segments (iliac to adductor hiatus), one of the most commonly used tests is Valsalva's maneuver. In a prospective study done in normal subjects using a duplex scanner, van Bem-

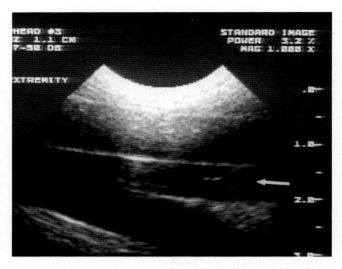

FIGURE 10.20. The valve shown is in the proximal superficial femoral vein and is closed. Note the relatively long portion of the two cusps that are fully coapted (see text).

melen and co-workers (45) showed that a reverse flow velocity of greater than 30 cm/sec was necessary to ensure valve closure. It was possible with the Valsalva maneuver to achieve these velocities in the common femoral vein in 90% of the subjects studied. However, this velocity could not be sustained for lower segments of the venous system because of the presence of intact valves. In practice, the presence of even one competent valve in the superficial femoral vein would prevent the successful use of this test for competence of valves at a lower level. It was also noted that limb compression was rarely strong enough to generate velocities that were sufficiently rapid to promote valve closure. Thus, it appears that this widely used method has little to support it in clinical practice.

The best method of testing valve competence is to use a pneumatic cuff around the limb, which can be rapidly inflated, creating a transvalvular pressure gradient to promote reverse flow. If one uses such an approach, it is necessary to use pressures of 80 mm Hg or higher to achieve reverse velocities consistently greater than 25 cm/sec and promote valve closure.

In practice, the procedure can be used to evaluate valvular function at all levels of the limb. For the proximal venous segments (iliac and proximal superficial femoral vein), Valsalva's maneuver can be used. If no reflux is detected in the superficial femoral vein, this may be consistent with valvular competence, or it may mean that the presence of a competent valve has prevented detection of incompetent leaflets at a lower level. When this occurs, it is necessary to use the cuff inflation and deflation method. We use a 24-cm cuff for the thigh, a 12-cm cuff for the calf, and a 7-cm cuff for the foot. It is also important to test the patient in the upright position, which is the posture during

which the most important pressure and flow changes normally occur (46,47).

When the pneumatic cuff is rapidly inflated, the transducer of the duplex scanner is placed cephalad to the cuff to document reflux. The changes in the direction of flow that occur with cuff deflation simulate muscle relaxation and provide the most reproducible results in terms of valve closure. The time to valve closure after deflation of the cuff for the tested venous segments is shown in Fig. 10.21. The advantage of this method is that it permits a truly segmental evaluation to be performed and should become the standard method of study of patients with the postthrombotic syndrome.

A further study of the role of duplex scanning for the documentation of segmental valvular reflux was conducted by van Ramshorst and colleagues (28). The method used was that by van Bemmelen and associates (49) described previously. This study was performed on 42 legs of 21 healthy subjects and 44 legs of patients with primary varicose veins. The findings indicated that duration of time before valve closure was significantly shorter in the more distal venous segments. The studies showed that 95% of the values were less than the following:

- Common femoral vein, 0.88 second
- Superficial femoral vein, 0.8 second
- Popliteal vein, 0.28 second
- Posterior tibial vein (calf and ankle), 0.12 second
- For the superficial veins, the 95th percentile was 0.5 second for all veins regardless of the location.

These studies further refine the criteria for the distinction between normal valve function and chronic venous valvular incompetence.

Because duplex scanning appears to be a satisfactory method of documenting both the presence and location of valvular incompetence, how should these studies be compared with photoplethysmography, which is commonly used for this purpose? Van Bemmelen and co-workers (47) examined the roles of duplex scanning and photoplethysmography in studying patients with chronic venous insufficiency. The study included 151 consecutive legs with suspected chronic venous insufficiency. The clinical presentation was as follows: 34% had a previous history of deep venous thrombosis, 26% had undergone previous superficial venous surgery, and 11% had active or healed ulceration. The findings with the two methods can be summarized as follows:

1. The photoplethysmographic findings were normal in 57% of the legs and indicated deep venous disease in 22%.
2. With duplex scanning, abnormal venous segments were found in 93% of the legs.
3. It appeared that the photoplethysmography was no better in predicting the presence of multilevel valvular incompetence than the presence of visible skin changes, which are the hallmark of the postthrombotic syndrome.

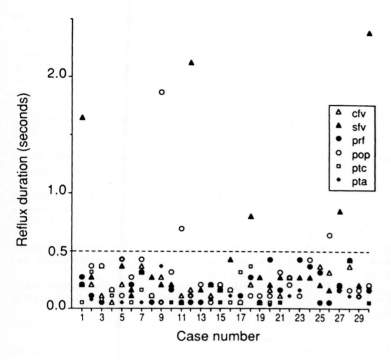

FIGURE 10.21. Duration from time of cuff release until closure of the venous valves in the common femoral vein *(cfv)*, superficial femoral vein *(sfv)*, profunda femoris *(prf)*, popliteal vein *(pop)*, posterior tibial in the calf *(ptc)*, and posterior tibial ankle *(pta)*. These data are from the limbs of 32 normal subjects. (From van Bemmelen PS, Bedford G, Strandness DE Jr. Quantitative segmental evaluation of venous valvular reflux with ultrasonic duplex scanning. *J Vasc Surg* 1989;10:425–431, with permission.)

4. It appeared that the use of a tourniquet in conjunction with photoplethysmography was of little value in localizing venous incompetence within the superficial or deep venous system.

The evaluation of chronic occlusion can be readily made by duplex scanning, but it is impossible to assess its effect on function without doing studies such as venous outflow plethysmography (8,17). Venous outflows are reduced in the presence of chronic venous occlusion but do not appear to bear a good relationship to the clinical picture except in cases of venous claudication. With venous claudication, the venous outflow through the collaterals does not permit rapid emptying. This results in the venous volume in the limb increasing rapidly, which leads to the pain that develops.

With regard to long-term outcome, Johnson and associates examined the relationships between changes in the deep venous system and the development of the postthrombotic syndrome (48). Seventy-eight patients were followed for a median of 3 years. Patients underwent regular follow-up studies. Forty-one percent of the limbs had features compatible with the diagnosis of postthrombotic syndrome. Those with this chronic problem had more than three times the odds of having combined obstruction and valvular incompetence.

REFERENCES

1. Cranley JJ, Canos AJ, Sull WJ. The diagnosis of deep venous thrombosis: fallibility of clinical symptoms and signs. *Arch Surg* 1976;111:34–36.
2. Haeger K. Problems of acute venous thrombosis. I. The interpretation of symptoms and signs. *Angiology* 1969;20:219–223.
3. Kakkar VV, Howe CT, Flanc C, et al. Natural history of postoperative deep venous thrombosis. *Lancet* 1969;2:230–232.
4. Markel A, Manzo RA, Bergelin RO, et al. Pattern and distribution of thrombi in acute venous thrombosis. *Arch Surg* 1992;127:305–309.
5. Browse NL, Clemenson G, Thomas ML. Is the postphlebitic leg always postphlebitic? Relation between phlebographic appearance and late sequelae. *Br Med J* 1981;281:1167–1170.
6. Cockett FB, Jones DFE. The ankle blow-out syndrome: a new approach to the varicose ulcer problem. *Lancet* 1953;1:17–23.
7. Strandness DE, Jr., Langlois Y, Cramer M, et al. Long-term sequelae of acute venous thrombosis. *JAMA* 1983;250:1289–1292.
8. Killewich LA, Martin R, Cramer M, et al. Pathophysiology of venous claudication. *J Vasc Surg* 1984;1:507–511.
9. Killewich LA, Bedford GR, Beach KW. Spontaneous lysis of deep venous thrombi: rate and outcome. *J Vasc Surg* 1989;9:89–97.
10. Sumner DS, Baker DW, Strandness DE Jr. The ultrasonic velocity detector in a clinical study of venous disease. *Arch Surg* 1968;97:75–80.
11. Barnes RW. Doppler ultrasonic diagnosis of venous disease. In: Bernstein EF, ed. *Noninvasive diagnostic techniques in vascular disease,* 2nd ed. St. Louis: CV Mosby, 1985:724–729.
12. Yao JST, Blackburn D. Doppler venous survey. In: Kempczinski RF, Yao JST, eds. *Practical noninvasive vascular diagnosis.* 2nd ed. Chicago: Year Book Medical Publishers, 1987:392–406.
13. Bauer GA. A venographic study of thromboembolic problems. *Acta Chir Scand* 1940;61[Suppl 84]:1–75.
14. Bauer G. Diagnosis and management of peripheral venous disease. *Am J Med Sci* 1957;23:713–723.
15. Rabinov K, Paulin S. Roentgen diagnosis of venous thrombosis in the leg. *Arch Surg* 1972;104:134–144.
16. Athanasoulis CA. Phlebography for the diagnosis of deep vein thrombosis and pulmonary embolism. DHEW Publ. No. (NIH) 76–866. 1975:62–76.

17. Sullivan ED, Peter DJ, Cranley JJ. Real-time B-mode ultrasound. *J Vasc Surg* 1984;1:465–471.

18. Langsfeld M, Hershey FB, Thorpe L, et al. Duplex B-mode imaging for the diagnosis of deep venous thrombosis. *Arch Surg* 1987;122:587–591.

19. Lensing AWA, Prandoni P, Brandjes D, et al. Detection of deep vein thrombosis by real time B-mode ultrasonography. *N Engl J Med* 1989;320:342–345.

20. Killewich LA, Bedford GR, Beach KW, et al. Diagnosis of deep venous thrombosis: a prospective study comparing duplex scanning to contrast venography. *Circulation* 1989;79:810–814.

21. Coehlo JCU, Sigel B, Ryve JC, et al. B-mode sonography of blood clots. *J Clin Ultrasound* 1982;10:323–327.

22. Alanen A, Kormano M. Correlation of the echogenicity and structure of clotted blood. *J Ultrasound Med* 1985;4:421–425.

23. Cronan JJ, Dorman GS, Scola FH, et al. Deep venous thrombosis: ultrasound assessment using vein compression. *Radiology* 1987;162:191–194.

24. Atri M, Herba MJ, Reinhold C, et al. Accuracy of sonography in the evaluation of calf deep vein thrombosis in both postoperative surveillance and symptomatic patients. *Am J Roentgenol* 1996;166:1361–1367.

25. Markel A, Goldman M, Coldwell DM, et al. Follow-up of percutaneous placed inferior vena cava filters by duplex scanning. *J Vasc Inv* 1992;16:74–78.

26. Markel A, Manzo RA, Bergelin RO, et al. Valvular reflux after deep vein thrombosis: incidence and time of occurrence. *J Vasc Surg* 1992;15:377–384.

27. Meissner MH, Manzo RA, Bergelin RO, et al. Deep venous insufficiency: the relationship between lysis and subsequent reflux. *J Vasc Surg* 1993;22:358–367.

28. van Ramshorst B, van Bemmelen PS, Hoeneveld H, et al. *The development of valvular incompetence after deep vein thrombosis: a follow-up study with duplex scanning.* Medical Thesis, Rijksuniversiteit Utrecht, 1992, ISBN-90-393-0461-0.

29. Goldhaber SZ, Buring JE, Lipnick RJ, et al. Pooled analyses of randomized trials of streptokinase and heparin in phlebographically documented acute deep venous thrombosis. *Am J Med* 1984;76:393–397.

30. Kakkar VV, Howe CT, Laws JW, et al. Late results of treatment of deep vein thrombosis. *Br Med J* 1969;1:810–811.

31. Kakkar VV, Lawrence D. Hemodynamic and clinical assessment after therapy for acute deep vein thrombosis. *Am J Surg* 1985;150:54–63.

32. Albrechtsson U, Anderson J, Einarsson E, et al. Streptokinase treatment of deep venous thrombosis and the postthrombotic syndrome. *Arch Surg* 1981;116:33–37.

33. Markel A, Manzo RA, Strandness DE Jr. The potential role of thrombolytic therapy in venous thrombosis. *Arch Intern Med* 1992;152:1265–1267.

34. Mewissen MW, Seabrook GR, Meissner MH, et al. Catheter-directed thrombolysis for lower extremity deep venous thrombosis: report of a national multicenter registry. *Radiology* 1999;211:39-49.

35. Meissner MH, Manzo RA, Bergelin RO, et al. Venous diameter and compliance after deep venous thrombosis. *Thrombos Haemostas* 1994;72:372–376.

36. Hjelmstedt A. Pressure decrease in the dorsal veins on walking in persons with and without thrombosis. *Acta Chir Scand* 1968;134:531–539.

37. Hobbs JT. The post-thrombotic syndrome. In: Hobbs JT, ed. *The treatment of venous disorders.* Philadelphia: JB Lippincott, 1977:253–271.

38. Abramowitz HB, Queral LA, Flinn WR, et al. The use of photoplethysmography in the assessment of venous insufficiency: a comparison to venous pressure measurements. *Surgery* 1979;86:434–440.

39. Killewich LA, Martin R, Cramer M, et al. An objective assessment of the physiological changes in the post-thrombotic syndrome. *Arch Surg* 1985;120:424–426.

40. Sumner DS, Baker DW, Strandness DE Jr. The ultrasonic velocity detector in a clinical study of venous disease. *Arch Surg* 1968;37:75–80.

41. Ludbrook J, Beale G. Femoral venous valves in relation to varicose veins. *Lancet* 1962;1:79–81.

42. Basmajian JV. Distribution of valves in femoral, external iliac and common iliac veins and their relationship to varicose veins. *Surg Gynecol Obstet* 1952;85:537–542.

43. Dodd H, Cockett FB. *The pathology and surgery of the veins of the lower limb.* Edinburgh: Churchill Livingstone, 1976.

44. Dodd H, Cockett FB. The surgical anatomy of the veins of the lower limb. In: *The pathology and surgery of the veins of the lower limb.* Edinburgh: Churchill Livingstone, 1976:18–49.

45. van Bemmelen PS, Beach KW, Bedford G, et al. The mechanism of venous valve closure: its relationship to the velocity of reverse flow. *Arch Surg* 1990;125:617–619.

46. van Bemmelen PS, Bedford G, Strandness DE Jr. Quantitative segmental evaluation of venous valvular reflux with ultrasonic duplex scanning. *J Vasc Surg* 1989;10:425–431.

47. van Bemmelen PS, van Ramshorst B, Eikelboom BC. Photoplethysmography reexamined: lack of correlation with duplex scanning. *Surgery* 1992;112:544–548.

48. Johnson BF, Manzo RA, Bergelin RO, et al. Relationship between changes in the deep venous system and the development of the postthrombotic syndrome after an acute episode of lower limb deep vein thrombosis: a one- to six-year follow-up. *J Vasc Surg* 1995;21:307–313.

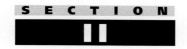

STUDY TECHNIQUE AND INTERPRETATION

11

EXTRACRANIAL ARTERIAL SYSTEM

JEAN F. PRIMOZICH

When duplex scanning was developed and applied to patients, the first area to be studied was the carotid artery. The arteries in the neck were not only easily accessible to this form of energy but also were very important in the pathogenesis of stroke. In addition, arteriography was frequently done to document the location and extent of the disease. The field has progressed rapidly in this area, to the point at which diagnostic arteriographic studies are rarely needed. In addition, it is clear that an accurate evaluation of the carotid bifurcation by ultrasound may be all that is needed before carotid endarterectomy (CEA) (1).

It has become increasingly evident that studies done for this location are not always as accurate as they should be. This may be surprising given the amount of time and effort devoted to this area, but it is a fact of life. It is recommended that the reader not only review the pertinent aspects of the disease process as it occurs but also take the time to master the details that will be covered here. The literature on this subject is voluminous and to some extent confusing. In this chapter, the University of Washington approach will be emphasized. However, it is acknowledged that other approaches may also work well, as long as certain fundamentals are understood and the study procedures strictly followed.

We will start with a review of some of the basic anatomy because without this knowledge, the rest of the procedures used will have little meaning or relevance.

ANATOMY

Common Carotid Artery

The first three large branches of the aorta are the brachiocephalic (innominate) artery, the left common carotid artery (CCA) and the left subclavian artery (SA). The brachiocephalic artery branches into the right CCA and the right SA just under the clavicle. The origin of the right CCA and right SA and the distal end of the brachiocephalic artery are accessible using a lower frequency transducer (5 MHz). The origins of the left CCA and SA are more difficult to image during a routine examination as they originate

off of the aorta. It may be necessary to get information about the origins of these arteries during the course of an examination. Significant disease is not common at the origins of these vessels, but it is possible to infer lesions by noting the flow patterns from a proximal location in these arteries.

At the upper border of the thyroid cartilage (Adam's apple), which is approximately at the level of the C4 vertebra, the common carotid bifurcates into the internal carotid artery (ICA) and the external carotid artery (ECA). The level of the bifurcation may vary from as high as C1 to as low as C6 in some people but lies at about the level of C3 or C4 in most patients. The carotid bifurcation is the most important site to study because it is here that atherosclerosis most commonly occurs.

The carotid bifurcation is unique in humans. It is here that a fusiform dilatation known as the *carotid bulb* is found. The exact location and length of the bulb varies among patients and may include the ECA and exclude the CCA or other variations, but the configuration is usually symmetric within a patient. Because of the variations of the bulb, it is important to specify its exact location for each patient, for example, "the bulb in this patient is located in the distal CCA and the proximal ICA," rather than simply using the general term *bulb* to define a specific location (Fig. 11.1). Unique flow patterns occur as a result of the dilatation and the bifurcation angle that need to be noted during the scan. This is not only important for the examination to be done properly, but it is of importance to the surgeon.

Internal Carotid Artery

The internal carotid artery returns to a normal caliber vessel beyond the bulb. The caliber of the mid ICA is approximately half the diameter of the bulb. There are no branches off the ICA in the neck. The distal cervical ICA may be tortuous, kinked, or looped, which creates difficulty when attempting to follow its course with the transducer. Once inside the skull, the ICA makes an S-shaped curve, which is known as the *carotid siphon*. The routine cerebrovascular

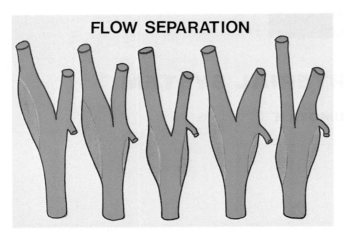

FLOW SEPARATION

FIGURE 11.1. Variations of the location and extent of the carotid bulb. The most common configurations are the two at the *left* of the figure. The *blue areas* represent predictable regions of flow separation as a result of the dilatation. Spectral waveforms from these regions will demonstrate normal disturbed flow patterns.

duplex examination does not directly study the siphon region of the ICA; however, flow changes in the ICA may indirectly indicate disease in this region. The first *major* branch of the ICA, proximal to the bifurcation of the middle cerebral artery (MCA) and anterior cerebral artery (ACA), is the ophthalmic artery (OA), which supplies the eye, although there are some smaller branches in the siphon region. The anatomy of the circle of Willis is detailed in Chapter 12, but a thorough understanding and appreciation of it is critical when performing a carotid study because it is a major collateral source in the presence of severe bifurcation disease.

External Carotid Artery

The ECA, the sister branch of the ICA at the bifurcation, supplies the muscles and skin of the face and scalp. The ECA lies medial and anterior to the ICA, which is located more posterior and lateral. The ECA, in contrast to the ICA, has numerous branches in the neck. The first branch of the ECA, and the one that is seen most often, is the superior thyroid artery (STA). The STA originates at or near the bifurcation or, more rarely, from the distal CCA. The superficial temporal artery, which can be palpated in front of the ear, is the distal end of the ECA. It is important to familiarize oneself with the ECA branches, even though they may not all be visualized during the scan. The ECA may serve as a collateral blood supply to the brain in the presence of a severe ICA stenosis or occlusion.

Vertebral Artery

The vertebral artery is the first branch off of the SA. It follows a relatively straight cephalad course in the neck for a

short distance and then usually enters the C6 vertebra. It then passes through the transverse processes of the cervical vertebrae. At the base of the skull, the vertebral artery traverses the C1 vertebra in a tortuous fashion, called the *horizontal segment*, and then passes into the skull through the foramen magnum. At this location it joins the other vertebral artery and becomes the basilar artery. The basilar artery terminates after a short distance into the two posterior cerebral arteries that make up the posterior portion of the circle of Willis. The posterior cerebral arteries supply the posterior territory of the brain and, through communicating vessels, connect to the anterior part of the circle.

Subclavian Artery

As noted previously, the left SA arises from the aortic arch normally, with the right taking its origin from the innominate artery. Because disease at the origin of the SA is so frequent, it must be included in every study done. As will be noted later, disease at this location may lead to reverse flow in the vertebral artery.

Collateral Pathways

Collateral pathways are essential to supply the brain with necessary blood flow in the presence of severe carotid artery disease that may prevent potential devastating symptoms of stroke or transient ischemic attacks. The blood flow is rerouted, as a result of a pressure differential, through alternate channels and in directions that may be opposite normal. Blood flow may increase in one system as a result of compensation for the loss of flow in another area. Collateralization directly affects the normally expected blood flow characteristics detected during a cerebrovascular examination. A working knowledge of the important collateral pathways, in addition to the routine carotid anatomy, and of the ways in which the flow velocity may be affected is fundamental to understanding and interpreting the results of a carotid duplex examination.

The major ICA collateral pathways include four of the eight branches of the ECA, distal ICA branches, the vertebral basilar system, and the circle of Willis. The ECA branches that anastomose to the ICA are the ascending pharyngeal, the facial, the inferior maxillary, and the superficial temporal artery. The occipital artery communicates directly with the vertebral artery. The important distal ICA branches are the supraorbital, the medial frontal, and the nasal artery that branch from the ophthalmic artery above the eye and communicate with the distal ECA branches. The circle of Willis allows anterior-to-posterior and right-to-left communication of blood flow through a small circuit of arteries connected by communicating vessels within the brain. And finally, the vertebral-basilar system may supply flow to the anterior portion of the brain through patent communicating arteries in the circle (2).

EXAMINATION TIME

A complete carotid duplex examination, including the vertebral and subclavian arteries, may require anywhere from 15 to 90 minutes to complete. The time is dependent on experience, the extent of the disease, the skill of the technique, and patient cooperation. The time it takes to complete the examination will decrease with experience, which is good news for technologists in busy clinical laboratories. However, even an experienced technologist will run across a difficult study that requires more time to sort out. The average time for an examination is 1 hour, which includes a preliminary interview, bruit auscultation, and blood pressure measurements.

EQUIPMENT

Instrumentation

Color and power Doppler facilitate the ease of locating and following vessels and can aid in localizing areas of interest. However, neither of these modalities has been shown to improve the accuracy of spectral waveform analysis, which is what is required to classify disease. Any standard duplex system that includes high-resolution B-mode imaging, pulsed Doppler, and a frequency spectrum analyzer is adequate to do a complete examination.

Scanheads

The carotid arteries are located 2 to 3 cm deep to the skin surface, with the exception of the most proximal CCA or vertebral artery and the distal ICA, which may dive deeper. Therefore, depth is not an issue when selecting a scanhead. The higher-frequency scanheads that range from 5 to 12 MHz center frequency may be used. The higher-frequency transducers of 7.5 to 12 MHz are more preferable for imaging the bifurcation region, and a 5 MHz transducer may be needed for the distal ICA, the origin of the CCA, and the vertebral and subclavian arteries. Some of the more recent transducer designs have multiple imaging frequencies, allowing the operator to change frequencies using the same transducer, which accommodates the deeper vessels without having to change scanheads.

The pulsed Doppler frequency may be the same as or different from the imaging frequency. The pulsed Doppler frequency should be between 4.5 and 10 MHz. The frequency of the Doppler is critical when using specific frequency shifts for classifying disease. The original classifications for ICA stenosis were generated using a 5-MHz Doppler frequency. Therefore, if a Doppler frequency other than 5 MHz is used to generate Doppler frequency shifts for classification, the original criteria values must be recalculated using the new center frequency.

Any type of scanhead design can be used, such as mechanical sector, linear array, or phased array. The linear array imaging format is particularly useful for the CCA and the bifurcation region, where the vessels are reasonably parallel to the skin surface. Some manipulation of the scanhead, like the heel-and-toe maneuver, may be necessary to obtain perpendicular imaging angles as the vessel curves away from the transducer. A curved array or the smaller footprint design of a phased array, both with a sector-type imaging format, may be more successfully used in the regions of the distal ICA and the vessels in the supraclavicular region.

Documentation Devices

A black-and-white printer or a matrix camera is necessary for making hard copy prints of both the spectral waveforms and the B-mode images. A color printer is optional if the instrument includes color imaging. Because the color prints are more expensive, it is recommended that black-and-white prints be used for the standard examination documentation of spectral waveforms and images and the color prints be reserved for regions of special interest. The multiple-image format available with the color printer will save on the amount of prints needed to document an examination, but the images may be too small to appreciate pertinent information, such as the location of the Doppler line and angle cursor or to read the velocity values.

A tape recorder with a microphone for documenting voice narration of the examination is essential for storing and reviewing the real-time portion of the study. Newer instruments may supply a computer disk method of data storage, which will allow rapid retrieval of images for review or for hard-copy printing.

Additional Supplies

A stethoscope, a continuous wave (CW) Doppler, a standard blood pressure cuff, and an aneroid sphygmomanometer are necessary for documenting brachial blood pressures, which must be a part of every examination.

A foam donut or a rolled-up or folded towel placed under the patient's neck is useful for proper positioning and support of the head. The neck support also allows the appropriate scanhead placement for optimizing imaging windows as well as providing comfort for the patient. In addition, a pillow or foam pad placed under the patient's knees will relieve the stress on the lower back, especially if the examination is difficult and time-consuming.

BEGINNING THE EXAMINATION

Patient Interview and Explanation of the Examination

The primary concern of the operator should be that the patient feels comfortable and is willing to cooperate during the examination. The symptoms of cerebrovascular disease can be frightening for the patients, who often do not have a good understanding of what is happening to them. Therefore, a brief explanation of the procedure and a reassurance of the harmless and painless nature of the technique are worthwhile. In addition, a short interview of the clinical symptoms is helpful and adds insight into the reason for referral. Knowing the symptoms can direct the technologist to concentrate on specific areas of interest while doing the routine examination. Other relevant medical history, including smoking history, hypertension, diabetes, heart disease, medications, and elevated cholesterol or triglyceride levels, is optional but may also be included in the interview.

Listening for bruits is optional but can be a good practice because it provides some additional information. It should include the low neck, over the bulb and distal to the bifurcation. The location of the bruit or murmur is noted on the report form, for example, cardiac, subclavian, low, mid, or high in the neck. Particular attention is paid to the mid neck region, which corresponds to the carotid bifurcation. An isolated bruit heard at any location should be thoroughly investigated to identify the source.

Blood Pressure Measurements

Bilateral brachial blood pressures are taken with a stethoscope and a CW Doppler and are a standard part of the cerebrovascular duplex examination. The stethoscope provides the measurement of the systolic and diastolic pressures. The Doppler measures only the systolic pressure, which is more accurate than the stethoscope pressure. A difference in blood pressure of 20 mm Hg between arms is significant with a stenosis in a more proximal vessel, usually the origin of the subclavian on the side of the lower pressure. There may be a difference in the audible character of the Doppler signal recorded from the two sides, which provides further confirmation of the presence of disease in the SA. Bilateral SA stenosis may result in similar, but symmetrically reduced, brachial pressures that can give a false impression of lower systemic pressure. This finding can be suspected if particular attention is paid to the character of the signals recorded from the brachial arteries. (See Chapter 16.)

Positioning (Patient, Technologist, and Scanner)

The patient is supine with the head resting flat on the bed, in a foam donut or with a rolled-up towel under the neck for support. The use of a pillow is discouraged unless the patient has difficulty breathing or cannot lie flat because of preexisting back problems. A pillow raises the head too much, which creates less flexibility of movement and shortens the length of the neck, both of which interfere with obtaining the most optimal imaging windows. A towel or a tissue is tucked into the neck of the patient's clothing for protection, or a patient gown may be provided.

The technologist is seated at the head of the bed with the scanner to the left, near enough so that the operator may reach the most frequently used controls with ease. The technologist should be seated slightly lower than the bed, with the elbow of the scanning arm resting on the patient bed for support and the last two fingers of the scanning hand resting gently on the patient's shoulder. This position decreases the stress on the technologist's back and arm during the examination. A stable scanning position for the arm is essential when trying to obtain difficult signals. The patient's chin is slightly hyperextended and turned toward the contralateral side at about a 45-degree angle from the midline. The head position may be changed as the examination proceeds to optimize and access the best imaging window.

This method may not work in all laboratories and may need to be altered according to space and technologist preference.

SCANNING TECHNIQUE

Scan Views

The cerebrovascular examination includes both longitudinal and transverse scans of the vessels. The longitudinal views are the most important for collection of the Doppler information. A transverse scan of the vessels, beginning at the most proximal CCA, is helpful when starting the scan. This view helps the technologist to visualize the proper orientation of the scanhead relative to the arteries and to become familiar with the patient anatomy, especially in the area of the bifurcation and the distal ICA, where tortuosity is inevitable. Transverse views often provide the most revealing images of eccentric plaques or lumen diameter. It is important to realize that several imaging windows may be necessary to obtain optimal cross-sectional views. Doppler velocity waveforms should *never* be evaluated from a cross-sectional view because the Doppler angle is unknown or close to perpendicular to the flow direction, which generates useless Doppler velocity information. Color Doppler images of vessels in cross-section can be deceiving because the angle and the direction of the flow relative to the transducer are unknown.

Most of the scan is accomplished using a longitudinal/sagittal view, which permits the most favorable Doppler angles for recording the velocity data and for color Doppler imaging. Caution must be exercised when visualizing plaque from a longitudinal view because the image plane is dissecting the vessel with a finite slice of some thickness based on the transducer design. Most plaque develops eccentrically; therefore, one longitudinal view will show only a portion of the plaque, which can be deceiving (Fig. 11.2). However, rotating the scanhead around the long axis

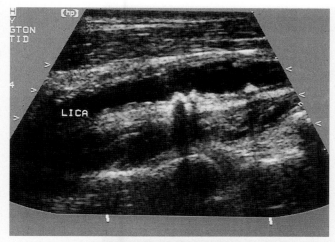

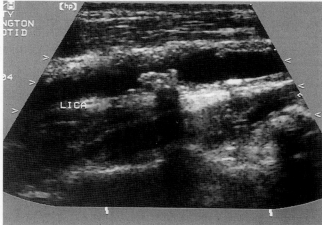

FIGURE 11.2. Two B-mode images taken from the same location in an internal carotid artery from slightly different scanhead orientations. Note that each image appears different, illustrating the eccentric nature of atherosclerotic carotid plaques.

of the artery or sliding the scanhead side to side with small movements will aid the technologist in appreciating the complex nature of the plaque. In addition, rotating the scanhead to the transverse view at the same location is essential for evaluating the characteristics and location of plaque. Measurements of the lumen or vessel dimension from either the longitudinal or the transverse view in complex disease is fraught with problems and should be discouraged as a means of accurately predicting diameter reduction.

From the longitudinal view, the sample volume of the pulsed Doppler should be swept smoothly throughout the length of the vessels, especially in the area of the bifurcation, searching for areas of increased velocity or flow disturbance. Spot checking the velocity information, or sampling sporadically from random locations, should be avoided. A systematic technique of "listening" with the Doppler sample volume throughout the entire course of the vessels will eliminate errors caused by insufficient sampling. Subtle areas of flow disturbance or increased velocity may go unde-

tected with random sampling of the sample volume. Neither the B-mode nor the color Doppler image will reliably pinpoint the area of *maximal* velocity or disturbance. Color Doppler and the B-mode images are helpful in localizing a particular area of interest that needs more specific, in-depth investigation with the pulsed Doppler sample volume. Color Doppler imaging is helpful as a roadmap to follow the path of the vessels in a relatively smooth, efficient fashion. However, color should not replace the standard technique of moving the sample volume through the vessels and directly evaluating each segment.

Different Angles for Different Modalities

Optimal B-mode images are obtained at angles that are different from those used for adequate spectral or color Doppler images. A perpendicular angle between the imaging beam and a surface, such as the vessel wall, produces the brightest reflection. The brightness of the reflection decreases as the angle of approach decreases relative to the surface. Therefore, the most optimal imaging angle is 90 degrees (perpendicular) to the surface of the artery (Fig. 11.3, *right*). On the other hand, the angle that produces the highest frequency Doppler signal is zero degrees, or parallel to the flow direction. Unfortunately, it is difficult to achieve parallel Doppler angles to the flow direction in most of the cerebrovascular vessels. Therefore, larger angles up to 60 degrees, between the vessel axis and the Doppler beam, must be used to obtain velocity information (3). Therefore, the same view used to create an applicable Doppler signal may not yield the highest resolution B-mode image (Fig. 11.3, *left*). Most ultrasound instruments have fixed imaging elements with a steerable Doppler beam. The operator must manipulate the scanhead in some fashion to optimize the image angle separately from the Doppler or color Doppler angle in the same location. Some ultrasound instruments allow the operator to steer electronically the image beams independently of the Doppler beam and thus allow optimization of both modalities simultaneously (Fig. 11.3). In all cases, every effort should be made to create the most applicable angle for each separate modality.

Scanning Windows

To begin, the patient's head should be turned to the contralateral side at a 45-degree angle from the midline with the chin slightly hyperextended. Placing the scanhead in an anteroposterior approach with the head in this position will yield the most proximal segment of the CCA and the cervical portion of the vertebral artery, both of which will be seen lying parallel to the skin surface (Fig. 11.4). The vertebral artery will appear deeper and slightly lateral to the CCA. The scanhead can then be pointed under the clavicle to follow the CCA more proximally toward the origin and then rotated 90 degrees to locate the subclavian. Some pres-

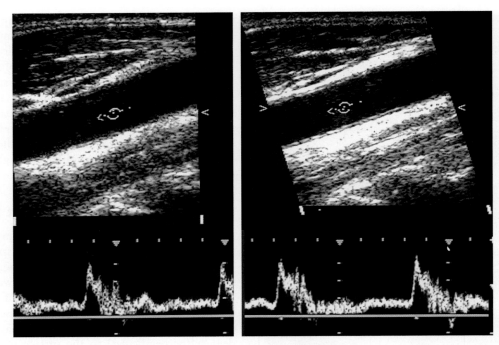

FIGURE 11.3. The **left figure** illustrates a suboptimal angle to the vessel walls, but a more optimal Doppler angle to the direction of flow. In the **right figure**, the image has been mechanically "steered" to intersect the vessel walls at a more optimal angle (perpendicular) while maintaining the same Doppler angle to flow, thereby allowing optimal information with both modalities simultaneously. Note the appearance of the double-line stripe of the normal arterial wall in the **right figure**, which is not appreciated in the **left figure**.

sure with the scanhead is necessary to image under the clavicle. As the scan continues more proximally toward the bifurcation, the scanhead should gradually slide to a lateral or posterolateral approach for the best view of the bifurcation and to follow the ICA to the most distal location in the neck. The most successful approach from which to image the bifurcation in the "tuning fork" configuration is from the posterior location, behind the muscle. Although it is

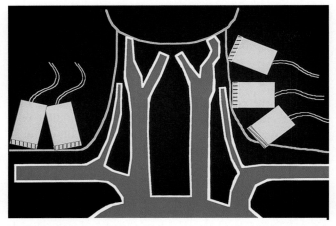

FIGURE 11.4. Typical scanhead placement to obtain Doppler and image information for all sites in a complete extracranial carotid duplex examination.

not necessary to see the bifurcation in this configuration to do a complete examination, it is always a bonus when it appears. It is important to identify both the ICA and the ECA as they branch from the CCA, even if they do not appear in the same image. To follow the ICA more distally, it may be necessary to reposition the scanhead by tilting under the mandible (Fig. 11.4, *upper right*). With the scanhead in this location, the ICA will be seen diving deep and away from the transducer and can easily be followed for several more critical centimeters. The patient's head may be rotated farther to the side or closer to the midline during the course of the examination in order to adjust the location of the vessels in the image. Rotating the head further to the contralateral side with the scanhead in a posterior approach will increase the depth of the vessels in the image. Conversely, rotating the head closer to the midline with the scanhead in a more anteroposterior approach will decrease the depth of the vessels in the image. The anteroposterior approach is *not* recommended for most of the examination.

SCANNING SEQUENCE: FINDING THE DISEASE

The cerebrovascular duplex examination can be thought of in two parts per side. The first segment of the examination involves a complete survey of the vessels and an assessment of the anatomy and the presence or absence of disease and its location. No spectral waveforms are taken for documentation during this initial surveillance. The technologist is free to move the sample volume around, to become familiar with the anatomy and the disease, to investigate the flow patterns through each vessel, and to select sites pertinent for documentation. It is this portion of the examination that is the most time-consuming. Once this investigation is completed, the technologist will then methodically return to preselected standard sites identified from the initial survey. Using the standard protocol that is discussed in the next section (e.g., correct angle, sample volume placement, Doppler gain), the technologist will record the velocity spectral waveforms that most accurately depict the representative flow patterns of the carotid system and the disease. Using the two-step method for scanning each side helps to delineate which data are important for documentation and interpretation and which information can be excluded. Ultimately, the technique saves time and potential errors of omission.

This section describes the investigative stage of the examination, that is, how to identify the appropriate vessels, to distinguish normal from abnormal, to profile disease, to define tortuosity, and to describe wall and plaque characteristics.

Normal Vessels and Locations

Common Carotid Artery

The common carotid is a relatively easy vessel to locate in the neck. Typically, most of the length of the CCA lies parallel to the skin surface and is 1 to 2 cm deep. The most proximal CCA (CCAp) is the region that includes the origin and the first third of the vessel. The CCAp is seen coursing toward the skin surface and then curving so that it is parallel to the transducer face. This section may be difficult to follow with the scanhead. The curve creates expected flow disturbances seen in the spectral waveforms that should not be mistaken for abnormal spectral broadening secondary to disease. It is often difficult to place the angle cursor so that it is parallel to the walls in a curve; consequently, a variety of estimated velocity measurements are possible from the same location. The origin of the right CCA and the right SA are easily accessible to the scanhead as they branch from the brachiocephalic artery and are routinely scanned. The left CCA and SA, originating deep and directly off of the aorta, are not usually scanned in a routine examination. An attempt to scan them should be made in the presence of suspected disease, for example, an unexplained bruit, an abnormal signal, or poststenotic turbulence in the mid CCA. A lower-frequency transducer will help to locate the origins of these vessels, although in some cases, it may not be possible to identify them. Marked flow disturbances near the origins of the vessels are common. In

addition, appropriate alignment of the angle cursor parallel to the vessel walls may be difficult to obtain; therefore, interpretation of the velocity measurements may be questionable.

The CCA straightens out beyond the curve in the midsection (CCAm) and becomes parallel to the skin surface. The walls of the CCA should appear smooth and uniform. Significant atherosclerosis rarely involves the CCA. However, it is common to see some increase in thickness of the intima-media stripe, which most likely represents a fibrous lesion. The sample volume should be scanned through the region, assessing for any changes in the flow velocity patterns.

The location of the distal CCA (CCAd) is the continuation of the scan to the bifurcation. Here, the vessel may dilate, as it becomes the bulb. Atherosclerosis may develop here and extend into the ICA and ECA. The exact location of velocity changes may be difficult to pinpoint in the presence of plaque and vessel overlap seen in the image. A transverse view helps to identify the anatomy more precisely relative to the velocity changes.

The scan from the origin to the CCAd should be relatively quick, and color flow is advantageous. The scanning technique involves imaging a segment of vessel, sweeping the sample volume through the segment, and then moving the scanhead more proximally to an overlapping, continuous image of the vessel. The procedure is repeated through the length of the vessel.

Proper Identification of the Internal and External Carotid Arteries

The proper identification of the ICA and ECA is the most critical task of a cerebrovascular duplex examination. Although these arteries may be obvious in some scans, in most, their identification is an important and difficult challenge. There is not one sure-fire method of distinguishing these two vessels; however, using a combination of features helps to ensure their accurate identification.

Anatomic Location

The usual anatomic configuration of the vessels of the bifurcation is that the ICA is located lateral and posterior in the neck, whereas the ECA is medial and slightly more anterior. The relative location of these two vessels in the image will change as the scanhead is moved from an anteroposterior approach to a lateral or posterior approach. It is important to identify landmark locations, like the thyroid, to use for setting up appropriate directions within the image, such as medial from lateral. In addition, the vessels may be transposed anatomically from the bifurcation. Simply relying on the anatomy in the image to distinguish the vessels is fraught with nuances that can be detrimental to the correct identification of the ICA and ECA, but it can be helpful if other methods are in question.

Hemodynamic Flow Changes and Resistance

The ICA supplies the low-resistance vascular bed of the brain. The ICA waveform reflects the distal low resistance with flow above the zero baseline throughout the cardiac cycle, specifically at end-diastole. Normally, the systolic velocity is lower in the ICA than in the ECA, with a slower acceleration to systole, resulting in a more rounded systolic peak of the waveform. The ECA waveform reflects the high-resistance vascular bed of the muscles and skin of the face and scalp. The ECA typically has a faster acceleration to systole, a higher peak systolic velocity (PSV) as a result of its smaller diameter and peripheral outflow, and end-

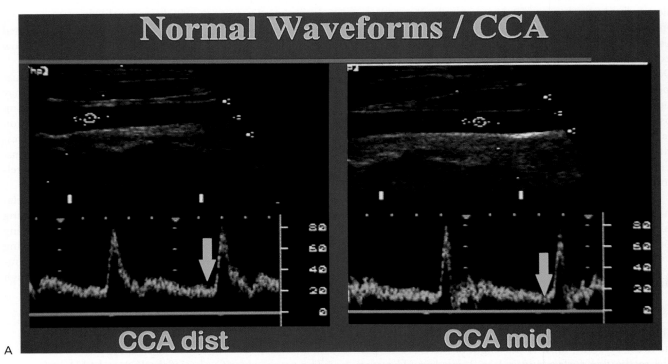

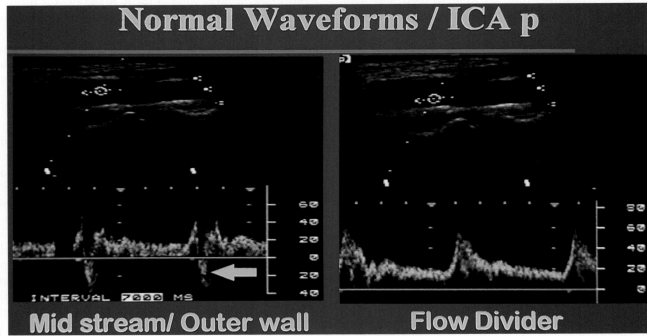

FIGURE 11.5. A–D: Normal spectral waveforms (see text).

diastolic velocity (EDV) that is at or near the zero baseline. In addition, the ECA may have a flow reversal component in late systole or early diastole that is a reflected wave from the high distal resistance. The waveforms from the ICA and the ECA demonstrate the changing distal resistance in both normal and abnormal conditions (Fig. 11.5C).

Therefore, to evaluate the differences, a *direct comparison of the waveforms* from the two suspected vessels is critical before using the resistance characteristics (waveform shapes) for identification. *Never assume the identification of an ICA or ECA before comparing the characteristics of both vessels.*

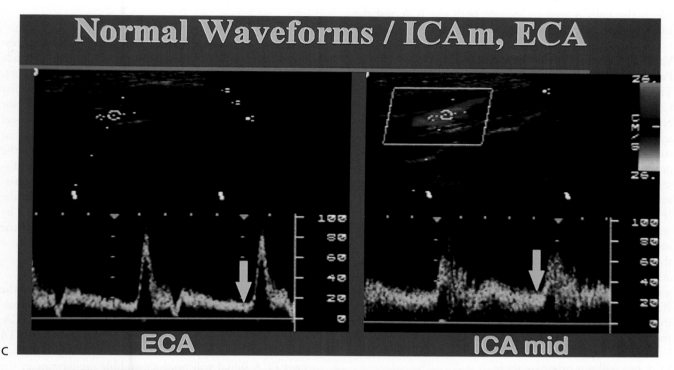

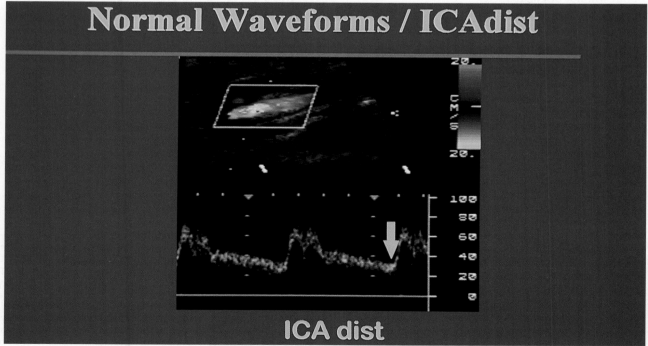

FIGURE 11.5. A–D (*Continued*)

Size of the Vessels

The ICA usually has a larger cross-sectional area at the origin when compared with the ECA in the transverse view as a result of the presence of the carotid bulb. The two vessels become similar in diameter beyond the bulb. As stated previously, the location of the bulb may vary to include the ECA or exclude both the ICA and ECA, in which case, the origin of the two vessels may be similar in size. In cases in which the bulb is seen to include both the ICA and the ECA, both vessels will taper as one scans more distally.

Variable Location of the Bulb and Related Flow Patterns

The most common location of the bulb includes the distal CCA and the most proximal portion of the ICA (Fig. 11.1). Normal flow disturbances, known as *boundary layer* or *flow separation*, occur as a result of the dilatation. Recognizing the location of the disturbances can be helpful in distinguishing the ICA from the ECA (see Normal Flow Patterns). The boundary layer separation is seen as a transient reversal of flow along the posterolateral portion of the bulb (Fig. 11.5B, *left*) The reversal is seen in the color display as well as in the spectral waveforms (Fig. 11.6). Therefore, identifying flow separation may be helpful in distinguishing the ICA. Identifying the location in the flow separation relative to the flow divider will assist in pointing out the origin of the ECA. If the bulb includes both the ECA and the ICA, the flow separation will be seen in both vessels, and this can be deceiving. In addition, if the bulb includes only the distal CCA, there will be accompanying flow disturbances that will radiate into the normal-caliber ICA and ECA but will not originate there.

Presence of Branches

There are eight branches of the ECA in the neck. The STA is the first and most commonly visualized branch. The STA usually originates from the most proximal ECA but may arise from the distal CCA. Other ECA branches may be seen as well, especially when using color Doppler. The identification of branches is usually verification of the ECA, because the ICA has no branches in the neck.

Two Vessels Defined by Color

Color Doppler imaging defines the appearance of two vessels and the presence of branches more clearly than B-mode imaging alone. In addition, the hemodynamic differences, that is, the resistance created by the different distal vascular beds of the ECA and ICA, are also recognized in the color display. The ICA will have continuous color in the vessel throughout the cardiac cycle, decreasing at diastole or reversing in the area of flow separation. Whereas, in the ECA, the color will decrease significantly or completely disappear in diastole, depending on the amount of distal resistance. These changes may not always be evident, that is, the hemodynamics of the ECA and the ICA will be altered by both normal and abnormal changes in the resistance of the distal vascular beds.

Superficial Temporal Tap

The superficial temporal tap is a technique that relies on the fact that the superficial temporal artery, which can be palpated in front of the ear, is the distal portion of the ECA. In theory, gentle, rapid compressions of the ipsilateral STA with a finger of the opposite hand while listening to the suspected ECA signal will produce audible oscillations of the

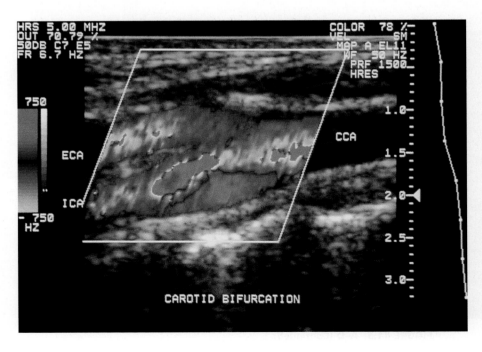

FIGURE 11.6. Color image of a carotid bifurcation including the bulb in the proximal internal carotid artery. The image is taken near peak systole. The transient flow reversal of boundary layer separation is seen as the region of *dark blue* at the outer wall of the bulb. Aliasing of the color Doppler frequency is seen as the *aqua blue* regions in the midstream of the common and internal carotid arteries.

Doppler signal. These oscillations are heard and displayed on the spectral waveform if the vessel in question is the ECA. No oscillations will be noted if the suspected vessel is the ICA. At first glance, this seems a foolproof method by which to distinguish these vessels. Unfortunately, this method is not foolproof. It should be used with considerable caution and not relied on as the sole method of distinguishing the ECA from the ICA. Some circumstances exist that will create erroneous results using the STA tap method: (a) ECA collateralization in the presence of a chronic arterial lesion in the ICA will invalidate this method, and the ECA will not respond; (b) the ICA, as well as the ECA, may respond to the compressions if the back-pressure of the oscillations is strong enough; (3) the STA may not be accurately palpated or adequately compressed, and consequently, the ECA will not respond; (d) the scanhead, the patient, and the bed may all be vibrated with the use of overly enthusiastic compressions, in which case, any Doppler signal will erroneously appear to oscillate. The STA compression maneuver should be used when the other methods fail, rather than as the primary approach to distinguishing the two vessels.

Normal Flow Patterns

Common Carotid Artery

The CCA is evaluated throughout its length for the presence of visible plaque, tortuosity, and any focal changes in the velocity. An isolated high-grade stenosis is rare in the CCA, but a thorough search of the vessel with the sample volume is always recommended.

The origin of the CCA may easily be evaluated on the right as it branches off of the brachiocephalic artery. It is more difficult, if not impossible, to obtain a signal from the left CCA origin. A lower-frequency transducer with a smaller footprint in a substernal approach may be useful. Flow disturbances may be noted at or near the origin of the CCA as a result of the branch angle and the curvature of the vessel as it leaves the chest cavity. These disturbances are to be expected and are normal. An assessment of the visual appearance of the vessel helps to sort out complicated and questionable waveforms.

A spectral waveform should always be obtained from the CCAm as it becomes relatively parallel to the skin surface in the image and more easily accessible with the scanhead. This location should be at least 2 cm proximal to the bifurcation. The CCAm waveform is typically of low resistance because about 70% of the blood flow goes to the ICA (Fig. 11.5A, *right*). Therefore, the EDV of the CCA will be above the zero baseline. Both the waveforms from the CCAm should be symmetric in shape and EDV. The CCAm signal is the most representative signal from this vessel; it is usually devoid of disturbances originating because of branch points, curves, and dilatations seen in the CCAp and the

CCAd. *It is for this reason that the CCAm signal is used for comparison to a similar waveform from the contralateral side in the case of a total ICA occlusion and also to calculate the ICA/CCA ratio (4).*

Important information about disease, which is remote from the bifurcation, may be suspected from changes occurring in the CCA waveforms. Significant disease, more proximally or distally in the ipsilateral system or in the contralateral system, will change the hemodynamics of the CCAm and result in asymmetry of the waveforms. In the case of a total occlusion or a very high-grade stenosis of the ICA, the blood flow is directed through the ECA, and the ipsilateral CCA will adopt the peripheral character of the ECA. In contrast, the contralateral CCA may have increased flow in end-diastole as a result of the body's effort to compensate for reduced flow to the brain. A patent anterior communicating artery can be attributed to this phenomenon. Therefore, a direct comparison of the two CCAm waveforms is valuable. In the case of a chronic ICA occlusion, the end-diastolic component of both CCAm waveforms may appear normal and symmetric because of collateralization. In addition, the CCA waveforms may appear peripheral in character and symmetric in the presence of some cardiac conditions.

The waveform from the CCAd, the site just proximal to the bifurcation, will change in character and velocity, by comparison (Fig. 11.5A, *left*). At this location, the CCA begins to dilate into the bulb; consequently, the normal PSV may decrease, and the waveform will have a slightly different character compared with the more proximal CCA waveform. The CCAd waveform may display higher end-diastolic velocities and/or flow disturbances as a result of the dilatation.

External Carotid Artery

Clinically, the ECA is not a very important artery. It supplies the face and scalp and is generally not a source of emboli to the brain; however, it is invaluable in the accurate identification of the ICA. As previously defined, the ECA waveform has a fast acceleration to systole, that is, sharp upstroke, a prominent dichrotic wave in late systole or early diastole, and velocity that is near or at the zero baseline in end-diastole (Fig. 11.5C, *left*). The PSV of the ECA is normally higher than the ICA because it is a smaller, peripheral vessel. The ECA may adopt the characteristics of the ICA in end-diastole as the resistance in the face and scalp decreases with temperature change and/or in the presence of disease (see Proper Identification of the Internal and External Carotid Arteries, earlier).

Carotid Bulb and Proximal Internal Carotid Artery

The carotid bulb is usually located in the proximal portion of the ICA and the distal CCA; however, the bulb location can vary, and reference to the image will clearly define the location. The normal flow patterns in the carotid bulb are complicated because of the dilatation and the branch angle of the bifurcation. These anatomic features create boundary layer separation and secondary helical flow patterns. Spectral waveforms from this area reflect these normal, yet complex flow changes (Fig. 11.5B).

A characteristic pattern of velocity waveforms is seen as the sample volume is moved across the proximal ICA and bulb. Near the wall of the flow divider of the bifurcation, there is a unidirectional forward flow velocity throughout the cardiac cycle (Fig. 11.5B, *right*). Near midstream, there is a transient reversal at peak systole, which is also seen near the outer wall opposite the flow divider (Fig. 11.5B, *left*). The flow velocity in end-diastole will drop to zero near the outer wall. The waveform changes represent normal flow disturbances and should be documented as such. The typical flow disturbances, along with the absence of visible plaque in the bulb, confirm the interpretation of "normal carotid bulb" (5).

Mid-Internal Carotid Artery

The mid-internal carotid artery (ICAm) waveform is taken distal to the normally placed bulb, where the vessel diameter becomes smaller. The typical flow pattern is of low resistance, with end-diastolic flow velocity well above the zero baseline (Fig. 11.5C, *right*). The PSV may be slightly higher than in the ICAp owing to the decrease in the diameter. The flow disturbances from the carotid bulb may travel into the ICAm and should be considered as normal spectral broadening. These relatively minor disturbances are not appreciated in the color display.

Distal Internal Carotid Artery

The distal ICA (ICAd) is that segment of the vessel that is *at least 3 cm* distal to the bifurcation and well above the area of a stenosis. The typical waveform from the ICAd is of low resistance and may have slightly higher velocity as a result of the decreasing diameter of the vessel (Fig. 11.5D). The flow disturbances of the bulb may extend as far as the ICAd but will be less pronounced than in the ICAm.

Atherosclerosis usually develops in the first 1 to 2 cm of the ICA and is rarely found isolated in the ICAd. The ICA, in this location, typically dives away from the transducer. It may be tortuous and exceedingly difficult to visualize owing to poor imaging angles. Color flow imaging is extremely helpful to follow the tortuosity because of more favorable Doppler angles. Extreme vigilance is necessary when taking velocity waveforms from the distal ICA to prevent inappropriate or inaccurate Doppler angle measurements that lead to overestimation of velocity increase and misdiagnosis of stenosis. The Doppler sample volume and use of color Doppler are helpful "pathfinders" in the case of a poorly visualized vessel.

Steering the Doppler line or color box straight down or to the right of the screen (caudad), rather than to the left (cephalad), can be extremely helpful when trying to obtain more appropriate angles for spectral waveform analysis.

There are rare cases in which true stenosis is detected in the ICAd. Fibromuscular dysplasia (FMD) is a rare disease found most commonly in young women. It is commonly a bilateral disease that is characterized by a series of fibrotic and hyperplastic lesions in the media of the arterial wall of the distal ICA and the renal arteries. It can also occur in the intima or adventitia. Although histologically different from atherosclerosis, the hemodynamic effects of these two disease processes are indistinguishable using spectral waveforms. One distinction between atherosclerosis and FMD, in addition to location, is that in FMD, there are usually a series of stenoses rather than one focal jet (Fig. 11.7). This condition is referred to as the "string of beads" seen on angiography. The method of duplex documentation is the same for both diseases; however, more waveforms are necessary to describe the multiple lesions of FMD clearly.

Vertebral Artery

The origins of the vertebral artery are the most common site of disease but lie deep under the clavicle and may be difficult to access. The vertebral artery is most commonly interrogated further distally in the neck, from an anteroposterior window, as it threads through the transverse processes of the cervical spine (Fig. 11.8, *left*). It is usually seen deeper but adjacent to the vertebral vein. Color Doppler is helpful to locate the vessel, but spectral Doppler must be used to verify it. A spectral waveform from the mid neck site yields information about direction of flow, waveform shape, and velocity but does not rule out disease at the origin. On rare occasions, a stenosis may be found in the cervical portion of the vertebral artery associated with cervical osteoarthritis.

The vertebral arteries may be small, asymmetric in size, and inaccessible. The typical spectral waveform from a vertebral artery is of low resistance, similar to the ICA (Fig. 11.8, *left*). Normal flow disturbances as a result of the branch angle may be detected at the origin (Fig. 11.8, *right*). The vertebral artery is assessed for direction of flow (i.e., antegrade, retrograde, or oscillating) and for any obvious abnormalities in the flow. Proper identification of direction of the flow is especially important in the presence of subclavian stenosis or occlusion because the vertebral flow may reverse to supply the arm. This is particularly important information in the presence of significant disease in the anterior circulation, that is, the bifurcations (6).

Subclavian Artery

The SA is classically peripheral in character. It should exhibit a typical triphasic waveform similar to that of a

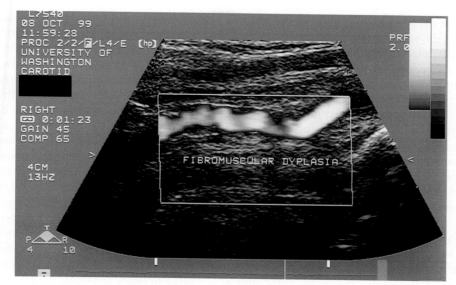

FIGURE 11.7. Fibromuscular dysplasia in a distal internal carotid artery is seen as a series of stenoses in this power Doppler image.

femoral artery, that is, a forward systolic component, a reversal component in late systole or early diastole, and a second forward phase in late diastole. The second forward phase may be lost in older patients as the vessels become stiffer and less compliant with age, but the reversal phase will be maintained. Loss of the reversal component is significant with the presence of disease and will be verified with a decrease in brachial blood pressure.

Profile of Stenosis

Identifying stenosis is accomplished in different ways: (a) the audible and spectral waveform characteristics, (b) the changes in the color Doppler display, and (c) the B-mode image. Although all of these methods help to focus on the area of disease, the Doppler sample volume is ultimately used to pinpoint the site of maximum velocity increase or disturbance.

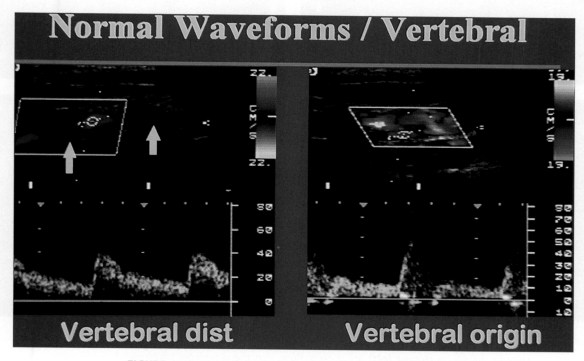

FIGURE 11.8. Normal spectral waveforms from a vertebral artery.

The classification of the percentage of diameter reduction *is only accurate using the Doppler spectral waveforms.*

The technologist must carefully move the sample volume through the area of interest, when identifying a stenosis, to detail the hemodynamic changes and to discover the site of maximum stenosis. Neither the color Doppler image nor the B-mode can be accurately relied on to distinguish precisely the site of the maximum velocity increase.

The stenosis profile is a collection of velocity waveforms that define the hemodynamic changes that occur through a stenosis. For proper interpretation, it is necessary to record each of the waveforms in the series. The proper profile of stenosis consists of the following waveforms (Fig. 11.9):

Prestenotic waveform. A signal taken in the normal artery proximal to the stenosis. The waveform may or may not show disturbance or spectral broadening, which is dependent on the shape of the lesion. A smooth entry into a stenosis will have fewer disturbances than an irregular wall (Fig 11.9, *upper left*).

Stenotic waveform. The signal taken at the site of maximum systolic velocity increase or at the site of most disturbed flow (Fig 11.9, *upper right*). This is the waveform from which the classification for disease will be determined. The color flow pattern in this location may demonstrate the increase in velocity (frequency shift) as a desaturated jet of color or an area of color aliasing; however, it will not precisely define the exact site of maximum velocity increase. It is important to note that the same color pattern (i.e., increased frequency shift) is also seen in the presence of an acute Doppler angle between the transducer and the direction of flow, as in a tortuous vessel. Once the area is located in color, the Doppler sample volume is then used to tease out the appropriate velocity changes, which can be frustrating if the jet is small compared with the sample volume or in the presence of dense calcification. The sample volume may need to be moved through the area multiple times in order to locate the signal.

Poststenotic waveform. This signal is taken from the area just distal to the site of the maximum velocity recording

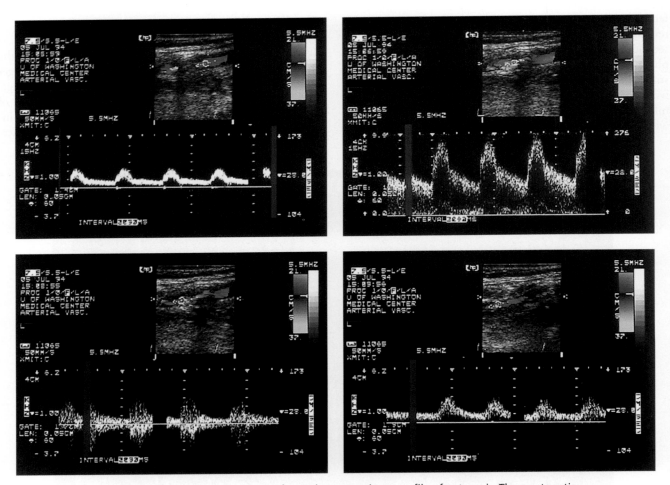

FIGURE 11.9. Doppler spectral waveforms demonstrating a profile of a stenosis. The prestenotic waveform **(upper left)**, the stenosis (i.e., the maximum velocity) **(upper right)**, and the poststenotic waveform **(lower left)** are shown. Note that the waveform taken distal to the poststenotic turbulence **(lower right)** appears relatively free of turbulence.

and reflects the chaotic nature of turbulent flow. Post-stenotic turbulence is seen in the spectral display as bidirectional flow, marked spectral broadening, and decreasing velocities as the sample volume is moved further distal from the stenosis (Fig 11.9, *lower left*). It may be difficult to define clearly or measure a representative velocity from the poststenotic turbulence because of the disturbed, oscillatory, or spiked appearance of the waveform. However, it is important for interpretation to record this signal and include it in the complement of waveforms, which validate the stenosis. The audible Doppler signal is unique, sounding like "water bubbling in a tube." The color flow pattern of poststenotic turbulence appears as an area of multihued colors, representing complex flow velocities and directional changes that often result in aliasing. Locating this region helps to delineate more precisely the end of the stenosis and indicates the highest velocity must be more proximal. The poststenotic turbulence may extend for several centimeters beyond the stenosis, decreasing in intensity. The abnormal-appearing waveform will normalize and not be identifiable at some distance beyond the stenosis (Fig. 11.9, *lower right*).

A color bruit may be seen in the tissue surrounding the poststenotic region. A bruit is seen at systole as speckled regions of dark red and blue in the tissue. It is a result of the turbulence causing the walls to vibrate, which in turn causes the tissue to vibrate at a low frequency. The tissue movement is detected by the Doppler and displayed in the image. Not all stenoses have associated bruits; however, the presence of bruits indicates that the stenosis is at least a 50% diameter reduction (Fig. 11.10).

Assessing Areas of Tortuosity

Tortuous vessels are simply a fact of life when scanning the carotid arteries. Normal flow disturbances are to be expected and anticipated as a result of the curves in the vessels. The disturbances will occur distal to the curve along the inner wall and will dissipate after a short distance downstream. The normal disturbances and eddies that develop distal to the curve are seen as rapid up-and-down oscillations and spikes in the spectral waveform, as seen in Fig. 11.11. In the color flow, they are represented as patches of directional color change (blue) in late systole that disappear in diastole.

It is difficult to know how to adjust the Doppler angle cursor and to know where to place the pulsed Doppler sample volume when assessing velocity in a curved vessel. In a straight vessel, the angle cursor is adjusted so that it is parallel to the vessel wall, representing the long axis. In a curved vessel, this is not as straight forward to perform. It is common to hear increased frequencies when scanning through curves because of acute Doppler angles relative to the changing directions of the blood flow and not as a result of increased velocity. The perceived peak velocities recorded in a curve can vary as much as 100% in the same location simply by varying the angle measurement relative to the

walls, each time believing that it is parallel. The inner wall of the curve is most easily used to align the angle cursor in an attempt to make it parallel; however, this method is not foolproof and will most certainly create variations in perceived velocity measurements in the curve. It is important to remember that blood flow is much more complicated than what angle-adjusted velocity and the Doppler equation would imply. It is very easy to overestimate the amount of narrowing in a curve as a result of this phenomenon. Caution is suggested when adjusting the angle cursor in a curve and the use of other clues to identify a true stenosis, e.g., poststenotic turbulence, is recommended.

In addition, it is often difficult to obtain the standard angle measurement (60 degrees) in or distal to a tortuosity, where the vessel may dive directly away from or toward the scanhead. In these cases, an angle measurement that is easiest to obtain and that is less than 60 degrees is recommended and *always with the angle cursor aligned parallel to the vessel walls*. The nonprotocol angle should be documented and reused for consistency in follow-up examinations of the same location. The velocity that is recorded using the smaller angle may not be accurately used with the criteria for diameter reduction because those values were validated using a 60-degree angle. Fortunately, tortuosity usually occurs in the most distal portion of the ICA, which is not the typical location of atherosclerosis. *The examiner must be continually cautious and vigilant when scanning tortuous vessels.*

Assessment and Characterization of Wall and Plaque

The presence of plaque in the vessel without a focal velocity increase is the method by which we can categorize the less than 50% diameter-reducing stenosis. The spectral waveforms are the most accurate method of classifying the greater than 50% diameter-reducing stenosis.

Multiple Windows

Because of the eccentric shape of atherosclerotic plaques, it is essential that multiple scan planes and windows be used to assess the presence and the character of the plaques (Fig. 11.2). The most successful window used to view the carotid bifurcation is with the scanhead in the lateral to posterior position on the neck, behind the sternocleidomastoid muscle. When a plaque is seen, the examiner must make every effort to view it from other approaches. It is difficult to obtain more than one acceptable view of the bifurcation owing to its location in the neck, but every attempt must be made.

Transverse and Longitudinal Views

Although the longitudinal view is the best view for obtaining spectral waveforms and color images, it is not the best or only

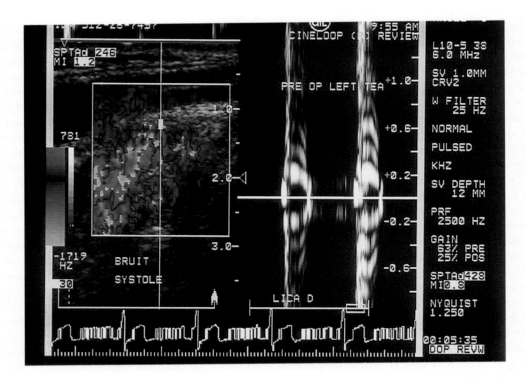

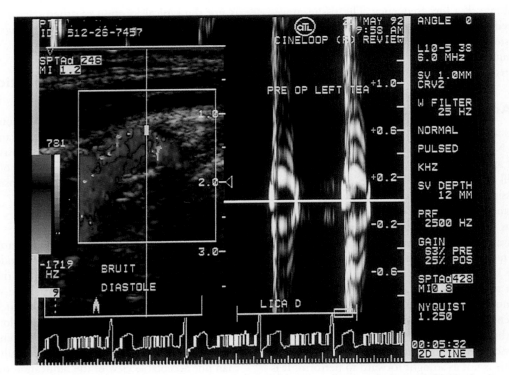

FIGURE 11.10. A carotid bruit seen in systole *(top left)* and not in diastole *(lower left)*. The bruit is also seen in the spectral display on the *right* as a low-frequency, bidirectional signal with associated harmonics appearing during systole.

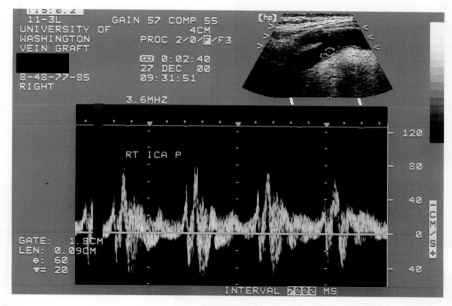

FIGURE 11.11. Spectral waveform taken downstream from a curve in a vessel. The up-and-down character of the waveform throughout systole is caused by the circular motion of eddies that develops as a result of the curve and is considered normal and expected. It is difficult to measure angle-adjusted peak systolic velocity in the presence of this type of waveform.

view for assessing the B-mode image of the plaque. Longitudinal and transverse views should be obtained for appropriate interpretation of the plaque, its size, and its location.

Perpendicular Angles to All Surfaces

The most optimal imaging angle is with the scan lines perpendicular to the surface of interest to obtain the brightest echo. As the imaging angle to the surface becomes smaller, the brightness of the echo decreases. Therefore, it is important to attempt to image all surfaces at perpendicular angles to compare echogenicity or to determine the presence or absence of an echo. At angles other than 90 degrees, a softly echogenic surface or plaque could certainly be missed. It is important to remember that the best Doppler angles are not the most optimal imaging angles. Some ultrasound instruments allow the image to be steered, unlike the fixed "straight down" linear array image, and this is independent of the Doppler steer. Thus, the same image may be optimized for both image and Doppler (Fig. 11.3). Without this instrumentation, the scanhead must be physically manipulated on the skin surface so that the Doppler angle and the image angles are optimized for the same site.

Assessing Plaque Character

Normal Walls

Normal vessel walls, typically best visualized in the CCA, should demonstrate the typical double line, as noted by Pignoli. The double line represents the thickness of the intima and media and is best seen when the image scan lines are perpendicular to the far wall of the vessel, as in Fig. 11.3, *right*.

They may not be appreciated at imaging angles that are less than perpendicular. The first line represents the interface between the blood and the intimal surface; the second, brighter line represents the interface between the intima–media complex and the adventitia. The double line is easily seen in the CCA and extends into the normal bulb, ICA, and ECA. However, it is often difficult to appreciate the double line in the ICA because of the difficulty obtaining perpendicular angles to the curved walls of the bulb and the diving distal vessel. Over time, the intima thickens, and the double lines appear more widely separated with more echoes in the region between the lines. Ultimately, as disease progresses, the lines become indistinguishable, and mounds of echogenic material (i.e., plaque) can be seen along the walls.

Plaque

The plaque character is evaluated using echogenicity or brightness of the echoes and texture or pattern of the echogenicity. The plaque is identified as either homogeneous or heterogeneous. A homogeneous plaque is one in which there is uniform echogenicity and texture throughout (Fig. 11.12). This pattern is seen in a fibrous lesion, often in the CCA. A heterogeneous plaque has mixed areas of brightness and textures (Fig. 11.13). The most brightly echogenic areas in the plaque are usually associated with calcium, which is dense and reflects most of the ultrasound. The bright areas are accompanied by an acoustic shadow that obscures visualization of any feature beneath it, making that area impossible to assess. Because of its dense nature, calcified plaques may obstruct or dampen the Doppler signal, at times making it difficult to obtain signals through

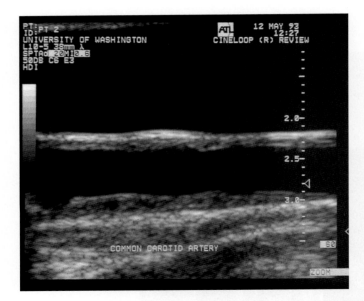

FIGURE 11.12. A homogeneous plaque of uniform density and texture, along the walls of a common carotid artery.

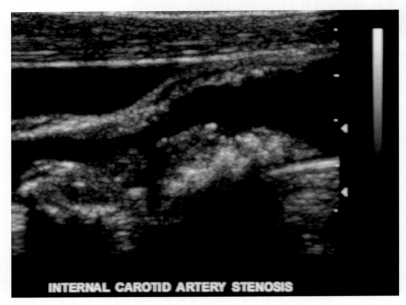

FIGURE 11.13. A heterogeneous plaque in an internal carotid artery. The brightest areas most likely correspond to calcified regions. There are several anechoic regions within the plaque.

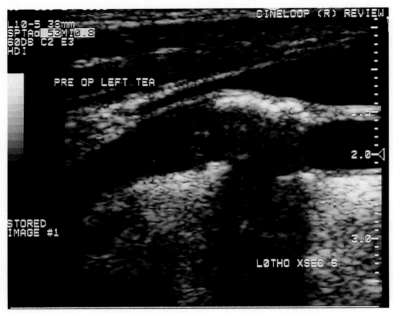

FIGURE 11.14. This image shows a densely calcified plaque in the near wall of an internal carotid artery with accompanying acoustic shadow obscuring and altering the image and Doppler details beneath it.

important areas of stenosis. Manipulating the scanhead to another approach may help to acquire Doppler signals from this area and to visualize the region below it. Some plaques are so densely calcified that Doppler signals are impossible to obtain (Fig. 11.14). In this case, assessing the flow velocity for the presence of poststenotic turbulence in a more distal segment may be the only clue to the presence of a high-grade stenosis.

In addition to brightly echogenic regions in the heterogeneous plaque, there will be areas with little or no ultra-sonic signal. Anechoic or softly echogenic regions within the plaque have been associated with hemorrhage, lipid, and necrotic tissue. It is impossible to distinguish the differences among these tissue types with ultrasound, which should be avoided (7).

Assessing the Surface Character

The surface character of the plaque is classified either as smooth or irregular, based on the appearance in the B-mode image. In the most obvious cases, this distinction can be

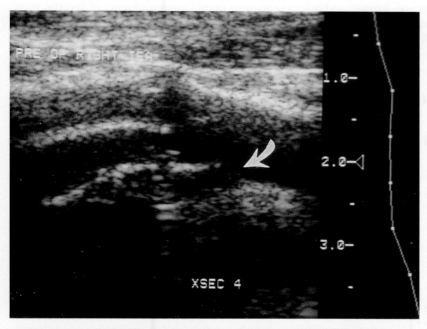

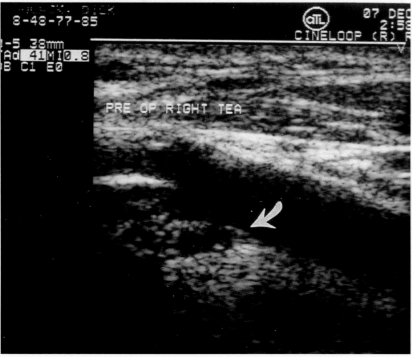

FIGURE 11.15. Two B-mode images that have been taken from similar locations in an internal carotid artery with a significant, complex plaque seen on the far wall. Each of the images has been taken from a different view by manipulation of the scanhead relative to the vessel orientation. The *arrow* in the **top image** points to an area that appears to be without a surface interface and that may be mistaken for an ulcerative region. The *arrow* in the **bottom image** shows the same location, with the scanhead approaching from a different and more favorable angle to visualize the surface interface in the questionable region.

accomplished with ease. A smooth surface should be surveyed over the entire length using perpendicular angles to ensure that the surface is continuous. An irregular surface is considered one in which an uneven or jagged appearance is seen on the B-mode image. It is impossible to distinguish by ultrasound a plaque surface that is truly irregular or ulcerated (i.e., one in which the fibrous cap or lining has broken down and the plaque constituents are exposed) from an unbroken and bumpy surface with hills and valleys, particularly when all of the imaging angles are not optimum (Fig. 11.15). B-mode imaging cannot reliably identify plaque ulceration with any consistency and should not be used for that purpose. Caution must be exercised when describing and interpreting images of plaque surfaces, taking into account that an irregular surface does not imply ulceration.

SCANNING SEQUENCE: CLASSIFYING THE DISEASE

Consistent Protocol for Collecting Spectral Waveforms

A standardized, consistent protocol is essential to document the spectral waveforms to ensure uniformity and repro-ducibility. The resultant velocity measurements are then used for interpretation and classification of the disease state. The criteria for ICA diameter reduction presented in this chapter were validated compared with angiography using waveforms that were generated using the following standardized protocol. Deviations from the standard protocol should always be well documented so that the study can be re-created at a later date for quality assurance and for adequate interpretation by someone other than the examiner.

Standard Anatomic Sites

Each examination should consist of a set of spectral waveforms and corresponding images from standard locations along the length of the carotid arteries (Fig. 11.16). These sites can and should be adjusted for each patient to embody and define each individual patient's disease pattern and are representative of the hemodynamic flow patterns present. Although each carotid system and disease pattern is slightly different, it is valuable to have well-defined locations for uniformity of data collection. It may be necessary and is recommended to gather additional spectral waveforms, along with the standard sites, to demonstrate complex and diffuse carotid disease. A routine cerebrovascular examination includes a complete set of waveforms *from both sides,*

Recording Sites

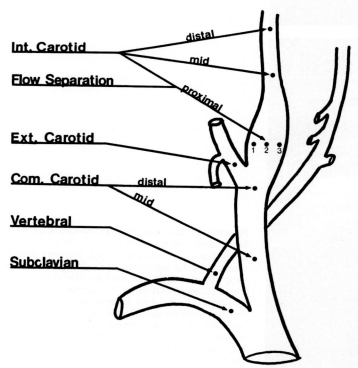

FIGURE 11.16. Standard locations in the extracranial arterial system for recording velocity data for a routine examination. Note that multiple signals may be taken from areas with more complex flow patterns, such as the carotid bulb, to demonstrate the different flow patterns that may be present and significant to the interpretation.

which will be essential for comparison of flow dynamics and for follow-up of contralateral disease.

Standard Doppler Angle to the Vessel Axis

All velocity spectral waveforms used for classification must be generated using a *consistent* angle between the Doppler line and the vessel axis for both frequency and angle-adjusted velocity measurements. The criteria developed at the University of Washington (UW) were created and validated using a 60-degree angle of the Doppler relative to the vessel axis (3). The vessel axis can be defined as an imaginary line drawn in the center of the vessel that parallels the walls. The angle cursor should be aligned along the imaginary line. In cases of tortuosity, in which a 60-degree angle is difficult to obtain, the waveform should be taken using an angle of less than 60 degrees, with the angle cursor aligned as described and clearly documented. Angles of greater than 60 degrees should *never* be used to obtain velocity spectral waveforms for analysis. The percentage of error is large in the velocity calculation when small changes are made to large angles. This error is due to the rapidly

changing cosine function of angles greater than 60 degrees. In addition, there is evidence that the measured, angle-adjusted velocity is different if variable angles are used from the same location (Fig. 11.17). Unfortunately, this inconsistency (i.e., overestimation of the peak velocity) is highly significant when using angles of greater than 60 degrees. Although the error in peak velocity measurement is less with angles of less than 60 degrees, it remains significant and inconsistent with the Doppler equation (see also Troubleshooting Errors in Velocity Measurements). Therefore, it is recommended that a consistent angle be used whenever possible. All angles must be appropriately documented for reference and reused for consistency in follow-up studies. In addition, the direction of the Doppler beam relative to the flow direction must be duplicated at all follow-up studies.

Sample Volume Placed Center Stream

When Doppler signals are taken for final analysis, as a general rule, the sample volume is placed in the center of the vessel flow channel in an effort to obtain the maximum of the velocity profile across the lumen. The sample volume is generally kept as small as possible to detect discrete changes

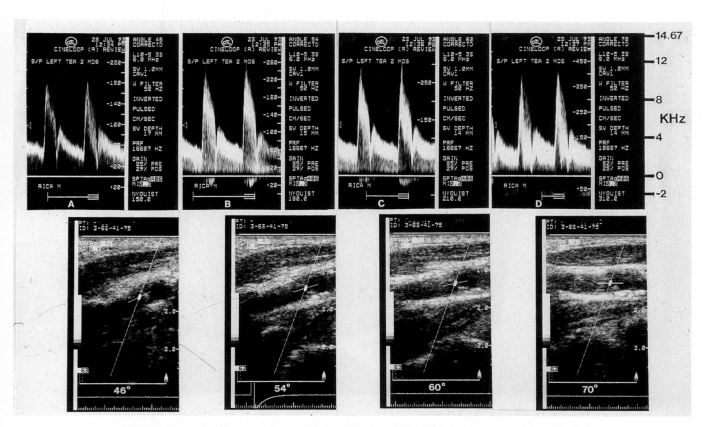

FIGURE 11.17. Velocity spectral waveforms taken from the same location in a stenotic internal carotid artery from four different angles (from *left to right*, 46, 54, 60 and 70 degrees). The measured peak systolic velocities, respectively, are 180, 250, 300, and 450 cm/sec. The apparent increase in velocity is not what is predicted by the Doppler equation.

in the velocity information; however, it may be made larger to search for small, illusive velocity jets or total occlusion that may be difficult to verify with a smaller sample volume.

Standard Doppler Gain Setting

The Doppler gain should be adjusted to a consistent threshold for each signal that is collected for final analysis. The PSV and the spectral broadening displayed in the spectral waveforms are directly affected by gain adjustment (Fig. 11.18). Too much Doppler gain will increase the amount of spectral broadening displayed as well as the measurement of peak velocity. Too little gain will decrease the measured peak velocity, and some spectral broadening will be lost from the display. A standard method by which the gain can be adjusted follows: (a) obtain the signal of interest, (b) turn the gain control to a position of over-gain where there is "noise" clearly seen in the background, and (c) turn the gain control down to a level at which there are a few "speckles" of noise in the background, but *not* to a level at which the background is completely black. For uniformity, each signal taken for analysis should be taken using this gain threshold method.

Considerations for Using the University of Washington Criteria for Internal Carotid Artery Diameter Reduction

There are different criteria for classifying percentage of diameter reduction in the ICA. Before applying any method of classifying disease, the method and the technique must be completely understood in terms of how and under what conditions the criteria were generated. These requirements are necessary to reproduce similar reported results.

Measuring the Waveforms

The angle-adjusted velocity calculations rely on a consistent measurement of the maximum PSV and EDV (Fig. 11.19). The PSV measurement should represent the peak of the systolic velocity acceleration through a segment of the artery in the appropriate direction of flow. The measurement of the appropriate peak may be confused by flow disturbances that occur later in systole (Fig. 11.11). The flow disturbances are seen as rapid oscillations of the spectral waveform, representing flow toward and away from the transducer, rather than accelerated velocity down the vessel. The disturbances

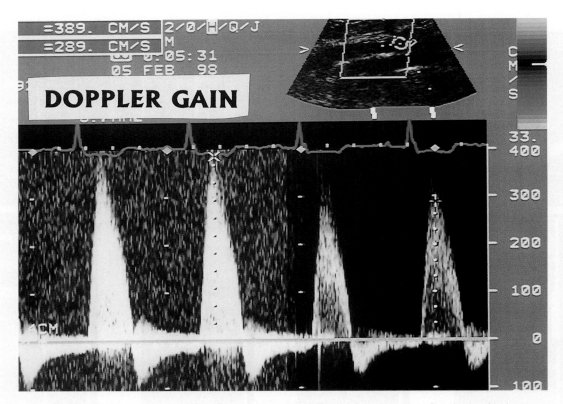

FIGURE 11.18. Two spectral waveforms taken with different Doppler gain adjustments demonstrating the effect on the measurement of peak systolic velocity. The waveform on the *left* is clearly "overgained," as demonstrated by the noise in the background and the brightness of the waveform obscuring the spectral character. The peak systolic velocity in this waveform is falsely measured at 389 cm/sec. The same waveform is shown on the *right* with the gain adjusted appropriately, and the velocity measures 289 cm/sec.

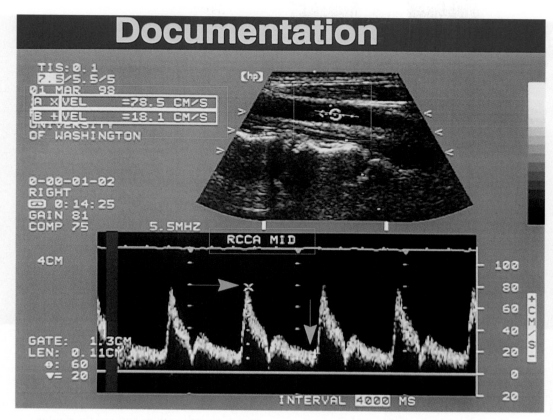

FIGURE 11.19. A spectral waveform showing the appropriate location for measuring peak systolic and end-diastolic velocity as indicated by the *arrows*. Note the clear image of the vessel, with the sample volume and angle cursor placement readily seen from the corresponding location from which the waveform was generated.

most certainly represent circular flow movement that may be created by eddies or vortices in areas like the normal carotid bulb, around carotid plaques, at branches and bifurcations, and distal to tortuosities and curves. The disturbances are seen in the waveform after peak systole, as the velocity slows down. Typically, the peak systolic measurement is taken at the end of the primary systolic acceleration slope, rather than at the spikes in late systole. Critical, clinical decisions are based on the measurement of PSV, and to be consistent, it would seem important that the measurement be taken at the same time in the cardiac cycle from each spectral waveform. There are a host of other technical and physiologic conditions that will affect the measurement of PSV. These considerations will be covered in a separate section (Troubleshooting Errors in Velocity Measurements) at the end of this chapter.

The peak EDV measurement is the value typically used to classify the patients with the most significant disease (i.e., greater than 80% diameter reduction) and is, therefore, a critical measurement (8). The EDV measurement is more clearly defined and identified than PSV. The measurement of EDV is made in the waveform 10 milliseconds before the upstroke of the next systole (Fig. 11.19).

Standard Angle Measurement

As previously stated, a consistent angle measurement of 60 degrees was used for collecting the spectral waveforms when the criteria were being validated. Some have suggested using off-axis color jets seen within the flow pattern and/or off-axis color flow channel walls for adjusting the angle cursor rather than using the vessel walls. There are no validated modified criteria that use this altered technique.

Criteria Used for Three Centimeters of the Internal Carotid Artery

The criteria can only be used accurately for spectral waveforms taken from the first 3 cm of the ICA (Fig. 11.20). Atherosclerosis typically will develop within the first 2 cm and rarely will be found in the more distal ICA. In addition, the vessel becomes smaller in diameter and often becomes tortuous and/or deep. These changes in vessel orientation and size create difficulty in visualizing the vessels walls and, hence, in aligning the angle cursor. Dramatic errors in velocity calculation can occur, falsely indicating the presence of disease. Therefore, the criteria cannot be used with accuracy in the distal ICA. The presence of poststenotic tur-

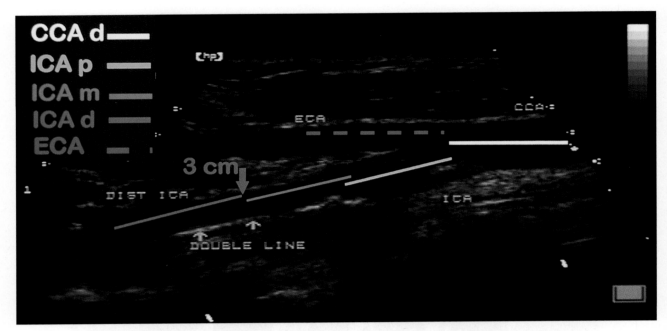

FIGURE 11.20. Standard sites in the carotid bifurcation. Note that the distal internal carotid artery (*DIST ICA*) is typically identified as the region at least 3 cm distal to the origin of the vessel.

bulence and the visualization of plaque must verify elevated velocity that is considered significant with stenosis in the distal ICA. The presence of tortuosity must definitely be ruled out or be suggested as a possible cause for the apparent velocity increase.

The criteria cannot be used to classify disease in the CCA, ECA, or vertebral arteries (see Common and External Carotid Artery Stenosis).

Using the Criteria for Classifying Internal Carotid Artery Stenosis

Note that measurement of percentage of diameter reduction has been derived from angiographic measurements of the stenosis that were retrospectively correlated with spectral waveforms and then prospectively tested. The classifications were not created from direct measurement of the vessels as seen on the B-mode images. The UW criteria were developed using the bulb as the reference artery for measuring the percentage of diameter reduction of the ICA stenosis as in the European Carotid Stenosis Trial (Fig. 11.21). The North American Symptomatic Carotid Endarterectomy Trial (NASCET) method of measurement uses the distal ICA as the reference artery to determine percentage of diameter reduction, similar to the American Carotid Asymptomatic Study (ACAS). (See Chapter 6.)

Normal

The classification of normal is derived from a PSV of less than 125 cm/sec in the ICA and no visible plaque or wall changes seen in the B-mode image. The vessel walls should appear smooth with or without the double line. The velocity waveforms from a normal carotid bulb will display typical flow disturbances (boundary layer separation) as a result of the dilatation and the secondary helical flow patterns from the bifurcation angle. It is imperative to learn to anticipate and recognize these reproducible flow disturbances and to use them to help define geometric changes in the normal vessels.

1% to 15% Diameter Reduction

This category was originally created to deal with minor changes in the wall of the carotid bulb that were not sufficient to make a discrete measurement of the degree of diameter reduction by arteriography. It is defined as minimal spectral broadening with a PSV of less than 125 cm/sec.

16% to 49% Diameter Reduction

Marked spectral broadening throughout the cardiac cycle (i.e., no systolic "window") and PSV of less than 125 cm/sec are the hallmark of this category. For a trained ear, this may also be detected as a harsh, raspy audible Doppler signal with no increase in the frequency shift.

What Is Spectral Broadening and Where Does It Come From?

Spectral broadening is defined as a distribution of the frequency content at each spectral sample, that is, every 10 mil-

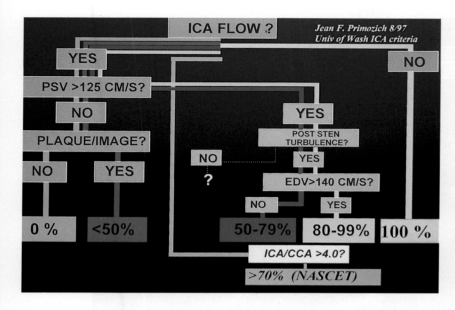

FIGURE 11.21. Criteria algorithm for classifying percentage of diameter reduction in the internal carotid artery (ICA), derived from using the bulb and proximal ICA as the reference vessel. Note that the categories of 1% to 15% and 16% to 49% have been combined into a 1% to 50% diameter reduction. The *blue line* and *box* refer to measurement of more than 70% diameter reduction, which is derived using the distal ICA as the reference vessel (North American Symptomatic Carotid Endarterectomy Trial).

liseconds. It could be called the "grass" that occurs under the outer envelope of the waveform and can extend into diastole.

Unfortunately, spectral broadening is not specific to the presence of minimal disease. It can occur as a result of other reasons, the most important of which may be the instrument technology. Some reasons for spectral broadening include the following: (a) the use of a large sample volume relative to a small vessel, thereby sampling across the entire velocity profile; (b) the placement of the sample volume too near the wall, detecting the slower velocities at the wall; and (c) the use of a large-aperture, multielement Doppler transducer like the present-day linear array scanheads (5).

The present-day linear array scanheads have a much wider slice thickness from which the imaging and Doppler information are generated. The larger thickness creates a larger area of spectral sampling for the pulsed Doppler in width dimension. The larger sampling area produces normal broadening of the spectral waveform as a result of sampling a larger area of the velocity profile rather than being secondary to disease.

In addition, the mechanical sector transducer used a single element with a fixed focus to obtain frequency information. This means that the Doppler information was generated from a single angle of approach. The linear array technology uses multiple elements in series, which creates a wider Doppler aperture from which the frequency information is generated. The benefit of using multiple elements is the ability to steer the beam for ease of use. Unfortunately, this type of technology is not without tradeoffs. The result of using multiple elements means that the Doppler frequency shifts are being detected from many different incident angles at once, not simply from the single Doppler line that is displayed on the image. Hence, there is a broadening of the spectrum, even from normal vessels, because of mul-

tiple frequency shifts being generated at once rather than as a result of disturbed flow. This phenomenon is referred to as *intrinsic spectral broadening*. It is for this same reason that the wide-aperture Doppler of the linear array scanhead has been shown to overestimate the peak velocity measured from the spectral waveforms approximately 16% to 60% (9). Most significantly, intrinsic spectral broadening affects our ability to "angle correct" and to obtain reproducible velocity measurements from the same site at different angles (see Troubleshooting Errors in Velocity Measurements).

For this reason and others, the use of spectral broadening to classify disease in the less than 50% categories appears to be far too subjective and much less reliable with the linear array technology than with the original mechanical sector scanheads. Although this concept has not been properly documented, it has been noted by technologists familiar with the previously validated protocol. Spectral broadening should not be dismissed as irrelevant if it is present in a waveform but not highly weighted when attempting to classify disease into these categories.

The original categories that encompass the less than 50% diameter reduction category (i.e., 1% to 15%, 16% to 49%) have traditionally been distinguished by the degree of spectral broadening occurring under the systolic peak of the velocity spectral waveform. PSV measurements in these categories are always less than 125 cm/sec. For completeness, they have been defined here; however, they have since been combined to become one category referred to as *less than 50% diameter reduction*.

Less than 50% Diameter Reduction

The B-mode image is highly sensitive and probably more reliable for identifying and classifying disease in the less than 50% category. In the minimal to moderate range of

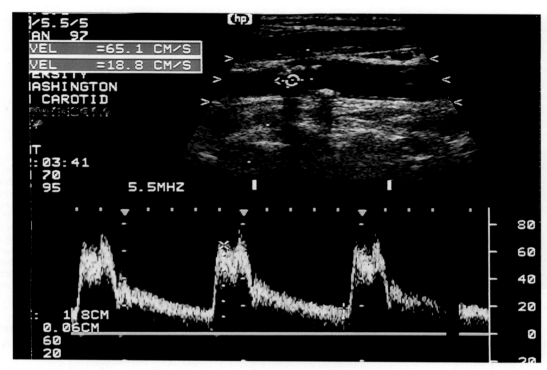

FIGURE 11.22. This lesion would be classified as less than 50% diameter reduction. Note that the spectral waveform is relatively free of spectral broadening, and the peak systolic velocity is less than 125 cm/sec; however, there is clear evidence of calcified plaque noted in the B-mode image.

disease, the plaques, wall, and lumens are more clearly defined in the B-mode image than are the typical complex plaques of the higher-grade lesions. Therefore, the classification of a less than 50% diameter reduction is made by the combined findings of visible plaque in the B-mode image, with or without spectral broadening and a PSV of less than 125 cm/sec (Fig. 11.22).

There is no typical color pattern associated with a less than 50% diameter-reducing stenosis. Spectral broadening as displayed in the spectral waveform will not be appreciated in the color display.

More than 50% Diameter Reduction

Clinically, these are the most critical of all of the classifications of disease. The Doppler spectral waveform is definitely the most accurate method of defining the disease once the luminal narrowing progresses beyond 50% and the plaque becomes more complicated. Unlike the lesser degrees of stenosis, for which the image has been shown to be of more value for classification, the image has not proved useful in classifying disease for the more significant lesions. These categories are rooted in the presence of a focal increase in PSV at the site of maximal narrowing and, as the disease progresses, an increase in EDV. A representative

waveform from the poststenotic turbulence should also be included in the complement of signals gathered for appropriate interpretation of a true velocity increase. A thorough scan with the sample volume through the region of interest, from the prestenotic zone through the stenosis and into the poststenotic zone, will ensure that the maximum velocity has been recorded for interpretation purposes. Neither the B-mode image nor the color displays will pinpoint the maximum velocity precisely.

Color Doppler imaging will not distinguish a 50% to 79% stenosis from an 80% to 99% stenosis. The color patterns should focus the technologist on the area of the stenosis. It may indicate that the lesion is greater than 50% because of the presence of typical color pattern of poststenotic turbulence. However, the real investigations for the maximum velocity must be accomplished with the sample volume sweep through the area.

50% to 79% Diameter Reduction

A PSV of at least 125 cm/sec (4 kHz with 5 mHz Doppler) and EDV of less than 140 cm/sec (4.5 kHz with a 5 mHz Doppler) are significant with a 50% to 79% diameter-reducing lesion. Spectral broadening is usually associated with this stenosis category as a result of the sample volume being large compared with the narrow lumen size, and encompassing a portion of the poststenotic region in addition to the velocity jet in the sample. Spectral broadening is not, however, required for interpretation. Multiple velocities and flow directions will be encountered; hence, spec-

tral broadening is usually seen in these waveforms. If the sample volume is placed precisely in the fastest, most organized area of the flow jet, it is possible to have increased velocity without the presence of spectral broadening (Fig. 11.23).

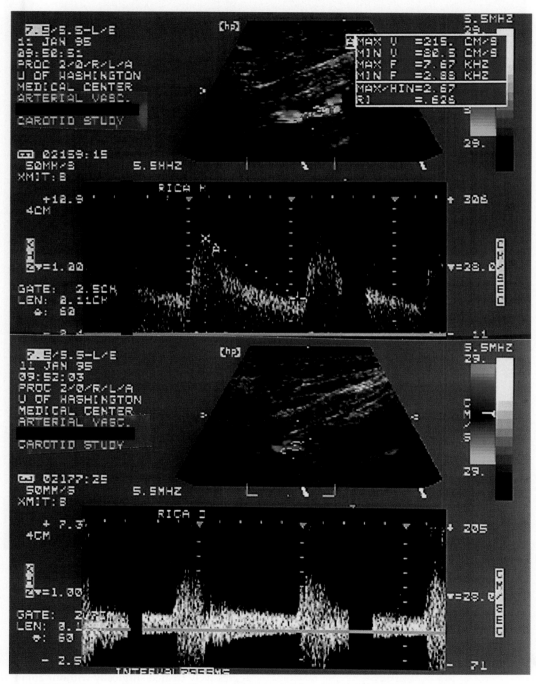

FIGURE 11.23. A 50% to 79% diameter-reducing lesion. The peak systolic velocity is 215 cm/sec, and the end-diastolic velocity is 80 cm/sec. Note that there is no spectral broadening associated with the jet of the stenosis in the **upper image**. The **lower image** shows the typical waveform of poststenotic turbulence that verifies the velocity increase.

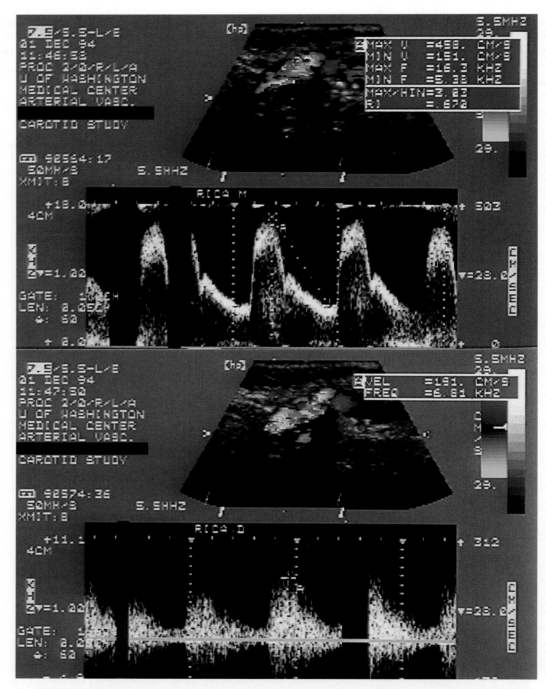

FIGURE 11.24. An 80% to 99% diameter-reducing stenosis. The end-diastolic velocity is 151 cm/sec, and the peak systolic velocity is 458 cm/sec. Note that there is no spectral broadening associated with the jet of the stenosis. The lower spectral waveform demonstrates the post-stenotic turbulence associated with the stenosis and marks the end of the stenosis.

80% to 99% Diameter Reduction

The 80% to 99% category of disease is extremely important to identify accurately and to distinguish from the 50% to 79% category. Asymptomatic patients who have a more than 80% diameter-reducing stenosis are being more aggressively treated surgically without angiography for verification (1). It can be difficult and often time-consuming for the technologist to search for the maximum velocity in these highly significant lesions. There may be multiple different velocities identified within a stenosis; however, the one used for the classification must clearly be the highest PSV and EDV.

This category is defined by an EDV exceeding or equal to 140 cm/sec (4.5 KHz at 5 MHz Doppler frequency), followed by poststenotic turbulence. The spectral waveform should clearly show the end-diastolic portion, which is measured at 10 milliseconds preceding the upstroke of the next systole (Fig. 11.24). The PSV is no longer an issue for classification with these waveforms because it has obviously exceeded 125 cm/sec. The PSV is, however, important for the calculation of the ICA/CCA ratio. It is important if the PSV becomes elevated to a level that exceeds the limits of the PRF and is "aliased" or wrapped around the scale, and the peak is not visible. The PSV can be impossible to measure accurately for the ICA/CCA ratio, which is used to define a greater than 70% (NASCET) stenosis. The EDV is more reliably measured and therefore a more dependable measurement in this case.

More than 70% Diameter Reduction (NASCET Measurement)

The NASCET results created a demand for a new category of disease, that is, 70% to 99% diameter reduction. The study showed that symptomatic patients with a greater than 70% diameter reduction benefited from CEA compared with medical therapy. The trial identified the severity of the disease on angiography by using the distal cervical ICA as the reference vessel for calculating ICA stenosis. As has been stated, the UW and European Carotid Surgery Trial (ECST) used the bulb as the reference site. Therefore, a NASCET criterion of greater than 70% was developed to define this decision category from information derived from a standard duplex study. The category is defined by calculating a ratio of the PSV of the ICA to the PSV of the CCA. A ratio of 4.0 or greater indicates a 70% or greater diameter reduction. Therefore, if an absolute peak velocity signal falls into the 50% to 79% diameter category (i.e. at least 125 cm/sec and less than 140 cm/sec EDV), an ICA/CCA ratio will be calculated to identify a 70% to 99% (NASCET) stenosis, and this value will also be included in the final interpretation (Fig. 11.21; see Chapter 6).

Similarly, the ACAS identified a group of asymptomatic patients with a stenosis of 60% or more, based on the similar angiographic measurement as NASCET, who benefited from endarterectomy compared with medical therapy. A similar study was done to identify this category, 60% to 99%, using the information generated from a routine clinical carotid duplex examination. An ICA/CCA ratio of more than 3.2 to 3.5 provided the best overall accuracy to define this category of disease. This value may also be incorporated in the final interpretation.

Considerations for Using the ICA/CCA Ratio

The values that are used to calculate the ICA/CCA ratio are well defined and specific. The ICA value is the PSV at the maximum velocity increase in the proximal or mid ICA or the distal CCA. The CCA velocity is taken from the CCAm, which is defined as at least 2 cm proximal to the bifurcation. *Both the ICA and the CCA velocity waveforms must be obtained using the standard angle of 60 degrees.* The CCA is easily visualized and fairly parallel to the skin surface in this location. If the CCA signal is taken from a location that is too proximal in the vessel, there is a risk for curvature or tortuosity that causes flow disturbances in the waveforms, making the measurement of the PSV difficult and questionable. The CCAm velocity is taken from a disease-free portion of the vessel.

Internal Carotid Artery Occlusion

The identification of a total ICA occlusion is often a difficult task for even the most experienced of examiners. The difficulty arises as a result of the inability to appreciate easily the occluded vessel on the B-mode image. The finding of an ICA occlusion is, of course, an important interpretation because the subsequent follow-up and therapy of the patient will depend on the results. Color Doppler should not be relied on as the sole means of identifying an ICA occlusion, although it can be helpful, additive information. The most accurate means of identifying a total ICA occlusion is by assessing the global hemodynamic changes that occur in the bilateral extracranial carotid system as a result of the occlusion. The following list is a description of the hemodynamic changes that occur as a result of a total ICA occlusion. Each of these flow changes should be documented for appropriate interpretation (Fig. 11.25).

1. The CCAm on the side of the occlusion will attach the characteristics of a high-resistance vessel, rather than the normal low-resistance character, as a result of the blood flow being directed through the ECA system. The ipsilateral CCA waveform will have an EDV that is at or near the zero baseline (Fig 11.25, *lower left*). Because the waveform characteristics of the CCA change as it approaches the dilated bifurcation region, it is important to assess the diastolic component in the CCAm, at least 2 cm proximal to bifurcation. Unfortunately, flow to zero may not be present in the patient who has a chronic ICA occlusion. In this patient, the EDV may be similar to that of the contralateral side as a result of intervening collateralization of the ECA and decreased distal resistance. Bilateral flow to zero could certainly be a finding in the presence of bilateral ICA occlusions, which is rare, but may also be associated with a more proximal cardiac condition.

2. The contralateral CCAm waveform, at about the same level in the neck, can exhibit increased EDV as a result of

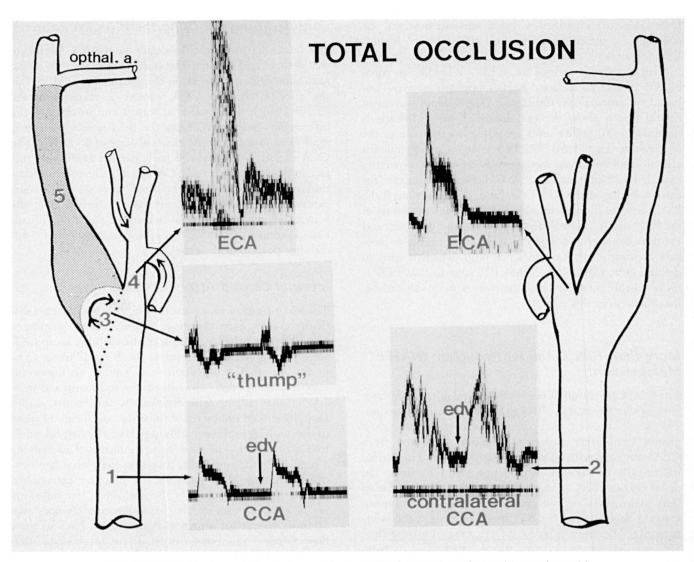

FIGURE 11.25. The hemodynamic changes that occur in the presence of a total internal carotid artery occlusion (refer to text).

compensatory flow (Fig. 11.25, *lower right*). An asymmetry of the flow patterns in the EDV will be present when compared with the ipsilateral CCA, unless the occlusion is chronic. As is always the case, a direct bilateral comparison of the spectral waveforms from the CCAP to CCAm can offer additional hemodynamic clues about the entire carotid system and, more importantly, about the condition of the more distal bifurcation vessels.

3. Scanning through the CCA and into the suspected ICA, a "thumping" sound may be heard or recorded with the Doppler at the stump of the vessel (Fig. 11.25, *middle left*). The stump, or pocket, at the origin of the vessel is often created when it occludes. The spectral waveform of the thump will appear damped and markedly attenuated, indicating no essential forward flow and a brief transient

reversal. The flow reversal is seen in the color display as a transient area of blue at the stump (Fig. 11.26). The reversal is a result of the blood flow striking against the occlusion and then immediately changing direction, similar to the effect of a water hammer. Unfortunately, this finding is not unique to occlusions and may not always be present. Dense calcification at the origin of the ICA, not associated with an occlusion, may attenuate the Doppler signal and mimic this signal.

4. Increased flow will be seen throughout the entire contralateral carotid system as mentioned in number 2. The increased flow boosts the normally occurring velocity of the contralateral ICA. Erroneous overestimation of the degree of narrowing in the ICA may occur. Modified ICA criteria by Fugitani may be used more reliably to classify severe ICA

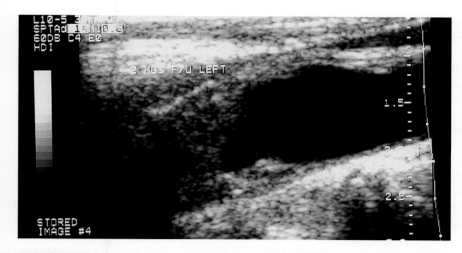

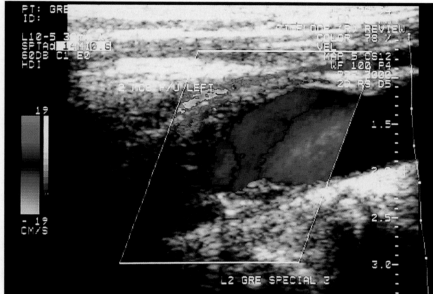

FIGURE 11.26. B-mode and color image of a total internal carotid artery occlusion with a stump. Note that the color appears to demonstrate a transient flow directional change as a result of the occlusion.

disease contralateral to an ICA occlusion (10). Using these criteria, a 50% to 79% diameter reduction is defined as PSV of at least 140 cm/sec and EDV of less than 155 cm/sec; an 80% to 99% diameter reduction is defined as an EDV of 155 cm/sec or greater. These criteria were produced using protocol similar to that used in the original UW criteria, in particular, using a 60-degree Doppler angle.

5. An increase in the flow through the ipsilateral ECA, as a result of the occlusion, will create higher velocities than would normally be expected (Fig. 11.25, *upper left*). Consequently, an overestimation of disease in the ECA may be expected. If the ECA is severely stenotic, it may lose its normal peripheral character and begin to appear similar to that of a stenotic ICA. Critical misidentification of the vessels can occur. It is important to note that in this case, the ECA will usually continue to have a sharp systolic upstroke, unlike a typical ICA.

6. An ICA will occlude from the origin at the bifurcation to the first major branch, which is the ophthalmic artery (Fig. 11.25, *left drawing*). Therefore, no flow should be detected in what is identified as the ICA in the neck. If flow is detected in the distal ICA, especially very low flow, damped velocity waveform, or poststenotic turbulence, the ICA is not occluded. Decreased flow in the distal ICA, in addition to the previously listed, hemodynamic findings should arouse suspicion of a high-grade stenosis that was not initially detected. In this case, the flow changes of the stenosis are mimicking that of a total occlusion. A thorough search through the plaque, concentrating on locating a high-velocity flow jet, should follow. The search can be tedious and time-consuming, especially in the presence of a highly calcified plaque that is dramatically attenuating the ultrasound transmission. In addition to a high-velocity jet, another troublesome scenario can be the presence of a

"string sign" stenosis, named for its appearance on the angiogram. In this case, a near-occlusive lesion may be present that displays uncharacteristically low, rather than elevated, velocity. In fact, the velocity may be lower than the thresholds of detection of the spectral or color Doppler. The aforementioned hemodynamic findings in the presence of the lack of any sign of flow after thorough search should be interpreted as a "suspected" high-grade stenosis or "preocclusive" stenosis. This kind of information is invaluable for the radiologist, who may decide, in light of the duplex report, to do a "trickle flow" angiogram, which involves obtaining late films to watch for delayed flow. Late films may not be part of a standard angiogram if a string sign is not suspected, and the vessel may erroneously appear to be occluded.

Common and External Carotid Artery Stenosis

The strict velocity criteria used to classify disease in the ICA are not used for classifying disease in the CCA or the ECA. The criteria were validated for use in the ICA only. Hemodynamically significant atherosclerotic disease is rarely found in the CCA. Thickened, fibrous plaques with relatively smooth surfaces are most often encountered in the CCA. These lesions are easily identified on the B-mode image and are usually not clinically important. Disease in the ECA is often seen, but is usually not of clinical import, unless the ECA is serving as a collateral source for an occluded ICA. The presence of any visual change in the vessel walls, for example, thickening or irregularity, should trigger a more intense search with the pulsed Doppler for flow changes that might be accompanying.

Significant stenosis in the ECA and CCA is typically identified by the presence of plaque seen in the B-mode image or the presence of a focal velocity increase of at least 100% compared with the prestenotic segment, followed by poststenotic turbulence. The CCA and the ECA can be classified into one of four categories of disease: (a) normal—no velocity increase and no visible plaque in the B-mode image; (b) less than 50% diameter reduction, with the presence of plaque, wall thickening, or irregularity with or without flow disturbance and no focal velocity increase; (c) greater than 50% diameter reduction, with a focal velocity increase of at least 100% compared with the prestenotic velocity, accompanied by poststenotic turbulence and the presence of plaque on the B-mode image; or (d) total occlusion—a clearly identifiable vessel with no Doppler signal located.

Abnormal Vertebral Artery

Stenosis of the vertebral artery is usually found at the origin and is rarely found in the more distal, cervical portion. Clinical identification of stenosis in the vertebral artery can add to the comprehensive analysis of the patient symptoms, overall hemodynamics, and subsequent therapy. For clinical purposes, vertebral artery stenosis is divided into two large categories: less than 50% and greater than 50% diameter reduction. A stenosis of greater than 50% is classified like the CCA and the ECA: a focal velocity increase of at least 100% followed by poststenotic turbulence. A totally occluded vertebral artery is often difficult to identify with confidence because of the location of the vessel. The examiner must be absolutely certain that the Doppler-silent vessel is the vertebral and not another branch of the SA or a vein with low flow. Color Doppler imaging can be helpful in locating the vertebral artery if it is not occluded, but the lack of color in a questionable occlusion must be carefully assessed and color set-ups adequately adjusted. The Doppler signal will absolutely distinguish the low-resistance vertebral signal from the high-resistance signals of the other subclavian branches.

In addition to the presence of stenosis in the vertebral artery, the duplex scan should demonstrate that flow is in the normal antegrade direction. Flow in the vertebral artery that is found to be in the retrograde direction is significant with a stenosis or occlusion in the subclavian or innominate artery proximal to the vertebral origin. Reverse flow in the vertebral artery to supply the arm is a normal collateral pathway in the presence of subclavian stenosis or occlusion. A significant decrease in the brachial pressure (more than 20 mm Hg) on the side of the suspected flow reversal helps to verify this finding. In most cases, the reversal does not lead to symptoms.

Another abnormal vertebral artery flow pattern may be detected, which is often initially difficult to appreciate or understand. The flow pattern is referred to as *to-and-fro flow*. Because of pressure differentials between the brain and the arm, in the presence of an SA occlusion or stenosis, the blood flow in the vertebral artery appears to slosh back and forth, changing direction during the cardiac cycle. The Doppler signal and the color flow pattern appear similar to venous flow and can be confusing. In these patients, a reactive hyperemia test with the cuff inflated over the brachial artery may be performed to detect directional flow changes after a period of ischemia.

Abnormal Subclavian Artery

Most SA stenoses are found at or near the origin, which on the left side is difficult to access with the scanhead during a routine examination, owing to depth and location of the vessel under the clavicle. A lower-frequency scanhead with a smaller footprint may be needed. A focal increase in velocity, the loss of the reversal component of the normally occurring triphasic waveform, and the presence of poststenotic turbulence identify a greater than 50% diameter-reducing stenosis. A decrease in the brachial pressure of at least 20 mm Hg in the ipsilateral arm verifies a hemodynamically significant stenosis. The correct interpretation of these duplex scan results is "the presence of a pressure-reducing subclavian stenosis." For completeness, this interpretation should also be accompanied by the more clinically important vertebral artery interpretation in regard to direction of flow (see Chapter 6).

Duplex Information for Preoperative Examinations

The use of angiograms to document carotid artery stenosis has decreased in recent years as a result of the outstanding accuracy of the carotid duplex examination in identifying the presence of carotid artery disease and estimating the amount of stenosis. Angiography, in many facilities, is reserved for those duplex cases with difficult or questionable results, or for cases in which more information about the cerebral circulation is required. Transcranial Doppler studies have, in fact, replaced some of those cases, reducing the need for angiography even more. For this reason, surgeons are relying solely on the results of the carotid duplex scan for preparation of the surgical procedure and for valuable information, previously available with angiograms, concerning the anatomy and the amount and extent of the disease of the carotid bifurcation.

An accurate estimate of the percentage of diameter reduction that has been determined by velocity measurements from the duplex examination is of foremost interest to the surgeon. As stated previously, these measurements must represent the true hemodynamic picture of the flow patterns within the vessels. The surgeon must rely on the examination to supply complete and appropriate data for proper interpretation of the results. The decision to operate on a patient may depend solely on the duplex results, and the responsibility lies with the technologist to produce a complete and technically adequate examination. The data form should include comments concerning the technologist's confidence in the examination results or variation from the normally expected protocol that may affect the interpretation. These comments are invaluable for the interpreting physician to sort out difficult or questionable results. Conversely, reporting positive confidence in the results, along with complete and appropriate documentation, is equally helpful to the surgeon when decisions concerning the patient's therapy are in question.

Technically, numerous pieces of surgically valuable information can be garnered from the duplex examination in light of the fact that an angiogram is not available. The technologist should be aware that the patient is a candidate for surgery and be prepared to report results that will be useful for the procedure.

Knowing the relative location in the neck of the level of the bifurcation will direct the surgeon's attention to the general area of the disease. Most carotid bifurcations are found at the level of the thyroid cartilage, which is about in the mid neck and easily accessible to the surgical procedure. Some bifurcations may be located higher in the neck, closer to the mandible, and likely creating a more difficult surgical access. A bifurcation that was difficult to access at the time of the duplex examination because of its distal location will probably also be difficult to access during the operation. Accessing an extremely low bifurcation may also be a challenge to the surgeon if not made aware preoperatively. Therefore, noting at the time of the duplex examination the location of the bifurcation and the ease of accessibility can prepare the surgeon for potential problems related to uncommon anatomy.

Typically, atherosclerosis develops at the carotid bifurcation, extending into the ICA for 1 to 2 cm. If the plaque extends more distally in the ICA, it may be a problem to achieve an adequate and smooth endpoint for the endarterectomy. Plaque that extends too far distally into the ICA may prevent the surgeon from performing the operation. The problem may be exacerbated by an abnormally high-level bifurcation. In addition, the plaque often begins more proximally in the distal CCA. Surgically, CCA plaque may be a problem in that it may be a site of thrombus or platelet formation or debris production after clamp placement and removal. Commenting about the bifurcation, measuring the relative location to the bifurcation, and making a drawing of the plaque location can be an invaluable aid to understanding the extent of the problem and to warn of potential problems.

Describing the plaque character in general terms can also be helpful. The presence of marked areas of brightly echogenic material may indicate a densely calcified plaque that may be hard to cut through at the time of the endarterectomy. Conversely, softly echogenic material may be a plaque that is friable and fragile and difficult to remove at the time of the surgery. Although a precise identification of plaque character still eludes ultrasound in general, we have some basic knowledge about levels of echogenicity of plaques that may relate to certain identifiable features.

The surgeon relies on the fact that the distal ICA remains essentially free of arterial disease to achieve a good endpoint of the endarterectomy. Therefore, comments in the duplex report concerning the condition of the distal ICA increase the surgeon's confidence in a successful procedure. The distal ICA should be free of disease with smooth walls and a relatively straight vessel (Fig. 11.20). The presence of disease in the distal artery, a relatively small vessel diameter, inability or difficulty following the vessel more distally in the neck, and obvious tortuosity are descriptive comments that are invaluable.

Finally, a comment in the duplex results concerning the relative size of the carotid arteries is advisable, particularly with patients who have small-diameter vessels. A small artery may need to have a patch closure after endarterectomy rather than a primary closure.

SCANNING POSTOPERATIVE AND POSTENDOVASCULAR PROCEDURES

Identifying recurrent stenosis is the major goal of the duplex scan after any interventional procedure (11). In addition, the follow-up examination documents progression of disease in the contralateral carotid system. Importantly, it may also document a decrease in the velocity of the contralateral side as a result of the restoration of normal flow to the ipsilateral carotid. The endarterectomy arteriotomy is either closed primarily or by using a patch of vein or prosthetic material. In addition, the use of stents has been added to the battery of procedures used to treat carotid bifurcation disease. Knowledge of the type of procedure performed prepares the technologist for obvious and predictable changes in the examination that are common to each procedure. The standard, *bilateral* cerebrovascular duplex examination should be performed, regardless of the interventional method. Appreciating the change in appearance of the arteries and paying particular attention to potentially problematic locations in the vessels that are specific for each procedure are paramount in follow-up examinations.

Duplex Results after Carotid Endarterectomy (CEA) with Primary Closure Arteriotomy

Simply defined, CEA involves an anterior wall incision of the artery, that is, the arteriotomy, originating proximal to the disease in the mid and distal CCA and continuing through the ICA beyond the disease. The plaque is dissected out, along with some of the media of the wall. The vessel is then closed using Prolene sutures to seal the arteriotomy.

A recurrent stenosis after endarterectomy most often begins at either the proximal or distal end of the arteriotomy. The recurrent stenosis is not a new growth of atherosclerosis, but instead is myointimal hyperplasia, which represents the arterial wall response to injury. Recurrent stenosis occurs in 10% to 20% of patients after primary closure CEA. Myointimal hyperplasia occurs within the first 2 years after the surgical procedure and tends to become a stable, fibrous lesion that is usually asymptomatic and rarely exceeds more than 80% diameter reduction. The recurrent stenosis may also be seen to regress over time.

The duplex findings of a recurrent stenosis are interesting to note. The lesion is composed of low-density, uniform echoes with relatively smooth surfaces. Calcification is not seen in a true hyperplastic lesion. An extended area of moderately increased velocity may be identified throughout the length of the endarterectomy, often not followed by the classic poststenotic turbulence. This finding may be interpreted as a smooth-surfaced, tapered lesion rather than that of a more typical, irregularly shaped atherosclerotic lesion. The diameter reduction, as classified by the spectral waveforms, rarely exceeds 50% to 79%. Total occlusion of the ICA due to the hyperplasia is rare after this surgical procedure. The recurrent stenosis may be complicated by the growth of atherosclerosis many years after the procedure.

The typical duplex findings following primary closure CEA follow.

1. A prominent lip or shelf may be seen in the far wall of the CCA at the proximal transection site of the endarterectomy (Fig. 11.27, *top image*). The location and height of the shelf depend on the extent of preexisting disease and the tacking procedure that was done at the time of the endarterectomy. The shelf is readily apparent in the early preoperative studies. However, if the follow-up study is done after an extended period of time following the CEA, the shelf may not be appreciated because of regrowth of the arterial wall in the endarterectomized site (Fig. 11.27, *lower three images*) .

Dramatic flow disturbances will be seen distal to a thick shelf owing to the dramatic change in diameter of the vessel. These flow changes must be anticipated and documented in a similar fashion as those disturbances found in the normally occurring bulb (i.e., sample across the vessel to identify the typical flow patterns). The flow disturbances may decrease or disappear over time owing to remodeling of the vessel wall and a loss of the dramatic diameter changes as the vessel wall fills in.

2. A suture line may be routinely seen beginning in the mid to distal CCA and extending into the ICA marking the arteriotomy. The sutures are most easily seen from the anteroposterior window. The suture line is identified as a series of small, brightly echogenic, regularly spaced echoes, either dashes or dots, along the near wall of the vessel and sometimes crossing the lumen. It may take some manipulation of the scanhead to locate these markers. The first suture, found usually within 1 cm proximal to the shelf, can be routinely identified at each visit and can be used as an internal marker for follow-up studies (Fig. 11.27, *top image*).

3. As the vessel wall heals, within the first 1 to 3 months after surgery, a new echogenic layer will develop at the endarterectomy site, most predominantly seen along the far wall. Over time, the wall may demonstrate the typical double-line appearance of a normal vessel (Fig. 11.27, *second image from top*) .The new layer is most probably made up of medial smooth muscle cells and collagen. The distance between the two lines may increase over time and will eventually stabilize (Fig. 11.27, *lower three images*). The original shelf in the CCA may disappear as this regrowth occurs.

4. Stainless-steel clips, used to control small bleeder vessels during the operation, may be seen in the tissue surrounding the vessel. Characteristically, the clips appear highly echogenic, accompanied by a white reflective shadow beneath them. The importance of this finding is that the shadow may be so profound that it will obscure both the image and the color display.

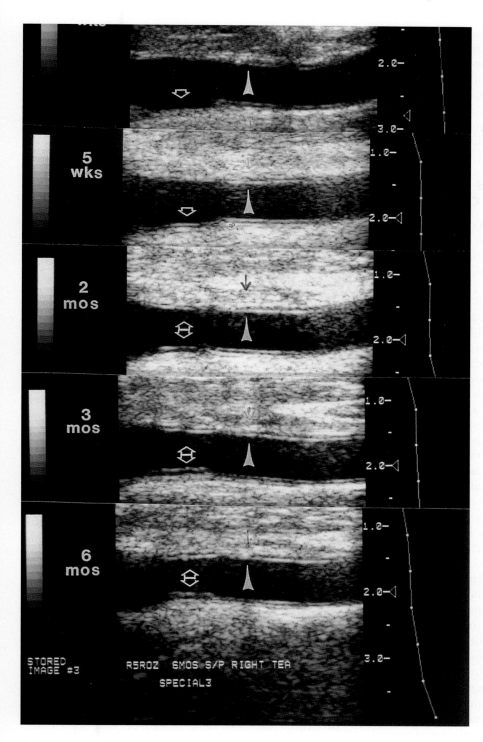

FIGURE 11.27. These images demonstrate the proximal site of a carotid endarterectomy (CEA) and the changes in the wall over time *(open arrow)* (from *top to bottom*, respectively, 1.5 weeks, 5 weeks, 2 months, 3 months, and 6 months). The *solid arrow* marks the first suture for reference in all images, seen most clearly as the bright echo in the **top image**. The shelf of the remaining wall, marking the beginning of the CEA, is seen on the far wall, most clearly in the **top image** (see text).

5. Small flaps of tissue may be seen along the wall in the region of the endarterectomy. These flaps, often difficult to visualize in the B-mode image without some manipulation of the scanhead, may be moving in the flow stream. The presence of the flap should be verified from both the longitudinal and transverse views. If small flaps are present, they will be seen predominantly in the first few weeks after the procedure. They appear to reattach to the wall and disappear in the early stages of healing after surgery. Because of this early attachment, the flaps are not usually seen at routine follow-up visits of 3 or 6 months. Unless the flap is large and obstructive or causing marked disturbance in the flow, it does not appear to be a clinically worrisome problem.

6. Dramatic curves or kinks may be seen at the distal end of the endarterectomy in the ICA. The kink creates dramatic flow changes, such as apparent velocity increases because of acute Doppler angles or disturbed flow. The kink may remodel or smooth out over time, and the associated flow changes may become less dramatic. It is often difficult to distinguish the disturbed flow patterns of the kink from those of a true recurrent stenosis or a distal flap as a result of difficulty measuring reliable Doppler angles.

Duplex Results after Carotid Endarterectomy with Patch Closure

The patch is used to increase the diameter of the vessel in an attempt to avoid narrowing as a result of recurrent stenosis. Autologous vein or prosthetic material may be used for the patch. The critical areas of restenosis are the proximal and distal ends of the endarterectomy.

The patched area is seen on the B-mode image as a dilatation in the area of the mid CCA and extending into the ICA. The extent and size of the dilatation is variable depending on the surgical technique. If PTFE is used, the typical bright double-line interfaces of this material may be identified on the near wall. A Dacron patch will appear as a thick, bright interface, and a vein patch may not be ultrasonically discernible from the wall. If a Dacron or PTFE patch is being examined with the ultrasound during or within 48 hours after surgery, the patch area may be difficult to image because of air trapped within the walls of the graft that prevents the transmission of the ultrasound.

Dramatic flow disturbances as a result of the change in the diameter will normally be seen in the patched area. The flow changes should be documented with multiple waveforms taken across the diameter of the lumen. Because of the flow disturbances, PSV may be difficult or impossible to measure accurately, in which case, a comment about the disturbance may be enough for documentation. Over time, the dilatation may begin to fill in or thicken, and the flow changes will minimize and eventually may disappear as the flow lumen becomes more uniform in size.

The color display in this area will reflect the marked disturbances in the flow patterns, similar to the spectral waveforms. A mixture of red and blue, reflecting the dramatic hemodynamic flow directional changes, will be seen throughout the cardiac cycle. A continuous forward flow channel may be seen throughout the cardiac cycle in the central portion of the vessel, with transient areas of reversal disappearing in diastole along the walls. The flow disturbances may be so dramatic that they radiate upstream into the ICA and the ECA, making isolated assessment of the waveforms from these vessels complicated to interpret.

Carotid and Subclavian Bypass Graft

The primary purpose of this procedure is to supply flow to the SA secondary to the presence of an occlusion or a tight stenosis at the origin. This procedure may also be used, however rarely, to supply flow to the carotid system when a proximal lesion in that vessel exists. Verifying the appropriate direction of flow in the graft is an important result of the duplex assessment.

Dacron or PTFE material may be used for the graft. The characteristic B-mode appearance of Dacron is a brightly echogenic surface, potentially with rings, as compared with PTFE, which has a brightly echogenic double-line appearance.

Severe angles at the anastomotic sites, especially the subclavian attachment, create difficulty in obtaining reliable velocity measurements. In addition, marked flow disturbances may be noted normally. Scanning may be difficult because of the limited and inflexible angles of approach with the scanhead. The entire graft should be examined with the pulsed Doppler, with particular attention paid to the anastomotic sites.

Duplex Results after Carotid Stent Placement

The area of transition between the native artery and the ends of the stent, both proximal and distal, should show minimal or no change in velocity. Therefore, it is necessary to document flow velocity just proximal to the stent, in the stent at both the proximal and distal ends of the stent, and just distal to the end of the stent (Fig. 11.28). If a focal velocity increase is present in any of these areas, document the waveform with the highest PSV. Then, provide a waveform from a distal site demonstrating poststenotic changes. Multiple samples of the velocity within the stent are necessary to verify uniform flow velocity throughout. The minimal number of sampling sites will depend on the location and the length of the stent. If the stent extends from the distal CCA into the ICA, at least three of the velocity samples should be taken from inside the stent, specifically in the distal CCA, the proximal ICA, and the mid ICA. If the stent begins at the orifice of the ICA, at least two of the velocity samples should be taken from inside the stent, specifically in the proximal and mid ICA. Additional samples are encouraged if there is a stenosis or if there are complicated flow patterns present. Regardless of how many signals are taken, the flow patterns within the stent should be well represented. More samples are better than not enough samples. Signals, such as poststenotic turbulence, may be required for validation of representative flow.

It is vitally important to scan the native vessel distal to the stent and to document representative flow velocity. The presence of tortuosity or dramatic changes in the vessel walls must be investigated and documented. The location of the stent relative to the walls may be an important finding in the presence of flow disturbance or velocity increase.

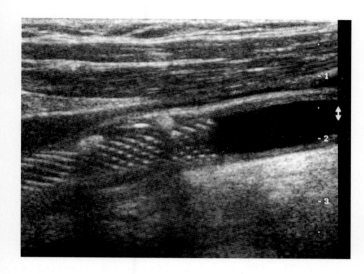

FIGURE 11.28. B-mode image of a carotid stent. The stent mesh pattern is readily apparent in the image. It is important to identify the ends of the stent as they relate to the flow velocities. The distal end of the stent is not seen in this image.

TROUBLESHOOTING ERRORS IN VELOCITY MEASUREMENTS

The measurements of peak systolic and EDV are key elements to the accurate classification of disease in the ICA. Because these measurements are critical to the interpretation, it is of value to list the most common reasons for measurement error. These potential errors are especially important when borderline velocity values occur between categories of disease and when the critical, clinical decisions are being made based on the interpretation of the duplex scan. As always, other clues to the presence of disease, like poststenotic turbulence, should be used along with the velocity measurements.

The errors can be considered in three categories: (a) angle adjustment, (b) technical problems, and (c) physiologic considerations.

ANGLE-RELATED ISSUES

Angle Cursor Not Aligned to the Vessel Walls

The angle cursor represents the axis of the vessel and the direction in which we assume the blood flow to be moving. Therefore, the angle cursor should be aligned so that it is parallel to the walls of the vessel. The Doppler line represents the direction of the ultrasound as it intersects the vessel axis. The angle between the angle cursor and the Doppler line is the Doppler angle that is used by the instrument to compute velocity. The instrument does not "see" the vessel walls and cannot "correct" orientation of the cursor. Therefore, the tasks of the technologist are to (a) adjust the angle cursor so that it properly represents the direction of the vessel walls (i.e., the axis of the vessel and the theoretic direction of the blood flow) and then (b) adjust the Doppler line so that the desired Doppler angle is obtained.

If the angle cursor is not parallel to the walls, a velocity will still be calculated; however, it will be meaningless to standard Doppler methods and the validated criteria—*it will be in error* (Fig. 11.29). Velocities derived with the angle cursor incorrectly aligned to the vessel walls must not be considered for interpretation. The data collection should be repeated, especially if the erroneous velocity values correspond to borderline or critical, clinical decision criteria.

Technologist tip: The best method of ensuring that the angle cursor is aligned appropriately in the vessel is first to adjust the cursor in the midstream to a position believed to represent the vessel axis (parallel to the walls) and then to move the cursor up to the near wall and down to the far wall, making certain that the cursor lies parallel to the wall in each location. If the cursor is not parallel, readjust the cursor alignment or adjust the vessel walls within the image,

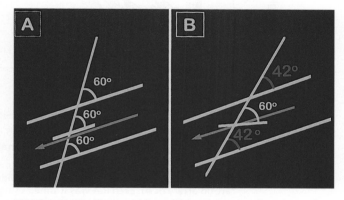

FIGURE 11.29. The graphic on **A** demonstrates the appropriate alignment of the angle cursor parallel to the vessel walls at 60 degrees. The graphic on **B** demonstrates inappropriate placement of the angle cursor. In this case, the instrument will use the cosine of 60 degrees (the angle between the Doppler line and the angle cursor) and the frequency shift from 42 degrees (the angle formed by the Doppler line and the axis of the vessel) to calculate a velocity value that will not be correct.

by doing a heel-and-toe maneuver with the scanhead, until the cursor is perfectly aligned. Repeat the cursor movement to the walls to confirm alignment. Then, return the cursor to midstream, adjust the Doppler line to create the desired Doppler angle, and take the signal.

Inconsistent Angle Measurements

There is evidence to show that velocity taken from different angles of incidence (aligned appropriately to the vessel walls) at the same site in the vessel will yield different values (Fig. 11.17). This finding is not what is predicted by the Doppler equation, which we rely on for our calculations. The Doppler equation implies that velocity taken at any angle from the same site should be the same if the angle is aligned correctly relative to the vessel walls. The reason for the differences most likely is a function of the multielement

linear array technology. It appears that these instruments display multiple frequency shifts at each sample site as a result of using a series of elements rather than one element as the mechanical sector transducer. The configuration of elements creates intrinsic spectral broadening, which in turn affects the measured velocity at each different angle. This is not an error that can be easily fixed because it is a result of instrument design. The issue must be dealt with at the technical level during each examination. Doppler angles must be consistent for each absolute velocity measurement and for ratio calculations. If not, errors will occur that will ultimately affect the interpretation of disease and potentially the patient's therapy.

The measured velocity appears to increase as the angle increases, and the differences become more pronounced when the velocity increases with increased narrowing (Fig. 11.30). The differences in velocity are not as striking at

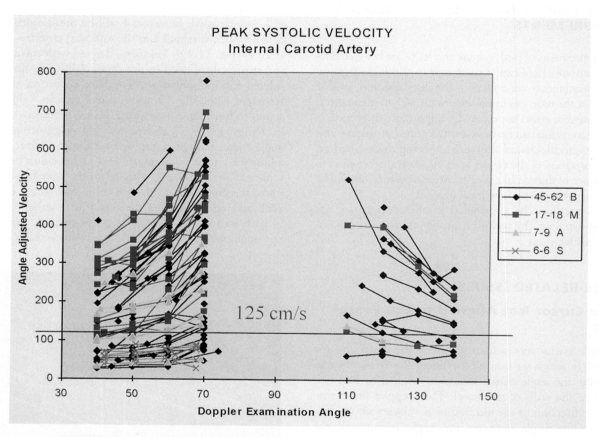

FIGURE 11.30. Each line represents an individual study of the most diseased site in an internal carotid artery (ICA). Each ICA was scanned using four different angles, 40, 50, 60, and 70 degrees, as in Fig. 11.17, and peak systolic velocity was measured, as seen by the *dots* on each line. Six technologists, in five different laboratories, using four different instruments performed the study. The series on the *right* were taken with the Doppler line pointed caudad and on the *left*, cephalad. The horizontal line represents 125 cm/sec (the criteria for 50% diameter reduction). There is a trend in all cases for the perceived measured velocity to increase as the angle increases, most markedly above 60 degrees. Note especially that the error in velocity increases dramatically in those patients with the highest velocity at 40 degrees. Note also the increase in velocity between 40 and 60 degrees.

angles below 40 degrees but become quite obvious in angles above 40 degrees and unacceptable at angles above 60 degrees. The errors are present in normal vessels and markedly present in abnormal vessels. Therefore, a measured velocity taken at 40 degrees from a stenotic ICA would be lower than if the velocity were taken at 60 degrees from the same site. A measured velocity from a normal CCA taken at 40 degrees would be lower than a velocity taken at the same site at 60 degrees. The difference would significantly affect the calculation of the ICA/CCA ratio that is used to distinguish patients who need endarterectomy.

The criteria described in this chapter were developed and validated using a 60-degree Doppler angle. The velocities are estimated assuming the blood velocity is parallel to the vessel walls. Velocities, particularly stenotic velocities, that are taken using angles of less than 60 degrees are comparatively lower because of the previously mentioned error in measurement. Therefore, these velocities cannot be used accurately with the criteria. A nonprotocol angle used to gather a signal for analysis must be documented and considered when interpreting the results of the study. The differences become especially critical in cases in which the velocity values may be on or near critical borderlines between categories. Velocities acquired using angles greater than 60 degrees are significantly and erroneously elevated compared with those of angles of 60 degrees and should be considered ineligible for classification. The velocity data must be repeated using more acceptable angle adjustments.

Poor Visualization of Vessel Walls and Angle Adjustment

Velocities that are acquired from vessels whose walls are poorly visualized as a result of image quality, calcification, depth, and so forth should be considered suspicious. The measured velocity is potentially erroneous and misleading because the angle cursor may not be aligned correctly and cannot be defined. Every attempt should be made to improve the image so that the vessel walls can be seen clearly. Color can be useful as a pathfinder in defining the direction of vessels and the walls. Complex plaque may obscure visualization of the walls and make angle measurement difficult or impossible.

Tortuosity

As previously described, tortuosity, or curvature of the vessel, poses a particularly difficult task when aligning the angle cursor for three reasons: (a) the predetermined protocol angle cannot be obtained as a result of the vessel orientation, (b) the curvaceous nature of the vessel makes angle alignment with the walls difficult, and (c) the curves produce complex normal changes within the flow stream, some of which we see displayed in the spectral waveforms and a lot of which cannot be adequately appreciated with the instrumentation.

Every attempt should be made to obtain the protocol angle in a tortuous vessel either by a readjustment of the Doppler beam to approach the vessel differently or by adjustment of the vessel within the image relative to the Doppler line. However, if the protocol angle cannot be achieved, the most optimal angle below 60 degrees should be used, making certain that the cursor is appropriately aligned to the walls at the new angle. The nonprotocol angle should be documented in the records so that it may be considered in the interpretation and used for follow-up studies at the same location.

Angle alignment is controversial when the spectral sample is taken at the curve, and the resultant velocity should be deemed suspicious. It is difficult to define the axis of the vessel (cursor parallel to walls) around a curve, and each operator may see it differently. Therefore, many different perceived velocity values can be obtained from the same location, none of which represents the true velocity. The inner wall of the curve is a standard reference; however, it may be difficult to define as well. A written comment on the data form regarding velocity measurements taken from a curved vessel will be helpful for the interpretation and for future reference. It may be difficult to rule in or out significant stenosis or to classify disease accurately in the presence of a tortuosity.

Finally, flow directions change rapidly as a result of a curve or kink, and normal flow disturbances develop downstream. Our instrumentation may detect some of the directional changes as oscillations or disturbances in the waveforms but may not detect the subtle changes in the directions of flow. For this reason and the question of angle measurement, the velocities from tortuous vessels become complex to understand, but not necessarily abnormal. The flow changes and angle alignment issues must be anticipated at and distal to curves and the measured velocity values interpreted with caution.

TECHNICAL PROBLEMS
Doppler Gain Adjustment

The Doppler gain adjustment will affect the measurement of peak velocity and the amount of spectral broadening. Displaying too much gain increases the measurement of peak velocity and the amount of spectral broadening that is displayed. Displaying too little gain decreases the perceived peak velocity measurement, and spectral information is dropped out (Fig. 11.18).

Measurement of the Highest Velocity in a Stenosis

The flow patterns in a stenosis are complex, and many different velocities will be detected throughout its length. The classification criteria rely on the measurement of the maximum velocity increase associated with the stenosis, which, in some cases, may be just distal to what visually appears to be the narrowest area. The jet extends beyond the stricture and continues to increase for a short distance in the post-stricture site. Therefore, the highest velocity may actually be detected distal to the narrowest-appearing portion of the plaque. Only a thorough investigation through the stenosis with the pulsed Doppler sample volume will yield this value. Neither the B-mode image nor the color Doppler will define this exact location precisely.

Aliasing of the Spectral Waveform

Aliasing of the spectral waveform occurs when the sampling rate is not high enough to detect the frequency shift, that is, when the pulse repetition frequency is too low. The waveform appears to wrap around the spectral display, with the peaks coming from the lower or upper edge of the opposite direction. Shifting the zero baseline and increasing the pulse repetition frequency usually eliminate the problem and illuminate the true peak. If the velocity (i.e., frequency shift) is too high and aliasing cannot be eliminated, the true peak velocity may not be measured accurately because it will be obscured in the disturbance. Also, if there is marked disturbance in both directions and aliasing in one or both directions, the true peak may be hidden in the disturbance that is coming from the top of the display. In this case, the peak is in question again and cannot be measured adequately. A comment on the data sheet by the technologist will alert the interpreter to this problem. Because this problem would occur in a stenosis with markedly elevated velocity, the absolute measurement of PSV may not be as important as the measurement of EDV, which is usually obvious and can be accurately measured.

Automated Velocity Measurements

Most of the ultrasound instruments have a method of automatically defining the outer envelope of the spectral waveform and displaying the values of PSV and EDV on the screen. The measurement is triggered from a level of noise detected by the spectrum analyzer that is factory set in the system. For the most part, this method will work and measure what appear to be the maximum velocity values. However, in the presence of a noisy signal, which is often the case in a high-grade stenosis, the mechanism may trigger on noise rather than the true value, and errors in velocity measurement will occur. The technologist must be vigilant of this problem and manually override an erroneous measurement with the measurement calipers provided on the instrument.

PHYSIOLOGIC CONSIDERATIONS
Decreased Cardiac Output

The PSV measurements are affected by a decrease in the overall cardiac output. The effects of decreased flow would be appreciated as an overall, symmetric decrease in velocity in the carotid waveforms bilaterally, beginning as low as the CCAp signals. If decreased cardiac output is suspected, the velocity that is measured in the ICA, especially a stenotic ICA, will be lower than would normally be expected, and the absolute velocity criteria may not be directly applicable. However, because the flow in the entire system is decreased, the ICA/CCA ratio may still apply and be used for identifying the level of disease.

Arrhythmia

Arrhythmia results in a peak-to-peak variability of the measurement of the spectral waveforms, which can result in misleading and inconsistent velocity measurements. The standard rule for measuring waveforms in a patient with arrhythmia is to take the measurement from an average or most commonly occurring peak—not the highest and not the lowest. The same method of selection should be used for all measurements in the study and for future follow-up. It may be helpful to run the recording device at a lower speed to display more waveforms in the frozen image and to demonstrate the arrhythmia more clearly for the interpretation.

Proximal or Distal Disease

The presence of significant disease in either the more proximal vessels, (e.g., CCA origin or innominate artery) or the more distal arteries (e.g., the carotid siphon or the circle of Willis) may decrease the overall velocity within the cervical carotid system. Hence, the measured PSV in the ICA in the presence of one of these situations would be lower than normal. A stenosis may appear to be less narrow based on the velocity that is measured, or the stenosis may be masked altogether. An assessment and comparison of the flow patterns from side to side will help to define the problem. Here again, as in the case of decreased cardiac outflow, the ICA/CCA ratio may be the best way to define the amount of disease in the ICA.

In addition, looking at the global hemodynamics of the cervical carotids can illuminate disease remote from the bifurcation. Noting overall flow changes or asymmetric flow changes from side to side may indirectly point to an unknown problem or etiology that is not part of or accessible to the routine cerebrovascular duplex scan in the proximal or distal vessels. These findings may be significant to the patient's therapy, and further testing may be necessary to define the specific source of the difference.

Contralateral Disease

As mentioned previously (see Internal Carotid Artery Occlusion), an ipsilateral occlusion or high-grade stenosis of the ICA may cause an increase in the flow rate in the contralateral side owing to collateralization through the anterior communicating artery. Consequently, the PSV in the contralateral ICA may be erroneously elevated, and overestimation of the disease status is possible. The increased flow rate will be noted in the CCA and the ECA. It is important to scan the contralateral carotid after a surgical or endovascular procedure to assess any changes in the velocity in the ICA that may affect the interpretation of disease.

Eddies and Disturbances in the Flow

Disturbances in the typical flow patterns can occur for many reasons. Curves, branches, dilatations, bifurcations, and the presence of disease can create flow disturbances, which will be detected by the pulsed Doppler and displayed in the spectral waveform. The disturbances should be anticipated and appreciated in the waveforms when scanning these areas. The disturbances occur later in the cardiac cycle after the acceleration of peak systole and may extend into diastole (Fig. 11.11). They appear as secondary spikes or peaks in the waveform that appear to oscillate up and down, sometimes crossing the zero baseline. The peak of the disturbances often increases to twice the normal-appearing velocity. The spikes can be deceiving, and it is tempting to measure them as the representative PSV. These disturbances represent circular, rotational flow moving toward and away from the transducer and not velocity, which is parallel to the vessel walls. Therefore, the peak of an eddy is not what is routinely measured. The velocity measurement from disturbance that occurs late in systole is due to high-frequency shifts as the eddy rotates rapidly toward and then away from the transducer through the sample volume. Eddies can be measured at much higher velocities than the true systolic velocity when angle correction is applied.

The disturbances may not be readily apparent in the waveform if the Doppler gain is set too high. Displaying too much gain tends to blur the oscillatory features together, and the jagged nature of the disturbance cannot be seen. Decreasing the gain will illuminate the disturbed character of the waveform and allow the operator to deliberate where the acceleration peak is located. In addition, increasing the speed of the recording device will stretch the waveform out over a longer time period, illuminating the waveform character more clearly. The "up-and-down" character of the spikes and disturbance becomes readily apparent. If the waveform is markedly disturbed and a true systolic peak cannot be identified, it is better practice to decline measurement and simply describe the waveform character, rather than risk a measurement that is in error.

REFERENCES

1. Dawson DL, Zierler RE, Strandness DE Jr, et al. The role of duplex scanning and arteriography before endarterectomy: a prospective study. *J Vasc Surg* 1993;18:673–683.
2. Roederer GO, Langlois YE, Strandness DR Jr. Cerebral arterial flow and cerebral vascular insufficiency. In: Condon RE, DeCosse J, eds. *Surgical Care II*. Philadelphia: Lea and Febiger, 1985:199–234.
3. Phillips DJ, Beach KW, Primozich J, et al. Should results of ultrasound Doppler criteria be reported in units of frequency or velocity? *Ultrasound Med Biol* 1989;15:205–212.
4. Moneta GL, Edwards JM, Chitwood RW, et al. Correlation of North American Symptomatic Carotid Endarterectomy Trial (NASCET) angiographic definition of 70%–99% internal carotid stenosis with duplex scanning. *J Vasc Surg* 1992;17:152–160.
5. Phillips DJ, Greene FM Jr, Langlois YE, et al. Flow velocity patterns in the carotid bifurcation of young, presumed normal subjects. *Ultrasound Med Biol* 1983;9:33–49.
6. Bornstein NM, Norris JW. Subclavian steal: a harmless hemodynamic phenomenon. *Lancet* 1986;2:203–205.
7. Hatsukami TS, Thackeray BD, Primozich JF, et al. Echolucent regions in carotid plaque: preliminary analysis comparing three-dimensional histologic reconstructions to sonographic findings. *Ultrasound Med Biol* 1994;20:743–749.
8. Roederer GO, Langlois AT, Jager K, et al. A simple parameter for accurate classification of severe carotid stenosis. *Bruit* 1989;3:174–178.
9. Daigle RJ, Stavros AT, Lee RM. Overestimation of velocity and frequency values with multielement linear array Doppler. *J Vasc Tech* 1990;14:206–213.
10. Fujitani RM, Mills JL, Wang LM, et al. The effect of unilateral internal carotid artery occlusion upon contralateral duplex study criteria for accurate interpretation. *J Vasc Surg* 1992;16:459–468.
11. Nicholls SC, Phillips DJ, Bergelin RO, et al. Carotid endarterectomy: relationship of outcome to early restenosis. *J Vasc Surg* 1985;2:375–381.

12

TRANSCRANIAL DOPPLER:
THE BASIC EXAMINATION

WATSON B. SMITH

Rune Aaslid first described the use of transcranial Doppler (TCD) in the study of the intracranial circulation, which permitted access to the intracranial circulation not previously studied by ultrasonic methods (1,2). This was made possible by using low-frequency ultrasound and higher power levels to gain access to the circle of Willis through the temporal bone (3). This region of the skull is fortunately thin enough in most patients to permit access. As noted later, this approach permitted evaluation of the arteries of the mid-anterior circulation. Access to the carotid siphon and vertebrobasilar arteries became possible through the orbit and foramen magnum, respectively. It is prudent to use lower power when the ultrasound beam is directed through the orbit and the retina (4).

The circle of Willis is a very complex network that is critically important for supplying blood to the various parts of the brain. Unfortunately, the circle is not functionally intact in all people, which may severely limit its use as a collateral source of blood to ischemic areas of the brain. It has been shown in necropsy studies of patients who have died from a stroke that the circle is incomplete in most cases (5,6). Theoretically, TCD could be a valuable method of studying the entire circle, but this is not without problems (4,7). The applications of this method have been evolving since its introduction, and they continue to evolve as new data become available.

Some of the obvious concerns registered about this method have been answered in part. For example, can velocity data be equated with the perfusion of an area? The answer to this question is both yes and no. It is necessary to define the circumstances under which the studies are carried out and what information is desired. For example, it appears that a reduction in flow across an area of stenosis of the middle cerebral artery (MCA) may or may not be associated with a perfusion abnormality (8). The brain's ability to autoregulate its blood flow will determine whether the neural tissue can function normally (6,9).

An interesting piece of information that is relevant to function may be seen in those cases with high-grade stenoses or occlusions of the carotid artery in the neck. If the MCA flow velocity is within a normal range, one can assume that adequate blood flow is present through the collaterals to supply this area. Another subject that is being explored is the brain's ability to increase flow when given a vasodilatory challenge, such as carbon dioxide. This information is being used more frequently to determine whether an extracranial–intracranial bypass graft is necessary to provide blood to an area whose reserve is exhausted because of inadequate inflow through the collaterals (6,9).

One of the most frequent applications of TCD is the study of the problem of vasospasm after an episode of subarachnoid hemorrhage (4,7). TCD can be used to follow the events after such a bleed and to predict whether vasospasm is occurring, thus permitting an aggressive approach to its management. In this setting, the findings of interest are a progressive increase in flow velocity to the MCA.

One of the most common causes of stroke is thought to be emboli arising from the carotid bifurcation, and TCD permits an opportunity to detect these emboli in their course to the MCA. There is no doubt that emboli can be detected with TCD, although the ability to identify the exact type by their "ultrasonic signature" remains elusive. Requests for monitoring of emboli are becoming more common, but in our experience, the yield is relatively low. It is our impression that considerably more data will be required before the role of TCD in monitoring emboli is fully defined (10). However, as will be noted later, it is clear that for this application, TCD can be used to great advantage.

TCD is a noninvasive method for evaluating cerebral hemodynamics with pulsed Doppler, color flow duplex scanning, or both (11). Even with recent advances in color flow imaging capabilities, TCD remains an advanced duplex technique that requires intricate knowledge of the structural anatomy, course of the cerebral vessels, and normal and abnormal cerebral hemodynamics as well as skill with color Doppler optimization.

The original nonimaging method used a 2-MHz pulsed range-gated bidirectional Doppler with a real-time spectral display. Its accuracy was highly dependent on the user's knowledge of the anatomy. Proper usage requires strict adherence to correct sample volume depth and flow direction and the ability to trace the vessels and their spatial direction as ascertained by probe angulation. This method still plays an important role in specialized and advanced procedures that require fixed head gear for bilateral or intraoperative monitoring and remains the method of choice for performing head-rotation studies (for mechanical compression of vertebral arteries) and for carbon dioxide reactivity examinations.

Color flow duplex imaging (CDI), which is now possible through the temporal bone with improved instrumentation, eliminates some of the pitfalls of the original technique by allowing more accurate vessel identification with the use of the color flow and B-mode image. With this method, one is still unable to visualize vessel walls because of attenuation from temporal bone and the small size of the vessels. However, the B-mode penetration and imaging are usually adequate to use bony structures and other landmarks, such as the sphenoid wing, the petrous ridge, and the cerebral peduncles, for more positive vessel identification.

EQUIPMENT NEEDED

TCD with CDI requires a low frequency (2 to 2.5 MHz) small-footprint (phased array) transducer to penetrate the small acoustic window, which is usually (but not always) present as a thin spot in the temporal bone just superior to the zygomatic arch.

All diagnostic information is derived from the spectral waveforms, and the equipment should have the ability to measure peak systolic velocity (PSV) and end-diastolic velocity (EDV), from which the mean velocity (MV) and pulsatility index (PI) can be calculated.

EQUIPMENT SETTINGS

A large sample volume size (5 mm) is used to locate and insonate the small basal arteries and focal stenoses, which can be difficult to locate. Sensitivity to low flow can be especially important for locating vessels in abnormal exam-

inations, in which velocities may be very low distal to severe stenosis or occlusion. Subsequently, low PRF or wall filter and high color frame averaging settings may help in locating the vessels.

PATIENT AND TECHNOLOGIST POSITIONING

Long examination times (30 to 90 minutes) and the small size of vessels, which requires fine motor movement of the hand, make it important to maximize patient and technologist position for comfort. The equipment should be positioned close to the patient to avoid long reaches to the controls, which can cause the operator to lose a difficult signal. Stabilizing the hand and probe on the bed or on the patient helps considerably.

The operator may scan from the head of the bed in a manner similar to that preferred by many users for a standard carotid or vertebral artery examination in an outpatient setting. It is also advantageous to practice scanning from the side of the bed, as is required in many portable inpatient or intensive care unit settings. The patient is positioned supine for transtemporal and transorbital approaches and is turned onto one side for the transoccipital approach.

EXAMINATION PROCEDURE

Four steps are taken at each of the three examination sites. The first step is to *locate the acoustic window*, which is sometimes the most difficult and important step of the examination. Studies show that older patients and women tend to have hyperosteosis of the temporal bone; subsequently, the transtemporal acoustic window may be poor, small, difficult to locate, or even absent. This is more common in elderly women and occurs in about 10% of cases. With CDI, the acoustic window, if present, appears as a sonolucent oval on B-mode image. If no window is present, the oval will appear fuzzy with no discernible bony landmarks (Fig. 12.1).

The second step is *vessel identification*. Four criteria are used for vessel identification: depth, flow direction, waveform contour and velocity, and spatial and anatomic position.

The third step consists of *insonating each artery at 0 .5-cm intervals*, searching for abnormalities. Step four is *documenting normal and abnormal findings*, usually with videotape, hard copy, or both. Representative PSVs and EDVs are measured for each segment, from which they can then be used to calculate the MV and PI, which are used for interpretation. Locations of spectral abnormalities such as bruits and turbulence are also recorded.

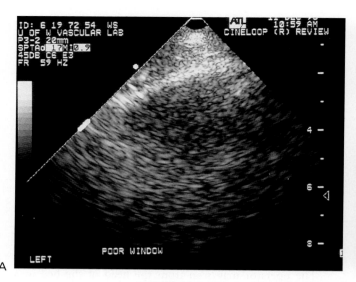

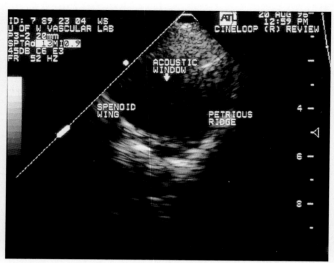

FIGURE 12.1. Side-to-side comparison of good **(A)** and poor **(B)** acoustical windows.

WINDOWS AND LANDMARKS

The *transtemporal approach* is used to evaluate the MCA, anterior cerebral artery (ACA), posterior cerebral artery (PCA), and terminal internal carotid artery (ICA). The anterior and posterior communicating arteries are very small and are not usually seen unless they are functioning as collateral pathways.

To locate the acoustic window with CDI, the transducer is placed flat on the temple just above the zygomatic arch, and the B-mode image is used to locate the small thin spot usually present in the temporal bone. When there is a good window, the operator should be able to visualize bony structures such as the sphenoid wing and the petrous ridge. Cerebral peduncles and midline structures such as the falx cerebri can often be appreciated (Fig. 12.2).

For vessel identification, all waveforms seen through the transtemporal approach should have the same contour as a normal ICA, as in standard extracranial carotid studies. The MCA is positively identified by its shallow depth (4 to 6 cm); its flow direction toward the transducer (red), and its anatomic course paralleling the lesser wing of the sphenoid bone. The average MV for the MCA is 60 cm/sec. The ACA is located at deeper depths (6 to 8 cm), its normal flow direction is away from the probe (blue), and it is anterior to the proximal MCA. It is short in length, and its average MV is 50 cm/sec. The PCA is also found at deeper depths (6 to 8 cm), but it has a more posterior location and is seen to course around the brain stem with flow direction toward the probe in its P1 segments (red) and with flow away from the probe (blue) in its P2 segments.

The average PCA MV is 40 cm/sec. When evaluating hemodynamics through the transtemporal approach, it is essential to recognize and remember that the MCA MV (60 cm/sec) should always be greater than the ACA MV (50 cm/sec), which is greater than the PCA MV (40 cm/sec) in

a normal patient. Changes in this relationship are used to identify collateral pathways.

The *transoccipital approach* uses the natural opening at the base of the skull, the foramen magnum to locate intracranial vertebral arteries, and the basilar artery. The probe is placed at the base of skull, with the patient's head tilted forward; the acoustic window is again seen as a somewhat smaller sonolucent oval. The bony structure of the atlas can be used as a B-mode landmark. All waveforms should look like normal extracranial vertebral arteries. Vertebral arteries are at shallow depths (5 to 8 cm), with normal flow direction away from probe (blue). The anterior spinal branches are sometimes seen flowing toward the transducer with a higher pulsatility and more resistive waveform, much like extracranial external carotid arteries (ECAs). The basilar artery can be found at deeper depths (8 to 10 cm) and often appears to be aligned with a dominant vertebral artery.

The *transorbital approach* is used to evaluate ophthalmic artery flow direction and carotid siphon through the optic canal. Ophthalmic artery waveforms should be similar to ECAs. The ophthalmic artery is at shallow depths (4.5 to 6 cm). The carotid siphon is deeper (6.5 to 7 cm), with waveforms like those of the ICA. Flow direction is not meaningful at the carotid siphon because it is possible to locate the paracellar (toward the probe), the genu (dual directional), or the supraclinoid segments of the carotid siphon. Although this technique has been used through the orbit for many years throughout the world with no reports of side effects, no diagnostic use of ultrasound through the orbit has been granted U.S. Food and Drug Administration approval, and it is prudent to minimize acoustic exposure by decreasing power output and intensity and reducing scanning time when possible.

Table 12.1 shows the characteristics, locations, and velocity values for the basilar arteries of the brain.

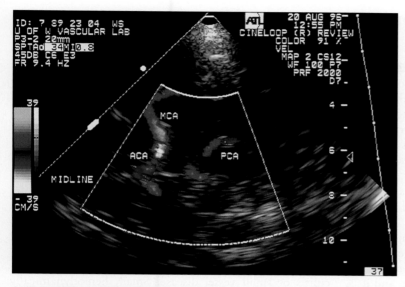

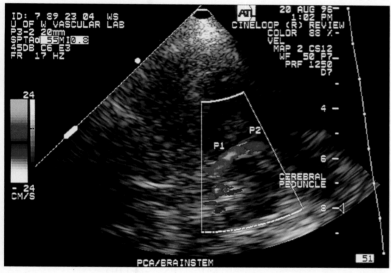

FIGURE 12.2. Color flow images of intracranial arteries along with usual anatomic landmarks.

TABLE 12.1. TRANSCRANIAL DOPPLER VESSEL IDENTIFICATION SUMMARY CHART

Artery	Window	Depth (cm)	Normal flow direction	Average MV (cm/sec)	B-mode landmarks
MCA	Transtemporal	4–6	Toward	60	Sphenoid wing
ACA	Transtemporal	6–8	Away	50	
PCA-1	Transtemporal	6–8	Toward	40	Cerebral peduncle
PCA-2	Transtemporal	6–8	Away	40	Cerebral peduncle
Vertebral	Foramen magnum	5–8	Away	30–40	Atlas
Basilar	Foramen magnum	8–10	Away	30–40	
Opthalmic	Transorbital	4.5–6	Toward	Variable	Optic canal
Siphon	Transorbital	6.5–7	Dual directional	Variable	

MCA, middle cerebral artery; ACA, anterior cerebral artery; PCA, posterior cerebral artery.

TECHNICAL PITFALLS AND SOURCES OF ERROR

The acoustic window should be located and optimized by first using the B-mode image alone without color flow Doppler. If one spends a few minutes obtaining the best possible B-mode image of the acoustic window and bony landmarks, the correct special positions of the arteries can be more accurately assessed, which minimizes errors in vessel identification and ensures that the best acoustic window is located.

After the acoustic window has been optimized and the color flow is turned on, a whole new set of potential pitfalls arises.

One simple error is inverting the color map, which can make directional information confusing. There is generally no need to invert the color map with TCD examinations.

Sensitivity to high or low flow can be a problem, and it is important to make sure that pulse repetition frequency (PRF) settings are appropriate. If the PRF is set too high, low-flow velocities will not be displayed; if the color PRF is too low, the aliasing will make directional information difficult to appreciate.

If color or Doppler gain and power are too low, the system will not display information that may be present.

One can maximize frame rate and its potential pitfalls by using a shallow image depth. Using smaller color flow boxes will also help keep the frame rate at manageable levels.

Although it is sometimes possible to insonate both hemispheres from one temporal window, this is a potential source of error, and it is recommended that each hemisphere be evaluated separately from its ipsilateral window.

Incomplete data are sometimes a potential pitfall. This can and does occur in difficult studies, but this error can be minimized by strict adherence to protocol. Be sure to document PSV and EDV for each sample depth and to document additional images of any flow disturbances or waveform changes. Increasing the pulsed wave sample volume size can also lead to errors because it is possible to insonate more than one artery or depth if a large sample volume is used.

Poor understanding of the normal intracranial anatomy and flow directions, the many possible variations in the circle of Willis, and the potential collateral pathways is also a common source of error.

One must also be aware of the three-dimensionality of the vessels, which can sometimes be confounded by tortuosity.

PATHOLOGY

TCD is useful for describing collateral pathways and adequacy of collaterals, identifying and quantifying intracranial stenosis, identifying and quantifying vasospasm, and locating large arteriovenous malformations, which can be done by identifying high flow and low pulsatility in the supplying vessels.

It is important to keep in mind that TCD is not a reliable tool for detecting intracranial aneurysms. Giant aneurysms may be seen, but small or distal aneurysms, which may not be in the scan plane, will not be detected. TCD does not detect subarachnoid hemorrhage.

Because current instruments cannot yet visualize vessel walls on B-mode image, it is important to remember that TCD is an almost purely color flow Doppler hemodynamic examination. Subsequently, vessel occlusion remains a difficult TCD diagnosis. Intracranial occlusions may sometimes be inferred from secondary findings, but if one cannot locate a vessel, it may be because of technical limitations. TCD is also not sensitive to vasculitis or small vessel disease. Small, hemodynamically insignificant arteriovenous malformations that do not alter Doppler flow patterns may also not be detected.

INTERPRETATION

Keep in mind that TCD is a test of ranges and comparisons with absolutes because many factors influence cerebral hemodynamics. Prior knowledge of the status of the extracranial circulation is imperative for correct interpretation of TCD findings. If there are no angiograms, a standard carotid or vertebral artery duplex examination is usually recommended and performed before a TCD examination. The formulas used to calculate MV and PI from PSV and EDV are as follows:

$$MV = \frac{(PSV - EDV)}{3 + EDV}$$

$$PI = \frac{(PSV - EDV)}{MV}$$

The Four-Point Interpretation Criteria for Middle Cerebral Artery Stenosis and Vasospasm

We use four-point interpretation criteria to locate and grade MCA stenosis. The four criteria are MV, Doppler waveform and spectral analysis, PI, and a hemispheric index.

Stenosis is located by its *focal* velocity increase. An MV of more than 80 cm/sec that is localized to one to two sample depths with at least 30 cm/sec difference when compared with adjacent normal segment identifies the lesion (Fig. 12.3).

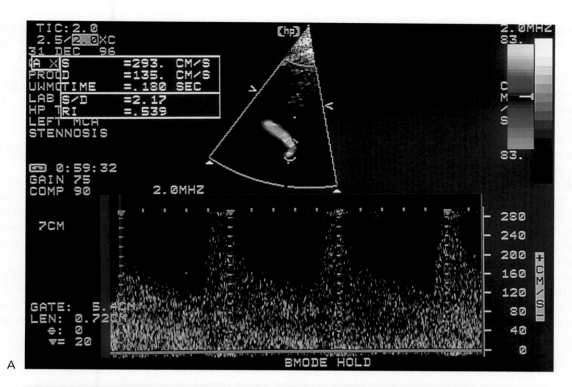

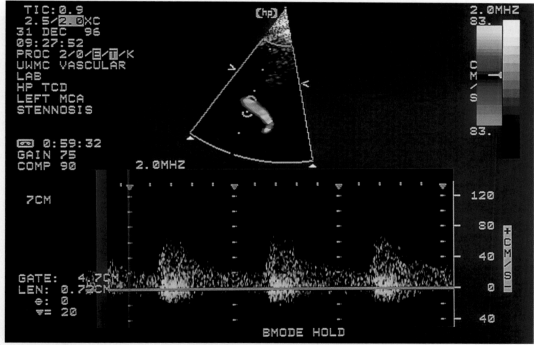

FIGURE. 12.3. Velocities at the site of a middle cerebral artery stenosis **(A)** and their decline distal to the lesion **(B)**.

Aaslid validated these criteria for quantifying vasospasm based on MV at the point of stenosis. An MV of 120 cm/sec is consistent with mild angiographic vasospasm, 120 to 150 cm/sec is mild to moderate, 150 to 200 cm/sec is moderate, and more than 200 cm/sec is consistent with severe vasospasm.

Analysis of the spectral waveform for location of bruits and waveform changes can be used to identify and locate a significant lesion. Doppler bruits are common in the basal arteries, however, especially in younger populations with global high flow, and thus may not indicate an abnormality. Bruits or changes in waveform contour are often localized and can pinpoint the lesion's location. Severe flow restriction lesions have a slow acceleration and decreased pulsatility distal to their location; PI measurements of less than 0.5 are abnormal.

A hemispheric index or MCA/ICA velocity ratio can be used to correct for global high-flow or low-flow states. ICA MVs are obtained by angling the same low-frequency transducer to a standard 5-cm depth from the angle of the jaw,

and a ratio is made with the highest MCA velocity. ICA velocities are only useful with normal ECAs; hence, this technique should not be used if there is ECA stenosis. Hemispheric indices of 1 to 3 are normal, 3 to 5 are consistent with mild MCA stenosis, 5 to 7 are moderate, and more than 7 indicate severe MCA stenosis.

Collateralization

Differentiating the high velocities associated with collateralization from the high velocities associated with stenosis is a potential pitfall. Keep in mind that the comparatively high-flow velocities in collateral channels will be found *throughout* the collateral vessels and will be present at all depths appropriate for that vessel.

The best identifying feature of *crossover collaterals* is a 25% higher velocity in the ACA contralateral to the ICA lesion, which is present as flow is increased to supply the larger territory (Fig. 12.4). Reversed flow direction is usu-

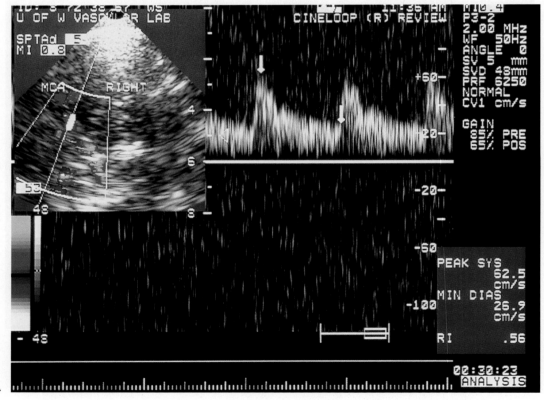

FIGURE 12.4. Crossover collateralization can be identified by the increase in flow velocity and change in direction of flow. **A** shows the normal direction, whereas **B** shows the reverse flow and increases noted in both the peak and end-diastolic flow velocities.

ally present in the ipsilateral ACA. It is common to find a prominent color flow or Doppler bruit midline, where the high flow is forced through the comparatively smaller anterior communicating artery. This also may create an effectual stenosis, which sometimes appears as a focal velocity increase at midline in the position of the anterior communicating artery.

- *Posterior to anterior collaterals* are identified by an ipsilateral PCA MV that is greater than the MCA velocity (Fig. 12.5). There may also be a bruit and focal high velocity at the posterior communicating artery.
- *External to internal collateralization* is identified by reversed or alternating flow direction in the ophthalmic artery (Fig. 12.6).

It is possible to give an estimation of the *adequacy of collaterals* by observing low and normal MCA velocities and pulsatility. If both right and left MCAs are symmetric and have normal velocity and pulsatility, collaterals are assumed to be adequate (Fig. 12.7). Asymmetry and abnormal velocity and pulsatility may be useful for differentiating ischemic from embolic events.

Interpretation Pitfalls and Sources of Error

Common sources of error are the poor understanding of potential collateral pathways and not recognizing the possible variations of the circle of Willis. Another source of error is lack of information about presence or absence of disease in extracranial vessels. Global low flow may be secondary to low blood pressure or cardiac output, advanced age of patient, or distal small vessel disease. Global high flow may be secondary to hypertension, volume depletion, young age of patient, vasodilators, or head injury.

One can mistake the high velocities associated with stenosis, which are focal and localized to one to two sample depths, for the high velocities that are associated with collateral flow. Remember that collateral flow is seen throughout the supplying vessel.

(Text continues on page 243.)

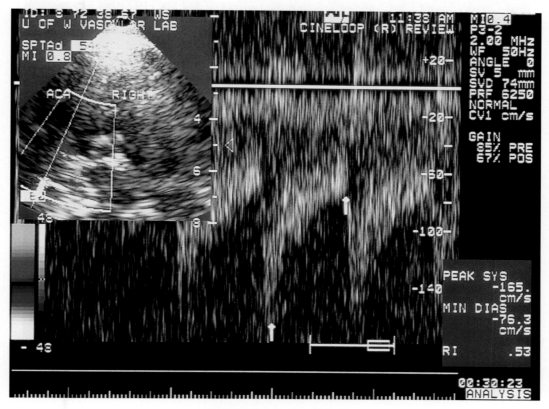

FIGURE 12.4. B *(Continued)*

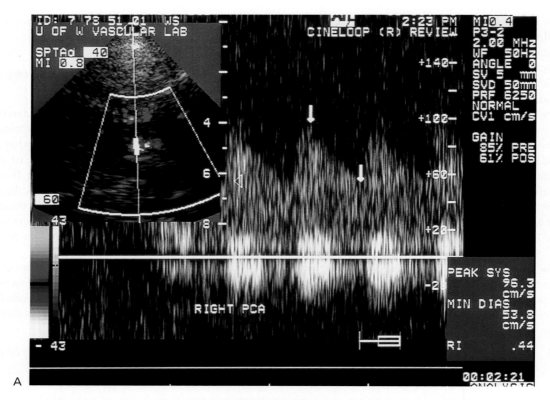

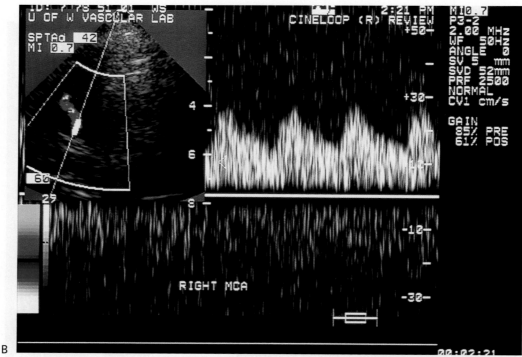

FIGURE 12.5. A posterior cerebral artery **(A)** velocity greater than the ipsilateral middle cerebral artery **(B)** indicates posterior-to-anterior circulation through a posterior communicating artery.

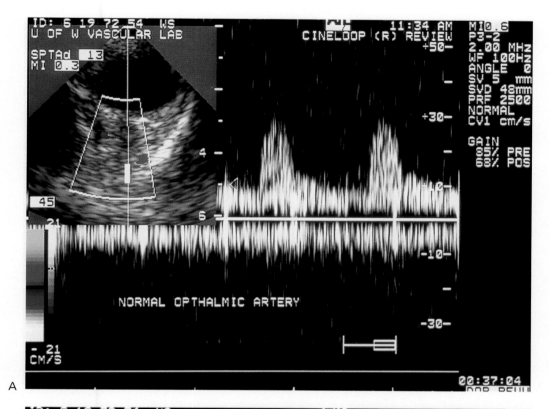

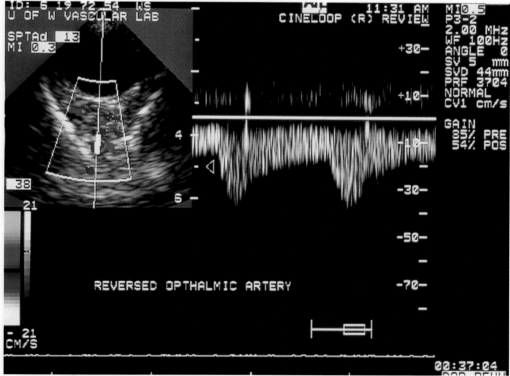

FIGURE 12.6. A: Panel shows the normal direction of flow in the ophthalmic artery. In **B**, a reverse flow is observed.

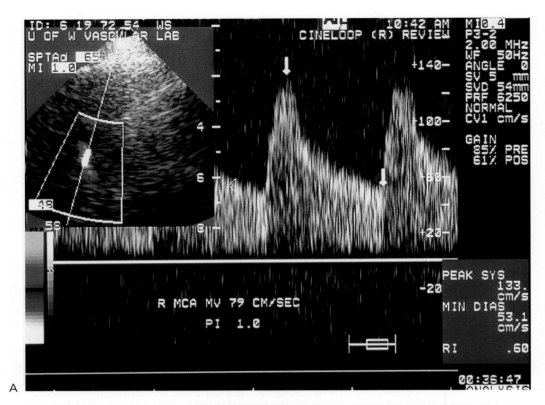

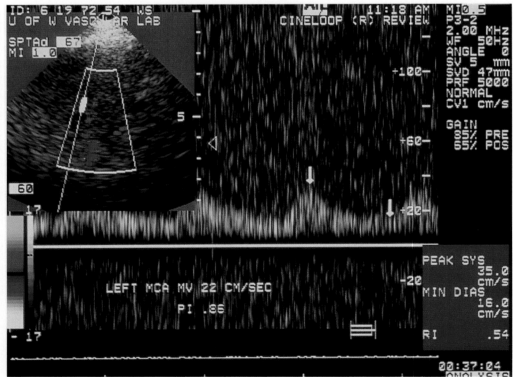

FIGURE 12.7. A: A normal right middle cerebral artery (MCA) velocity of 74 cm/sec is seen. In contrast, in **B**, the mean velocity in the left MCA is only 22 cm/sec, suggesting poor collateralization to this side.

CONCLUSIONS

Advances in color flow technology have reduced some of the pitfalls of TCD. TCD in the hands of an experienced observer is especially useful in the evaluation of stroke and neurosurgical patients.

REFERENCES

1. Baumgartner RW, Mattle HP, Aaslid R. Transcranial color-coded duplex sonography, magnetic resonance angiography, and computed tomography angiography: methods, applications, advantages, and limitations. *JCU J Clin Ultrasound* 1995;23:89–111.
2. Aaslid R, Marler JR. Non-invasive transcranial Doppler ultrasound recording of flow velocity in basal cerebral arteries. *J Neurosurg* 1982;57:769–774.
3. Otis S, Rush M, Boyajian R. Contrast-enhanced transcranial imaging: results of an American phase-two study. *Stroke* 1995;26:203–209.
4. Otis S, Ringelstein EB. Transcranial Doppler sonography. In: Zweibel WJ, ed. *Introduction to vascular ultrasonography.* Philadelphia: WB Saunders, 1993:145–171.
5. Marx F. An arteriographic demonstration. *Acta Radiol* 1949;31:155–160.
6. Wiener LM, Berry RG. Intracranial circulation in carotid occlusion. *Trans Am Neurol Assoc* 1964;89:161–164.
7. Aaslid R, Huber P, Nornes H. Evaluation of cerebrovascular spasm with transcranial Doppler ultrasound. *J Neurosurg* 1984;60:37.
8. Röther J, Schwartz A, Wentz KU, et al. Middle cerebral artery stenoses: assessment by magnetic resonance angiography and transcranial Doppler ultrasound. *Cerebrovasc Dis* 1994;4:273–279.
9. Ringelstein EB, Grosse W, Matentzoglu S, et al. Non-invasive assessment of the cerebral vasomotor reactivity by means of transcranial Doppler sonography during hypo and hypercapnia. *Klin Wochenschr* 1986;64:194–195.
10. Ringelstein EB, Droste DW, Babikian VL, et al. Consensus on microembolus detection by TCD. *Stroke* 1998;29:725–729.
11. Byrd S. An overview of transcranial color flow imaging: a technique comparison. *Ultrasound Q* 1998;13:197–210.

13

TRANSCRANIAL DOPPLER MONITORING FOR CAROTID ENDARTERECTOMY

WATSON B. SMITH

One area that has always been a source of concern and controversy is the role of any intraoperative method of monitoring during carotid endarterectomy (CEA). The problem is that, in skilled hands, the stroke rate associated with this procedure is extremely low, ranging from 2% to 5% depending on the indications for operation. To our knowledge, there are no studies documenting the potential advantages of any form of monitoring during the operation, and given the low complication rate, it would take a very large randomized trial to document the advantages of one method over another. There is also some controversy over the type of anesthesia because it is possible to use direct observation and monitor for symptoms if local anesthesia is used.

The approaches used vary from no monitoring to the universal use of a shunt. Monitoring is primarily used to either infer or document the status of the ipsilateral hemisphere during the time the carotid artery is occluded. For those who routinely use shunts, this would appear to be irrelevant as long as the shunt provides sufficient nutrient flow during cross-clamping. However, shunts are not free of problems, and a good monitoring method can also evaluate the shunt for complications. On two occasions, we have observed atheroma within the shunt—presumably scooped up when the proximal end of the shunt was placed in the common carotid artery. Although neither of these episodes led to an ischemic event, this was true only because the potential embolic material did not enter the circulation distal to the shunt.

There are different applications of the various methods, and this section covers how we use these procedures at the University of Washington. The procedures are reviewed in terms of application:

1. Transcranial Doppler (TCD). Before the operation, the patient is studied to document the presence or absence of a transtemporal acoustic window and to measure baseline velocities for the middle cerebral artery (MCA). The probe is fixed to the patient's head with headgear before induction of anesthesia (Fig. 13.1). It is possible for the technologist and the monitor to be placed at the side, out of the way of the anesthesiologist. Mean velocities are then noted before and after induction of anesthesia. Because the audible Doppler signal can be heard in real time, it is possible for surgeons to monitor the MCA Doppler signal continuously themselves during various stages of the procedure. This is particularly important during the dissection of the carotid bulb, when emboli may be dislodged. These Doppler emboli can be appreciated both audibly and on the spectral display as a transient, high-amplitude "chirp."

2. EEG. We have used this method to document hemispheric perfusion during the period of cross-clamping. If there are no changes during a 2-minute period of occlusion, we usually proceed without a shunt unless there are dramatic changes in the TCD findings.

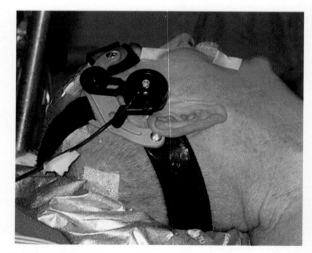

FIGURE 13.1. Photograph of a patient in position for carotid endarterectomy, with headgear in place

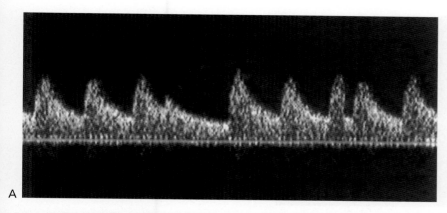

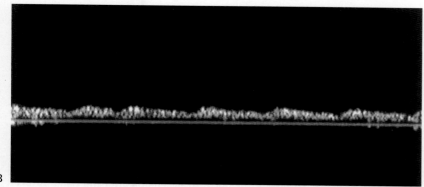

FIGURE 13.2. Images of middle cerebral artery baseline **(A)** and postclamping waveforms and velocities **(B)**.

3. Stump pressure. For years, we have utilized this in a general way to document collateral pressure when the common and external carotid arteries are clamped. Although some have published guidelines for pressures and shunting, this remains an open and disputed question even today. The pressures at which some use shunts range from less than 25 mm Hg to less than 50 mm Hg. We also pay attention to the pulsatility of the visualized waveform because this may also provide some indirect evidence of collateral adequacy in the ipsilateral hemisphere.

The criteria used to document the need for a shunt include a fall in the power of the electroencephalogram (EEG) and a drop in the MCA velocity to less than 40% of the baseline level recorded before the induction of anesthesia (Fig. 13.2). It is *critically important* to note the detection of embolic signatures during mobilization of the carotid bulb (Fig. 13.3A). As Ackerstaff and colleagues have shown, the detection of more than 10 emboli during this period of time is associated with an increase in magnetic resonance imaging–detected changes in the brain after the procedure (1–4).

When the clamps are removed from the carotid artery, a burst of air emboli is often detected (Fig. 13.3B). These emboli should occur only at this time and are recognized by their high-amplitude chirping sounds. Emboli that occur after this period of time are thought to be platelet aggregates that may or may not be a sign of problems within the endarterectomized segment (5–7). If they decrease during the time of closure, this is a good sign. However, we have adopted the practice of leaving the headgear in place and monitoring the MCA status in the recovery room as well. When emboli are detected at this time, the level of concern must go up. It may be necessary to bring a duplex scanner to the recovery room and evaluate the endarterectomized segment directly for thrombosis or occlusion. If Doppler emboli continue to increase in frequency, it may be necessary to return the patient to the operating room for exploration.

There are four potential causes of neurologic complications during the performance of CEA: hypoperfusion, embolization, perioperative thrombosis, and hyperperfusion syndrome or intracranial hemorrhage.

HYPOPERFUSION

In theory, if the circle of Willis is anatomically and functionally intact, one should be able to clamp the internal carotid artery with little or no decrease in perfusion to the ipsilateral hemisphere. However, as noted earlier, the circle is frequently not as one would hope. The most common anomaly is the lack of adequate posterior communicating arteries. Although one would hope that four-vessel angiography and perhaps TCD singly or together might provide

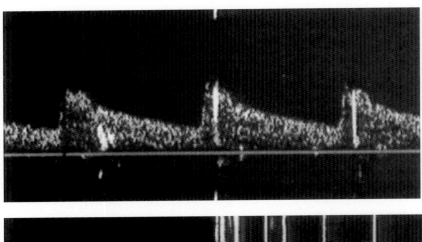

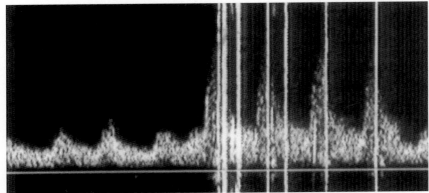

FIGURE 13.3. A: Example of particulate emboli. **B:** Air emboli after the clamp is taken off.

accurate preoperative information on the adequacy of the circle from a functional standpoint, this is not the case. The matter is complicated further by the occlusive lesions themselves, which may involve one or more extracranial and intracranial arteries to varying degrees. In addition, it is well known that the brain can autoregulate its blood flow and keep it at normal levels even to mean pressures of 50 mm Hg. However, it is not at all clear that one can reliably depend on this in patients who are hypertensive. Do they autoregulate to the same levels? This is impossible to predict. To estimate cerebral blood flow, the EEG has been used, assuming the electrical activity accurately reflects cerebral perfusion. The EEG has been used both in its traditional manner with multiple leads or as a "power" monitor for each of the hemispheres. It is also important to remember that the EEG may not reflect what goes on at the subcortical level of the brain.

Given these considerations, what might one depend on to assess the state of perfusion other than the EEG? Obviously, a direct measure of cerebral blood flow, such as using ^{133}Xe, may be the best method, but this is cumbersome to perform and is not widely used. The most direct method is to examine a target vessel, such as the MCA, and assume that flow here is a marker for the rest of the brain. The

MCA is the best target vessel because it is in this vascular distribution that most strokes occur after endarterectomy. If MCA velocity does not decrease with clamping of the internal carotid artery, it would appear to be a good assumption that cerebral blood flow is adequate. The question is, at what level of a decrease in MCA velocity is one able to perform the procedure without a shunt? It has been recommended that if the mean MCA velocity remains above 40% of the baseline level noted before the induction of anesthesia, perfusion is adequate. This, combined with no change in the EEG, would appear to be adequate evidence for not requiring a shunt. In our experience, problems related to hypoperfusion are uncommon causes of neurologic complications. Although there is no doubt that this can occur, it is not a major complication in our experience. A key factor is maintenance of adequate perfusion pressure during the operation. Hypotension in the setting of even temporary occlusion of the internal carotid artery must be avoided.

Embolization is clearly the most important cause of stroke. It may occur during dissection, during cross-clamping, with insertion of a shunt, and after removal of the clamps at the end of the procedure. TCD is the best method for detecting emboli. As noted earlier, Ackerstaff and his group have convincingly shown the relationship between emboli occurring during mobilization of the bulb and postoperative stroke (1–4). Once emboli are detected during dissection, the surgeon can be warned of the occurrence and can be more careful in mobilizing the carotid bulb.

The most distressful time is during and after declamping of the internal carotid artery. Although not universal, the release of microbubbles is very common, and they are recognized by their chirping sound and the high amplitude echo that is displayed. It should be noted that if one uses a patch, microbubbles are commonly released with declamping. After one is convinced that the operation is complete and there are no defects seen with intraoperative duplex scanning of the endarterectomized segment and no further Doppler emboli, one can be fairly certain that there are no residual problems. However, platelet thrombi can develop in the endarterectomized segment in the absence of a technical defect and give rise to postoperative ischemic events. For this reason, TCD monitoring is continued in the recovery room. Detection of emboli at this time, particularly if they are increasing in number, can be worrisome and should prompt a duplex scan to document the status of the operated segment. In some cases, returning the patient to the operating room may be the best way of resolving the issue and revealing the cause of the ongoing microembolization.

Perioperative thrombosis of the internal carotid artery is a dreaded complication with a high incidence of ischemic problems. To minimize this possibility, intraoperative duplex is now routinely employed to detect technical problems that may lead to thrombosis. This is covered in a separate section. It is our impression that the thrombotic event is often complicated by associated embolization from the developing thrombus.

The hyperfusion syndrome is another complication that must be avoided, if at all possible. TCD may be helpful here because it is a reflection of the increase in blood flow to the brain that may lead to severe headaches and, if not controlled, intracranial hemorrhage. This has not been a problem at our institution, possibly because of the much better anesthesia and blood pressure control after completion of the procedure. All of our patients are placed in the intensive care unit for at least one night. TCD is particularly helpful if the marked increase in MCA blood flow is associated with the appearance of headache and a problem with blood pressure control.

ADVANTAGES AND DISADVANTAGES OF TRANSCRANIAL DOPPLER

The major advantages of TCD are its noninvasive character and the availability of information concerning blood flow to the MCA at all times before, during, and after the procedure. The data are in real-time and are instantaneously available to the surgeon. If one chooses to use a shunt, its performance can be evaluated, and if the shunt flow is affected, this is known

immediately. A major function of the method is its detection of particulate matter that may be released during the procedure. It is true, however, that short of air emboli that occur with declamping, the Doppler signature of the detected signal does not necessarily provide information on the nature of the material. This could be of great importance, but at present we are left with the impression that all emboli are potentially harmful and should be avoided if at all possible.

One of the limitations of TCD monitoring is the lack of a suitable transtemporal acoustic window. Fortunately, this can be determined before the procedure. The other disadvantage is that it requires an experienced technologist to fix the headgear correctly on the MCA. This, however, may be of some advantage because before the application of the headgear, a survey is done of the circle of Willis that can identify active collateral pathways, and information of importance (e.g., MCA or carotid siphon stenosis) may be noted at the time of the baseline examination. Although these lesions are an uncommon problem with extracranial disease, TCD may also be helpful in that case.

The headgear must be properly fixed to avoid movement during the operation. This has not been a problem to date, but a technologist remains present during the entire procedure to ensure that this does not occur. Proper placement of the headgear has not interfered with the conduct of the anesthesia. In addition, the technologist must be certain that the signal being recorded is from the MCA. The technique for identifying the MCA is covered in Chapter 12.

If no emboli are detected during the procedure and during declamping, normalization of the MCA velocity and waveform is expected. However, mean velocities are often higher than noted before the procedure, and this may indicate hyperemia. The increase in mean velocity can be measured if the issue of hyperperfusion arises in the postoperative period. A 150% increase in the mean velocity from baseline levels that persists for longer than 15 minutes is consistent with hyperemia. If Doppler emboli are detected in the perioperative period, it is important to determine their rate. It is our practice to count them over a 15-minute period. If they increase, it is necessary to stay in the operating room until one is certain that there is not an explanation for this occurrence. As noted earlier, we also survey the patient in the recovery room to assess both the MCA velocity and the occurrence of embolic events. When emboli are detected at this time, this is worrisome, and we recommend re-scanning the operated area by duplex. If duplex is not available, the patient can be returned to the operating room to document the basis of the problem.

REFERENCES

1. Ackerstaff RGA, Jansen C, Moll FL. Carotid endarterectomy and intraoperative emboli detection: correlation of clinical, transcra-

nial Doppler, and magnetic resonance findings. *Echocardiogr J Cardiovasc Ultrasound Allied Tech* 1996;13:543–550.

2. Ackerstaff RGA, Jansen C, Moll FL, et al. Regarding "The significance of microemboli detection by means of transcranial Doppler ultrasonography monitoring in carotid endarterectomy" [Reply]. *J Vasc Surg* 1996;23:735–736.

3. Van Zuilen EV, Moll FL, Vermeulen FEE, et al. Detection of cerebral microemboli by means of transcranial Doppler monitoring before and after carotid endarterectomy. *Stroke* 1995;26:210–213.

4. Jansen C, Ramos LMP, Van Heesewijk JPM, et al. Impact of microembolism and hemodynamic changes in the brain during carotid endarterectomy. *Stroke* 1994;25:992–997.

5. Dagirmanjian A, Davis DA, Rothfus WE, et al. Silent cerebral microemboli occurring during carotid angiography: frequency as determined with Doppler sonography. *Am J Roentgenol* 1993;161:1037–1040.

6. Ries S, Schminke U, Daffertshofer M, et al. High intensity transient signals and carotid artery disease. *Cerebrovasc Dis* 1995;5:124–127.

7. Silvestrini M, Troisi E, Cupini LM, et al. Transcranial Doppler assessment of the functional effects of symptomatic carotid stenosis. *Neurology* 1994;44:1910–1914.

## 14

INTRAOPERATIVE DUPLEX EVALUATION

KAREN A. GATES

With the availability of scanning systems with suitable scanheads that can comfortably be used in the wound, it has now become possible to carry out studies in the operating room to detect problems that might compromise the clinical outcome (1–6). With arterial reconstructions, problems may develop that lead to immediate thrombosis, release of emboli, or defects that at some time in the future might lead to failure of the procedure. The major procedures in which intraoperative monitoring is performed are carotid endarterectomy, peripheral vein grafts, and intraabdominal procedures such as renal artery or mesenteric artery reconstructions. The nature of the evaluation is dependent on the anatomic site being corrected and the potential problems.

It has been our policy to have the technologist come to the operating room during the times we need to obtain optimal information concerning a reconstruction. The probe for use in the operating field should be small, with a small footprint to allow its placement in the depths of the wound and to be able to scan the entire area of the reconstruction. The technologist can optimize the gain settings and the color Doppler and record information that is key to our evaluating the outcome. The technologist also records the data for the permanent record, indicating the source of the documentation and what if anything was done to correct a problem that might have developed. Although not a routine practice, we take the scanner to the recovery room or intensive care area if there are any concerns about the success or failure of the procedure. The findings at this time have on occasion resulted in an immediate return of the patient to the operating room to correct a problem.

CAROTID ENDARTERECTOMY

Carotid endarterectomy is carried out in a standard fashion by most vascular surgeons both in this country and abroad. The procedure by necessity requires mobilization of the common carotid artery well below the bulb to beyond the lesion in the bulb and its possible extension into the inter-

nal carotid artery. After the mobilization has been completed and a decision to shunt or not has been made, the carotid artery is opened longitudinally, and the plaque is removed by dissecting it free from the outer third of the media. The surgeon then must decide whether a patch should be used and what type. Let us assume two scenarios that will need to be examined:

1. *Primary closure—no patch*. In this particular case, the entire endarterectomized segment can be examined with ultrasound. It is important to do this sequentially, as will be noted. There are three important anatomic sites that need to be seen ultrasonically and examined:
   a. The point in the common carotid artery at which the lesion is transected. This leaves a distinct shelf, which can be appreciated on B-mode imaging. The shelf at the site of the transection is easily seen. This can be examined in both the transverse and longitudinal planes.
   b. The velocity data proximal to, in, and distal to the endarterectomy site must be obtained in the longitudinal scan plane, moving the sample volume across the entire scan plane looking for "step-ups" in the peak systolic velocity that might signify an area of narrowing. A similar scan is done across the bulb into the internal carotid artery, paying particular attention to the point of transection of the plaque.
   c. The external carotid artery is also assessed from its origin for the first few centimeters, looking for residual plaque and areas of thrombosis.
2. *Patch closure*. If one uses a prosthetic patch such as Dacron or PTFE, it will be impossible to scan through the patch itself because of the air within the wall of the patch. Nonetheless, it is possible to scan along the sides of the artery either anterior or posterior to the patch to obtain the necessary information.

We are interested in documenting those factors that may compromise the immediate outcome of the procedure, including intraoperative thrombosis with either total occlu-

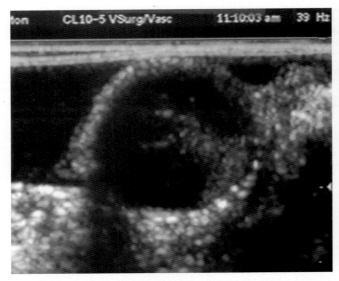

FIGURE 14.1. This cross-sectional B-mode image of the carotid bulb clearly shows what appears to be an intraluminal thrombus.

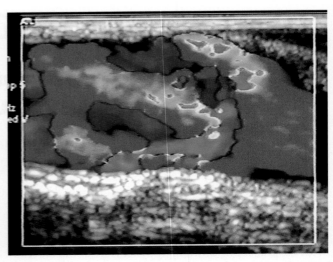

FIGURE 14.3. When color Doppler is added to the B-mode image seen in Fig. 14.1, the very disturbed flow pattern is evident.

sion or the release of embolic material to the brain. Because we also perform transcranial Doppler monitoring of the middle cerebral artery, emboli released from the site of repair are immediately recognized. The manner in which this is done and interpreted is covered in Chapter 13. In addition, there is always some concern about the creation of a stenosis at the distal end of the arteriotomy site or at the site of plaque transection in the common carotid artery.

Example 1. When the endarterectomy was completed, a transverse scan of the bulb region revealed a large web-like structure that had the homogeneous appearance of a platelet thrombus (Fig. 14.1). After this "thrombotic" material was removed, the identical cross-sectional view showed the area to be free of material (Fig. 14.2). It was also possible with color Doppler to see the relationship between the visualized thrombus and flow (Fig. 14.3). A longitudinal color flow map of the same region showed it to be normal (Fig. 14.4).

Example 2. This case, shown in Figs. 14.5 and 14.6, illustrates both the subtleties of the examination and how interpretation may be difficult. In Fig. 14.5, flow across the proximal shelf taken at 10:27 AM was by color flow normal, and the peak systolic velocities were in the range of 60

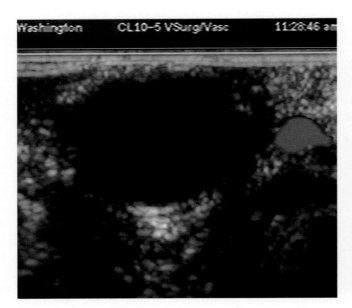

FIGURE 14.2. After removal of the thrombus, the area is free of any intraluminal defects.

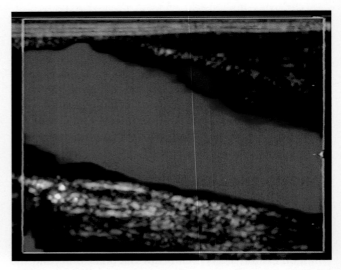

FIGURE 14.4. The color Doppler flow map after removal of the thrombus has returned to normal.

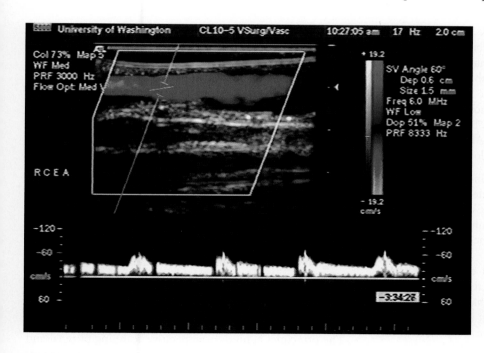

FIGURE 14.5. This longitudinal scan across the proximal shelf taken at 10:27 AM was normal.

cm/sec. Three minutes later, the picture changed, with the peak systolic velocity now in the 150 cm/sec range along with a very discrete area of flow increase seen in color. This was not repaired at the time of operation, but the area thrombosed in the postoperative period, requiring reoperation.

Although detection of areas of residual narrowing is a key element in the scanning process, we are also interested

in detecting thrombi (usually platelets) that may form in the endarterectomized segment and that may be a source of emboli to the brain and a nidus for postoperative thrombosis. Whenever these are detected, they must be corrected. Because transcranial Doppler monitoring is also being done, the detection of ongoing emboli after closure of the artery should alert the surgeon to the fact that the origin of these may be a forming thrombus at the site of plaque removal. We consider these findings to be critically impor-

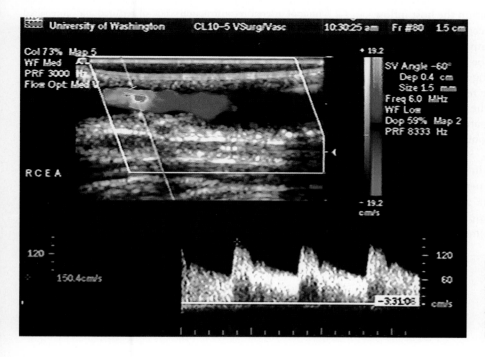

FIGURE 14.6. Taken only a few minutes after that in Fig. 14.5, the same area shows a very focal increase in flow velocity. This area was not repaired, and the artery thrombosed in the postoperative period, requiring return to the operating room.

tant, demanding immediate correction. This may require reopening of the carotid bulb to correct any defects that may be seen. However, it is now clear that platelet thrombi can occur in the absence of any detectable technical problem.

We can often determine with ease those cases that need to be reopened at the time of operation, but there are some cases in which the decision is not easy. Although it is difficult to generalize, our policies are as follows:

- The finding of a thrombus at any point along the reconstruction must be corrected immediately.
- If there is a large step-up in the peak systolic velocity at the distal end of the closure, this should be treated at the time. This is most likely to occur when a patch has not been used.
- A prominent shelf on the proximal end of the arteriotomy where the plaque was transsected is not reopened if there is not an associated velocity change that is severe. If the velocity at the shelf is twice that just proximal, this probably should be repaired, but there are no hard or fast rules concerning this.
- With the current high-resolution scanners, we often see fronds "waving" in the breeze of an operated segment. These should not be attended to because they are not a problem unless they are associated with a large velocity change across the area.

LOWER EXTREMITY BYPASS GRAFTING

The problems that can occur in the lower extremity bypass graft are largely related to technical problems at either anastomosis or in the main body of the graft. However, it is possible on occasion to detect a problem within the host inflow and outflow arteries that will need correction. For example, the site of placement of a vascular clamp should always be scanned to detect problems that might be related to fracture of a plaque. The two types of grafting procedures commonly used are the *in situ* graft and the reversed saphenous graft. In the case of the *in situ* graft, the valves have to be lysed, and the venous branches of the graft need to be interrupted to prevent graft compromise from an arteriovenous fistula.

The scanning procedure is done in the longitudinal mode looking for velocity changes that may be secondary to a technical problem. The velocity data and the forward–reverse–forward flow characteristics are important. The angles of the proximal and distal anastomoses are often dif-

ficult to study, but the combination of the B-mode image along with velocity data can be helpful.

The arteriovenous shunts that occur with the *in situ* graft can be systematically located by the use of the duplex scanner but also with a continuous wave Doppler. Listening to the flow in the graft as it is sequentially occluded digitally will give the surgeon an idea of where and how big a venous branch may be. However, some small arteriovenous shunts may be missed, only to appear during the course of a postoperative surveillance study.

After a scan has been completed, it may be possible to confirm the duplex studies by intraoperative arteriography. However, if the intraoperative scan does not show any problems, we do not do the contrast studies. Unless one has a suite that allows the entire graft to be easily imaged, only the distal graft anastomosis can be regularly imaged by radiograph.

VISCERAL ARTERY RECONSTRUCTION

The principles behind intraoperative scanning of renal and mesenteric artery scanning are similar to those for bypass grafting of the limb. The major concern relates to the hemodynamic success of the reconstruction, be it by endarterectomy or bypass graft. In this particular area, immediate hemodynamic success is essential if organ preservation is to be obtained. This can be assessed by the flow patterns in the conduit, providing an immediate indication of the result.

REFERENCES

1. Bandyk DF, Mills JL, Gahtan V, et al. Intraoperative duplex scanning of arterial reconstructions: fate of repaired and unrepaired defects. *J Vasc Surg* 1994;20:426–432; discussion, 432–433.
2. Kinney EV, Seabrook GR, Kinney LY, et al. The importance of intraoperative detection of residual flow abnormalities after carotid endarterectomy. *J Vasc Surg* 1993;17:912–922.
3. Mills JL, Bandyk DF, Gahtan V, et al. The origin of infrainguinal vein graft stenosis: a prospective study based on duplex surveillance. *J Vasc Surg* 1995;21:16–22; discussion, 22–25.
4. Schwartz RA, Peterson GJ, Noland DA, et al. Intraoperative duplex scanning after carotid artery reconstruction: a valuable tool. *J Vasc Surg* 1988;7:604–624.
5. Lingenfelter DA, Fuller BC, Sullivan TM. Intraoperative assessment of carotid endarterectomy: a comparison of techniques. *Ann Vasc Surg* 1995;9:235–242.
6. Gilbertson JJ, Walsh DB, Zwolak RM, et al. A blinded comparison of angiography, angioscopy and duplex scanning in the intraoperative evaluation of in situ saphenous vein bypass grafts. *J Vasc Surg* 1992;15:121–127.

15

PERIPHERAL ARTERIAL EVALUATION

MOLLY J. ZACCARDI
KARI A. OLMSTED

The vascular diagnostic laboratory has come to play an increasingly important role in the evaluation of patients suspected of having or with known peripheral arterial disease. As a simple screening test for occlusive arterial disease, the clinical history, supported by assessment of the ankle/brachial index (ABI), is generally all that is needed (1–3). However, there are situations in which the clinical history and even the finding of a normal ABI require further investigation. These are patients who have exercise-induced pain in one or both limbs. If they do not have the classic walk–pain–rest cycle, they may be suffering from pseudoclaudication. In this situation, further testing may be in order to make this separation, and an exercise test may be needed (4,5). Other indications for study are those that occur before some form of intervention, be it endovascular or direct arterial surgery. In addition, there are increasing indications for follow-up surveillance studies to document the sites of recurrent problems that might threaten graft survival. We are also asked to document the presence of aneurysmal disease (true or false), evaluation of digital ischemia, and the thoracic outlet syndrome. The evaluation of patients with vein grafts or pseudoaneurysms is covered in chapters 17 and 18. In this chapter, we describe the basic testing procedures that we use to evaluate the arterial system in the upper and lower extremities. Surveillance of bypass grafts and treatment of pseudoaneurysms are described in detail in chapters 17 and 18.

LOWER EXTREMITY ARTERIAL EVALUATION

As noted previously, the initial testing includes ABI and an exercise test if the diagnosis of intermittent claudication is open to question. The ABI and exercise test require about 30 minutes for completion. If it has been decided that a complete bilateral arterial duplex is warranted, an additional hour will be required.

Equipment

The equipment required for the arterial evaluation consists of blood pressure cuffs, a handheld continuous wave (CW)

Doppler, treadmill, photoplethysmograph, sphygmomanometer, and a color duplex ultrasound system with printer and videotape for documentation. The blood pressure cuffs are 12 cm wide for the arm and 10 cm wide for the ankle; a variety of smaller cuffs are available for the toe. A 5-MHz transducer is the most suitable handheld CW Doppler for this evaluation. For the imaging portion of the examination, a low-frequency transducer in the range of 2 to 4 MHz is necessary for aortic and iliac evaluation. A mid-range transducer with a range of 4 to 8 MHz is ideal for the legs. This examination has been performed successfully without the use of color Doppler, but we have found that color greatly enhances the ability to visualize vessels (6) and therefore reduces the length of time of the arterial ultrasound examination.

Patient Preparation

There is no patient preparation for the initial screening tests. If a full duplex arterial examination is requested, it is preferable to schedule it in the morning after a 12-hour fast. Patients with insulin-dependent diabetes mellitus are not expected to fast but are asked to eat a small breakfast. This preparation reduces some of the difficulties caused by bowel gas in producing adequate ultrasound images of the aorta and iliac arteries.

Examination Technique

Ankle/Brachial Indices

The patient is required to rest supine for 5 minutes for blood pressures to stabilize. Blood pressure cuffs are placed on both arms and both ankles. Systolic pressures are recorded from both arms and both ankles (posterior and anterior tibial arteries) (3,7). If signals cannot be heard from the two tibial arteries, the peroneal artery systolic pressure is recorded. It is extremely important that all pressures be measured using the CW Doppler. Using the highest arm blood pressure and the highest tibial artery pressure, an index is calculated, as shown in the following example (ankle/arm index is the same as ABI):

Resting ABI	*Right*	*Left*
Brachial artery	120	118
Posterior tibial artery	100	98
Anterior tibial artery	110	100
Peroneal artery	90	86

$$ABI = \frac{\text{Highest ankle blood pressure}}{\text{Highest brachial blood pressure}}$$

$$= \frac{\overset{\text{Right}}{110 \text{ mm Hg}}}{120 \text{ mm Hg}} \qquad \frac{\overset{\text{Left}}{100 \text{ mm Hg}}}{120 \text{ mm Hg}}$$

$$= \quad 0.92 \qquad\qquad 0.83$$

At the time the pressures are measured, it is important to document the quality of the Doppler signal heard both from the brachial and the tibial arteries of the lower leg. The audible characteristics of the signals will indicate whether the flow patterns are normal or abnormal. The evaluation of subclavian arteries will be discussed in more detail in Chapter 16. It is not uncommon to record abnormally high ankle pressures when patients have diabetes mellitus. When this occurs, or if the pressures seem to be unusually high, it is necessary to measure the toe pressures using a photoplethysmograph. These patients often have medial wall calcification of the tibial and peroneal arteries, giving rise to this problem. In fact, it is good practice to measure toe pressures routinely in patients with diabetes to obviate this problem.

With experience, the technologist will eventually be able to interpret arterial flow signals on the basis of the audible characteristics alone. The normal flow pattern in the leg is triphasic (forward–reverse–forward) within each heart cycle. A biphasic flow signal without reverse flow is not a normal finding in the leg and indicates a proximal obstruction. However, a biphasic flow pattern in an upper extremity artery may be within normal limits. An absence of a reverse flow component in a normal arterial system reflects the lower resistance to flow. An arterial flow pattern in the arms or legs that is monophasic is always abnormal, reflecting the presence of a high-grade stenosis or occlusion proximal to the recording site. An example of a printout of the flow patterns is seen in Fig. 15.1.

If the ABI is abnormal and the patient is being considered for intervention, a full lower extremity arterial duplex ultrasound examination may be performed, at the request of the referring physician. If the patient has diabetes and the ankle arteries cannot be compressed, the patient unquestionably has medial calcification of the tibial and peroneal arteries (8). It is important to realize that the calcification that leads to this problem is within the media of the artery and not the intima. It is possible to have totally calcified arteries in this location that are not occluded by atherosclerosis. Another indicator of medial calcification is an ABI of more than 1.2 to 1.3. In this case, the ankle pressures are probably falsely elevated, and an effort should be made to measure the toe pressure. If the ABI is normal and the patient does not have diabetes mellitus we proceed to the exercise test. The toe pressure measurement and exercise test are described following the ABI criteria:

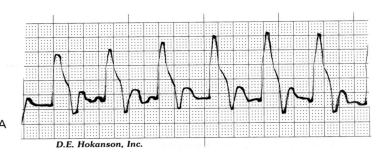

D.E. Hokanson, Inc.

Triphasic (Normal)

FIGURE 15.1. Normal and abnormal waveforms are shown in this illustration [triphasic **(A)**, biphasic **(B)**, and monophasic **(C)**].

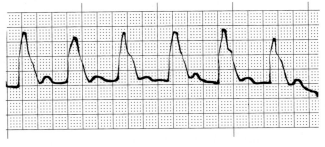

Biphasic (Abnormal in legs – normal in arms)

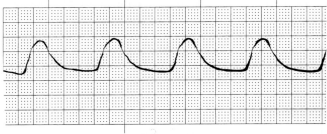
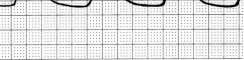

Monophasic (Abnormal)

A

B

C

Diagnostic Criteria: Ankle/Brachial Indices

- *Normal,* more than 0.95
- *Abnormal,* less than 0.95
- *Multilevel disease,* less than 0.50
- *Critical ischemia,* less than 0.30

Toe Pressure Measurements

A small blood pressure cuff is placed around the great toe. Using double-stick tape, adhere the photoplethysmograph transducer to the pad of the toe (Fig. 15.2). The toe pressure should be measured by a strip chart recorder and photoplethysmograph. When the digital pulse waveform is obtained, the cuff is inflated to suprasystolic pressure. As is true with measurement of the ankle pressures, the toe pressure is not recorded during cuff inflation but only during cuff deflation. The systolic pressure is the pressure recorded at the point the pulsatile flow is restored during cuff deflation.

Toe/Brachial Index	*Right*	*Left*
Brachial artery	120	118
First digit (great toe)	90	66
Second digit	86	60

$$\text{Toe/brachial index} = \frac{\text{Toe blood pressure}}{\text{Highest brachial blood pressure}}$$

	Right	Left
Toe/brachial index =	$\dfrac{90 \text{ mm Hg}}{120 \text{ mm Hg}}$	$\dfrac{66 \text{ mm Hg}}{120 \text{ mm Hg}}$
Toe/brachial index =	0.75	0.55

The criteria used for interpreting the toe/brachial index are as follows:

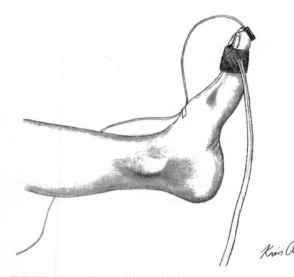

FIGURE 15.2. Photocell attached to the great toe to measure toe pressures.

Diagnostic Criteria: Toe/Brachial Indices

- *Normal,* more than 0.70
- *Abnormal,* less than 0.69

Exercise Test

An exercise test is indicated for three reasons: (a) to document the severity of the walking distance limitation; (b) to determine the extent of the ischemic response in terms of the magnitude of the postexercise pressure drop and time required for recovery to baseline levels; and (c) to determine whether the walking-induced pain is secondary to arterial disease or other causes, such as neurospinal disease. It should be noted that a patient may have true vascular claudication even with normal resting systolic limb blood pressures because a stenosis that is not significant at rest may become significant when the flow across it is increased in response to exercise.

The standard exercise test is performed with settings of 2 mph at 12% grade. These settings may be altered to accommodate the needs of the patient but must be documented. The patient is carefully screened to rule out exercise-induced angina or shortness of breath. Although we have not had a catastrophic event during this protocol, it is important to be cautious.

During the exercise test, the patient is asked to report any discomfort and to describe the symptoms during the exercise period. The time when the symptoms develop and the location of those symptoms must be documented. The standard exercise testing time does not exceed 5 minutes (Fig. 15.3). Immediately after the treadmill test, the patient lies back on the bed, and pressures are recorded within the first minute after exercise and then every 2 minutes until returning to within 10 mm Hg of the baseline pressure. An example of an exercise test is seen on the worksheet that follows.

Diagnostic Criteria: Exercise Treadmill Test

Normal. The exercise treadmill test is considered normal if the patient has a normal ABI before exercise and if the postexercise ankle systolic pressure falls less than 20% below the resting ankle pressure and returns to baseline within 3 minutes after the test is completed.

Abnormal. The exercise treadmill test is considered abnormal if the postexercise ankle systolic pressure falls greater than 20% of the baseline and requires longer than 3 minutes to recover. If the pressure fall is abnormal, it is important to continue recording the pressures until they have recovered to baseline levels. The length of time it takes to return to baseline is a good marker of the extent of the muscle ischemia that occurred with the walk (5). It is extremely important to record the absolute values of ankle systolic pressure after exercise and not the ABI, which is often done and is incorrect. With exercise, the arm systolic

UNIVERSITY OF WASHINGTON MEDICAL CENTER - VASCULAR DIAGNOSTIC SERVICE

LOWER EXTREMITY ARTERIAL EXERCISE EXAM   HISTORY _____

58 y/o m w/ history ® calf pain when walking

UH# _____

NAME _____

D.O.B. _____

REFERRED BY _____   PHONE _____

ADDRESS _____

SYSTOLIC PRESSURES	RIGHT	LEFT
BRACHIAL ARTERY	120	118
POSTERIOR TIBIAL ARTERY	110	112
ANTERIOR TIBIAL ARTERY	118	120
PERONEAL ARTERY	102	110
ANKLE/ARM INDEX	.98	>1.0

RISK FACTORS	
HTN	+
SMOKING	+
DIABETES	Ø
LIPIDS	?
CAD/PVD	?

EXERCISE TREADMILL: Speed __2__ mph Grade __12__ %

TIME	SYMPTOMS WITH EXERCISE
1:45	® calf tightness
3:00	® calf pain
:	
:	
:	

TOTAL WALK TIME: __4__ MIN. __30__ SEC.

STOPPED DUE TO: _calf pain_

POST EXERCISE PRESSURES			
RT PT	TIME	LT PT	∠ARM
50	1 MIN	90	148
72	2 MIN	110	136
92	4 MIN		120
110	6 MIN		120
	8 MIN		
	10 MIN		
	12 MIN		

	RIGHT	LEFT
TECH		
TAPE #		

PHONE/PRELIMINARY REPORT IN CHART_____

DICTATED_____

DR. SIGNATURE/DISTRIBUTION_____

FIGURE 15.3. The technologist collects the following data when performing an exercise test.

pressure will increase in proportion to the workload (9). Thus, it is not proper to relate the pressure increase at the arm level to the pressure changes that occur at the ankle.

Lower Extremity Arterial Duplex Examination

Throughout the arterial duplex examination, a 60-degree angle of insonation to the long axis of the artery is used to record Doppler signals. In cases of very tortuous vessels, angle correction may be used but requires an angle of 60 degrees or less. The entire length of the vessels will be inter-rogated by "sweeping" the Doppler sample volume throughout the vessel. Areas of plaque, calcification, or dilatation are noted and recorded. It is important to remember that one cannot use the B-mode image to determine the degree of narrowing produced by a plaque. Evaluation of aneurysms is described later in chapter 22 in more detail. Doppler velocity changes (spectral broadening and velocity increase) are documented wherever they are noted. The criteria for disease classification are based on these data. At any site of velocity increase, both the prestenotic and poststenotic signals are recorded. The criteria for disease classification are based on the change of the flow velocity from the normal segment to the abnormal segment. Any vessel segment in which flow cannot be detected is assumed to be occluded. It is also important to note the length of the arterial segment in which flow cannot be detected. The site at which patency is restored will be the point where the reentry collaterals will be found. Equipment settings should be adjusted at the abdominal, femoral, and tibial levels as the flow velocities gradually decrease from the proximal iliac to distal tibial arteries. Jager and colleagues described the flow velocities that were found in a group of healthy volunteers to demonstrate this finding, as follows (10):

Artery	Peak Systolic Velocity ±SD(cm/sec)
External iliac	119.3±21.7
Common femoral	114.1±24.9
Superficial femoral (proximal)	90.8±13.6
Superficial femoral (distal)	93.6±14.1
Popliteal	68.8±13.5

With the patient in the supine position, a low-frequency transducer is placed below the xyphoid process and angled cephalad. The proximal abdominal aorta can be seen in long axis with visualization of the celiac trunk and proximal mesenteric artery (Fig. 15.4). A recording and hard-copy print are made from specific sites at each level as indicated by the worksheet in Fig. 15.5.

The proximal abdominal aorta is evaluated both by B-mode and Doppler. The transducer is angled distally to evaluate the distal abdominal aorta. The transducer at the level of the umbilicus is placed in an oblique approach (patient's left side) to visualize the aortic bifurcation (Fig. 15.6). It is very important to sweep the sample volume slowly through the bifurcation and proximal common iliac arteries. The transducer is placed at the level of the iliac crest to evaluate the middle common iliac and proximal external iliac arteries. This usually requires applying considerable probe pressure. In many cases, the internal iliac artery can be seen from this view and can be assessed. The internal iliac artery is used as a landmark to separate the common from the external iliac artery. Otherwise, the contour "dip" helps differentiate the vessel segments (Fig. 15.7).

Changing to the mid-range transducer, the transducer is placed in the groin and pointed in a cephalad direction to assess the distal external iliac and common femoral arterial segments. Slide the transducer down the leg to encounter the junction of the profunda femoris and superficial femoral arteries (Fig. 15.8). The profunda femoris is normally evaluated in the first 3 or 4 cm, at which point it begins to descend more deeply into the thigh. The attention is then back to the superficial femoral artery, which is followed down to the level of the knee. When the superficial femoral artery passes through Hunter's canal, it assumes a deeper position, which may be difficult to assess with the patient in the supine position. At this point, the patient may need to be placed in the prone position to assess the distal superficial femoral and popliteal arteries. As the popliteal artery is scanned in a longitudinal mode, the first vessel to be encountered is the anterior tibial artery (Fig. 15.9).

After the origin of the anterior tibial artery has been identified and interrogated, the technologist places the transducer at the level of the ankle, posterior to the medial malleolus, to visualize the posterior tibial artery. It is possible to follow the posterior tibial artery throughout its entire

(*Text continues on page 260.*)

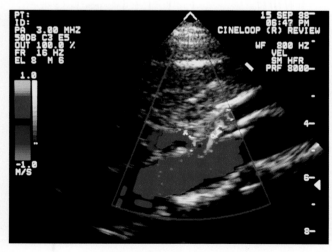

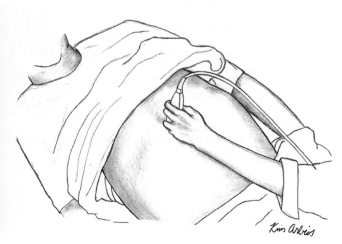

FIGURE 15.4. Transducer placement just below the xyphoid process, angled cephalad, to produce a typical image of the proximal aorta.

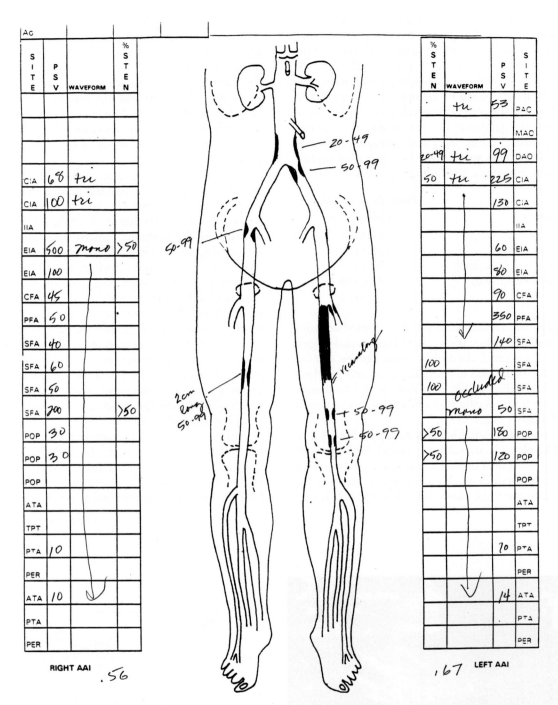

FIGURE 15.5. Data for the peripheral arterial duplex are documented on the worksheet.

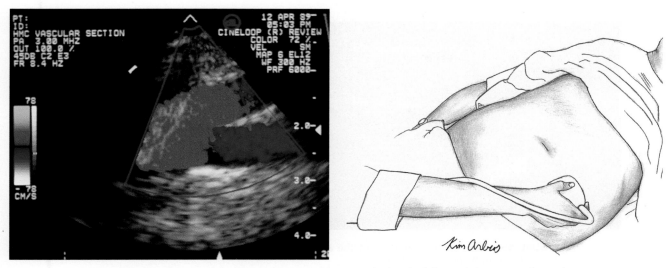

FIGURE 15.6. The transducer is positioned oblique at the level of the umbilicus to evaluate the distal aorta and common iliac bifurcation.

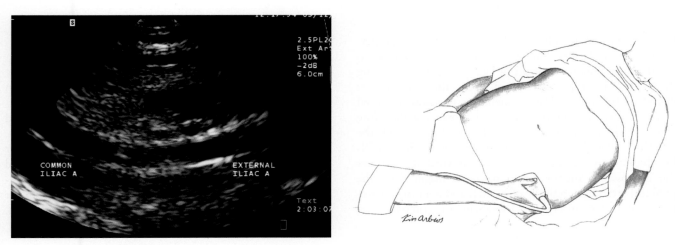

FIGURE 15.7. The transducer is placed at the iliac crest and tilted medially to visualize the common and external iliac arteries.

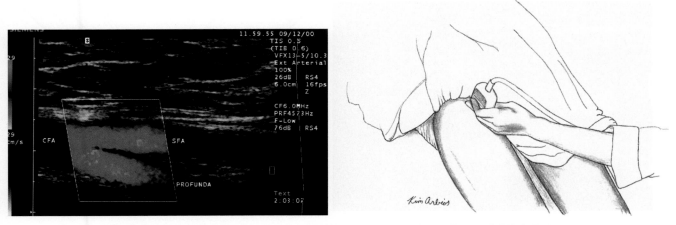

FIGURE 15.8. Placing the transducer at the groin, the common femoral artery bifurcation is easily visualized.

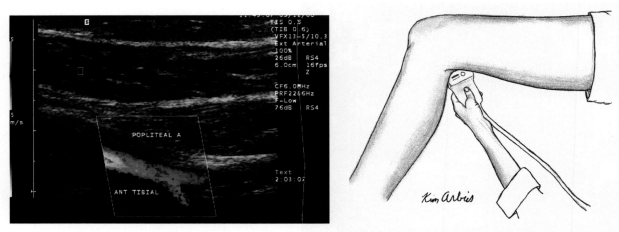

FIGURE 15.9. The proximal portion of the anterior tibial artery can be easily evaluated as it branches from the popliteal artery.

length up to and including the bifurcation of the tibial/peroneal trunk in the proximal calf. The paired veins help identify the tibial arteries, as noted in Fig. 15.10. After scanning the length of the posterior tibial artery, the transducer is placed posterior to the lateral malleolus to assess the distal peroneal artery. Sliding the transducer proximally, the entire length of the peroneal artery is evaluated. Finally, with the transducer placed anterior on the ankle, it is possible to follow the anterior tibial artery to the level at which it penetrates the interosseous membrane to reach its origin from the popliteal artery. An example of normal and abnormal waveforms can be seen in Fig. 15.11 following the criteria.

Diagnostic Criteria: Lower Extremity Arterial Disease

The principle elements to take into consideration when interpreting findings collected in the lower extremity arterial duplex evaluation are peak systolic flow velocity and arterial waveform contour.

Color flow is extremely helpful as a pathfinder and for demonstrating flow patterns associated with turbulence and poststenotic turbulence (6,11). The most important criterion to estimate the degree of narrowing is the change in the peak systolic velocity at the site of the stenosis. In addition,

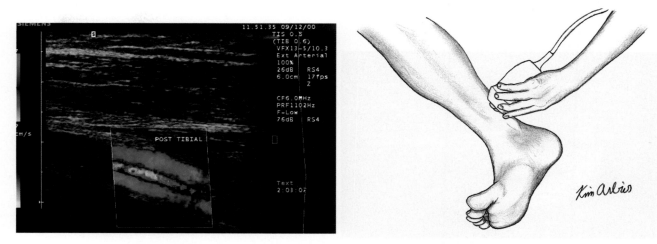

FIGURE 15.10. The tibial artery is identified by the adjacent paired tibial veins.

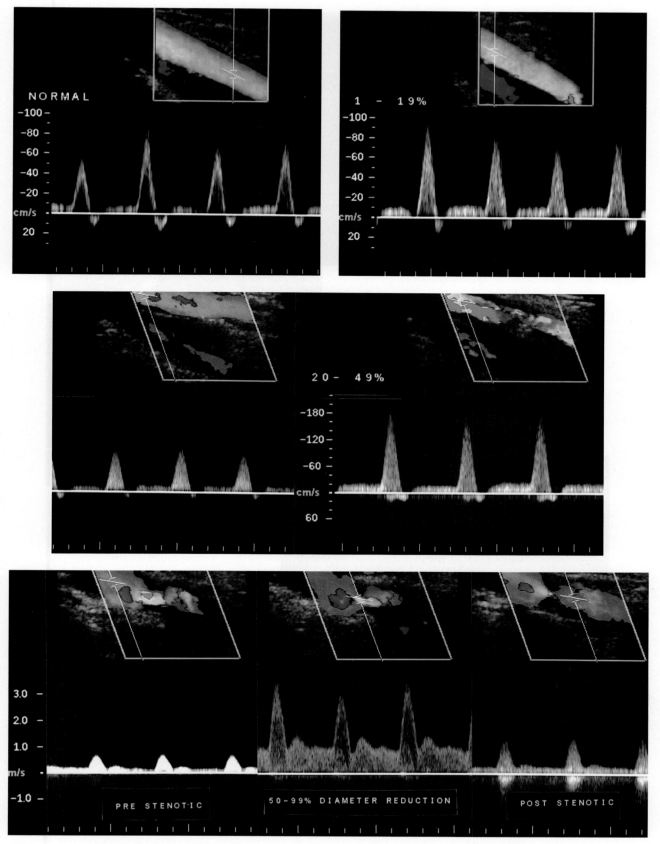

FIGURE 15.11. These waveforms are examples of the five different peripheral arterial categories. *(Continued on next page)*

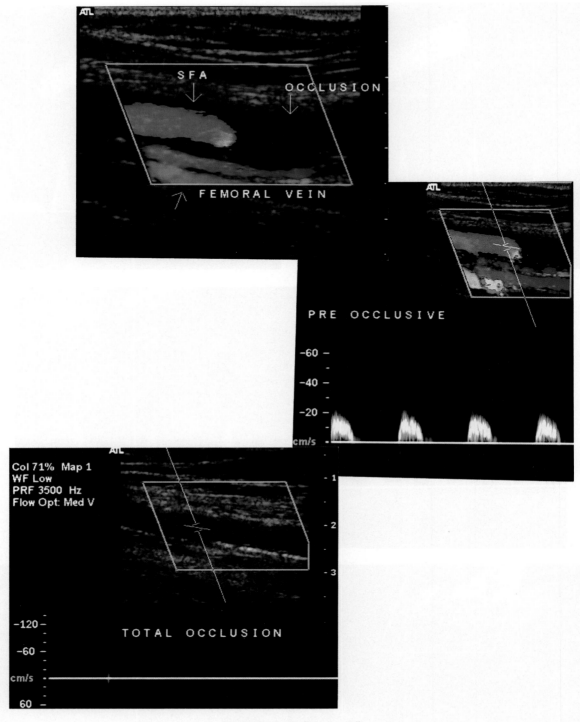

FIGURE 15.11. (Continued)

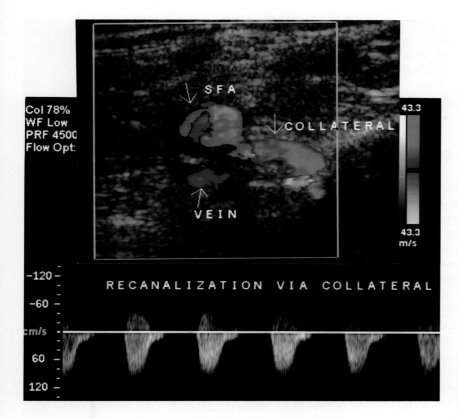

FIGURE 15.11. *(Continued)*

TABLE 15.1 CATEGORICAL CRITERIA FOR ARTERIAL DISEASE IN THE LOWER EXTREMITIES

Diameter reduction (%)	Waveform criteria
0	Peak systolic velocity within normal limits Clear window underpeak systole Reverse flow present
1–19	Peak systolic velocity within normal limits Spectral broadening present Reverse flow present
20–49	Peak systolic velocity increase (but not more than 100% from previous segment) Reverse flow present No poststenotic flow
50–99	Peak systolic velocity increase (more than 100% from previous arterial segment) Absence of reverse flow Poststenotic flow present
Occluded Reconstitution	Absence of Doppler signals Retrograde flow in collateral artery at site of vessel entry

Assuming all velocity data are collected at an angle of 60 degrees to the long axis of the artery.

it is known that there is a loss of the reverse flow component when a hemodynamically significant stenosis is found. In cases that may appear borderline, poststenotic flow and the appearance of a color bruit are useful indicators of a hemodynamically significant narrowing. Table 15.1 describes the criteria we use to categorize arterial disease in the lower extremities.

Pitfalls with Peripheral Arterial Duplex

The results of a complete, well-visualized duplex examination compare very well with independently read arteriograms (12). In our laboratory, the numbers of requests for arterial duplex examinations are increasing. At the time of this writing, about 13% of examinations requested are for assessment of peripheral arterial disease. There are some limitations resulting from pitfalls, which need to be addressed.

The abdominal vessels may be difficult to assess because of bowel gas. In addition, the iliac arteries may be difficult to access in obese patients. The common iliac artery normally dives deep into the pelvis, and the external iliac artery curves upward to the common femoral arterial segment. The origin of the common iliac artery is often difficult to visualize. Another approach is to use the umbilicus as a window, with the transducer angled caudally and to the right or left. This also allows visualization of one iliac artery at a time (Fig. 15.12).

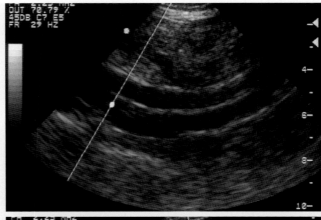

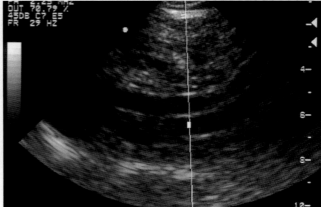

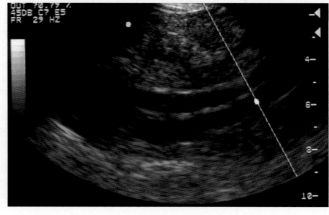

FIGURE 15.13. An appropriate angle of insonance is often difficult to achieve in the iliac artery, as is seen in these examples.

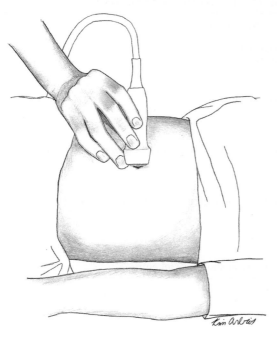

FIGURE 15.12. The iliac vessels can be visualized by placing the transducer at the umbilicus.

This anatomy may create a problem when attempting to maintain the artery at a 60-degree angle of insonance for the velocity studies. Tilting the transducer head during the scan may assist in the accurate evaluation of these arteries (Fig. 15.13). To minimize the problem of bowel gas, patients are scheduled for studies in the morning after a 12-hour fast. If bowel gas is seen, it may be displaced from the site of insonation by placing the patient in reverse Trendelenburg's position. It may also be necessary to apply considerable transducer pressure manually to displace the gas.

Many patients have dense calcification, especially in the tibial arteries. At times, we are unable to penetrate these segments with ultrasound. If the flow pattern and velocity have not changed greatly from one segment to another, we assume the vessel is patent throughout that segment. On the other hand, if the flow pattern is normal proximally and is monophasic distal to the calcification or displays a significant reduction in the flow velocity, we would report probable obstruction.

Flow direction must be noted throughout the examination. It is possible for a vessel to be tightly narrowed or occluded in a short segment and to have retrograde filling through collaterals. An example of this can be seen in Fig. 15.14. It is also possible for a vessel to have a tight focal lesion and a normal waveform distally (Fig. 15.15). For this reason, the entire vessel segment must be evaluated with Doppler.

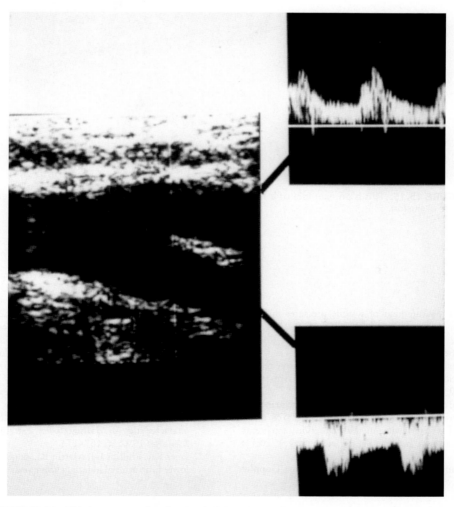

FIGURE 15.14. This is an example of an occluded common femoral artery with retrograde filling through the profunda femoris artery to supply the superficial femoral artery.

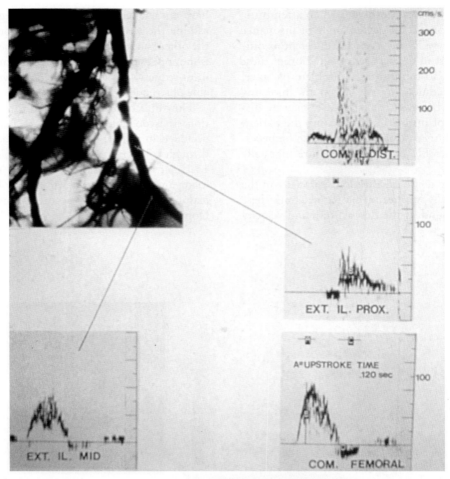

FIGURE 15.15. This is an example of a flow pattern that has normalized distal to a tight stenosis or occlusion.

REFERENCES

1. Carter SA. Clinical measurement of systolic pressures in limbs with arterial occlusive disease. *JAMA* 1969;207:1869–1874.
2. Carter SA. Arterial auscultation in peripheral vascular disease. *JAMA* 1981;246:1682–1686.
3. Marinelli MR, Beach KW, Glass MJ, et al. Noninvasive testing vs. clinical evaluation of arterial disease: a prospective study. *JAMA* 1979;241:2031–2034.
4. Carter SA. Response of ankle systolic pressure to leg exercise in mild or questionable arterial disease. *N Engl J Med* 1972;287:578–582.
5. Strandness DE Jr. Exercise testing in the evaluation of patients undergoing direct arterial surgery. *J Cardiovasc Surg* 1970;11:192–200.
6. Hatsukami TS, Primozich JP, Zierler RE, et al. Color Doppler imaging of lower extremity arterial disease: a prospective validation study. *J Vasc Surg* 1992;16:527–533.
7. Knox RA, Strandness DE Jr. Clinical assessment of peripheral arterial disease. *Semin Ultrasound* 1981;2:264–275.
8. Orchard TJ, Strandness DE Jr. Assessment of peripheral vascular disease in diabetes. *Circulation* 1993;88:819–828.
9. Stahler CS, Strandness DE Jr. Ankle blood pressure response to graded treadmill exercise. *Angiology* 1967;18:237–241.
10. Jager KA, Ricketts HJ, Strandness DE Jr. Duplex scanning for the evaluation of lower limb arterial disease. In: Bernstein EF, ed. *Vascular diagnosis*, 4th ed. St. Louis: CV Mosby, 1985:619.
11. Hatsukami TS, Primozich J, Zierler RE, et al. Color Doppler characteristics in normal lower extremity arteries. *Ultrasound Med Biol* 1992;16:167–171.
12. Jager KA, Phillips DJ, Martin RL, et al. Noninvasive mapping of lower limb arterial lesions. *Ultrasound Med Biol* 1985;1:515–521.

## 16

UPPER EXTREMITY ARTERIAL EVALUATION

MOLLY J. ZACCARDI

Diseases that affect the arterial supply of the upper extremity are relatively rare. Even though atherosclerosis is the most common arterial disorder in Western society, its involvement of the arteries distal to the origin of the subclavian artery is very rare. In fact, the senior author of this text has operated on only two patients with lesions in the brachial artery in more than 30 years of practice. However, as noted in the chapters on lower extremity arterial disease and extracranial arterial disease, we always attempt to evaluate the status of the origin of the subclavian artery as a routine part of our studies. This is done initially by simple assessment of the arm systolic pressures. If there is a gradient between the two arms of more than 15 mm Hg, it is likely that there is a stenosis or occlusion on the side of the lower pressure. In this situation, we carry out a duplex evaluation of the subclavian artery to assess if the artery is narrowed or totally occluded. The request for an upper extremity arterial evaluation may be for either acute or chronic problems, as listed (1):

- *Acute*: suspected embolic event (thrombotic events are extremely uncommon)
- *Chronic*: cold sensitivity—primary or secondary Raynaud's disease; thoracic outlet syndrome–vascular versus neurogenic; documentation of subclavian steal syndrome; suspected vasculitis

Each of these problems requires specific study protocols to document the status of the circulation. The ultrasound duplex studies are designed to document the status of the large and medium-sized arteries (all have proper names). To evaluate acute arterial occlusions, the studies must be able to separate problems that involve the large and medium-sized arteries from those that may be found in the digital arteries. The thoracic outlet syndrome and the subclavian steal syndrome involve the arteries at the thoracic outlet and their branches. To evaluate cold sensitivity and suspected vasculitis, the involvement of the circulation is often at the small arteries and arteriolar level. As will be shown, our ability to document the fact that the large and medium-sized arteries are free of disease will help focus our attention on

the small arteries and arterioles at the sites of involvement. Documentation of subclavian steal is described in detail in chapter 11.

EQUIPMENT

The equipment required for the upper extremity arterial examination includes a 12-cm blood pressure cuff for the arm pressure and a 10-cm blood pressure cuff for use at the wrist to measure the systolic pressure from the radial and ulnar arteries. A 3- to 4-cm cuff is used for the assessment of digit pressures. The upper arm and wrist pressures are taken using 5-MHz continuous wave (CW) handheld Doppler. Digit pressures can on occasion be measured using the handheld CW Doppler, but in general, the photoplethysmograph (PPG) with strip chart recorder is more accurate, providing better documentation and more information relative to the circulation to the digits. An immersable thermometer and basin are needed for the cold-sensitivity test. For evaluation of the large and medium-sized arteries, a duplex ultrasound system with mid-range transmitting frequencies (4 to 8 MHz) is adequate. Some ultrasound systems offer a small phase array scanhead that allows better visualization of the subclavian and innominate arteries in the region of the clavicle.

EXAMINATION PROTOCOL

No preparation is required of the patient. The initial assessment is done with the patient supine. Allow the patient to rest for 5 minutes to allow the blood pressures to stabilize.

A systolic pressure measurement is taken from the upper arm (brachial artery) and at the wrist (radial and ulnar arteries). Normally, there is not a recordable gradient between any of these sites. These data provide information concerning the large and medium-sized arteries and their contribution to the level of the wrist. In addi-

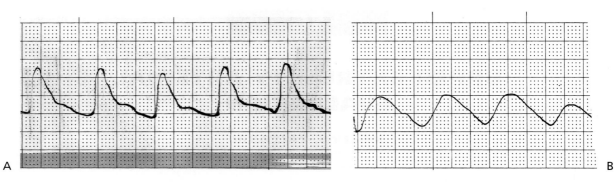

FIGURE 16.1. A: Normal digit pulse waveform. **B:** Pulse waveform with arterial obstruction at some site proximal to the recording site.

tion, by using the CW Doppler, it is possible to assess the characteristics of the velocity signals from any of the sites. If the patient is being evaluated for cold sensitivity or vasculitis, it will be necessary to include measurements of the digit systolic pressure.

The systolic pressures at the digit level are evaluated using a PPG (AC coupled) and a strip chart recorder. One advantage of the PPG is that it is possible to record the volume pulses from the tips of the digits, which may also be useful in documenting obstruction within the digit arteries themselves. The photocell is attached to the finger pad of the digit with double-sided tape. A digit volume pulse tracing is recorded at high speed to evaluate the shape of the waveform. An abnormal waveform will have a rounded peak, as opposed to the normal notched peak (Fig. 16.1). A digit blood pressure cuff is placed around the digit, avoiding the bony structure of the joint. At reduced chart recorder speed, the pulsations are recorded while the blood pressure cuff is inflated. When digit pulsations are obliterated, the cuff is slowly deflated until the pulsation returns. The pressure reading at this point is recorded as illustrated in Fig. 16.2. If the digit pressures are normal and the digit pulse waveforms are normal in contour, this study will be

reported as normal. This also confirms patency of major vessels proximal to the digits because a proximal obstruction would produce reduced digit pressures and abnormal waveforms from all digits.

If a pressure gradient is noted between arms (right to left) or from level to level (above elbow to below elbow), it is necessary to proceed with a duplex scan to identify sites of involvement.

The following arteries are easily assessed by duplex scanning:

- Innominate
- Subclavian
- Axillary
- Brachial
- Radial
- Ulnar

Although the innominate and subclavian arteries should be assessed by duplex scanning, those outside the thorax can be easily assessed by CW Doppler, B-mode imaging, pulsed Doppler, and color Doppler. The criteria we use for upper extremity arterial testing are listed next, followed by examples in Fig. 16.3:

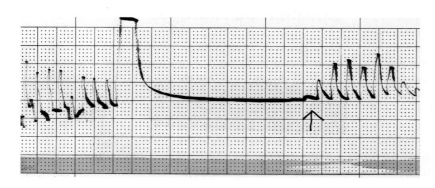

FIGURE 16.2. The digit systolic pressure is recorded at the onset of pulsations after deflating the blood pressure cuff.

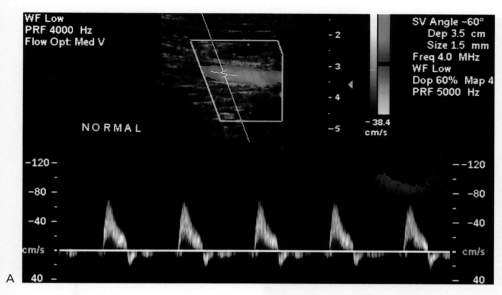

A

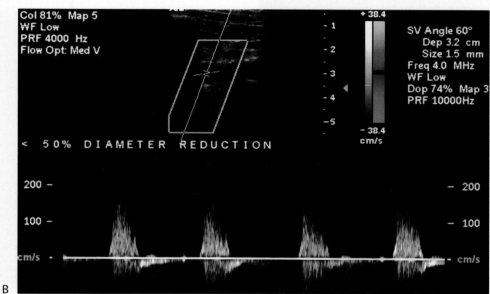

B

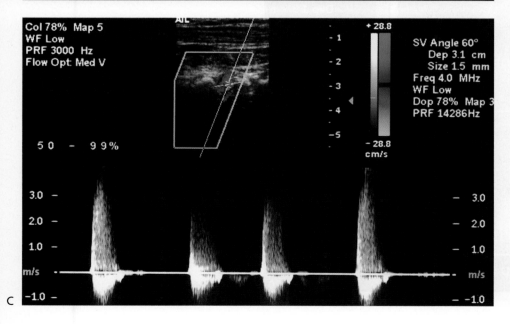

C

FIGURE 16.3. A–F: Examples of the categories of disease as diagnosed by velocity waveform for the upper extremity arteries. *(Continued on next page)*

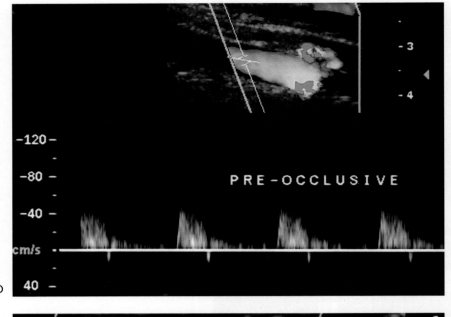

PRE-OCCLUSIVE

D

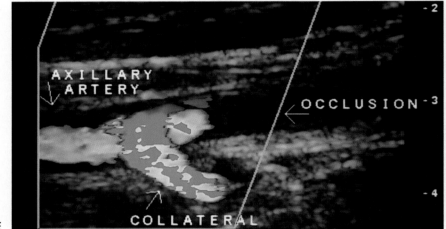

AXILLARY ARTERY

OCCLUSION

COLLATERAL

E

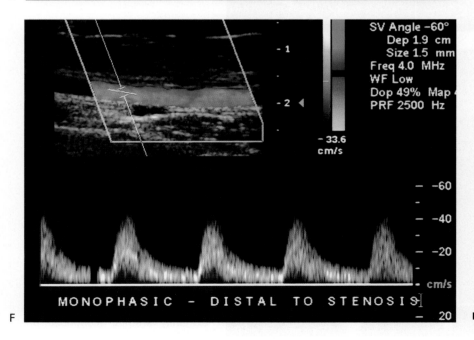

SV Angle −60°
Dep 1.9 cm
Size 1.5 mm
Freq 4.0 MHz
WF Low
Dop 49% Map
PRF 2500 Hz

− 33.6 cm/s

MONOPHASIC − DISTAL TO STENOSIS

F

FIGURE 16.3. *(Continued)*

DIAGNOSTIC VELOCITY WAVEFORM CRITERIA

- *Normal*: uniform waveforms; biphasic or triphasic waveforms; clear window beneath systolic peak
- *Less than 50% diameter reduction*: focal velocity increase; spectral broadening; possibly triphasic or biphasic flow
- *More than 50% diameter reduction*: focal velocity increase; loss of triphasic or biphasic velocity waveform; poststenotic flow (color bruit)
- *Occlusion*: no flow detected

If the subclavian, axillary, radial, and ulnar arteries are normal and the digit pressure is abnormal, it can be assumed that either the palmar or digit arteries are obstructed. It is not possible to image the digit arteries with currently available equipment. A worksheet describing normal and abnormal findings is included in Section IV.

THORACIC OUTLET TESTING

For this assessment, obstruction of the subclavian artery is ruled out by the pressure measurements described previously. If there is no evidence of a hemodynamically significant lesion of the subclavian artery, we proceed to the maneuvers that document the status of the subclavian artery when the

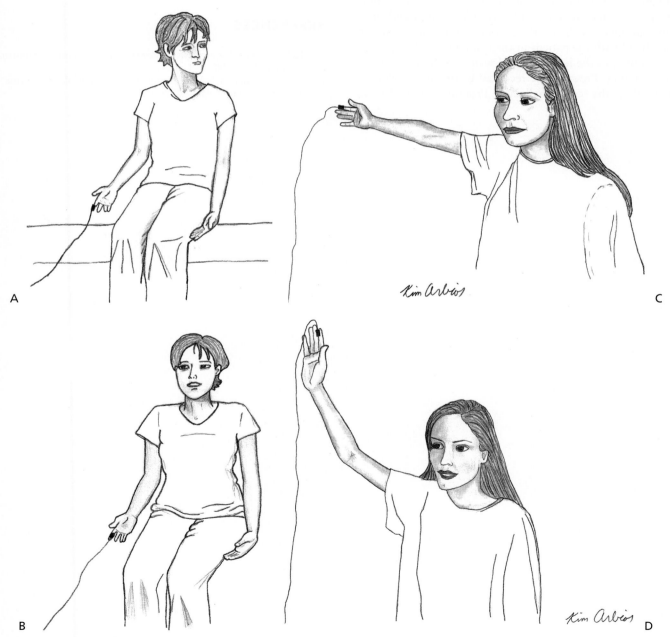

FIGURE 16.4. A–D: The different positions used to produce compression of the subclavian artery during the thoracic outlet test procedure.

arm is placed in different positions. The PPG is placed on a digit (as described earlier) to obtain a digit pulse waveform on the strip chart recorder. We then have the patient assume the position that causes pain so that we can test the effects of that position on the digit pulsations. If the digit pulses disappear, this signifies that at least in that position, the subclavian artery is temporarily occluded. A variety of positions have been suggested and used for this purpose. These positions are shown in Fig. 16.4. A worksheet indicating normal and abnormal findings is included in Section IV.

COLD-SENSITIVITY TESTING

Proximal obstruction must first be ruled out with the resting pressure measurements (2). Sample tracings and pressures are taken with the PPG from at least two digits on each hand with the patient in the resting state. The patient then immerses the hands in cold water (10 to 12°C) for 3 to 5 minutes. Pressures are recorded in the digits immediately after the cold challenge. Pressures often fall to unrecordable levels in patients with true cold sensitivity. A worksheet describing normal and abnormal findings is included in Section IV.

The interpretation of the results of this testing sequence is important. If the patient has normal digit pressures and waveforms at room temperature but these pressures decrease with cold exposure, this patient has primary Raynaud's disease, which is a benign disorder. If, on the other hand, abnormal digit pressures and waveforms are noted at rest, we suspect an underlying disorder, such as scleroderma, which results in occlusions of the digital and palmar arteries. These patients also have a drop in their digit pressures with cooling of the hand. Worksheets illustrating a normal and abnormal examination follow in Section IV.

REFERENCES

1. Machleder H. Vaso-occlusive disorders of the upper extremity. *Curr Probl Surg* 1988;25:1–67.
2. Neilsen SL, Lassen NA. Measurement of digital blood pressure after local cooling. *J Appl Physiol* 1977;43:907–910.

## 17

DETECTION AND TREATMENT OF IATROGENIC FALSE ANEURYSMS AND ARTERIOVENOUS FISTULAS WITH DUPLEX ULTRASOUND

WATSON B. SMITH

"Color duplex ultrasound (CDU) has emerged as the method choice for initial evaluation of iatrogenic vascular injury. These injuries usually result from puncture during invasive procedures including angiography, cardiac catheterization and catheter placement for intravascular monitoring and access" (1). Complication rates of 1% to 9% are reported in the literature, of which 64% are pseudoaneurysms, 15% are arteriovenous fistulas (AVFs), 11% are hemorrhage, and less than 1% lead to thrombosis or dissection. The femoral artery is the most common arterial access for these procedures and the most common site of injury. Less common sites are the axillary, brachial, radial, and carotid arteries.

PSEUDOANEURYSMS

CDU can readily distinguish pseudoaneurysms from other pulsatile masses in the groin. A pseudoaneurysm is connected to the artery by a "neck," or tract, through which there is the characteristic "to-and-fro" flow pattern. The mass has radial pulsation on B-mode image, with detectable flow within the mass (2) (Fig. 17.1).

ARTERIOVENOUS FISTULAS

AVFs occur when both the artery and the adjacent vein have been injured, resulting in a channel, which allows the high-pressure arterial blood to flow into the low-pressure venous system. This may occur with or without a concurrent pseudoaneurysm. AVFs are identified by the high-velocity, low-pulsatility arterial waveform in supplying vessels proximal to the AVF, the turbulent and pulsatile venous Doppler pattern, and a prominent color flow spectral Doppler bruit. A communicating channel can sometimes be visualized

between the vessels on B-mode or color flow image. Doppler waveforms in the opening itself have a characteristic high-velocity, low-pulsatility flow pattern (Fig. 17.2).

PITFALLS IN DUPLEX DIAGNOSIS

Hyperemic lymph nodes can sometimes be mistaken for pseudoaneurysms or AVFs, but they do not have the characteristic to-and-fro or high-velocity, low-pulsatility waveform characteristic of pseudoaneurysms or AVFs. They tend to have normal arterial and venous Doppler flow patterns. On B-mode image, lymph nodes usually have a parenchyma and/or hilum, much like a miniature kidney. The inferior epigastric artery, which branches from the proximal common femoral artery and courses superiorly toward the abdominal musculature, should not be mistaken for vascularized a needle tract. It will also have normal arterial and venous Doppler waveforms. True aneurysms are usually easy to differentiate from pseudoaneurysms because the vessel's course, walls, and lumen can usually be seen on color flow and B-mode images. True aneurysms often have a low-velocity Doppler waveform with a reversed flow component similar to those of a carotid bulb. Other masses, such as abscess and hematoma, do not have detectable Doppler flow and do not have radial pulsation on B-mode image or a communicating neck.

MANAGEMENT

Prevention is the best cure. The greatest risk associated with pseudoaneurysms is too short a period of manual compression regardless of the procedure performed.

A strong argument could be made for a *conservative approach* to asymptomatic pseudoaneurysms. The natural

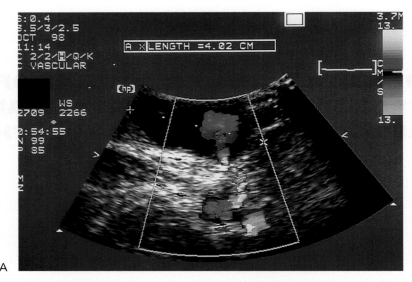

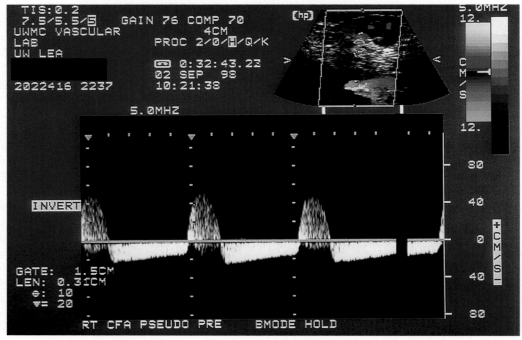

FIGURE 17.1. A: A typical pseudoaneurysm of the common femoral artery. **B:** The characteristic "to-and-fro" Doppler flow pattern that is seen in the communicating "neck."

history of iatrogenic, as opposed to traumatic, pseudoaneurysms is considered to be benign, and many may spontaneously thrombose. Studies have shown that as many as 89% of untreated pseudoaneurysms resolve in 5 to 90 days (3). However, no Duplex criteria have been shown clearly to be useful in predicting which pseudoaneurysms will resolve without treatment. There is general consensus in the literature that very large or expanding pseudoaneurysms, especially in patients who require ongoing anticoagulation, should be treated. For symptomatic pseudoaneurysms, *Duplex-guided compression therapy* or *thrombin injection* can

be safely done. Atypical or deep pseudoaneurysm configurations or pseudoaneurysms that have not responded to compression therapy or thrombin injection may require *surgical repair*.

The natural history of AVFs is largely unknown. Duplex velocities have not been shown to predict resolution.

Duplex-Guided Compression Therapy

Duplex-guided compression therapy has proved effective for treating pseudoaneurysms. During the 1990s, this

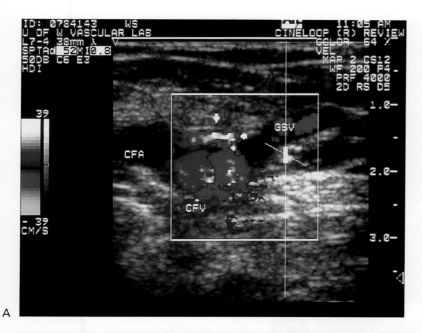

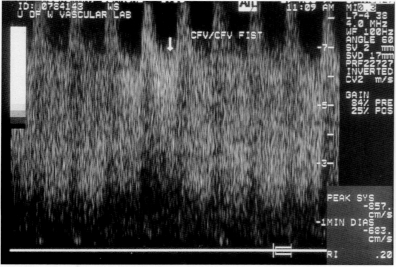

FIGURE 17.2. A: A common femoral arteriovenous fistula. **B:** A typical high-velocity, low-pulsatility Doppler waveform is present in a fistula.

method alone was the initial treatment of choice for pseudoaneurysms (4). However, there are several disadvantages to this technique, including patient and technologist discomfort and long procedure times. It is more difficult with atypical or incompressible pseudoaneurysms and when patients need to remain anticoagulated. Absolute contraindications are skin necrosis and signs of local infection.

Some cases in the literature have reported success in treating AVFs with compression, but in our experience, this has not been successful.

Duplex-Guided Thrombin Injection

More recently, Duplex-guided thrombin injection has been shown to be safe and effective (5–7). Several methods of

thrombin injection have been reported in the literature (7). Thrombin injection with a 21-gauge needle is most commonly used in conjunction with saline injection to visualize the tip of the needle; however, scoring the needle or injecting a small amount of thrombin from the needle tip may also aid in visualization (Fig. 17.3). Variations in the technique include thrombin dose, single or double syringes, and monitoring of the patient. Patients typically receive 500 to 1,000 units of bovine thrombin after the echogenic needle is visualized within the cavity. Most injections occur in a monitored setting, and at least two personnel are present to allow simultaneous visualization and injection of the pseudoaneurysm. There are several potential benefits of this technique. The rapid thrombosis of the pseudoaneurysm is better tolerated by the patient than the often long and painful compression

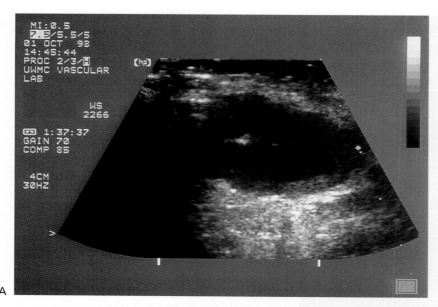

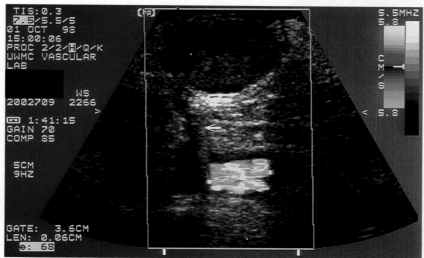

FIGURE 17.3. A: The tip of the needle within the pseudoaneurysm is shown before injection of the thrombin. **B:** The thrombosed pseudoaneurysm after thrombin injection.

times associated with compression therapy. It also avoids technologist muscular discomfort and prolonged use of ultrasound equipment. In addition, success rates may be superior to compression, decreasing the need for repeated study, treatment, or surgical intervention. Contraindications are similar to those for compression therapy, and pseudoaneurysms with skin necrosis or signs of local infection are best treated surgically. Compression and thrombin injection are not recommended for pseudoaneurysms associated with bypass grafts because there is likely to be an underlying defect in the graft that will require surgical repair.

REFERENCES

1. Berdejo G, Wengerter KR, Marin M, et al. Color flow duplex-guided manual occlusion of iatrogenic arteriovenous fistulas. *J Vasc Tech* 1995;19(2):79–83.

2. Carroll CA. Pulsatile groin masses in the postcatheterization patient. In: *RSNA Special Course in Ultrasound.* Department of Radiology, Duke University Medical Center, Durham, NC, 1996: 107–115.

3. Samuels D, Orron DE, Kessler A, et al. Femoral artery pseudoaneurysm: Doppler sonographic features predictive for spontaneous thrombosis. *J Clin Ultrasound* 1997;25 (9):497–500.

4. Hood DB, Mattos MA, Douglas MG, et al. Determinants of success of color-flow duplex-guided compression repair of femoral pseudoaneurysms. *Surgery* 1996;120(4):585–590.

5. Liau CS, Ho FM, Chen MF, et al. Treatment of iatrogenic femoral artery pseudoaneurysms with percutaneous thrombin injection. *J Vasc Surg* 1997;26(1):18–23.

6. Kang SS, Labropoulos N, Mansour MA, et al. Percutaneous ultrasound guided thrombin injection: a new method for treating postcatheterization femoral pseudoaneurysms. *J Vasc Surg* 1998;27(6): 1032–1038.

7. Kang SS, Labropoulos N, Mansour MA, et al. Expanded indications for ultrasound-guided thrombin injection of pseudoaneurysms. *J Vasc Surg* 2000;31(2):289–298.

## 18

VEIN GRAFT SURVEILLANCE

JEAN F. PRIMOZICH

Saphenous vein grafts are the most commonly used and durable conduits for bypassing areas of occlusion in the arteries of the lower limb. They have a better long-term patency rate and can be repaired if new lesions develop that threaten their patency. One of the remarkable developments in promoting long-term patency of vein grafts was the realization that if followed closely, particularly in the first year after implantation, the secondary patency rates could be kept in the range of 90% at 3 years (1–9). It also became clear that the most common problem that threatened the long-term patency of these grafts was myointimal proliferation. This process tended to develop early—within the first few months—and could be detected by its effect on velocity patterns within the grafts themselves.

The progress in using duplex as a monitor of change now appears to be well accepted. However, there are some aspects of the scanning procedure and its interpretation that need to be emphasized because progress continues to occur. For example, the role of the residual venous valve as a problem has been overemphasized (10).

The manner in which the scanning should be done and its interpretation are the subject of this section.

EQUIPMENT NEEDED

Lower extremity saphenous vein bypass grafts will be found at a range of depths. The depth of the bypass will depend on the type of graft, that is, *in situ* vein bypass or reversed saphenous vein (RSV) bypass, and the location of the anastomoses. Therefore, a range of transducer frequencies is necessary to scan the various types of grafts. A 5- to 7.5-MHz transducer will be the most commonly used scanhead for most of the femoral to popliteal RSV bypass grafts. The proximal portion of the graft will be relatively shallow in the groin and become fairly deep more distally because it is usually tunneled beneath the sartorius muscle in the thigh and then deep behind the knee to anastomose to the popliteal artery. If the leg is large, the distal thigh region of the graft may require a lower-frequency transducer to follow the graft course deep to the muscle. An *in situ* vein bypass, by

definition, is shallow throughout most of its length and can be scanned using a higher-frequency transducer, such as 7.5 to 12 MHz. The transducers that are designed for intraoperative use work well for most of the length of the *in situ* vein bypasses and yield excellent images because of superior near-field resolution.

Linear array transducer technology provides the best images for most vein grafts. A phased array transducer with 3- to 5-MHz frequency may be necessary if inflow disease is suspected in the abdomen and can be used for reversed saphenous vein grafts in the thigh if the leg is exceptionally large and the graft is deep.

The routine equipment also includes a continuous wave "pocket" Doppler with a 10-MHz transducer, a sphygmomanometer, and blood pressure cuffs with widths for both arm and ankle sizes, which are necessary for taking routine pressures used for ankle/arm indices. The typical items of transmission gel and towels, tissues, or wash clothes will also be necessary. Additionally, a tape measure and an indelible marking pen are helpful for identifying and marking pertinent graft features that will be tracked over time in subsequent studies.

PATIENT PREPARATION

The patients with vein grafts have most likely been seen in the vascular laboratory before operation for a baseline lower extremity duplex examination and are familiar with the typical lead in explanations of the safety, ease, and harmless nature of ultrasound. Because this is a surveillance examination, only the involved leg will be scanned, and the time to do the study will be decreased compared with the original full lower extremity examination. A short interview concerning new symptoms begins the examination and is helpful for interpretation of the results.

Bilateral brachial and ankle pressures are taken using a continuous-wave Doppler at each visit to follow the physiologic affects of the graft progress and to identify intervening progression of disease in the inflow and outflow vessels. A blood pressure is taken using both the posterior tibial and the dorsalis pedis arteries in the foot. In addition, a peroneal artery pressure is taken specifically if it is the single outflow of the vein graft or if the posterior tibial or dorsalis pedis artery pressures are abnormal, that is, lower than the arm pressure. An ankle/brachial index (ABI) is calculated using the highest of the two brachial pressures and the highest of the three tibial artery pressures. It is critical to take both brachial artery pressures because an occult subclavian stenosis may cause an abnormally low pressure, and this in turn will falsely elevate the ABI, which can be deceiving in the interpretation. Close attention should be paid to the brachial Doppler signals, specifically listening for differences from side to side or abnormal bilateral signals, which may indicate bilateral subclavian stenosis. In the presence of bilateral subclavian stenosis, an ABI would be in error and misleading.

Before studying the patient, a copy of the operative report or a verbal communication about the surgical procedure can prepare the technologist for how extensive an examination is required and about areas of particular importance to the examination.

PATIENT POSITIONING

The patient is studied supine, comfortably resting with pillows for the head. The position of the leg will vary slightly depending on the type of graft, that is, *in situ* or RSV, and the location of the anastomoses. An *in situ* bypass will be superficial and easily visualized for the most part as it follows the course of the saphenous vein along the medial aspect of the leg. Therefore, the scan will begin with the leg straight for the assessment of the inflow and the proximal anastomosis in the groin. The leg is then rotated out with the knee slightly bent and resting on a support, such as a rolled-up towel. The entire graft can be scanned from this position.

If the distal anastomosis is to the anterior tibial artery on the lateral side of the leg, the leg can be rotated back to the straight position or turned to the opposite side. A typical femoral-to-popliteal reversed saphenous vein graft may require more manipulation of the leg to access the entire graft because of the deep tunneling below the muscle in the distal thigh. Initially, similar to an *in situ* vein bypass, the leg is straight to scan the inflow and the proximal anastomosis in the groin. As the scan follows the graft down the thigh, the leg may need to be rotated outward, bending the knee slightly, to follow the deeper portion in the distal thigh to the anastomosis.

If the distal anastomosis is below the knee, there are several position options that work depending on the depth of the graft and the angle of the anastomosis. The distal graft may be followed entirely, with the scanhead approaching from the medial aspect of the leg and with the leg bent and resting on a support. Another option is to rotate the leg

back to the straight position with the knee bent and then scan from behind the knee following the natural course of the vessels. Finally, rolling the patient to the opposite side, with the legs slightly bent, or rolling the patient prone and scanning from the back of the knee will access the distal anastomosis. Some grafts may require some creativity to access them throughout their length. Every attempt should be made to see the complete length of the graft by whatever method that works. Do not be afraid to move, rotate, or bend the leg to a different position if the viewing window becomes obscured and the graft cannot be visualized.

GRAFT TYPES AND REVISION PROCEDURES

The type of graft placed relies on several important factors, the most critical being the extent and location of the arterial disease, as well as the condition and availability of the autologous vein. Before the duplex scan of graft, it is good practice to have a copy of the operative report that describes the surgery in detail, including the exact location of the anastomoses, the type of graft, and any intraoperative revisions or procedures. The surgical details, sometimes quite complex, facilitate the duplex scan and the interpretation of the results. In the absence of the operation notes, a verbal description of the critical details by the surgeon can be helpful. Each graft type and revision has specific characteristic, duplex findings that are unique. Understanding the procedures and anticipating the findings improves the results of the duplex scans.

The two most common procedures, both using autogenous vein, are the RSV graft and the *in situ* saphenous vein bypass (1–3). The saphenous vein may also be used in a nonreversed manner, that is, the transposed vein bypass graft. Each of these procedures has unique characteristics associated with it that require attention and that will affect the interpretation of the results. Alternative veins, including upper extremity cephalic or basilic veins, may be used if the saphenous veins are inadequate. The arm veins may be used independently or as a portion of a composite graft along with portions of saphenous vein or other arm vein. They are joined using an end-to-end anastomosis to create adequate length for the bypass.

In Situ Saphenous Vein Bypass

The *in situ* saphenous vein bypass uses the greater saphenous vein as it lies in its normal location in the leg. Because the valves will be directed opposite to the direction of the arterial flow, the leaflets are disrupted or cut using a valvulotome. The branches are ligated or tied off to prevent arteriovenous fistulas (AVFs). Leaving the vein in place allows the large end to be anastomosed to the large portion of the artery and the small end to the smaller distal artery (Figs. 18.1 and 18.2). Similarity of vessel size at the anastomoses

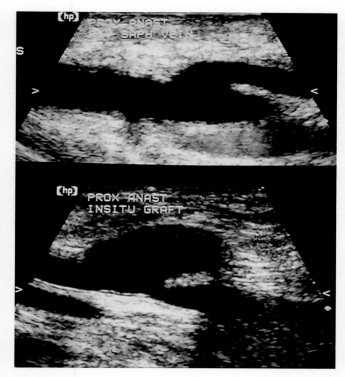

FIGURE 18.1. Proximal anastomoses of an *in situ* vein **(bottom)** and a reversed saphenous vein (RSV) **(top)** bypass. There is a similarity in the size of the *in situ* vein and the native artery compared with the size mismatch of the RSV bypass relative to the native artery.

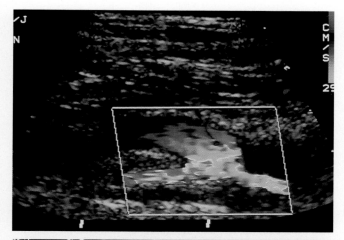

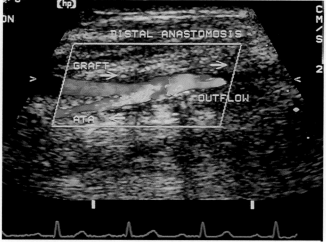

FIGURE 18.2. Color Doppler images of the distal anastomosis of a reversed saphenous vein bypass graft **(top)** and an *in situ* vein bypass **(bottom)**.

is an obvious advantage of this type of graft procedure in that the amount of flow disturbance is decreased. A disadvantage of the *in situ* vein bypass is that each disrupted valve site is a potential location for stenosis as a result of wall injury and the growth of intimal hyperplasia. In addition, a nondisrupted valve becomes a restriction to flow and threatens the graft patency almost immediately. An AVF can eventually lead to decreased flow in the graft and may need to be repaired. An intraoperative duplex scan may illuminate most of the technical problems immediately, and intraoperative repair may decrease the potential for future problems.

The largest part of an *in situ* vein bypass is easily visualized with ultrasound because of its mostly superficial location. Details of the vein walls are generally seen with more clarity than reversed saphenous vein grafts. The dilated valve sinuses are conspicuous and do not appear to "disappear" over time, as in the RSV bypass. The normal flow velocity in the graft tends to be lower in the proximal portion and increases more distally as a result of the typical anatomic decrease in vein size.

Reversed Saphenous Vein Bypass Graft

In this procedure, the saphenous vein is excised from the leg, branches are tied, and the vessel is reversed and placed

in the leg; the smaller end of the vein being more proximal and the larger end of the vein as the distal graft (Figs. 18.1 and 18.2). The valves are now lying in the same direction as the arterial flow and do not require disruption. Hence, no mechanical injury occurs to the walls, as compared with the *in situ* vein bypass. As a result of the increase in flow velocity in the arterialized vein bypass, it is expected that the valve leaflets are forced against the wall and subsequently become contiguous with it. The valve sinuses are often more evident in the images of the *in situ* vein bypass as compared with RSV bypasses. In the RSV bypass, the sinuses appear to be filled in, perhaps with the leaflets, and therefore not as obvious. In addition to becoming a part of the vein wall, the valve leaflets may "freeze" in the lumen, at times creating a stenosis. In some cases, the valves may appear functional, creating an increased velocity or flow disturbances detected with the pulsed Doppler (10). Valve sinuses are important areas on which to focus attention when doing a duplex scan of a vein graft.

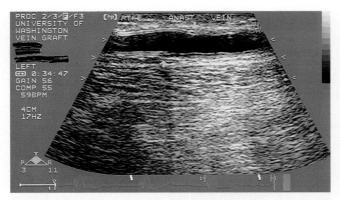

FIGURE 18.3. End-to-end anastomosis of an interposition PTFE graft and a vein graft. Note the bright double-line appearance of the PTFE on the *left* and the thickened vein wall on the *right* of the image represented by a single bright interface.

Most infrainguinal bypasses use autogenous vein. However, prosthetic grafts can also be used and are easily distinguished from native vein tissue and from each other by their unique, characteristic ultrasonic image patterns. PTFE has a typical bright double-line appearance in the ultrasound image (Fig. 18.3) whereas Dacron appears as a single, thick, bright interface (Fig. 18.4). A corrugated or rippled wall appearance may be noted if ringed material is used. The characteristic ultrasonic appearance of the prosthetic material is easily identified in patch revisions and is distinguished from vein patches that resemble the typical vein wall (Fig. 18.3).

Graft revisions are necessary in about one third of vein bypasses. An appreciation of the kind of revision, the location, and the material used for the repair is critical for complete and appropriate duplex surveillance. Some graft revisions, as a result of complicated anatomic and hemodynamic circumstances, can be quite creative and complex and difficult to sort out ultrasonically. Most graft repairs are straightforward, involving either patch angioplasty with or without excision of the lesion, extension or "jump" graft repair, or

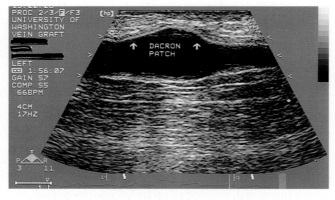

FIGURE 18.4. A Dacron patch angioplasty at the proximal end of a reversed saphenous vein bypass. The Dacron is distinguished by the uniformly thick bright interface. There is thickening of the deeper vein wall.

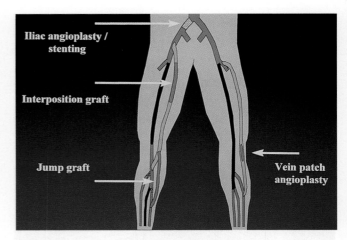

FIGURE 18.5. This drawing depicts the various kinds of graft revisions. The graft on the *left* represents a common femoral artery to distal popliteal artery bypass, with a proximal interposition graft repair and a distal extension or "jump" graft to the posterior tibial artery. The bypass on the right represents a profunda femoris artery to anterior tibial artery (ATA) bypass graft with a patch angioplasty repair of the mid-graft. Patch angioplasty repair is common at the anastomoses. An angioplasty, stent repair, bypass, or endarterectomy may be done in the inflow vessels.

interposition graft. New anastomotic sites and patch repairs become potential areas for intimal hyperplasia. An appreciation of the surgical technique helps to anticipate potentially confusing ultrasound findings, to locate areas requiring more intense study, and to interpret the final duplex results (Fig. 18.5).

SCANNING SEQUENCE

The graft is scanned in the longitudinal view to obtain the velocity spectral waveforms, which will be used to classify the amount of narrowing. Selective use of transverse views is extremely helpful to identify changes in dimension, intimal hyperplasia, valve leaflets and features, wall thickening, and/or directional changes. The scan should be dynamic, and the use of multiple views is encouraged in an attempt to sort out difficult situations. One critical area where the use of multiple views is encouraged is at the site of valve sinuses, especially in RSV grafts. In RSV grafts, both leaflets remain intact. In theory, the leaflets will be lying in the direction of the flow and are forced against the wall with the high arterial pressure and will not be visualized. In practice, the leaflets provide a challenge because they can be seen in many stages, such as frozen at various locations within the lumen, moving in the flow stream, or continuing to "function" with the pulsatility of the arterial flow (10). Anatomically, the leaflets do not lie parallel to the wall of the vein graft but extend out from the wall at angles and from two different directions as seen by the scanhead (Fig. 18.6). The viewing direction should be changed at suspected sinuses to

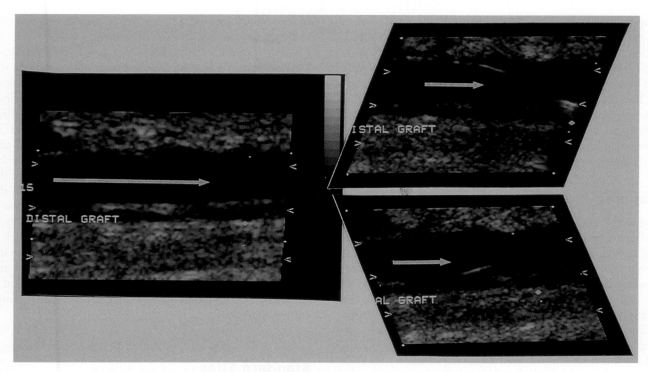

FIGURE 18.6. The image on the **left** shows the vein graft, with the image beams steered perpendicular to the walls, and the angled leaflets are not visible. At **top right**, the ultrasound image is steered to the left; at **bottom right**, the image is steered to the right, intersecting the surface of the leaflets at a perpendicular angle.

image more clearly each of the leaflets if they are present and especially if there is disturbance or increased velocity that is unaccounted for. An ultrasound scanner that allows the operator to steer the image beam independently while holding the scanhead motionless is ideal for assessing these valve features.

Color Doppler and color power imaging are useful tools to follow the course of the vein graft, especially as the graft dives deep under the muscle in the distal thigh. Changes in the color pattern should direct attention to an area that requires more in-depth investigation with the pulsed Doppler and the B-mode image. Color power, although not a necessity in the scan, is especially useful in defining the luminal dimensions in areas of narrowing or complex geometry. However, similar to color Doppler, color power is subject to "overgain" or "undergain," leading to false impressions of the lumen, walls, and valve leaflets. Color Doppler appears to obscure surfaces more than power imaging, yet color Doppler demonstrates flow dynamics and directional changes more obviously than power Doppler. For example, the typical color changes significant with flow separation can define an anastomosis when it is not obvious on the B-mode image or power image. In addition, both color Doppler and power Doppler are helpful in pinpointing small AVFs in *in situ* vein bypasses and the proximal outflow vessel with retrograde flow, which is a good marker of the distal anastomosis (Fig. 18.2, *lower image*). It is clear

that using a combination of the imaging modalities is necessary throughout the scan to define the subtle, yet important, features of the graft.

As with any duplex scan, the sample volume is swept through the vessels to identify subtle flow changes that are not obvious in the color display. Clearly, it is unnecessary to sample at every site along the length of the graft if the color is demonstrating the typical red-blue-red color characteristic of a triphasic flow pattern throughout. Conversely, distinct color changes, other than the normally expected triphasic pattern, demand further investigation with the pulsed Doppler sample volume to identify the source. Pulsed Doppler is used to obtain velocity waveforms at a standard angle of 60 degrees from sites along the graft, which define the representative flow changes. Velocity waveforms from areas of disturbance and stenosis are recorded, along with a reference signal in the normal graft segment preceding the stenotic site. The velocity ratio, by which stenosis is defined, is calculated from these two values.

Pertinent graft features necessary for sequential follow-up studies include anything that ultimately may affect the flow patterns or be responsible for stenosis. Valve features of interest include the presence of a sinus, leaflets, remnants of leaflets, or the mobility of the leaflets. Comments about the character of the wall, whether it is smooth, irregular, calcified, or thick, may be important at future studies if problems should develop at the site. Diameter changes in the vein graft will create expected changes in the velocity that are easily misinterpreted if not accompanied with an explanation. Alterations in graft geometry at anastomoses or revisions have distinct velocity changes and disturbances that can be attributed to directional changes rather than stenosis. Because the graft will be studied serially, the features and flow characteristics will be assessed for changes over time as well as on a one-visit basis. Prior knowledge of expected changes in the graft flow helps to make the appropriate interpretation of the results.

Mapping the Graft

The entire graft is scanned, including the inflow and the outflow vessels. The vein grafts will be of differing lengths and have different anastomotic sites, all of which is dependent on the extent and location of the native arterial disease. In addition, revisions may be done throughout the history of the graft that may change the character and length of the vein graft over time. Therefore, it is impossible to define strictly where exactly each site should be sampled because this will change with every graft. Because each graft is individual, it is invaluable to have a drawing of the leg for each visit in the patient record that shows the graft placement, the anastomoses, and revisions for quick reference. The drawing may also include markers of the locations of the velocity sampling sites, especially areas of stenosis, and other features of interest along the graft, such as valves, diameter changes, and so forth (Fig. 18.7). When doing surveillance studies, it

is important to reference the previous study in order to correlate similarities and characterize change.

Graft features are identified at each visit by the relative location from a known reference point, which may be the proximal end of a scar in the groin. The reference location, or *fiducial*, must be a fixed location that will not change during the surveillance time. Subsequent surgery may affect the fiducial location if the scar is extended or changed, in which case the location would have to be reassigned and documented. The fiducial location is indicated on the leg drawing for reference. During the scan, the locations of the features of interest are marked with an indelible pen on the skin surface. After the scan is complete, a tape measure is laid on the skin along the course of the graft, and each location is measured in reference to the fiducial point, which is point zero. The locations are also recorded on the drawing and used for further surveillance studies. A record of the exact feature locations can be invaluable to the surgeon if the choice is to do a revision of the graft without a preoperative angiogram.

Standard Sites

The vein graft is divided into general sections of investigation (Fig. 18.8), the relative length of which will vary for each individual bypass graft depending on the location of the anastomoses. A minimum of one representative velocity waveform is collected from each specific section. Additional waveforms are collected, and encouraged, within a section, if more pertinent velocity information is deemed important because of complex hemodynamics or multiple areas of stenosis. The combined velocity data create the hemodynamic picture by which the interpretation is made about the status of the graft.

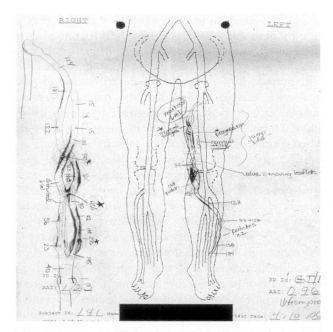

FIGURE 18.7. A sample of a drawing of a vein graft and multiple revisions and details that can be included in the patient chart for quick reference and updated after each study.

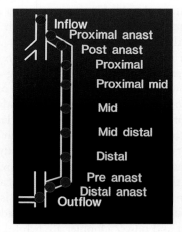

FIGURE 18.8. Representative areas of investigation from which representative velocity waveforms are taken to map the graft hemodynamics. Additional sites are recommended if further documentation is necessary.

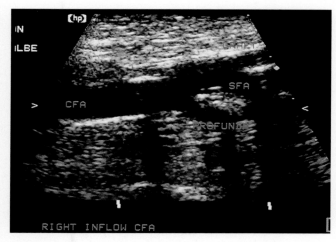

FIGURE 18.9. The graft anastomosis is at the origin of the superficial femoral artery (*SFA*) in this image. The profunda femoris artery is seen deeper to the native SFA.

Inflow

First to be scanned are the inflow vessels. The inflow vessels will vary depending on the placement of the proximal anastomosis. The usual location of the proximal anastomosis is the common femoral artery (CFA) just proximal to the bifurcation of the superficial femoral artery (SFA) and the profunda femoris artery (PFA). Therefore, the CFA and the distal external iliac artery are scanned as the inflow vessels. This general location of the anastomosis is variable, so that proper identification of anatomic landmarks becomes critical (Fig. 18.9). If the graft originates from the SFA at any location, the scan should always include the CFA and the PFA as well as the proximal SFA. The inflow vessels are assessed for progression of native arterial disease that, if

severe enough, could cause the graft to fail as a result of decreased inflow. The presence of plaque or wall changes is noted (Fig. 18.10).

At least one velocity waveform is taken from the inflow vessels to compare with the previous study. If a stenosis is present, the waveforms should represent the hemodynamics through the stenotic area, including prestenotic, stenotic, and poststenotic waveforms. The shape, characteristic flow pattern, and velocity are recorded. A significant decrease in velocity or a change in the waveform shape and flow characteristics may indicate disease progression in the more proximal vessels, and a more extensive study of them may be necessary. The typical waveform in the CFA is multiphasic with a sharp upstroke and reversal in early diastole. Known disease in more proximal vessels may change the waveform shape from normal; however, this finding would be noted at the first visit and would not be expected to change throughout the surveillance time unless there is disease progression. A change from a triphasic to a monophasic signal in the inflow vessels between visits should be noted as a significant change. In addition to inflow disease progression, this change may indicate significant disease development in the graft or outflow vessel and definitely requires intense investigation to search for the cause.

The inflow CFA may be the site of an additional surgical procedure, either at the time of the initial graft placement or later as a revision for progressing disease. Revisions, such as patches, endarterectomy, or angioplasty, alter the appearance of the vessel and require thorough investigation for changes such as restenosis or intimal flaps. The inflow vessel may also be the site of a clamp injury. Stenosis caused by a clamp injury occurs focally, proximal to the anastomosis, and is associated with wall thickening. It may be severe enough to threaten the graft flow.

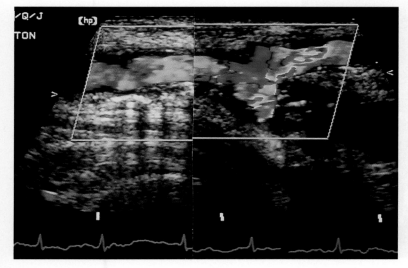

FIGURE 18.10. Proximal anastomosis extending from a moderately diseased common femoral artery. The origins of the superficial femoral artery and the profunda femoris artery can be seen deep to the graft.

Some grafts originate as far down the leg as the distal SFA or the popliteal artery and extend to a tibial artery. In these patients, a quick scan of the vessels from the groin to the proximal anastomosis ensures a complete study of the accessible inflow vessels.

Profunda Femoris Artery

Although the PFA is not the site of the proximal anastomosis in most infrainguinal bypass grafts, it is the major source of flow to the thigh. Documentation of the presence of flow or disease in the PFA is valuable information should the graft fail. The proximal anastomosis can originate from the PFA because of disease in the CFA and the SFA. Knowledge of this before the scan can be extremely helpful in that the anatomy may be confusing without known landmarks, especially if the SFA is occluded. The PFA can be distinguished from the SFA by its depth and direction away from the transducer in the image. In addition, the spectral waveform from the PFA typically has a lower-velocity, earlier-occurring reversal component as a result of the resistance in the thigh.

Proximal Anastomosis

The most common location for the proximal anastomosis is the CFA just proximal to the bifurcation of the SFA and PFA. The anastomosis is usually performed with an end-to-side connection that creates a geometric appearance similar to that of a carotid bifurcation with the dilatation of the carotid bulb (Fig. 18.9). The hood of the vein graft is sutured to an arteriotomy in the side of the CFA. Similar to the carotid bulb, the size of the dilated region and the angle at which the graft extends from the inflow artery can create dramatic, normal flow disturbances that should be anticipated. Similar to

a carotid bifurcation, these complex flow patterns can be difficult to interpret or measure the peak systolic velocity (PSV). The typical flow patterns from an anastomosis can become a signature of the region (Fig. 18.11) and can be used to identify its location. Appreciating the difference between these normal flow disturbances as a result of geometric changes and abnormal flow disturbances associated with stenosis is invaluable in interpreting any arterial examination that uses velocity spectral waveforms. It is meaningless to calculate a velocity ratio in the anastomosis because the PSV measurement is difficult to determine as a result of the flow disturbances and because of the size difference of the vessels. In addition, aligning the Doppler angle to the vessel walls can be questionable and the resultant velocity measurements deceiving. Hence, the amount of diameter reduction or the progression of disease must be determined by focal changes in the flow patterns (e.g., poststenotic turbulence), by a change in the waveform over time, and by an overall change in the graft hemodynamics.

It should be noted that the proximal anastomosis may also originate from the SFA or the PFA using an end-to-end anastomosis, like that used with an interposition graft (Figs. 18.3 and 18.5). In this procedure, the ends of the vein and the artery are connected in an overlapping fashion, creating a more "in-line" connection as compared with the angle of an end-to-side anastomosis. There will be little if any distortion in the flow patterns through the region. There may be a dilated region at the overlap and some angulation changes that will affect the velocity measurements accordingly. Sutures can be seen on both sides of the connection and are a hallmark of this type of procedure, as in an interposition graft.

The anastomoses, both proximal and distal, are primary sites for the development of intimal hyperplasia and stenosis. The dilated portion of the anastomosis may fill in with neointimal growth or laminated clot, similar in location to

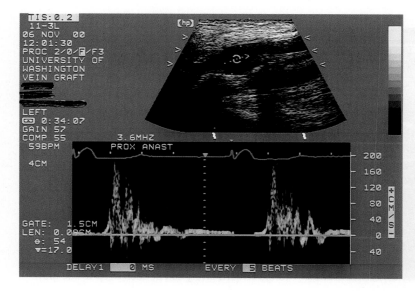

FIGURE 18.11. Spectral waveform from a proximal anastomosis of an interposition PTFE graft segment of an *in situ* vein bypass. Note the markedly disturbed flow characteristics of the spectral waveform as a result of the eddies created by the complex geometry of the area. It is difficult to determine an accurate angle measurement relative to the vessel walls. This fact, in addition to the marked disturbed flow pattern, makes the measurement of peak systolic velocity difficult and potentially misleading.

plaque growth in the carotid bulb. A comment in the report about the appearance of the thickening is important even though the growth may stop and become stable. The flow channel may become more uniform as the dilatation fills in, and as a result, the normal flow disturbances may disappear.

The amount of flow disturbance and the appearance of the anastomosis will be different in a RSV graft than in an *in situ* vein bypass. A RSV graft will have the small end of the vein attached to the large end of the artery. Consequently, there can be a significant size mismatch that, in turn, creates significant flow disturbances. There may be an expected velocity increase in the smaller graft just distal to the anastomosis. Conversely, an *in situ* vein bypass combines the large end of the vein with the large portion of the artery. There is not as much of a size difference; consequently, there may be minimal flow disturbance. The velocity may be low in the proximal end of an *in situ* bypass owing to the large diameter of the conduit.

Sutures are often seen in the anastomosis and can be used to verify its location (Fig. 18.12). They are seen in the image as brightly echogenic, evenly spaced dots or dashes along the wall or crossing the lumen. Sutures may not be seen from every view and are best visualized when the image beams are perpendicular to the surface. Some manipulation of the transducer or image beams may be necessary in order to appreciate them. Identifying sutures can be invaluable when searching for or verifying a revision site or an anastomosis that is not readily apparent.

Postanastomosis Graft Segment

The graft distal to the anastomosis, extending about 4 cm, is an important area for investigation because of neointimal hyperplasia growth extending from the anastomosis. Obvious wall thickening is not uncommon and is easily visualized. Because of the size mismatch in a RSV graft, there may be increased velocity as a result of the smaller conduit that may be difficult to distinguish from hyperplasia. The B-mode image helps to make the distinction. A small-diameter velocity increase will extend for a distance with no post-stenotic turbulence.

An *in situ* vein bypass has the larger end of the vein in this position, and the velocity is usually low as one scans from the proximal anastomosis. Often, there is a large valve sinus, normally occurring in the vein, just distal to the anastomosis. As a result of the dilatation, there is a normal flow disturbance and a decrease in the velocity. It is a good idea to investigate this sinus (and all other sinuses) for the presence of leaflet remnants that may be mobile or causing disturbance. The remnants typically disappear over time as they adhere to the wall.

Body of the Graft

The body of the graft can be considered in five evenly divided regions for examination purposes: proximal, proximal/mid, mid, mid/distal, and distal. (Fig. 18.8) The length of each of these sections depends on the total length of the graft. The arbitrary divisions allow the operator to define a general region of a feature or stenosis clearly, which permits better reproducibility of data and more precise comparison of details at specific sites in serial examinations. Additionally, the tape-measured distance from a reference mark allows for more precise resolution of location within each section.

The body of the graft should be scanned thoroughly with color Doppler and interrogated thoroughly with the pulsed Doppler. At least one representative velocity waveform should be collected along the length from each section and marked with the appropriate location. The PSV pattern differs with the procedure as one scans down the graft. A RSV graft displays higher velocity in the smaller, proximal end of the vein and lower velocity in the distal, larger end. Conversely, an *in situ* vein bypass has lower velocity in the more proximal portion that increases more distally.

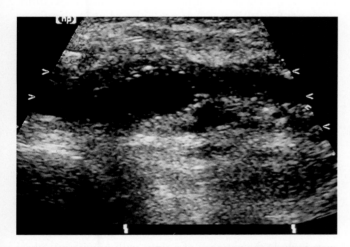

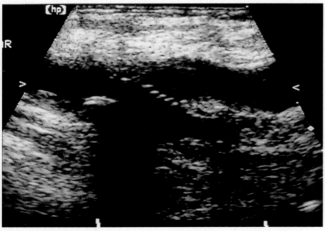

FIGURE 18.12. Sutures can be seen in both of these images of proximal anastomoses as brightly echogenic, evenly spaced dots or dashes.

The B-mode appearance of the graft body should be noted along with the sample velocity recordings. The walls of the graft appear smooth and may develop a double-line appearance over time (Fig. 18.13, *top*). Myointimal hyperplasia is not easily appreciated in the B-mode image in the early stages (Fig. 18.13, *bottom*; Fig. 18.14), owing to the softly echogenic nature of the tissue. As the graft ages, the surface becomes more echogenic and easier to define. In the early stages, it may be detected by the appearance of a color-filling defect that may be accompanied with a stenotic velocity signal.

Other features of the graft are worthy of comment and should be marked for surveillance over time.

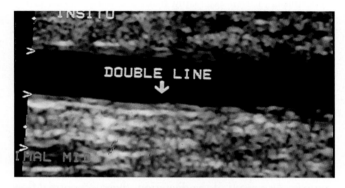

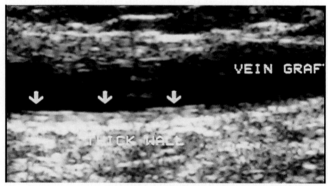

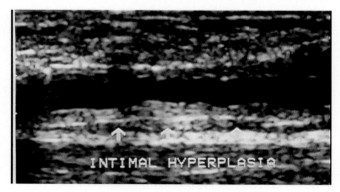

FIGURE 18.13. The **top image** shows the typical smooth, double-line appearance of a normal graft wall, representing the thickening of the intima and the media of the vein wall. The **middle image** shows a thickened vein graft wall with brightly echogenic material obscuring the double-line appearance. The **bottom image** shows a markedly thickened vein wall.

1. Fibrous wall thickening may be present at the first postoperative study because of the condition of the vein before surgery. Thickening of the wall may also develop over the course of the surveillance as result of the normal "arterialization" of the wall. Normally, this process stops within the first year as the vein heals. Calcification, seen as brightly echogenic areas of the wall accompanied by acoustic shadowing, may also be noted at the initial visit or may develop in older grafts.

2. Changes in the diameter of the vein (e.g. varicosities) along the length create interesting velocity patterns down the graft but are not usually detrimental to graft survival. Large changes in diameter are worth noting, if for no other reason than to use as anatomic landmarks along the graft. Thickening of the wall in the dilated areas is not uncommon and is most likely a result of the normal flow disturbances that occur. Rarely does the thickening interfere with the lumen.

3. Twists or kinks in the graft are important to note, in that they may also be associated with functional stenosis and can cause graft failure. Noted for the dramatic directional changes in the color flow or in the velocity spectrum, this graft feature is rare, but not unheard of. A significant twist or kink may need to be revised, commonly with an excision and reanastomosis or interposition graft. Grafts may twist, kink, or become compressed with rotation of the leg, which may not be initially noted in a routine examination. In this situation, the graft velocity either decreases or becomes focally stenotic as the leg is rotated into a specific position (Fig. 18.15) and returns to normal as the leg is moved back to the straight position. This condition is not common but is worth remembering.

4. Valves and valve features are the most common, noteworthy items in vein graft surveillance. Valves and the remnants of them may certainly be the nidus for stenosis either by the leaflets themselves or the growth of intimal hyperplasia as a result of the disturbances and injury. Features of note include the presence of a sinus with or without subsequent thickening, remnants of leaflets in *in situ* vein bypasses, complete leaflets in different arrangements in RSV grafts, and flow disturbances and velocity changes as a result of the presence and mobility of the leaflet or remnant. The presence of an uncut valve in an *in situ* vein bypass is a condition that should be identified immediately after placement. An uncut valve requires repair because it may create a major restriction to the flow in the graft (see Valves in Vein Grafts).

5. Separate from the vein graft, it is worth noting any fluid collection seen in the vicinity of the graft. Hematoma, seroma, and edema are easily seen on the B-mode image and are not uncommon to see in the first several months after the graft placement. Hematoma and seroma are seen as well-defined structures, either anechoic or softly echogenic, often with septations that may develop over time. They usually disappear over time as the fluid is reab-

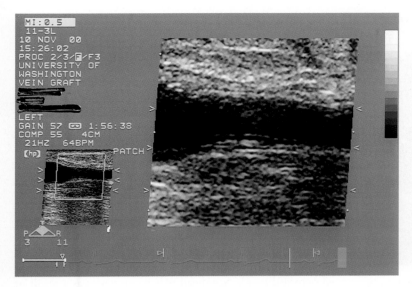

FIGURE 18.14. The thin echogenic interface of early intimal hyperplasia can be seen on the far wall covering an even brighter area of thickening distal to a vein patch.

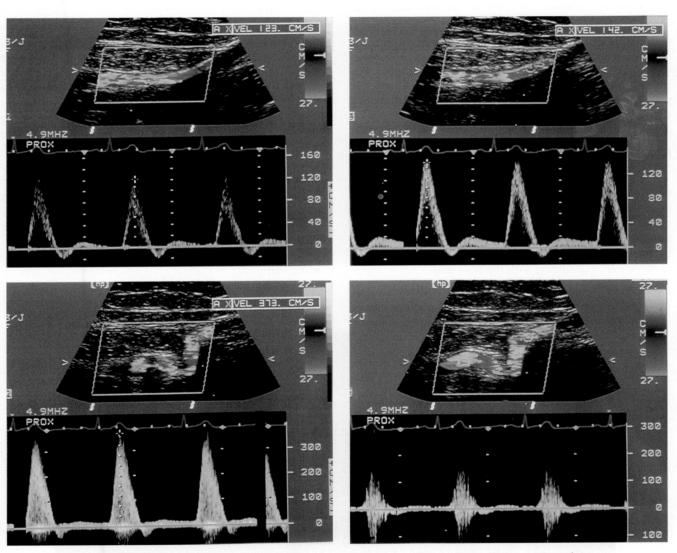

FIGURE 18.15. The images on the top represent the mid-portion of a reversed saphenous vein graft with the leg straight. The **top** waveforms represent normal velocity and waveforms from this region of the graft. The **bottom** images have been taken from the same location in the graft after the leg has rotated outward. The images show a marked kink in the graft, and the waveforms demonstrate elevated velocity **(bottom left)** with poststenotic turbulence **(bottom right)**.

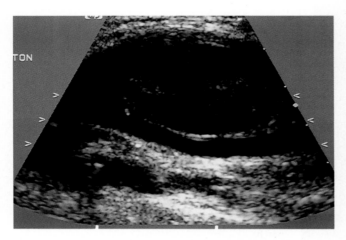

FIGURE 18.16. A large hematoma in the groin region following a proximal graft revision. The graft can be seen deep to the hematoma.

sorbed. Noting the size and location relative to the graft at each visit is important. A seroma (i.e., a serous fluid-filled structure) may linger or become larger over time and may need to be drained (Fig. 18.16).

Pre–Distal Anastomosis

The segment of the graft proximal to the distal anastomosis (about 4 cm) is similar to the region of the graft distal to the proximal anastomosis in that it is the site of potential neointimal growth that may threaten the graft. Therefore, thorough investigation is critical. The velocity is usually higher in *in situ* vein bypasses because of the small caliber of the vessel as compared with the RSV graft.

Distal Anastomosis

Most infrainguinal vein bypasses originate from the femoral artery and end either at the above-knee (AK) or below-knee (BK) popliteal artery. The distal anastomosis is notoriously more difficult to locate, especially in the BK location, than the proximal anastomosis because of the position and depth. Some grafts extend into the calf or to the ankle to one of the tibial arteries. The distal anastomosis of a distal tibial bypass is less difficult to locate because it is more superficial. Regardless of the location, the distal anastomosis must be investigated thoroughly because this is a common site for stenosis (Fig. 18.17).

The distal anastomosis of a femoral to BK popliteal bypass is usually found behind the knee proximal to the tibial peroneal trunk. Scanhead placement varies as a result of the relative and individual patient anatomy. A posterior approach, from above the knee to behind the knee and into the upper calf, may work with some grafts, whereas a medial approach, following the graft along the inside of the knee and into the upper calf, may work for others. Color Doppler is extremely helpful for following the course of the graft in this deep, distal region. Graft or wall features may not be easily identified because of the limited imaging potential; however, the Doppler velocity information should still be obtainable throughout. The angle at which the graft intersects the site of the anastomosis is often severe and requires quite a bit of manipulation of the scanhead in order to follow it. The severe angulation may place Doppler angles in question or make them difficult to measure accurately, and velocities may be difficult to interpret. Color serves as the most reliable means of sorting out this potential problem, in that the direction of the vessel can be more easily mapped.

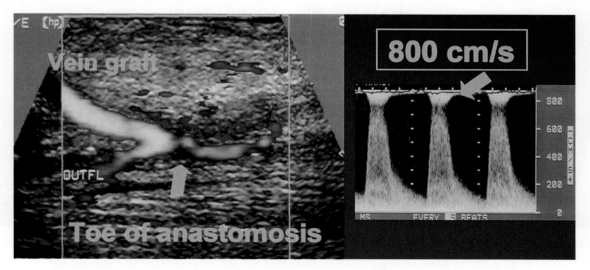

FIGURE 18.17. Power Doppler image of a high-grade stenosis at the distal end of the end-to-side distal anastomosis to the anterior tibial artery (ATA).

The end-to-side distal anastomosis has an appearance similar to the proximal anastomosis (Fig. 18.2). The exact location may not be easily identified, but using some helpful scanning tips will ensure the exact location. The anastomosis is usually a dilated area with normal flow disturbances similar to the proximal anastomosis. The identification of sutures verifies its location. The proximal outflow vessel may have retrograde flow up the leg, which can be a useful indicator of the exact location of the anastomosis (Fig. 18.2, *bottom*). Similar to the proximal anastomosis, flow velocities may be disturbed locally, and accurate measurement of PSV may be difficult. It is also impossible to calculate a meaningful velocity ratio, owing to the diameter changes and the disturbances. Therefore, as in any significant stenosis, looking for a focal velocity increase, followed by poststenotic turbulence with a decrease in flow downstream, is the best means to identify stenosis. Following the velocity changes serially is critical for demonstrating a progressive, significant stenosis. The new appearance of a color bruit may also be a significant indicator of progression of stenosis in an anastomosis. Noting the location of the stenosis relative to the sutures can be helpful in determining the reason for the stenosis.

Outflow Arteries

The outflow vessels are those to which the graft is delivering blood flow. They vary depending on the extent and location of distal arterial disease and may only be one tibial vessel. The popliteal artery, either AK or BK, is a common outflow vessel, although the tibial peroneal trunk and the three tibial vessels are also commonly used. As always, the vessels are interrogated for stenosis signified by a velocity increase followed by poststenotic turbulence. In the case of a RSV graft, there may be a large size differential between the graft and the outflow vessel, creating a normal elevated velocity.

Poststenotic turbulence accompanying the velocity increase helps to verify the presence of a stenosis. Also, a comparison of the velocity to that found further downstream may clear up the question of stenosis.

For completeness, it is a good idea to interrogate from the outflow popliteal artery, through the tibial peroneal trunk and into, at least, the origins of the tibial vessels, noting the velocity. If the outflow vessel is a single tibial artery, it is important to scan to the ankle, ensuring that there is no occult stenosis that may threaten the graft. Knowledge of the outflow velocity is helpful in determining whether progression has occurred in a graft lesion and whether the lesion is graft threatening and requires revision. Scanning the outflow and inflow arteries is essential in a surveillance study, especially after the first year of graft placement. Progression of atherosclerosis in the native arteries threatens the graft more than intragraft lesions after the first year. The outflow vessel walls may be densely calcified, which can be easily distinguished from the vein graft by the brightly echogenic surfaces. The velocity in a calcified outflow artery may be elevated normally as a result of the decrease in the compliance of the walls.

WAVEFORM TYPES FOUND IN GRAFTS

The hemodynamics of the graft can be observed in the waveform patterns that develop and change throughout the surveillance follow-up. An appreciation of the normally expected waveforms can then help distinguish which changes in the flow patterns are graft threatening. Knowledge of the reason for the graft placement (i.e., claudication or limb salvage) prepares the examiner to expect specific flow patterns as a result of the existing disease.

The normal waveforms, in a graft placed for claudication, will change in the graft as it is followed over time. In the initial postoperative period, which may be within days or a month of graft placement, the waveforms throughout the graft may be hyperemic, reflecting the increased flow (Fig. 18.18, *left*). After the first month, the velocity waveforms begin to have a multiphasic characteristic with flow reversal in early diastole, which becomes more pronounced in later studies and then stabilizes (Fig. 18.18, *right*). A graft placed for limb salvage or end-stage disease may exhibit hyperemic waveforms (end-diastolic flow above zero) throughout the follow-up period. A graft, previously identified with normal triphasic waveforms, found to have returned to hyperemic flow raises suspicion of abnormal changes somewhere in the system. A reason for the change must be sought. The presence of stenosis within the graft or in the inflow or outflow is usually the reason; however, an infection in the distal leg can also change the flow patterns. An awareness of the results of the previous study alerts the examiner to this significant change.

The presence of a low-resistance AVF in an *in situ* vein bypass will increase the flow velocity, especially in diastole, in the waveforms taken in the graft proximal to the fistula. The increased flow enhances normal disturbances at the anastomosis or at valve sites. Distal to the fistula, the waveform may return to the high-resistance, multiphasic character (Fig. 18.19). The changes may be subtle but are a good indicator of the presence of an AVF that should be identified and noted because it could lead to graft failure. The velocity waveform from the AVF has markedly increased flow in both systole and diastole and often is accompanied by a color bruit.

Disturbed flow occurs as a result of some normal, as well as abnormal, reasons. As previously mentioned, such circumstances as dilatations, anastomoses, and valve sinuses exhibit flow disturbances that should be anticipated and recognized. The waveform from normal flow disturbance exhibits a typical initial upstroke to systole, followed by oscillations toward and away from the transducer, often

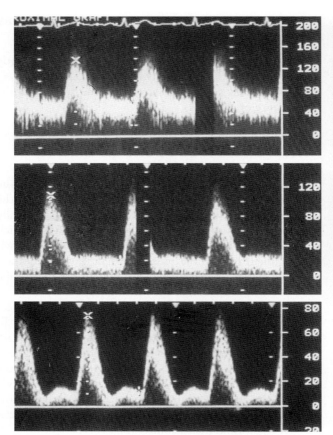

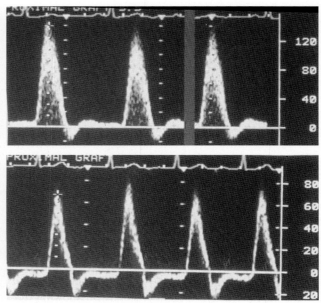

FIGURE 18.18. An array of waveforms encountered in vein grafts reflecting the subtle changes in the distal peripheral resistance following graft placement. The **top left image** is the most hyperemic, usually seen the first month after placement. The **top right image** is triphasic, reflecting increased peripheral resistance of the normal vascular bed.

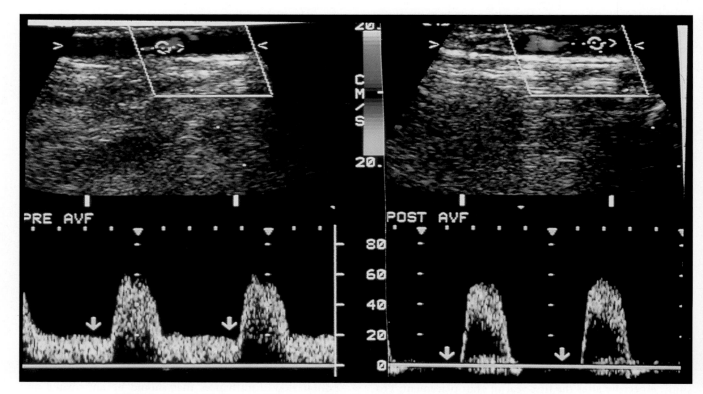

FIGURE 18.19. Velocity waveforms reflecting the presence of an AVF in an *in situ* vein bypass. The **left** waveform reflects the low resistance proximal to the AVF. The **right** waveform reflects the high resistance distal to the AVF.

crossing the zero baseline in late systole, most likely representing normal, rotational motion of eddies within the flow (Fig. 18.11). The extent and character of the disturbance depend on the source, along with the angle and direction from which the waveform was taken. The appearance of the disturbance will change if those conditions are changed. The disturbance is consistent and will not change over time unless something changes it, such as the development of stenosis or thickening of the area. PSV is difficult to establish in disturbed waveforms. It may be best for interpretation purposes to mark PSV as "unable to measure accurately because of disturbed flow" on the report form. Disturbed waveforms are typically seen in anastomoses and appear more disturbed with increased flow. The disturbance from the anastomosis extends downstream into the graft and is reflected in the velocity spectral waveforms for a distance (Fig. 18.20).

One waveform that is unique to RSV grafts is that found at the site of a "functioning" valve with and without reflux.

In the presence of a functioning valve, the waveform occurs only when there is a triphasic flow pattern and high enough velocity in the reverse direction to close the valve leaflets completely. A typical "click" is noted in the waveform at the time of valve closure and may be followed by reflux through the leaflets (Fig. 18.21). The presence and character of this waveform adapt to the overall changes in the flow patterns from one study to the next because they depend on a certain amount of reversed flow velocity to respond.

Stenotic waveforms are those with a PSV that is elevated compared with the previous normal graft segment. The sample volume is moved through the suspected region, seeking the maximal velocity increase and profiling the stenosis. The prestenotic signal is taken at a location 1 cm proximal to the jet in a normal graft segment. The stenotic signal is taken at the site of maximal velocity increase in the stenosis. The PSV measurement of the prestenotic signal, along with the stenotic PSV, is used to calculate the velocity ratio. As with any stenosis, it is important to identify the

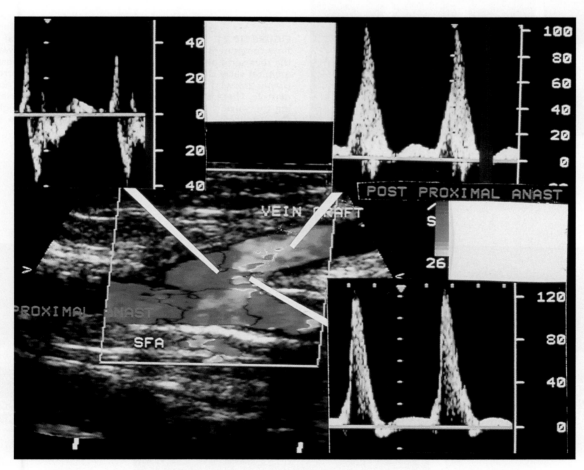

FIGURE 18.20. Waveforms from a normal proximal anastomosis reflecting the typical disturbance due to the branch angle and the dilatation and similar to a carotid bifurcation **(upper right)**. Note that the disturbance extends into the proximal graft, making the accurate measurement of peak systolic velocity difficult.

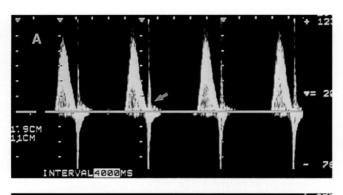

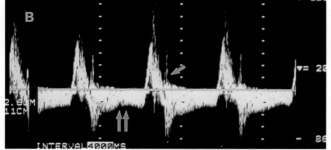

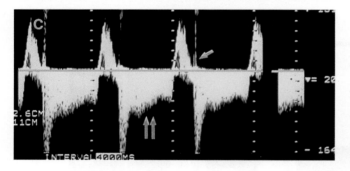

FIGURE 18.21. The **top** waveform reflects the normal forward flow component that opens the leaflets. Following forward flow, the reversed flow velocity will close the leaflets, and there will be a typical valve click on the spectral waveform as the narrow spike (*single arrow*). If the valve is competent, there will be no flow in diastole. There will be a period of elongated flow reversal following the valve click, sometimes with elevated velocity higher than the systolic velocity if the valve is incompetent (**middle** and **bottom** waveforms; *double arrow*).

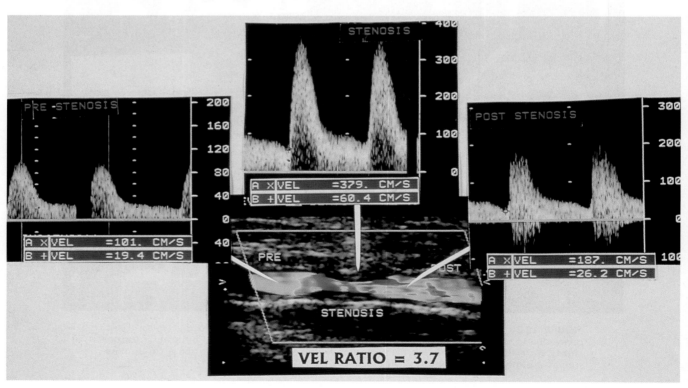

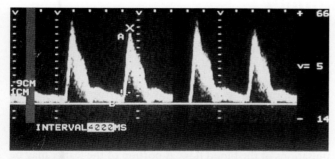

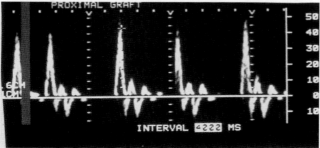

FIGURE 18.23. The staccato waveform **(bottom)** can be compared with the more normal-appearing waveform taken in the same graft 1 month earlier **(top)**. The preocclusive waveform is unique. Note the abrupt upstroke to systole, a narrow, shortened systolic peak, and multiple oscillatory, early reversal components.

poststenotic turbulence to mark the distal end of the lesion and to verify a genuine stenotic velocity increase. This signal is invaluable to the interpretation of the graft results (Fig. 18.22).

A monophasic signal in the graft, either initially or as a change in the serial follow-up examination, indicates that there has been a significant change (i.e. stenosis) that has developed either proximal or distal from the site of recording. The presence of monophasic waveforms in the graft is reason to scan carefully, including inflow and outflow, to identify the reason for the change.

A "staccato" waveform found in a graft suggests that the graft is in danger of occluding (Fig. 18.23). The staccato waveform is usually detected at the inflow vessel and is seen throughout the graft, decreasing in velocity in the more distal locations. It is significant with a distal lesion, either at the anastomosis or in the outflow, which has progressed dramatically. The severe stenosis acts as a powerful, local resistance to the flow that causes the unique waveform shape with the dramatic, rapid oscillations.

VALVES IN VEIN GRAFTS

The suspected valve area is imaged initially using a longitudinal view. Using a beam-steering feature or by manipulation of the scanhead (Fig. 18.6), multiple angles of insonation are used to locate potential leaflets that will lie at angles to the vessel wall. It is important to attempt to obtain perpendicular angles to the leaflet surface and therefore the brightest reflection. Once the longitudinal view is assessed, the transducer is turned 90 degrees to the vessel axis at the location in question to obtain transverse images. Similar to the long view, multiple angles of approach are used to investigate the sinus (Fig. 18.24). Color Doppler imaging is often helpful to pinpoint disturbances caused by dilatation of the sinus, the leaflets, or the reflux present at the leaflet site. Once the valve or feature is identified, the color is turned off to observe the B-mode characteristics of the valve. Doppler spectral waveforms are also gathered through the area of the sinus. M-mode tracings can be obtained to verify and document movement of the leaflets (Fig. 18.25).

The identification of a valve is based on the visualization of a sinus, a suspected leaflet, or a typical velocity waveform showing increased velocity, disturbance, a valve click of a functioning valve, or reflux through an incompetent valve. A valve sinus is defined as a uniform dilatation of the walls of the vein graft. A sinus location is difficult to identify clearly when the dilated portion of the sinus is filled in, creating a uniform-appearing flow channel seen in color flow. Careful cross-sectional B-mode imaging is helpful in defining the sinus region. An area of flow recirculation in the sinus may be seen in the color flow as patches of blue in the dilated portion along the wall. The recirculation is also recognized in the spectral display by the typical normal disturbance seen in the waveform, which is similar to but not as pronounced as that found in the carotid bulb. There may be a decrease in the velocity in the sinus if the dilatation is pronounced.

Valve leaflets are defined as thin, echogenic surfaces (interfaces) attached at the wall and extending into the vessel at an angle to the wall. Each leaflet of the pair is seen at a different and opposite angle to the transducer (Fig. 18.6). The beam-steering feature without moving the transducer on the skin surface is particularly helpful in defining the presence of the leaflets. Initially, the leaflets may not be visualized if the beam is directed in a straight up-and-down configuration, that is, perpendicular to the walls. It requires diligence on the part of the operator to identify precisely

FIGURE 18.22. A velocity profile of a vein graft stenosis, showing the prestenotic signal **(left)**, the maximum increased velocity within the stenosis **(middle)**, and the poststenotic turbulence **(right)**. The velocity ratio is 3.7, which indicates a more than 75% diameter reduction.

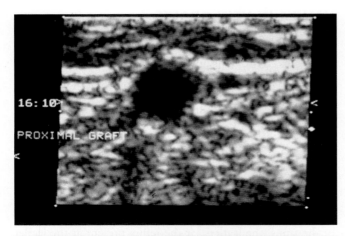

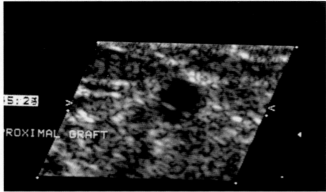

FIGURE 18.24. The vein graft is imaged in cross-section from two different angles to properly visualize the valve cusps.

the leaflets in the B-mode image. The presence of the leaflets is then verified using a transverse view. The three-dimensional configuration of the leaflets makes verification using multiple views a critical step in the identification valves.

Valve leaflets are classified as either frozen, moving, or functional. Frozen leaflets have no movement but appear to be extending into the lumen. A moving leaflet is one that appears to be moving or fluttering in the lumen with the pulsations of the blood flow. A portion of the leaflet may be moving, and a portion may be stationary. The movement is documented using an M-mode tracing (Fig. 18.25). Doppler spectral waveforms taken in the area may or may not demonstrate flow disturbance associated with the moving leaflet. The degree of movement may change over time, that is, the leaflet may become frozen or disappear into the wall over time.

The identification of a functioning valve, as defined by Tullis and colleagues (10), is based initially on either the characteristic Doppler waveform or the typical color flow pattern, followed by the subsequent visualization of the mobile valve leaflets on the B-mode image. The Doppler waveform consists of end-systolic valve closure and an audible Doppler click followed by no flow or varying degrees of reflux (Fig. 18.21). The color pattern is marked by an initial forward red systolic flow component followed by a lingering patch of blue, which represents the reflux. The rapidly moving valve leaflets are often difficult to identify on the B-mode image because of the fragile nature of the tissue, the rapid mobility of the leaflets, and the variable planes in which they lie. Multiple viewing planes are neces-

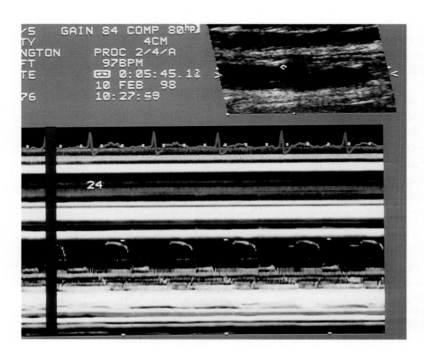

FIGURE 18.25. An M-mode trace of a competent valve in a reversed saphenous vein bypass graft. The leaflets are not visible in the B-mode image at the top of the figure.

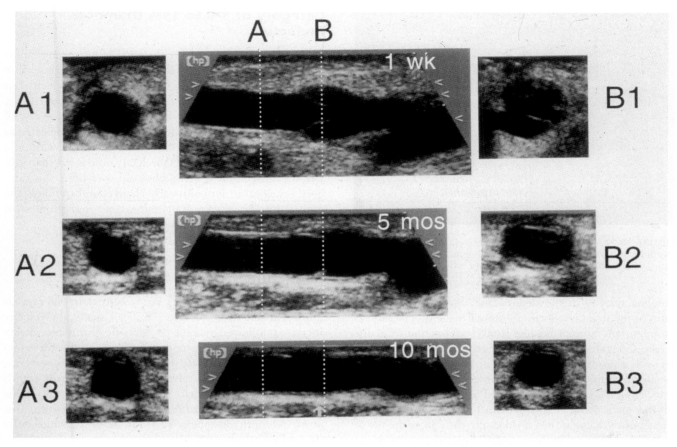

FIGURE. 18.26. A prominent valve sinus with frozen leaflets in a reversed saphenous vein bypass at 1 week (*top*), 5 months (*middle*), and 10 months (*bottom*) after graft placement (longitudinal views, *center column of images*). A cross-sectional view of the inflow at each visit is shown in the *first column of images on the left* (**A1–3**). A cross-sectional view through the region of the leaflets is shown in the *last column of images on the right* (**B1–3**). The leaflets appear to retract, and the dilated sinus disappears over time, with no apparent wall thickening at the site.

sary to isolate the leaflets, and an M-mode trace documents the movement. The leaflets are best identified in the transverse view. Velocity waveforms are sampled through the functioning valve to document the prevalve flow pattern, the valve including the click with or without reflux, and the postvalve region. Reflux occurs after closure because of the inability of the leaflets to remain closed during diastole. For a valve to be functional, there must be flow reversal, that is, distal resistance creating multiphasic flow patterns in the graft. Therefore, the function of the valve can be altered or obliterated from visit to visit by changes in the distal resistance.

All suspected valve areas are thoroughly inspected with the pulsed Doppler for any flow changes that may be present. Any change from the typical multiphasic waveform should be documented with a complete set of velocity spectral waveforms. Spectral waveforms should be sampled from the normal graft proximal to the sinus and in the sinus, including along the walls and distal to the sinus. Velocity

changes, disturbances in the flow pattern, valve click, reflux, and poststenotic flow patterns are recorded for documentation. An increased velocity may be seen through a functioning valve, followed by poststenotic turbulence; that is, the valve leaflets create a mild to moderate narrowing. Frozen valve leaflets can create a focal velocity increase associated with severe stenosis in the graft and may need to be repaired. The increased velocity, however, may also decrease over time as the leaflets retract and become a part of the wall. The sinus may also disappear in the image (Fig. 18.26).

DIAGNOSTIC CRITERIA

The purpose of vein graft surveillance is to identify potentially dangerous graft lesions that will decrease the graft velocity to a level that will cause the graft to thrombose (1,2,9). The criteria used to classify the graft lesions employ the

Vein Bypass Graft Surveillance
Interpretation Criteria*

Normal	>45 cm/s in smallest segment No spectral broadening
1-19%	*Visualized wall irregularities* *Minimal spectral broadening*
20-49%	Velocity ratio >2.0 and <2.5 PSV >45 cm/s and <150 cm/s
50-74%	Velocity ratio >2.5 and <3.5 PSV >150 cm/s, loss of reversal
75-99%	Velocity ratio >3.5 EDV >100 cm/s, loss of reversal
Occlusion	No audible Doppler signal Intraluminal echoes

*Bandyk, Sem Vasc Surg, 1993

FIGURE 18.27. Diagnostic criteria used to classify percentage of diameter reduction in infrainguinal vein bypasses. These criteria cannot be used accurately at anastomotic sites.

absolute velocity in the stenosis and, more importantly, a ratio of the stenotic velocity to normal velocity. The ratio is an important concept because it takes into account the differences in graft dimensions. Some grafts have a large diameter with a normally low overall graft velocity; others have a smaller dimension and a higher overall graft velocity. The velocity ratio is calculated using the PSV in a normal segment of the graft about 1 cm proximal to the stenosis. The prestenotic velocity is then divided into the PSV at the site of the maximal velocity in the stenosis. The ratio, along with the absolute velocity, is then used to classify the amount of diameter decrease. The criteria were developed by Bandyk and are currently used in our laboratory. The distinct categories permit the identification of severe stenosis as well as the stepwise tracking of the natural history of lesions as they change over time, either progressing or regressing. In addition to the criteria, there are other physiologic and physical conditions that are considered when making the decision to revise a graft that is in danger of occluding, including overall graft velocity, ABI, and the return of symptoms (Fig. 18.27).

Normal

It is difficult to identify a normal velocity value that universally defines all grafts because grafts vary in size from person to person, and the size varies within the graft from proximal to distal (Fig. 18.27). Therefore, appreciating the size of the conduit that is being scanned and considering the normal changes in diameter along the length of the graft help to characterize the normal velocity for each specific graft. In the presence of normal velocity, the walls and the lumen should be free of irregularity or protrusions that would be considered abnormal. The normal walls have a typical double-line appearance, in response to the arterialization of the vein wall, with thickening of the intima, media, or both to accommodate the arterial flow.

Category of 1% to 19% Diameter Reduction

The category of 1% to 19% diameter reduction or "minimal disease" is designed to identify areas of the vessel that have minor changes that do not affect the flow velocity but can be distinguished from a normal-appearing vessel (Fig. 18.27). The distinguishing feature of this category is wall irregularity, either seen in the B-mode image or detected as minimal disturbance in the flow velocity with or without a minimal velocity increase. The velocity ratio is less than 2.0. Because the patient is being observed over time, this category is helpful to pinpoint early changes and to follow the natural history of vein graft lesions that may progress to more severe stenosis and require revision.

Category of 20% to 49% Diameter Reduction

The hallmark of this category is a velocity ratio that exceeds 2.0 but is less than 2.5 (Fig. 18.27). Usually, the velocity increase is followed by some poststenotic disturbance. Every attempt should be made to identify the reason for the velocity change in the B-mode image (e.g., intimal hyperplasia, wall irregularity, frozen valve leaflet, kink, or tortuosity). It is important to note that, in our study, nearly all of the lesions that later required revision were detected at the first 1- to 3-month postoperative study, some of which were defined as 20% to 49% (2).

Category of 50% to 74% Diameter Reduction

In this category, the velocity is clearly increased in the stenotic jet, and there is always well-defined, poststenotic turbulence (Fig. 18.27). The velocity ratio is greater than 2.5 and less than 3.5. The B-mode image helps to define the reason for the stenosis. Frozen valve leaflets may create this amount of narrowing but may be difficult to identify in the image. Angled leaflet surfaces relative to the walls are not readily appreciated without a thorough investigation. It is important to distinguish between a valve leaflet stenosis and that of intimal hyperplasia, in that the natural history may be different for the two lesions (Fig. 18.28). Valve leaflet stenosis tends to be focal and, if detected early, may regress over time to become a moderate to minimal stenosis.

Category of 75% to 99% Diameter Reduction

This significant and severe lesion in the vein graft is defined by a velocity ratio that exceeds 3.5 with clear and well-defined poststenotic turbulence (Figs. 18.22 and 18.27). It is this lesion that may prompt a revision of the graft and that therefore needs to be identified accurately. Often, because of

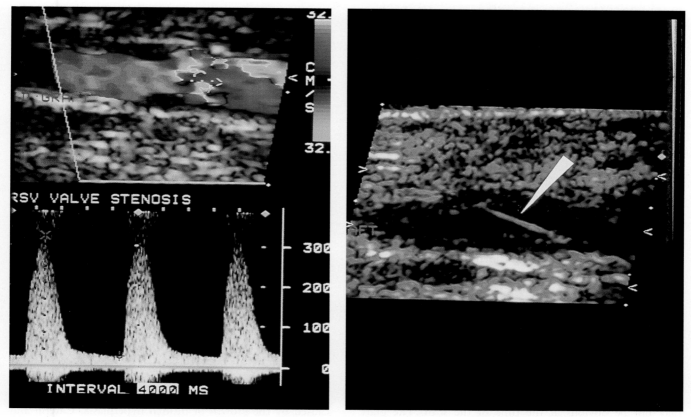

FIGURE 18.28. The image on the **right** shows the bright interface of the frozen valve leaflet. Note the image beams are steered to the left to detect the surface. The **upper left** image shows the color display of the leaflet stenosis and the **lower left** shows the spectral waveform from the stenosis (300 cm/s). The region was subsequently revised using a vein patch angioplasty.

the severity of the stenosis, the overall graft velocity may decrease along with the ABI, indicating a critical narrowing. Progression to this level of stenosis should be an indication that graft revision will be needed. This lesion is especially significant if there is also a change in the overall graft waveform shape to that of a monophasic signal or, more notably, if the waveforms in the graft become staccato along with the progression of the lesion. These changes are a clear indication that the graft is in threat of impending occlusion.

Total Occlusion

Total occlusion is identified by the lack of flow within the graft (Fig. 18.27). Because the graft is a continuous conduit with no branches, the occlusion will include the entire length and sometimes the outflow, thereby eliminating the need to scan the whole graft once occlusion has been established. Usually, the occlusion is easily identified at or after the proximal anastomosis (Fig. 18.29). It is important to scan the distal anastomosis and outflow for remaining flow because this could be of clinical import for future therapy or revision. The occlusion may or may not be heralded by a

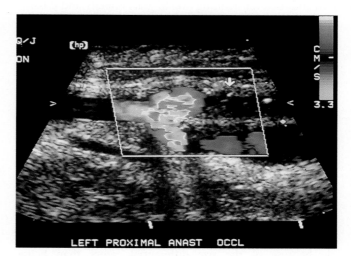

FIGURE 18.29. Occluded reversed saphenous vein bypass graft distal to the proximal anastomosis off the common femoral artery (CFA). Softly echogenic material is seen in the occluded graft (more superficial vessel), and the origin of the profunda femoris artery is seen extending from the CFA and deep to graft.

drop in the ankle pressure but will most certainly be characterized by a drop in the ABI after the occlusion.

Pitfalls of Vein Graft Duplex Scans

1. One of the best tools to aid in scanning vein grafts is prior knowledge of the exact surgical procedure that was performed. The type of graft that was used, the condition of the vein before placement, the exact location of the anastomoses, the type and location of revisions, and any other details of the procedure can be helpful when doing the duplex study. A copy of the operative notes or a verbal description can be used as a guide to direct the scan to specific areas that may require more thorough interrogation. Without a prior description of the surgical procedure, extra time and effort is spent sorting out technical details of graft geometry that may be easily explained away or that may be critically important to the interpretation. Vein grafts are often lumped under the common term "fem-pop bypass," which denotes that the bypass extends from the CFA to the popliteal artery, either AK or BK. A good number of vein grafts are just that and are obvious and easily scanned, even without prior knowledge. Unfortunately, as a result of the location and extent of the offending arterial disease or technical difficulties during the operation, a number of the grafts will have variations in the standard placement that may not be obvious at the time of the scan. The graft anatomy, therefore, becomes more complex and time-consuming to scan.

2. "Spot sampling," or taking Doppler samples at random locations in the graft rather than sampling representative signals smoothly throughout the length of the graft, can be the downfall of any type of duplex examination. The Doppler spectral waveforms that are generated from the scan and used for defining overall graft velocity and classification of narrowing should represent the hemodynamic character of the blood flow throughout the graft. Graft stenoses may be focal or subtle and can easily be missed by taking spot samples. The use of color, recognizing specific color patterns of valves and stenosis, is invaluable to highlight regions of interest for more in-depth interrogation. Using the B-mode image will help to define specific valve features and wall changes that color Doppler may mask.

3. Normal changes in diameter affect the velocity: smaller vessels have higher velocity, and wider vessels have lower velocity. Appreciating the changes in the diameter of the graft on the B-mode image can help to define the changes in velocity. In a RSV graft, the proximal vein may be quite small compared with the CFA and the dilated anastomosis. The velocity would be expected to be higher, simply because of the size differential rather than being misidentified as a stenosis.

4. The distal portion of a RSV graft to the BK popliteal is usually quite deep as it dives below the sartorius muscle in the thigh; it can be difficult to image and follow thor-

oughly to the distal anastomosis. Color Doppler is invaluable for scanning this portion of the graft. The B-mode image may not offer information about subtle features, but obvious stenosis will be evident in the color display. Bending the leg slightly, rotating it outward, and resting it on a pillow can create a more optimal window to the graft; however, it may appear slightly deeper in the image. Turning the patient prone and propping the ankle up can also be used in an attempt to follow the entire length of the graft. The distal anastomosis in these grafts may also be difficult to scan, owing to the depth or the sharp angle that may be created between the graft and the native artery. One must be suspicious of increased velocity in the area if the Doppler angle is not optimum or cannot be determined because of the acute angulation of the vessel into and out of the anastomosis.

5. Some grafts can be very superficial, lying just under the skin surface, at times. Pressure of the transducer may compress the graft and create an apparent velocity increase that may be misinterpreted as stenosis. Pulling up on the scanhead and relieving the pressure with a cushion of gel or a standoff, or rotating the scanhead to the side of the graft, can eliminate the problem.

6. Frozen valve leaflets may cause a functional stenosis identified by the typical increased velocity followed by poststenotic turbulence and may be confused with stenosis caused by the growth of intimal hyperplasia. Careful and meticulous imaging of the region, using multiple angles of approach and views, will illuminate the cause of the stenosis. The leaflet will be at an angle to the wall, with a thin, echogenic interface, and may be found in pairs. However, intimal hyperplasia is initially seen as softly echogenic thickening or mounding along the wall, which initially is not well defined. Over time, the surface interface becomes more easily defined as the mound thickens and is clearly distinguished from a leaflet. A valve stenosis may remain stable over time or may regress and become less significant as the leaflets shorten and become more contiguous with the wall.

7. A graft can fail if there is a significant decrease in either the inflow or the outflow vessels. Not recognizing ominous changes in the waveform characteristics of these vessels or not scanning the vessels thoroughly when there is an ill defined decrease in the overall graft flow can lead to a subsequent failure.

8. Velocity ratios should not be used in the anastomoses. Because of the often-dramatic changes in size from the anastomosis compared with the graft, the ratio becomes meaningless and invalid. Looking at the absolute velocity change and comparing it over time along with poststenotic turbulence will define a significant stenosis in the anastomosis. As always with graft scanning, an assessment of the overall graft velocity and the waveform shapes can help to determine whether progression has occurred or if the stenosis is significant.

REFERENCES

1. Bandyk DF, Schmitt DD, Seabrook GR, et al. Monitoring functional patency of *in situ* saphenous vein bypasses: the impact of a surveillance protocol and elective revision. *J Vasc Surg* 1989;9: 286–294.

2. Caps MT, Bergelin RO, Cantwell-Gab K, et al. Vein graft lesions: time of onset and rate of progression. *J Vasc Surg* 1995;22:466–474.

3. Idu MM, Buth J, Hop WCJ, et al. Vein graft surveillance: is graft revision without angiography justified and what criteria should be used? *J Vasc Surg* 1998;27:399–411.

4. Bandyk DF, Calligaro KD, Andros G, et al. Selective use of duplex ultrasound to replace preoperative arteriography for failing arterial vein grafts [discussion]. *J Vasc Surg* 1998;27:94–95.

5. Calligaro KD, Syrek JR, Dougherty MJ, et al. Selective use of duplex ultrasound to replace preoperative arteriography for failing arterial vein grafts. *J Vasc Surg* 1998;27:89–94.

6. Mills JL, Harris EJ, Taylor LM, et al. The importance of routine surveillance of distal bypass grafts with duplex scanning: a study of 379 reversed vein grafts. *J Vasc Surg* 1990;12:379–389.

7. Mattos MA, van Bemmelen PS, Hodgson KJ, et al. Does correction of stenoses identified with color duplex scanning improve infrainguinal graft patency? *J Vasc Surg* 1993;17:54–66.

8. Strandness DE Jr, Jing Ming J, Primozich JP, et al. A new approach to vein graft surveillance. *J Vasc Invest* 1999;4:1–7.

9. Bandyk DF. Postoperative surveillance of infrainguinal bypass. *Surg Clin North Am* 1990;70:71–75.

10. Tullis MJ, Primozich J, Strandness DE Jr. Detection of "functional" valves in reversed saphenous vein bypass grafts: identification with duplex ultrasonography. *J Vasc Surg* 1997;25:522–527.

## 19

RENAL ARTERY EVALUATION

KIM CANTWELL-GAB

One of the most difficult areas for study with ultrasound has been the renal arteries, their course to the kidney, and the parenchyma. Although the role of the renal artery in terms of producing hypertension has been known since the work of Goldblatt in 1934 (1), it has only been in recent years that we have been able to study the renal arteries directly and noninvasively (2–5). The renal arteries lie in the posterior abdomen, making them difficult to access without the availability of low-frequency transducers. In addition, the problem of bowel gas has always been a limiting factor for access, although it is possible by studying the patients in the morning after an overnight fast to minimize this problem. In addition, the use of alternate scanning approaches has also been a great help.

The potential value of using duplex ultrasound for this purpose is now clearly evident. We can reliably detect areas of narrowing and occlusion, making it possible to document the role of renal artery disease in the production of hypertension and ischemic renal failure (6,7). Another major role for duplex scanning is its use in documenting both renal artery disease progression and the evolution of the shrinking kidney (7,8).

There have been attempts to shorten the examination time and make it more acceptable for screening purposes. The proponents of this approach have been Stavros and co-workers (5). These authors and others proposed using an approach to the hilum of the kidney to document changes in the waveform shape of the renal artery velocity pattern to suggest the presence of renal artery narrowing (4,9). We do not believe this approach should be used if one takes the time to become familiar with the scanning method used for renal arteries.

The role of renal artery stenosis and occlusion in the development of ischemic renal failure is of great interest. Stents are being used more frequently to preserve patency and hopefully prevent progression to occlusion. We can document both the presence of renal artery stents and their effectiveness in restoring kidney blood flow to normal (10).

Another advantage of renal duplex studies is our ability to document the diagnosis of fibromuscular dysplasia (FMD). This disease is found in young to middle-aged women. It is recognized by its typical location in the mid-distal renal artery and by its typical string-of-beads appearance. It is also possible to follow the results of renal angioplasty by duplex scanning (11).

EQUIPMENT REQUIRED

To perform an abdominal vascular evaluation of any type, a high-resolution duplex scanner with a 2- to 4-MHz phased array or curved linear transducer is necessary to obtain adequate penetration to the depth of the aorta and the renal arteries. Color flow is extremely helpful when performing visceral vascular evaluations, but it is used only as a pathfinder and not a diagnostic tool. For the comfort of the patient, we suggest having a gel warmer available. Also needed are a blood pressure cuff, sphygmomanometer, and stethoscope to obtain bilateral blood pressures. In addition, it can be extremely beneficial to have a stretcher that has a reverse Trendelenburg's position, which will sometimes drop the bowel out of the scan plane and improve visualization of the left renal artery.

PATIENT PREPARATION

It is recommended that all patients undergoing an abdominal arterial evaluation remain fasting for at least 8 hours before the evaluation because this tends to reduce the amount of bowel gas, which blocks the transmission of ultrasound. It is recommended that the patients take their medications with a small amount of water. The exception to this type of preparation would be a patient who has brittle diabetes mellitus. In this case, it is suggested that the patient's referring physician be consulted as to what type of preparation would be permissible. At the University of Washington, we also suggest the patient eat a bland evening meal the day before the evaluation, avoid gum chewing, and if possible, decrease or stop smoking the morning of the examination to decrease the amount of air in the bowel.

SCANNING TECHNIQUES

Most of the visceral vessels may be visualized with the patient in the supine position. The transducer is placed in the subxiphoid position using a transverse orientation. The first vessels to be identified are the abdominal aorta and the inferior vena cava. Because of their close proximity, they should be seen simultaneously; at this point, the gain settings should be adjusted to document their echo-free lumens. The spine lies immediately posterior to the aorta, providing a highly reflective echo boundary. A normal finding may be reverberation artifact present along the anterior aspect of the vessels secondary to the reflective interface at the vessel walls. Continue scanning the aorta inferiorly until the common iliac bifurcation is identified, noting branch vessel origins, intimal changes, tortuosity, and any areas of dilatation and keeping in mind that, as the aorta courses inferiorly, it normally tapers, becoming smaller in caliber. With the aorta in a transverse orientation, anteroposterior and width measurements are made at three areas as well as any areas of concern. The three areas that must be documented are (a) supraceliac or suprarenal, (b) perirenal or juxtarenal, and (c) infrarenal to document whether aneurysmal changes are present above or below the level of the renal arteries (Fig. 19.1). The aorta is also evaluated in a sagittal or longitudinal view and can usually be identified as an anechoic tubular structure to the left of midline. The aorta is scanned from the supraceliac level to the common iliac bifurcation, noting any areas of tortuosity, intimal changes, and dilatation, with measurements made of the length of any dilatation or aneurysm.

Doppler evaluation of the aorta is performed with the vessel in a sagittal view, sweeping the Doppler sample volume through the entire length of the vessel. A small (1.5 to 2 mm) sample volume size at a 60-degree angle is used at all times (Fig. 19.2). Doppler spectral tracings are recorded at the suprarenal level, infrarenal level, and any areas of intimal change visualized on the B-mode image. The suprarenal aortic spectral signal has a sharp systolic upstroke and typically has forward flow above baseline throughout diastole because the vessel is primarily supplying a low-resistance vascular bed at this level. The velocities will range from 80 to 100 cm/sec (±20 cm/sec) at this level. After moving below the level of the renal arteries, the flow pattern will change to a high-resistance flow with a reverse flow component present and diastolic flow closer to or at the baseline secondary to the vessel primarily supplying a high-resistance peripheral vascular bed (Fig. 19.3). It is important to document the suprarenal or supraceliac aortic velocity because this velocity will be used to calculate ratios that determine the degree of stenosis in the renal arteries (discussed later).

After the abdominal aorta has been evaluated, return the transducer to the subxiphoid position with a transverse orientation and scan inferiorly until the first branch of the aorta is identified, which will be the celiac axis (Fig. 19.4). It originates from the anterior aspect of the aorta and is usually within the first 2 cm. The celiac artery is typically 1 cm in length, and its caliber varies from 5 to 10 mm in width. In most people, the celiac artery gives off three branch vessels: the common hepatic artery, the left gastric artery, and the splenic artery. Viewed in the appropriate plane, the image resembles a seagull in flight. It may be useful to use anatomic landmarks when attempting to locate these vessels, especially when extensive bowel gas is present. The common hepatic artery usually has a sharp takeoff from the celiac artery and may course at a 90-degree angle rightward toward the hilum of the liver. It follows the upper border of the pancreatic head and, at the duodenum, turns anteriorly to enter the hilum of the liver following the course of the main portal vein (becomes the proper hepatic artery). The proximal portion of the left gastric artery occasionally may be seen. It has an anterior and superior course from the celiac axis and turns leftward to provide the blood supply to the stomach and esophagus. It is not considered an abnormal finding if this vessel is not visualized. The splenic artery takes a horizontal and leftward course from the celiac axis and can be quite tortuous and difficult to follow, especially in elderly people. The splenic artery follows the upper margin of the pancreatic body posteriorly before entering the hilum of the spleen, with branches also providing a blood supply to the stomach and pancreas.

The second major branch vessel from the abdominal aorta is the superior mesenteric artery (SMA). This vessel also originates from the anterior surface of the aorta about

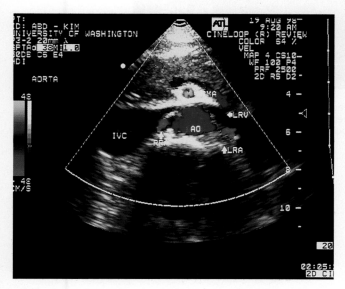

FIGURE 19.1. B-Mode image of transverse view of aorta, with origin of right renal artery *(RRA)* at the 10-o'clock position and left renal artery *(LRA)* at the 4-o'clock position. The left renal vein *(LRV)* crosses over the aorta between the superior mesenteric artery *(SMA)* and the aorta to enter the inferior vena cava *(IVC)*.

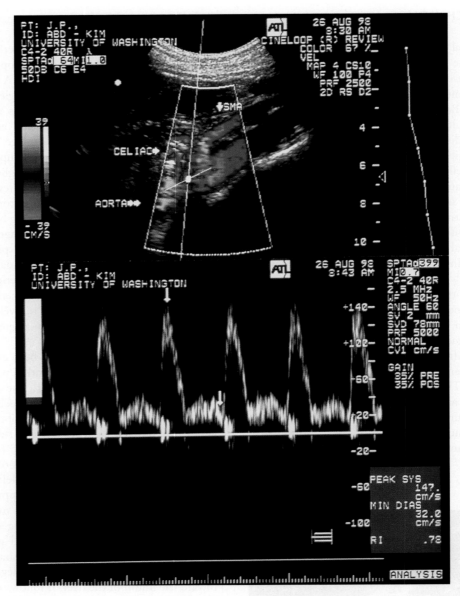

FIGURE 19.2. B-Mode image of sagittal view of aorta showing the origin of the celiac axis and the superior mesenteric artery *(SMA)*. Doppler spectral tracing showing aortic velocity obtained at the level of the SMA. Systolic and diastolic velocity are above baseline on the spectral tracing.

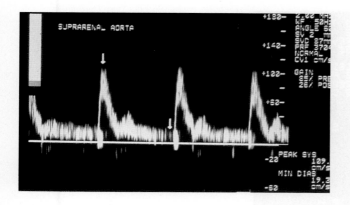

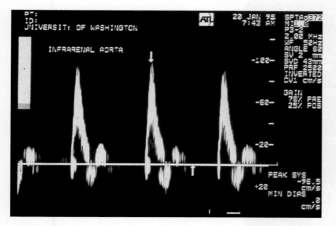

FIGURE 19.3. Doppler spectral tracing of aortic velocity. The suprarenal aortic spectral tracing shows systolic and diastolic velocity above baseline, whereas the infrarenal aortic spectral tracing shows systolic velocity above baseline and diastolic velocity at or below baseline.

1 to 2 cm below the celiac axis (distance varies significantly among patients). With the transducer in a transverse view, the SMA appears rounded and is surrounded by an echo-dense collar consisting of mesentery and fat. As the SMA begins its caudad course, it travels posterior to the pancreatic body and anterior to the uncinate process. It then continues inferiorly, paralleling the aorta; for this reason, it is easiest to evaluate in a sagittal or longitudinal view. There are several branches from the SMA along the entire length of the vessel that provides the blood supply primarily to the small bowel and the large bowel. (Just inferior to the SMA lie the renal arteries, which will be covered shortly.) The inferior mesenteric artery (IMA) is the last major branch to arise from the abdominal aorta before it bifurcates into the common iliac arteries. It originates from the anterior aspect of the aorta and runs leftward and inferiorly into the abdomen. The IMA provides blood supply to the distal portion of the colon. Failure to identify the IMA does not imply occlusion. The vessel is usually covered by the duodenum, often making it difficult to image.

Inferior to the SMA lie the renal arteries. They are usually evaluated in the transverse view because of their perpendicular relationship to the acoustic beam. The right renal artery tends to arise from the lateral aspect of the aorta (at the 10-o'clock position) and courses posterior to the inferior vena cava (retrocaval). The left renal artery arises from the lateral or posterolateral aspect of the aorta (at the 3- or 4-o'clock position). The renal arteries also course posterior to their companion renal veins. Doppler spectral

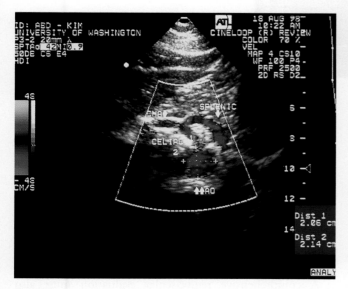

FIGURE 19.4. B-mode image of the aorta in transverse view showing celiac trunk (celiac artery, common hepatic artery, and splenic artery), which resembles a seagull in flight.

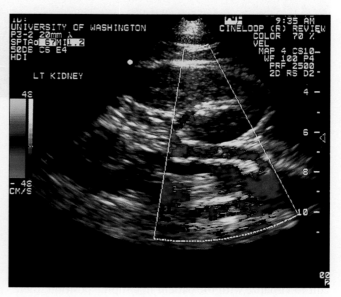

FIGURE 19.5. B-mode image of left renal artery *(red)* entire length, and pole-to-pole image of left kidney and left renal vein *(blue)*. The patient position was lateral oblique; coronal position for transducer.

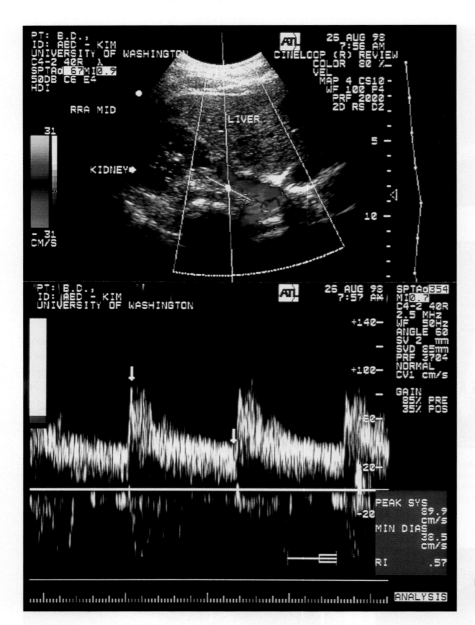

FIGURE 19.6. B-mode image of right kidney in cross-section and of right renal artery *(red)* with normal Doppler spectral tracing.

analysis consists of evaluating the renal arteries throughout their entire length using a small, 2-mm sample volume size as well as a low wall filter. The Doppler sample volume is swept through the artery, documenting velocities at the origin, proximal, middle, and distal portions of the vessel, with special attention given to any areas of intimal and/or velocity change (Fig. 19.5). The distal renal artery may be difficult to visualize with the patient in a supine position; therefore, a lateral decubitus or lateral posterior oblique position may be needed (Fig. 19.6). The right renal vessels may be best imaged with the transducer placed transversely over the right kidney and angled medially. The left renal vessels are

best visualized with the transducer placed in a transverse orientation in the midline of the abdomen, just inferior to the origination of the SMA. After identifying the main renal arteries, an attempt should be made to locate any accessory renal arteries (Fig. 19.7). The normal renal artery waveform should have a sharp systolic upstroke with a low-resistance forward flow throughout diastole because it is supplying a low-resistance vascular bed (Fig. 19.8).

A comprehensive renovascular evaluation must also include an examination of the parenchyma of the kidney. The renal hilar and segmental branches, parenchymal arteries (interlobar, arcuate, and at times interlobular arteries),

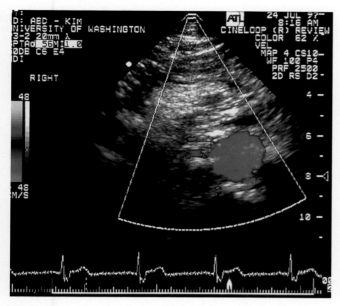

FIGURE 19.7. B-mode image of aorta in cross-section with an accessory right renal artery and main right renal artery.

renal parenchymal tissue and kidney length, and renal veins are also included in a complete renovascular evaluation.

Before or immediately after entering the hilus of the kidney, the renal artery divides into segmental or lobar branches. In practical terms, the renal hilum is where the blood flow enters the kidney. The renal sinus B-mode image appears as a compact area of homogeneous central echoes within the kidney sinus. The echo intensity is caused by hilar adipose tissue, blood vessels, and the collecting system. The renal hilar or segmental branches are evaluated with the kidney either in a longitudinal or transverse view using either the liver on the right or the spleen on the left as an acoustic window. To evaluate the multiple branches that are present at the hilar level, a large, 10-mm sample volume size is used at a 0-degree angle. To provide optimal evaluation of the waveform contour, a fast sweep speed (100 mm/sec) is used. This will spread the spectral waveform out over time and facilitate calculation of the hilar parameters. The normal Doppler waveform at the hilar level will appear similar to the distal renal artery; however, the velocities will be lower. There should be a dicrotic notch or early systolic component present in the waveform (Fig. 19.9).

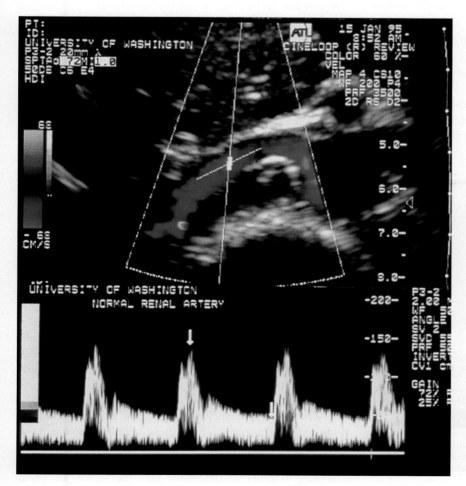

FIGURE 19.8. B-mode image of aorta in cross-section with right renal artery *(RRA)* origin *(red)* and proximal-middle artery *(blue)*, with normal Doppler spectral tracing showing sharp systolic upstroke and low-resistance diastolic flow pattern.

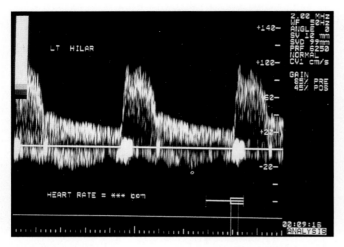

FIGURE 19.9. Doppler spectral tracing of normal hilar waveform showing sharp systolic upstroke, presence of a dicrotic notch, and normal acceleration time.

The following hilar parameters have been evaluated in the University of Washington Vascular Research project, "Natural History of Renal Artery Stenosis," but are not routinely performed in patients referred to the clinical vascular laboratory:

Acceleration time (AT). The AT is defined as the time interval from the onset of systolic flow to the initial peak and is reported in milliseconds. An AT of more than 100 milliseconds is considered abnormal.

Acceleration index (AI). The AI is the slope of the initial systolic acceleration on the Doppler waveform. This is calculated as the change in velocity between the onset of sys-

tole and the peak of systole (cm/sec) divided by the AT. An AI of less than 3.78 kHz/sec is considered to be abnormal.

Early systolic peak (ESP) or tardus parvus pattern. The ESP is best defined as the peak of the acceleration phase of the velocity waveform, which is followed by a short deceleration phase and a second acceleration phase before the true systolic peak. The absence of the normal ESP is considered an abnormal finding and is detectable by pattern recognition. However, distinguishing between the initial or compliance peak and the true systolic peak of the waveform can be difficult because of variations in the normal hilar waveform and changes secondary to patient respiration (Fig. 19.10).

The limitations and pitfalls of using the hilar evaluation to determine renal stenosis include:

- Inability to distinguish renal artery stenosis from renal artery occlusion
- Lack of sensitivity to a stenosis in an accessory renal artery or segmental branch
- Bilateral changes caused by lesions proximal to the renal arteries (i.e., aortic coarctation or stenosis), possibly giving false-positive results
- Inability to localize the site of the stenosis
- Lack of velocity information for serial follow-up evaluations
- Inability to identify a less than 60% stenosis

The parenchymal arteries that are evaluated during a renovascular examination are the interlobar and the arcuate arteries. Within the renal sinus, each segmental or lobar artery branches to form the interlobar arteries, which pass between the pyramids and branch into the arcuate arteries at the base of the pyramids, providing the blood supply to the cortex (Fig. 19.11). Surrounding the renal sinus, two distinct areas of the kidney parenchyma must be differentiated ultrasonographically: the medulla and the cortex. Differentiation between the cortex and medulla is easiest in thin patients and children; the medullary region is larger in children. Also, keep in mind that the diuretic status of the kidneys affects the detectability and ultrasonographic characteristics of the medulla. When there is an increase in diuresis, the pyramids become more prominent and anechoic and are easier to visualize. The corticomedullary junction is recognized by discrete, high-level, comma-shaped, specular echoes arching over the tops of the pyramids, which serve as a marker for cortical thickness (Fig. 19.12). The echogenicity of a normal adult renal cortex is comparable to that of the spleen or the liver at the same depth and is valid only in the absence of hepatic or splenic disease.

The parenchymal Doppler spectral evaluation is performed using a small (1.5 to 2 mm) sample volume size and a 0-degree angle. At the University of Washington, color flow or color power angiography is used to visualize the arteries in order to determine that the vessels are being

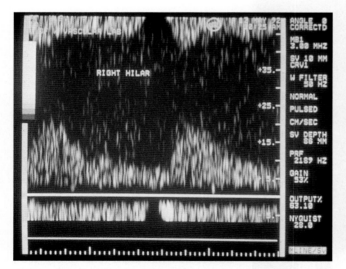

FIGURE 19.10. Doppler spectral tracing of abnormal hilar waveform, showing abnormal systolic upstroke (rounded and dampened), absence of true dicrotic notch, and delayed acceleration time.

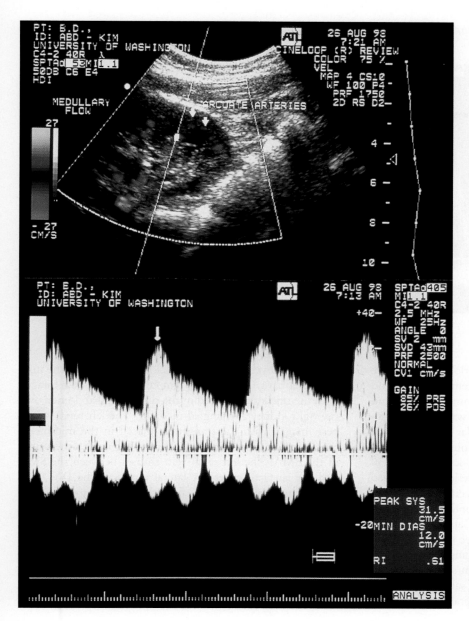

FIGURE 19.11. B-mode image of kidney parenchyma with Doppler sample volume (gate) placed in location where medullary velocities are obtained (interlobar artery). Normal Doppler spectral waveform of medullary flow.

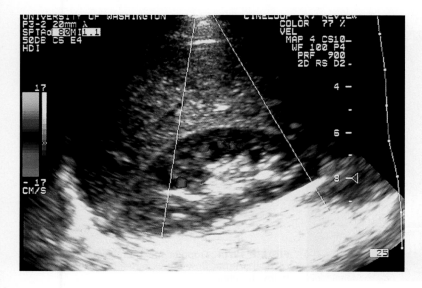

FIGURE 19.12. B-mode image of kidney parenchyma using color flow to determine cortical-medullary junction.

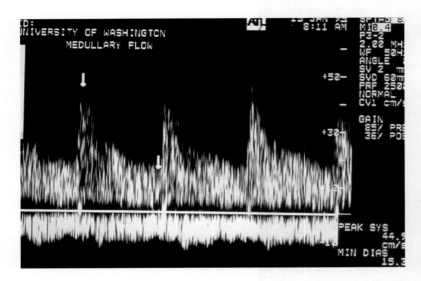

FIGURE 19.13. Doppler spectral waveform of normal medullary arterial flow above baseline and venous flow below baseline. Note the sharp systolic upstroke and low-resistance diastolic flow. The parenchymal flow patterns should be similar to renal artery flow patterns.

insonated at a 0-degree angle. The interlobar arteries are identified between the collecting system calyxes, and Doppler spectral tracings are obtained from the upper and lower poles of the kidneys. The Doppler waveform characteristics should appear similar to the hilar signal but will have lower velocities. Typically, we have found that, at a 0-degree angle, the normal peak systolic velocities average 30 to 40 cm/sec (Fig. 19.13). The arcuate arteries are identified in the cortical region, and Doppler spectral tracings are obtained from the upper and lower poles of the kidneys. The Doppler waveform characteristics should appear similar to the interlobar arteries but will have lower velocities. Typically, we have found that, at a 0-degree angle, the normal peak systolic velocities average 20 to 30 cm/sec (Fig. 19.14).

The renal veins are visualized at the same level as the renal arteries. The right renal vein is generally shorter than the left renal vein because of its close proximity to the inferior vena cava (IVC). The right renal vein is best imaged with the transducer placed in the right lateral abdomen over the right kidney and angled medially. The left renal vein is best imaged with the transducer placed in the midline of the abdomen (transverse orientation) inferior to the origin of the SMA. The left renal vein courses between the SMA and the aorta to enter the lateral aspect of the IVC. The renal veins typically have a pulsatile flow component present near their entry into the IVC secondary to the right atrial pressure and transmitted pulses. However, distally or at the hilar level, the renal veins should have phasic flow, the diameter of the vessel should change with respiration, and the lumen of the vessel should be anechoic (Fig. 19.15). Bilateral pulsatile flow in the kidney or in the renal vein near the pelvis or hilum of the kidney is usually due to

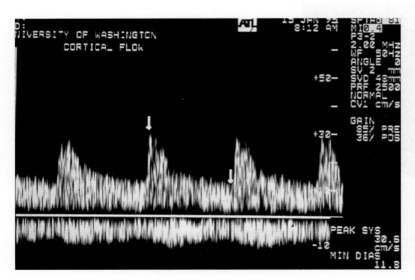

FIGURE 19.14. Doppler spectral waveform of normal cortical arterial flow above baseline and venous flow below baseline.

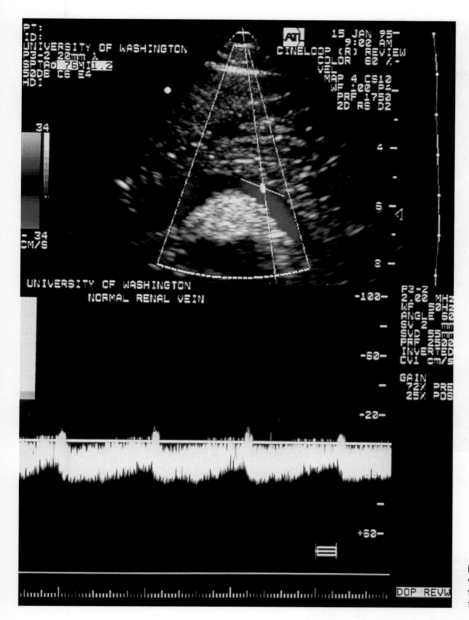

FIGURE 19.15. B-mode image of left renal vein and accompanying Doppler spectral tracing showing normal, phasic renal vein flow.

increased central venous pressure such as is found in patients with fluid overload, congestive heart failure, cardiomyopathy, or pulmonary edema (Figs. 19.16 and 19.17).

Routine evaluation of the kidneys and their parenchymal tissue should be performed in conjunction with evaluating the arterial and venous flow. The kidneys are located retroperitoneally under the costal margin. The right kidney lies slightly lower than the left because of the right lobe of the liver. During inspiration, the kidneys may move downward by as much as 2.5 cm; therefore, asking the patient to take a deep breath may improve the visualization of the kidneys. The normal kidney is about 10 to 12 cm long, 4.5 to 6 cm wide, and 3 to 4 cm thick (height). Generally, both kidneys

attain about the same dimensions; therefore, a difference of more than 1.5 to 2 cm between sides is significant. The kidneys are surrounded by three layers of supportive tissues. The innermost layer is the fibrous renal capsule, which covers the surface of the kidney. The second layer is a mass of perirenal fat. The third, or outermost, layer is the renal fascia, also referred to as *Gerota's fascia*. This dense, fibroareolar connective tissue encloses the kidney, the perirenal fat, and the adrenal gland and anchors these organs to surrounding structures (12,13). Using the liver as an acoustic window, the right kidney is best imaged with the patient in either a supine or left lateral decubitus position, scanning through the anterior axillary line, intercostally or subcostally. Using the spleen as an acoustic window, the left kidney is best imaged with the

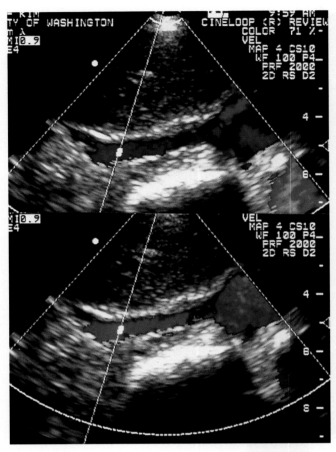

FIGURE 19.16. B-mode color image of right renal vein showing color flow patterns (forward–reverse) with abnormal pulsatile venous flow.

patient in a right lateral decubitus position, scanning through the posterior axillary line in an intercostal space. When the left upper pole cannot be identified because of rib or bowel gas interference, a fluid-filled stomach can be used as an acoustic window. However, it is recommended to wait until the end of the examination before having the patient fill the stomach with fluid because this causes extensive peristalsis. It is important to visualize some portion of the liver with the right kidney and the spleen with the left kidney because their echo amplitude can be compared with that of the renal parenchyma.

After identifying the most optimal view of the kidney, obtain three kidney length measurements from pole to pole using the renal capsule as a landmark (Fig. 19.18). When the kidney atrophies, the parenchymal tissue will become hyperechoic, which can make visualization of the kidney difficult (Fig. 19.19). The three kidney length measurements are averaged together and reported as one measurement on the patient report. What scanning approach was utilized in obtaining the kidney measurement is documented for follow-up evaluations, in addition to noting any possible difficulties in obtaining the measurements. The transducer is then rotated so that the kidney appears in a transverse view, and three kidney width measurements are obtained using the renal artery and renal vein as landmarks. The three kidney width measurements are averaged together and reported as one measurement on the patient report.

Cortical thickness measurements should be performed on every visit because it has been shown that the cortex thins as the patient develops renovascular disease. The cortical measurements are best obtained by visualizing the arcuate arter-

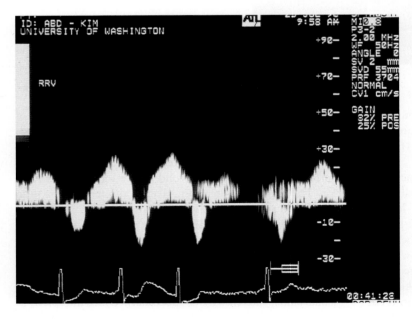

FIGURE 19.17. Doppler spectral waveform of abnormal pulsatile venous flow. Waveform appears similar to arterial pulsation.

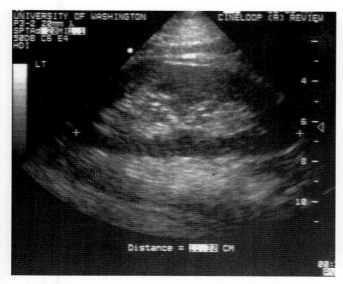

FIGURE 19.18. Pole-to-pole kidney length, normal example.

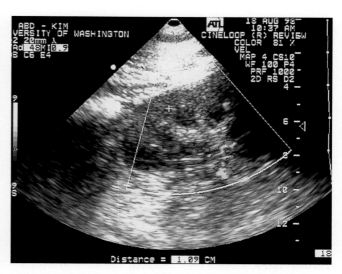

FIGURE 19.20. Cortical thickness measurement using the arcuate artery as a landmark for the corticomedullary junction.

ies as they arch over the tops of the pyramids (Fig. 19.20). Two cortical thickness measurements are taken from the upper and lower poles of the kidneys. The measurements are averaged together and reported as one measurement on the patient report. Normal cortical thickness is 1 to 1.5 cm when the arcuate arteries are used as a landmark for measuring.

INCIDENTAL OBSERVATIONS OF IMPORTANCE

Atherosclerotic involvement of the renal artery nearly always involves the origin and consists of a complicated ath-

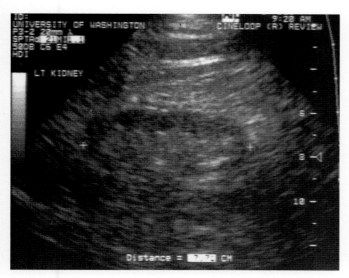

FIGURE 19.19. Pole-to-pole kidney length, abnormal length showing atrophied kidney with hyperechoic parenchymal tissue.

erosclerotic plaque. Calcification in these lesions is common. They can be recognized as highly echogenic structures with acoustic shadowing (Fig. 19.21).

Renal vein thrombosis may occur with renal carcinoma, nephrotic syndrome, trauma, renal transplantation, infant dehydration, and compression of the renal vein secondary to an extrinsic tumor. The renal vein will be dilated at a point proximal to the occlusion, and in many cases, thrombus may be visualized in the vessel lumen. In the acute phase, the thrombus may appear isoechoic to the surrounding blood, there will be no venous flow identified with the Doppler, and there will be an enlargement of the affected kidney with a loss of the normal renal architecture. In long-standing cases, the thrombus generally appears as an echogenic foci, and there may be abnormal, continuous venous flow identified with the Doppler.

Kidney Parenchymal Abnormalities

It is important for the vascular technologist or ultrasonographer performing the study to have a working knowledge of parenchymal abnormalities that will be seen on occasion. For a review of congenital anomalies, cystic diseases, obstructive uropathy, inflammatory diseases, infiltrative diseases, neoplasms, and renal failure, it is recommended that a general ultrasound textbook be consulted. In our clinical vascular laboratory, if we encounter changes in the kidney parenchyma not related to vascular disease, the referring physician is informed. These patients are then often scheduled for a general ultrasound examination or a computed tomography scan.

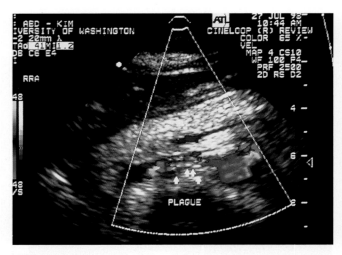

FIGURE 19.21. B-mode color image of the aorta in cross-section, with the right renal artery *(RRA)* sagittal view documenting echo-dense plaque along the posterior wall, beginning at the origin and extending to proximal level.

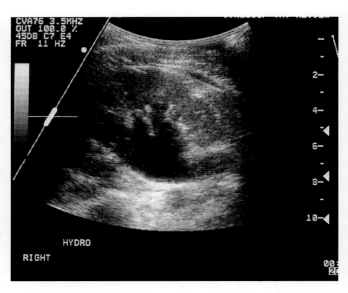

FIGURE 19.23. B-mode image of moderate hydronephrosis of right kidney. Note dilated calyxes.

Renal Cysts

Renal cysts are fairly common, and ultrasound is an excellent modality for separating a cystic from a solid lesion. The most frequent type of renal cyst is a simple serous fluid collection originating in the renal cortex (Fig. 19.22). Single cysts are more common, but they can be multiple, although they rarely number more than four per kidney. They have an epithelial lining and may contain some septation or loculation. These cysts can be located anywhere in the kidney, including the adjacent tissues of the renal pelvis (peripelvic cyst). For ultrasonographic differential diagnosis, these lesions must meet classic cyst criteria: (a) clear, smooth wall demarcation, especially a sharply defined far wall; (b) spheric or slightly ovoid

shape; (c) absence of internal echoes; and (d) acoustic enhancement beyond the cyst, as compared with the intensity of echoes of normal adjacent renal parenchyma.

Parapelvic cysts are located in the renal hilus and have no communication with the collecting system. Parapelvic cysts develop from lymphatic or other nonparenchymal tissues. In practice, however, the term is frequently applied incorrectly to describe renal cysts that originate near the hilus and extend anterior or posterior to the renal pelvis. Ultrasonographically, its hilar location should differentiate a pararenal cyst from a perirenal cyst.

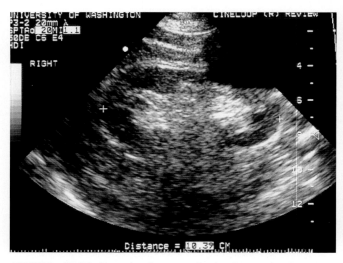

FIGURE 19.22. B-mode image of simple cystic structure attached to cortex of right kidney.

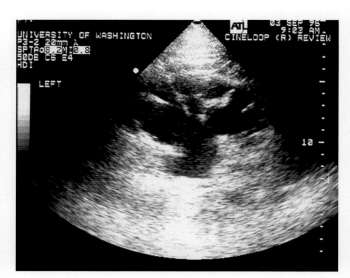

FIGURE 19.24. B-mode image of severe hydronephrosis of left kidney, with no functioning parenchyma tissue present due to surgical ligation of ureter.

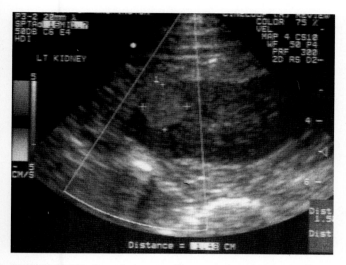

FIGURE 19.25. B-mode image of hypernephroma (renal cell carcinoma) of left kidney, stage II. Note the well-defined walls and hyperechoic echogenicity of mass. The anechoic areas surrounding mass are vascular flow.

Hydronephrosis

Hydronephrosis represents dilatation of the renal pelvis, calyceal structures, and infundibula and may have an intrinsic or extrinsic cause. The ultrasonographic hallmark of hydronephrosis is splaying, spreading, or ballooning of the central echo complex. It may be difficult to distinguish mild hydronephrosis from conditions that stimulate it, including normal variations, increased urine flow, inflammatory disease, renal cystic disease, and other causes, such as postsurgical dilatation and renal sinus lipomatosis. If hydronephrosis is identified, it is important to have the patient void and repeat the scan to avoid a misdiagnosis resulting from a full

bladder, overhydration, diuresis secondary to medications, and so forth (Figs. 19.23 and 19.24).

Renal Masses

It is important that the vascular technologist or ultrasonographer be able to identify any renal masses that may be seen. The report should note their location, describe the ultrasonographic appearance, and document whether the mass has vascular flow (Fig. 19.25). For the purpose of this chapter, further descriptions of renal masses are not covered.

DIAGNOSTIC CRITERIA FOR DISEASE CLASSIFICATION

Renal Arteries

The estimation of the percentage of diameter reduction of the renal arteries is based on the velocity at the site of narrowing and the renal/aortic ratio (RAR). To calculate the RAR, the highest peak systolic velocity (PSV) found in the renal artery is divided by the aortic PSV taken at or above the level of the SMA (suprarenal aortic velocity). The RAR should not be calculated and used for disease classification if the aortic velocity is less than 50 cm/sec because the RAR may be overestimated.

Normal

The normal renal artery waveform should have a sharp systolic upstroke with a low-resistance forward flow throughout diastole because it is supplying a low-resistance vascular bed. The renal artery along its length will have velocities of less than 180 cm/sec, with no focal velocity increase in flow or abnormal flow patterns, such as poststenotic turbulence.

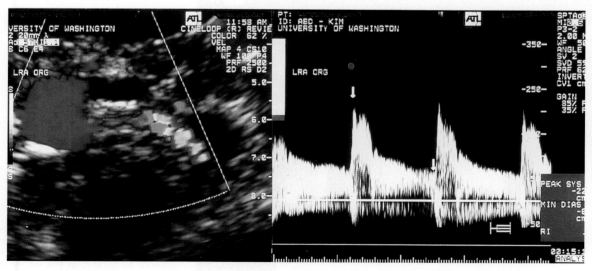

FIGURE 19.26. B-mode color image of the aorta in cross-section, with the left renal artery *(LRA)* sagittal view documenting echo-dense plaque along the anterior wall, beginning at the origin and extending to the proximal level. The accompanying Doppler spectral waveform shows peak systolic velocity of 228 cm/sec and end-diastolic velocity of 66 cm/sec.

Less than 60% Diameter Reduction

The renal artery will have a focal velocity increase present with velocities greater than or equal to 180 cm/sec, with abnormal flow patterns such as poststenotic turbulence. There may be plaque visualized on the B-mode image (Fig. 19.26). The RAR will be less than 3.5.

Greater than or Equal to 60% Diameter Reduction

The renal artery will have a focal velocity increase present with velocities greater than or equal to 180 cm/sec, with abnormal flow patterns such as poststenotic turbulence or a Doppler bruit. There may be plaque visualized on the B-mode image. The RAR will be greater than or equal to 3.5 (Fig. 19.27).

Occluded

There will be no arterial flow detected in the renal artery. The kidney length is typically less than 9 cm. If flow is detected in the kidney parenchyma, it is usually less than 10 cm/sec. *Note*: With the improvements in the gray-scale image on the duplex scanners, the presence and location of visualized plaque are now included in the description of the renal artery.

Renovascular Resistance

The diastolic/systolic ratio (DSR) is calculated to *estimate* renovascular resistance using the parenchymal flows obtained in the medulla and cortex of the kidneys. The end-diastolic velocity (EDV) is divided by the PSV to calculate the DSR.

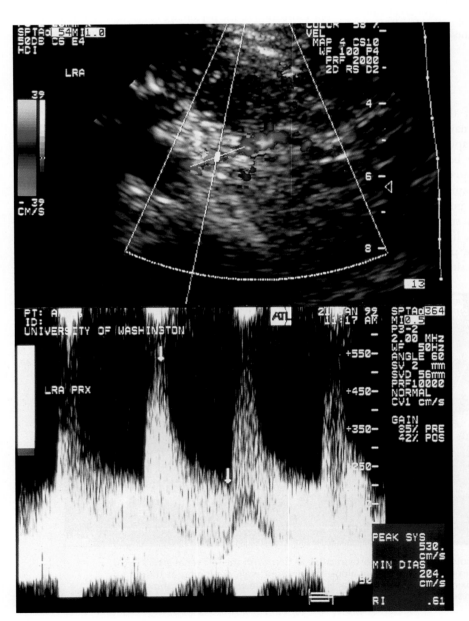

FIGURE 19.27. B-mode image of aorta (anechoic structure to the *left of color box*) with echogenic plaque present in aorta anterior to takeoff of the left renal artery. Doppler spectral waveform of the proximal left renal artery, showing peak systolic velocity of 530 cm/sec and end-diastolic velocity of 204 cm/sec (the patient's renal/aortic ratio *[RAR]* was 9.26).

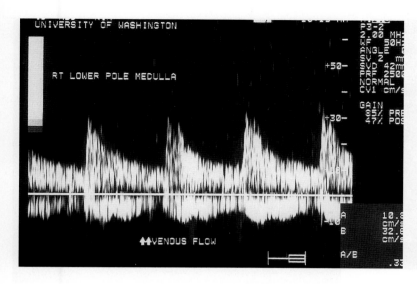

FIGURE 19.28. Doppler spectral waveform of normal renovascular resistance. The diastolic/systolic ratio *(DSR)* is 0.33.

- *Normal low renovascular resistance*: a DSR greater than or equal to 0.30 (Fig. 19.28)
- *Borderline increased renovascular resistance*: a DSR between 0.20 to 0.30
- *Increased renovascular resistance*: a DSR equal to or less than 0.20 (Fig. 19.29)

It has been shown in patients with severe renal artery stenosis that low renal cortical blood flow velocity is correlated with renal atrophy and elevations of serum creatinine. It was shown that patients who had renal cortical PSV of less than 15 cm/sec and EDV of less than 5 cm/sec had a higher incidence of renal atrophy (8).

Additional Notes Regarding Renal Evaluations

Renal Artery Bypass Grafts

Renal artery bypass grafts are evaluated following the same technique as a native renal artery, keeping in mind that the proximal anastomosis may be inferior or superior to the normal anatomic takeoff of the renal artery. It is important to obtain a copy of the operative report before beginning the duplex scan. Special attention should be paid to the proximal anastomosis site with transverse views used to obtain antero-posterior and width measurements because vein grafts tend to become aneurysmal over time (Fig. 19.30).

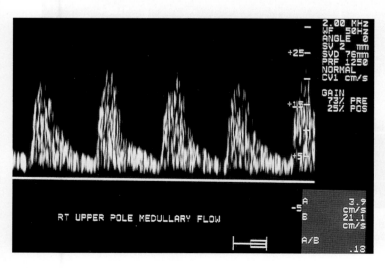

FIGURE 19.29. Doppler spectral waveform of abnormal renovascular resistance. The diastolic/systolic ratio *(DSR)* is 0.18.

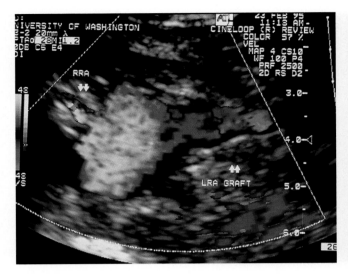

FIGURE 19.30. B-mode color image of the aorta in cross-section, with right renal artery *(RRA)* stenosis and dilatation of a left renal artery *(LRA)* bypass graft.

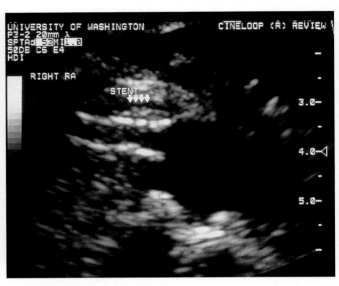

FIGURE 19.32. B-mode image of right renal artery stent (posterior wall extending into aorta).

Renal Artery Stents and Angioplasty

Stents and angioplasty are evaluated following the same technique as the native renal artery, distinguishing residual stenosis from recurrent stenosis (Fig. 19.31). Special attention is paid to the B-mode image, attempting to identify the exact location of the stent, which is easily visualized because of the bright reflections from the stents (Fig. 19.32).

It is important to document whether the stent extends into the aorta, and if so, how far. Any residual plaque or intraluminal echoes are noted for follow-up evaluation, which is helpful in distinguishing residual stenosis from recurrent stenosis.

Fibromuscular Dysplasia

FMD typically presents in the middle to distal portion of the renal artery, and the patient is most commonly a young or middle-aged woman. Therefore, special attention is directed to the middle and distal segments of the renal artery. Depending on the patient's body habitus, the classic string-of-beads appearance may be visualized on the B-mode image, but typically what is found is a long segment of diffuse narrowing (Fig. 19.33). If FMD is suspected, the mesenteric and carotid arteries should also be evaluated because the disease may be found there as well.

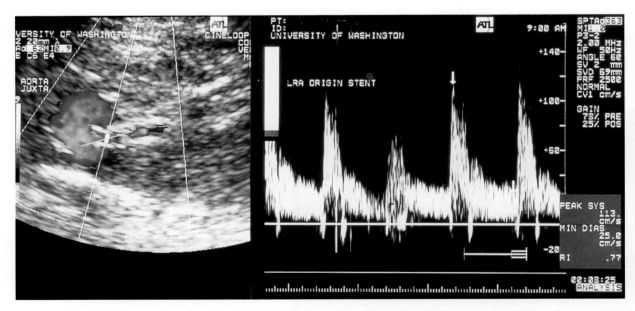

FIGURE 19.31. B-mode color image of the aorta, with left renal artery stent (bright echoes of stent struts) and accompanying normal Doppler spectral waveform.

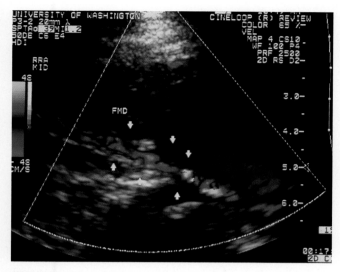

FIGURE 19.33. B-mode color image of fibromuscular dysplasia *(FMD)* of the middle right renal artery *(RRA)*. Note the mosaic color pattern due to multiple areas of narrowing.

LIMITATIONS AND PITFALLS

The limitations and pitfalls of the indirect or hilar evaluation have previously been covered. When performing the direct or transabdominal renovascular evaluation, there are also limitations that are encountered. Evaluating the entire renovascular system can be time-consuming. We allow 1 hour to perform the evaluation. This does not include the paperwork and analysis required for the evaluation, which can take up to 30 minutes to complete. About 5% of examinations will be incomplete because of depth of the vessels, bowel gas, uncooperative patients, respiratory motion due to severe cardiac or pulmonary problems, and inability to reposition the patient due to arterial lines, recent invasive procedures, and so forth. Performing a thorough renovascular evaluation does require meticulous technique, and the velocities may be underestimated or overestimated because of incorrect Doppler angles being used. Also, accessory vessels may not always be visualized using this approach.

REPORTING AND INTERPRETATION

Interpreting a renovascular duplex scan requires assessing all aspects of the duplex scan. The questions involved with interpreting a renovascular evaluation are as follows:

1. Does the aorta have any plaque, thrombus, or aneurysm formation? Is there normal flow throughout the aorta, with diastolic flow above the renal artery level?
2. Are the renal veins patent? What is the flow pattern?
3. Were the renal artery velocities greater than 180 cm/sec with poststenotic turbulence present?

4. Was there any plaque visualized at the ostium of the renal artery or at any other site?
5. What was the RAR?
6. Were the pole-to-pole kidney length measurements normal?
7. What were the parenchymal tissue characteristics; for example, was the tissue hyperechoic in one kidney versus the contralateral kidney?
8. Were there any cysts or masses present?
9. What was the cortical thickness?
10. Were the medullary and cortical velocities normal? Was the cortical PSV greater than 15 cm/sec? Was the cortical EDV greater than 5 cm/sec?

Following the above steps will allow you to interpret any renovascular evaluation whether it is a baseline or postintervention evaluation.

RENAL TRANSPLANTS (ALLOGRAFTS)

Renal transplants have become a standard treatment for chronic renal failure (14–16). The surgical procedure involves rotation of the donor kidney, placing it in the contralateral iliac fossa. The allograft renal artery usually has an end-to-side anastomosis. The renal artery may be anastomosed to the common iliac, hypogastric, or external iliac artery; hence, it is helpful to obtain an operative report before beginning the duplex scan. The renal vein is anastomosed end to side with the iliac vein. The renal hilar structures are medial to the renal parenchyma, but the surgical placement changes the orientation so that the renal pelvis is most anterior, the renal vein is posterior, and the renal artery is between them. The allograft ureter is anastomosed into the bladder above the normal ureteral orifice through a submucosal tunnel in the bladder wall. The tunnel creates a valve in the terminal bladder to prevent reflux of urine into the transplanted kidney. The patient's own kidneys and ureters are usually not removed. The superficial location of the transplanted kidney allows excellent ultrasonographic delineation of its anatomy and pathology.

After transplantation, the kidney may undergo normal renal hypertrophy. A duplex scan should be performed within the first 48 to 72 hours to determine shape and echo characteristics, establish baseline measurements and renal volume, and evaluate the renal and perirenal area to rule out hemorrhage or fluid. The patient is scanned in a supine position with a full, but not distended, urinary bladder. Images can often be obtained by scanning along the incision, angling toward the allograft and obtaining the images along the anatomic coronal plane. Immediate posttransplantation Doppler evaluation establishes the baseline for monitoring the response to immunosuppressive therapy, rules out vascular occlusion, and detects renal artery stenosis. A transplanted kidney should have similar waveform characteristics and velocities to a native kidney, with the exception that there may be a slight amount of turbulence at the anastomosis of the main renal artery with the inflow vessel (usually secondary to angle or vessel diameter discrepancies). Renal venous waveforms should be obtained from the renal parenchyma, renal hilus, and main renal vein and should have phasic flow present.

Rejection has been identified ultrasonographically by noting enlarged pyramids or decreased echogenicity (edema), congestion, and hemorrhage of the interstitial tissues. There may be hyperechogenicity of the cortex, which is thought to be related to ischemia and cellular infiltration of the cortex. Necrosis and liquefaction are seen as patchy anechoic areas in the parenchyma, usually in the polar regions. Parenchymal distortion and compression of the renal sinus echoes reflects the generalized edema, cellular infiltration, and vascular congestion of the rejecting renal allograft. A normal duplex evaluation does not rule out rejection.

In the early stages of rejection, Doppler evaluation has been of limited value. However, it can be useful in moderate to severe rejection, in which the edema causes increased resistance to flow. It is very useful in documenting a change in the pattern of blood flow, with a very sharp systolic upstroke and increased resistance noted in diastole and with flow closer to baseline.

Acute tubular necrosis (ATN) is the most common cause of acute posttransplantation renal failure and is more common in cadaver transplants. ATN usually resolves early in the postoperative period. Uncomplicated ATN is often reversible and can be treated by immediate use of diuretics and satisfactory hydration. The diagnosis is commonly one of exclusion. Associated with the ultrasonographic appearance of no changes seen within the renal parenchyma, a clinical history and laboratory values indicative of acute renal failure suggest the diagnosis of ATN.

Obstructive nephropathy occurs in 1% to 10% of transplant recipients. The causes of obstructive uropathy include ureteral necrosis, intrinsic blockage, stricture formation, and extrinsic pressure from any pelvis mass.

Renal vein thrombosis is predominately a postsurgical complication due to ischemic alteration of the vessel wall or placement of the graft into too tight a retroperitoneal space. The ultrasonographic parenchymal findings of acute renal vein thrombosis include immediate kidney enlargement, increased cortical thickness, sparsely distributed cortical echoes, diminished echogenicity of the renal cortex, indistinct corticomedullary junction, and hypoechoic regions within the renal parenchyma due to hemorrhage, dilated renal vein, or renal rupture. The primary documentation is done by performing a Doppler evaluation of the renal vein, which typically shows no venous flow. Intraluminal echoes may be present depending on the age of the thrombus (it may appear anechoic), and the vein proximal to the thrombus will be dilated.

Renal artery occlusion may be due to technical difficulties at the time of surgery or to severe rejection. If no arterial signals are obtained and technical factors have been excluded, arterial occlusion is probably present. Segmental infarction may be documented by the absence of arterial signals within one portion of the kidney when signals are normal elsewhere. Renal artery stenosis is documented following the same criteria as a native renal artery, with the exception that a renal/iliac ratio (RIR) may be used to determine the degree of stenosis because the common iliac artery has now become the inflow vessel for the renal artery. The literature varies concerning the RIR value, ranging from 3.0 to 3.5 for a greater than 60% diameter reduction. One of the reasons for this variation is the size discrepancy between the renal artery and the iliac artery.

REFERENCES

1. Goldblatt H, Lynch J, Hanzal RF, et al. Studies on experimental hypertension. I. The production of persistent elevation of systolic blood pressure by means of renal ischemia. *J Exp Med* 1934;59:347–379.
2. Hoffman U, Edwards JM, Carter S, et al. Role of duplex scanning for the detection of atherosclerotic renal artery disease. *Kidney Int* 1991;39:1232–1239.
3. Kohler TR, Zierler RE, Martin RL, et al. Noninvasive diagnosis of renal artery stenosis by ultrasonic duplex scanning. *J Vasc Surg* 1986;4:450–456.
4. Handa N, Fukuanga R, Etani H, et al. Efficacy of echo-Doppler examination for the evaluation of renovascular disease. *Ultrasound Med Biol* 1988;14:1–5.
5. Stavros AT, Parker SH, Yakes WF, et al. Segmental stenosis of the renal artery: pattern recognition of tardus and parvus abnormalities with duplex sonography [see Comments]. *Radiology* 1992;184:487–492.
6. Jacobsen HR. Ischemic renal disease: an overlooked clinical entity? *Kidney Int* 1988;34:729–743.
7. Caps MT, Perissinotto, C, Zierler RE, et al. Prospective study of atherosclerotic disease progression in the renal artery. *Circulation* 1998;98(25):2866–2872.
8. Caps MT, Zierler RE, Polissar NL, et al. Risk of atrophy in kidneys with atherosclerotic renal artery stenosis. *Kidney Int* 1998;53:735–742.
9. Martin B, Nanra RS, Wlodarczyk J, et al. Renal hilar Doppler analysis in the detection of renal artery stenosis. *J Vasc Technol* 1991;15:173–180.
10. Tullis MJ, Zierler RE, Glickerman DJ, et al. Results of percutaneous transluminal angioplasty for atherosclerotic renal artery stenosis: a follow-up study with duplex ultrasonography. *J Vasc Surg* 1997;25:46–54.
11. Edwards JM, Zaccardi MJ, Strandness DE Jr. A preliminary study of the role of duplex scanning in defining the adequacy of treatment of patients with renal artery fibromuscular dysplasia. *Vasc Surg* 1992;15:604–609.
12. Hagen-Ansert SL. *Kidneys and adrenal gland*. St. Louis: CV Mosby, 1989.
13. Kawamura DM. *Abdomen*, 3rd ed. Philadelphia: JB Lippincott, 1992.
14. Sorrell K, Blacksher DFM. Diagnosis of occlusive renal vein thrombosis in renal allografts by duplex ultrasonography. *J Vasc Technol* 1992;11916:123.
15. Peterson L, Blackburn D, Astleford P, et al. Duplex evaluation of renal transplant perfusion. *J Vasc Technol* 1989; 3:81–85.
16. Sollinger H. Renal transplant surgery. In: Johnson RFJ, ed. *Comprehensive clinical nephrology*, 1st ed. 2000:87.1–87.8.

20

PORTAL AND MESENTERIC CIRCULATION

MICHAEL BERTOGLIO

Diseases of the mesenteric circulation are infrequent but serious problems that may threaten the life of the patient. The problems present in two major ways, with the first and most catastrophic being acute superior mesenteric artery (SMA) occlusion. When this occurs, the patient develops a sudden, catastrophic, cramping abdominal pain. When the patient is first seen and the diagnosis is suspected, no time should be wasted pursuing a duplex study. Rapid restoration of blood flow is mandatory if gut viability is to be maintained and patient survival obtained. The urgency of the case requires immediate restoration of blood flow to the intestine.

If chronic mesenteric angina is suspected, duplex scanning can be of great value. It is well known that for this problem to develop, it is necessary for all three major arterial inputs to the small bowel to be involved (celiac, superior mesenteric, and inferior mesenteric arteries). This is because the collateral blood supply to the gut is so good that nearly all of its major arterial input will have to be compromised. As noted previously, the major inputs to the gut are the SMA, the celiac artery, and the inferior mesenteric artery. All three of these arteries are now accessible for study (1–4). A major advantage of this method is that it can be used for follow-up studies as well.

Use of the provocative feeding test to bring out subclinical cases of chronic mesenteric angina has been disappointing (1,2). Although we still do this test on request, we do not feel that it adds much to our evaluation of the celiac and mesenteric arteries.

Other areas of great clinical interest include the hepatic-portal system and the numerous problems that may involve the blood supply of both arterial and venous systems. The literature on this area is extensive, with topics ranging from cirrhosis of the liver, portosystemic shunts, the Budd-Chiari syndrome, and transplantation (5–15). The vascular laboratory is frequently called on to help sort out problems relating to each of the major areas. As will be noted, the proper use of the vascular diagnostic laboratory requires a good knowledge of the anatomy and of where the particular vessels of interest lie. For most of the applications, we are not asked to define an exact degree of narrowing for a particular vessel; an exception is the hepatic artery after transplantation because failure here occurs in 5% to 10% of patients. For this particular application, studies are often carried out on a regularly scheduled basis to document results.

PORTAL AND MESENTERIC SCAN

We ask that patients have nothing by mouth 12 hours before the scan. Diabetic patients are allowed to take a minimal breakfast and required medications. The transducers needed for mesenteric and portal studies are in general the same as for any abdominal scan. Our preferred scanheads are the low-frequency 2-MHz phased, 3-MHz curved linear, or a 5-MHz phased for a select group of thin patients. A small probe footprint is often helpful, especially when directing the sound beam under or between the ribs (Fig. 20.1). Increasing the color wall filter setting can help to diminish flash artifact from respiratory variation. As anyone who has been doing abdominal scans knows, these patients often have poor acoustic windows for a variety of reasons, including presence of bowel gas, body habitus, and poor access to the organ under investigation. Usually, we use a small sample volume (5 mm) to interrogate the vessels. However, if the patient has chronic obstructive pulmonary disease, the sample volume size may have to be increased. With the smaller sample volume and excessive motion of the rib cage and diaphragm, there may be loss of signal as it moves out of the field of flow. To insonate the portal vein a low Doppler wall filter is often helpful for detecting the low flow that may be present. We also find it helpful to have available a broad range of filter settings both for color wall and Doppler arterial settings.

We usually start out with the patient in a supine position, using a midline approach. Putting the patient in reverse Trendelenburg's position is often helpful to shift the bowels and any bowel gas to the lower abdomen. This

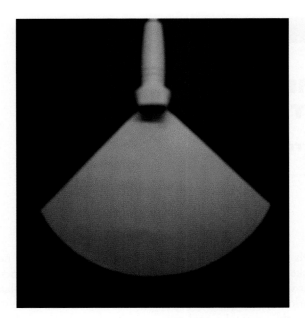

FIGURE 20.1. This transducer with a small footprint is ideal for scanning under or beneath the ribs and through the liver.

provides a better acoustic window for examining the arteries and veins of the upper abdomen. Using the left lateral decubitus position, we can use the liver as an ultrasonographic window (Fig. 20.2). For patients in the intensive care unit, a variety of scanning approaches may be necessary. We may be forced, because of all the equipment in place on and around the patient, to experiment to find the most suitable position for insonating the vessels of interest. The presence of bowel gas may also pose a problem in this setting.

SCANNING SEQUENCES

We use a midline subxiphoid approach to begin the mesenteric scan with a low-frequency transducer. Moving slightly to the left of midline, the aorta will come into view. We always scan the proximal and mid-segments of the abdominal aorta during a mesenteric scan to document the presence of narrowing and aneurysmal disease that might encroach on the orifices of the celiac and mesenteric arteries. Moving the probe more proximal and angling cephalad, the SMA and celiac artery will now come into view (Fig. 20.3). Before considering the abnormal findings with this disease, it is important to realize what the normal velocity waveforms look like when taken just beyond the orifices of these major arteries (Fig. 20.4). As noted in Fig. 20.4, the celiac artery supplies the liver and spleen, which have a very low resistance to flow; thus, the end-diastolic velocity should normally be above zero. With the SMA under fasting flow conditions, it is a high-resistance arterial bed. In this setting, there will be a brief period of reverse flow, as shown. The mesenteric arteries may come off at acute angles that will require angle correction to obtain accurate velocity signals. When a stenosis is apparent, a dramatic increase in the peak systolic velocity (PSV) is noted (Fig. 20.5). Poststenotic turbulence is often noted as well.

Normally, the celiac axis lies slightly cephalad to the origin of the SMA. One variant to note is the presence of a common origin for the celiac artery and SMA. By starting at the origin of the celiac artery, it is possible to trace the vessel to its branches into the splenic and common hepatic arteries. Increased velocities in the celiac axis can be due to compression by the median arcuate ligament (Fig. 20.6). When this is suspected, it is necessary for the patient to take

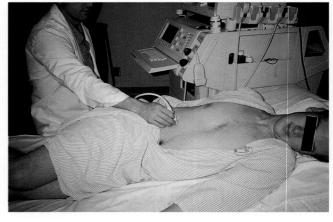

FIGURE 20.2. This illustrates the left lateral decubitus position, which is often used for portal mesenteric scanning.

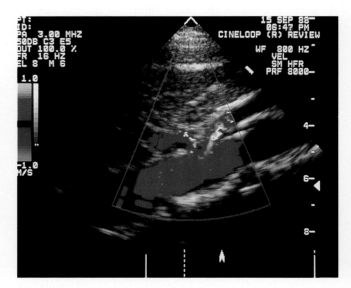

FIGURE 20.3. In this longitudinal color Doppler, both the celiac and superior mesenteric arteries come in view. When atherosclerosis affects these arteries, it is at the origin.

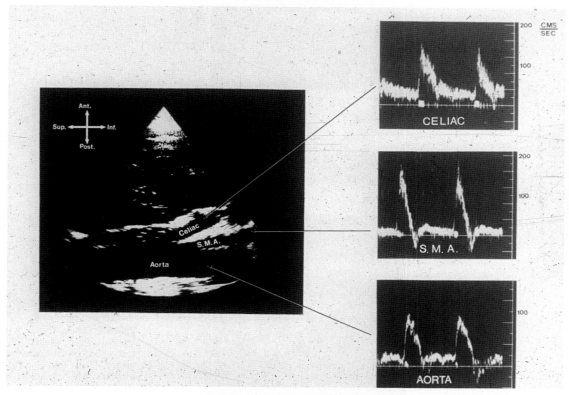

FIGURE 20.4. The normal velocity waveforms from the celiac and superior mesenteric arteries and aorta are shown. These were taken under fasting conditions. With the celiac artery, the end-diastolic flow is above the zero baseline. The superior mesenteric artery demonstrates a brief but definite reverse flow component.

a deep breath, with which the velocity in the celiac artery will normalize (Fig. 20.7).

The inferior vena cava (IVC) lies posterior to the liver on the posterior side of the peritoneal cavity. Normally, flow in the IVC is spontaneous and phasic with respiration. More cephalad segments of the IVC tend to be more pulsatile because of closer vicinity to the right heart. When scanning the IVC, we look for the following:

1. The phasic nature of the flow is important because very pulsatile velocity signals are often seen in patients with congestive heart failure.
2. If there is external compression of the IVC, a focal increase in velocity may be observed.
3. If the patient has had an IVC filter placed, we can determine its position and the flow through it (Fig. 20.8). On occasion, it is possible to visualize trapped thrombi in the cage.
4. If the IVC is occluded, it may appear as a small atretic vessel.
5. Thrombi may be seen on occasion. If they are chronic, they may appear as a bright echo.

To identify the extrahepatic portal vein, we return to the SMA and celiac axis, locating the common hepatic artery and following it to the porta hepatis, where the main portal vein is identified superior to the artery (Fig. 20.9). The extrahepatic portal segment is tortuous as it enters the liver; hence, it is important to tilt the scanhead to get a correct angle on the vein. Normal flow in the extrahepatic portal vein is spontaneous and toward the liver (hepatopetal). The normal flow pattern is semicontinuous with little respiratory variation. It is helpful to set the flow direction above the line in the same direction as the hepatic artery. Portal vein diameters exceeding 1.3 cm have been associated with portal hypertension (16). Normally, the hepatic artery may not be easy to detect. However, if it appears enlarged, the possibility of the existence of portal hypertension must be entertained. Moving caudally, the splenic vein–superior mesenteric vein confluence comes into view. An enlarged splenic vein is also associated with portal hypertension. Because a splenorenal shunt may be done, it is important to note the size of the splenic vein.

In the liver, the portal and hepatic veins and bile ducts all run in parallel. Their more echogenic shiny endothelial layer more easily identifies portal veins. The hepatic veins are more easily identified in a longitudinal view as they drain into the IVC. Hepatic veins are generally more

(*Text continues on page 324.*)

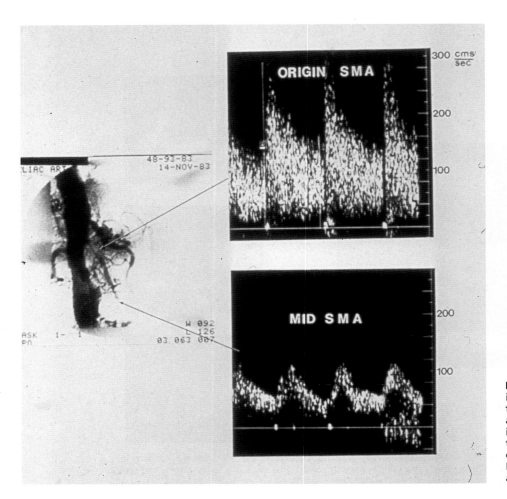

FIGURE 20.5. There is a dramatic increase in peak systolic velocity at the orifice of the superior mesenteric artery. The peak systolic velocity increase falls off rapidly, as shown by that recorded from the mid-segment of the superior mesenteric artery. Even at this level, the waveform is abnormal.

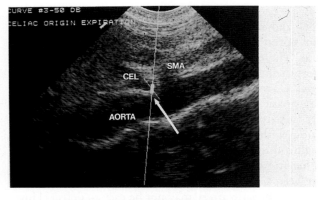

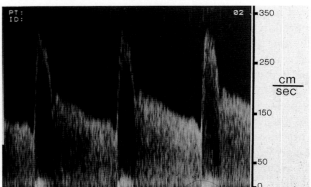

FIGURE 20.6. With compression of the celiac axis by the crus of the diaphragm, a high-velocity signal can be recorded from the celiac artery during expiration. This also creates a bruit, which can be heard.

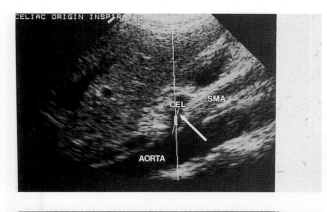

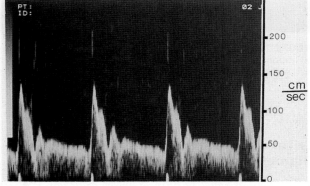

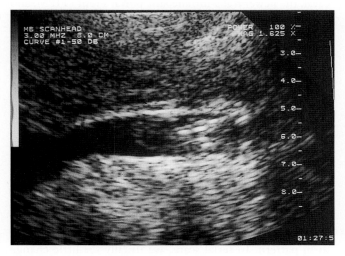

FIGURE 20.7. During inspiration, the high-velocity signal normalizes, and the audible bruit disappears.

FIGURE 20.8. This longitudinal B-mode image of the inferior vena cava clearly demonstrates the location of the Greenfield filter. A thrombus is visible both within the cage and attached to the distal end.

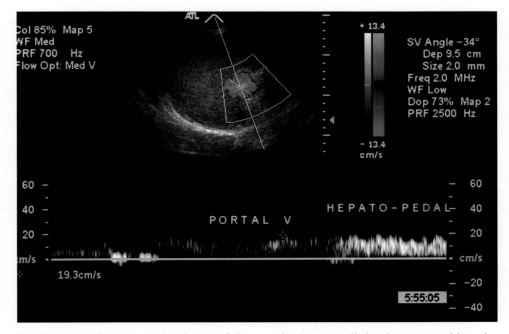

FIGURE 20.9. This cross-sectional view of the portal vein can easily be demonstrated by color Doppler.

pulsatile in terms of waveform signature than the portal vein. We are often asked to identify the patency of the hepatic veins when the Budd-Chiari syndrome is suspected.

Ultrasound has proved invaluable in identifying portosystemic shunts as well as the direction of flow. A variety of shunts are referred to us, including portacaval, mesocaval, the newer trans-intrahepatic portal shunt (TIPS), and splenorenal shunts.

Turbulent flow is normal for a working portacaval shunt. A midline approach using the liver as a window is often useful. TIPS are easily identified in the liver because of their bright edge.

Reflectors

High-velocity flow, sometimes more than 100 cm/sec, is normal for a TIPS, whereas velocities under 25 cm/sec are associated with worsening shunt function. Splenorenal shunts are best viewed from the flank, with a left side lateral decubitus position. As in the case of portacaval shunts, high-velocity turbulent flow is the normal waveform pattern. In serial scans, we usually see little change between visits; either the shunt is patent, or it is occluded. When a shunt is working, flow in the intrahepatic portal vein is usually hepatofugal because the venous flow channel takes the path of least resistance, out of the liver.

DIAGNOSTIC CRITERIA

As noted previously, for chronic mesenteric angina to develop, it is necessary to have involvement of all three potential inputs to the small bowel. These are the superior mesenteric, celiac, and inferior mesenteric arteries. Until we had color flow available and became more facile with studies of the abdominal aorta, it was often difficult to visualize the inferior mesenteric artery. It is now a routine part of our examination, but we have not established firm Doppler criteria for determining the degree of diameter reduction (Fig. 20.10). However, if a high-velocity signal is noted along with poststenotic turbulence or the appearance of a bruit, this is taken as sufficient evidence that it is severely narrowed.

A variety of velocity parameters have been developed for documenting the degree of narrowing of the superior mesenteric and celiac arteries. Although these criteria are adequate for classification purposes, it has been our experience that both of these major inputs to the small bowel must be severely narrowed or occluded before symptoms develop.

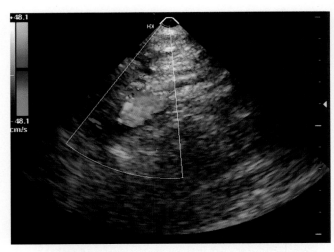

FIGURE 20.10. This longitudinal color Doppler view of the distal abdominal aorta delineates the origin of the inferior mesenteric artery. This is routinely looked for in patients who are suspected of having chronic mesenteric angina.

Criteria for Determining the Degree of Diameter Reduction

- *Less than or equal to 69% diameter reduction*: PSV less than 275 cm/sec in SMA, less than 200 cm/sec in celiac artery
- *70% to 99% diameter reduction*: PSV more than 275 cm/sec in SMA with poststenotic turbulence, more than 200 cm/sec in celiac artery
- *Occlusion*: absence of Doppler signal

Portal Vein

Normal Findings

1. Superior mesenteric vein: flow phasic with respiration, direction of flow toward the confluence of the main portal vein (hepatopetal)
2. Splenic vein: flow phasic with respiration, direction of flow toward the confluence of the main portal vein (hepatopetal)
3. Main portal vein: flow phasic with respiration but may be mildly continuous with low mean and peak velocity; some increase during inspiration. Velocities in the main portal vein can vary with posture, exercise, and dietary states. Flow direction will be toward the liver (hepatopetal).
4. Right and left portal veins: will have similar flow patterns to the main portal vein with hepatopetal flow. They branch to right and left lobes of liver.
5. Hepatic veins: have pulsatile components reflecting events in the right atrium. Flow is central toward the IVC, draining out of the liver.

6. IVC: pulsatile flow at hepatic vein level; flow is central toward the right atrium.
7. Liver parenchyma: echogenicity should be consistent, without calcification, tumors, or masses

There should be no fluid around the liver or in the peritoneal spaces.

Abnormal Findings

1. Loss of respiratory variation in superior mesenteric, splenic, and portal veins
2. Bidirectional or reversed flow in portal, splenic, or superior mesenteric vein
3. Diameter of the main portal vein greater than 13 mm
4. Absence of wall motion changes with respiration
5. Absence of venous flow in well-visualized vessels with intraluminal echoes, suggesting occlusion
6. Presence of portosystemic collaterals (coronary, paraesophageal, and umbilical veins, which may appear as a dilated tube structure at porta hepatis ("bull's eye" sign)
7. Extravascular abnormalities present, producing extrinsic compression on the vessels
8. Fluid present around the liver and peritoneal space, suggesting ascites

REFERENCES

1. Moneta GL, Cummings C, Castor J, et al. Duplex ultrasound demonstration of postprandial mesenteric hyperemia in splanchnic circulation collateral vessels. *J Vasc Technol* 1999;15:37–39.
2. Moneta GL, Yeager RA, Dalman R, et al. Duplex ultrasound criteria for diagnosis of splanchnic artery stenosis or occlusion. *J Vasc Surg* 1991;14:511.
3. Taylor DC, Moneta GL, Cramer MM, et al. Extrinsic compression of the celiac artery by the median ligament of the diaphragm: diagnosis by duplex ultrasound. *J Vasc Technol* 1987;11:236–238.
4. Bowersox JC, Zwolak RM, Walsh DB, et al. Duplex ultrasonography in the diagnosis of celiac and mesenteric artery occlusive disease. *J Vasc Surg* 1991;14:780
5. Delinqua M, Elerick C, Green D, et al. Use of Duplex Doppler sonography and color flow imaging to demonstrate hemodynamic changes before and after portosystemic shunts. *JDMS* 1994;10:7–11.
6. Lee R, Moneta G, Cummings C, et al. Duplex ultrasonography of the mesenteric arteries and portal venous system: a review of current applications. *Video Journal of Color Flow Imaging* 1992;2:61–76.
7. Johansen K, Paun M. Ultrasonography of the portal vein. *Surg Clin North Am* 1990;70:181–190.
8. Sorrell K. The role of color flow duplex ultrasonography in portosystemic shunts. *J Vasc Technol* 1995;18:285–293.
9. Helton WS, Montana M, Dwyer D, et al. Duplex sonography accurately assesses portacaval shunt patency. *J Vasc Surg* 1988;8:660–675.
10. Sorrell K, Vingan H, Asarias P, et al. The role of color flow duplex ultrasonography in transjugular intrahepatic portosystemic shunts (TIPS). *J Vasc Technol* 1993;17:235–241.
11. Wozney P, Zaioka A, Bron S, et al. Vascular complications after liver transplantation: a five year experience. *Am J Roentgenol* 1986;147:657–663.
12. Marder D, DeMariano G, Sumkin J, et al. Doppler ultrasound of the hepatic artery and vein performed daily in the first two weeks after orthotopic liver transplantation: useful for diagnosis of acute rejection. *Invest Radiol* 1996;31:173–179.
13. Bolondi L, Mazzioti A, Arienti V, et al. Ultrasonographic study of portal venous system in portal hypertension and after portosystemic shunt operations. *Surgery* 1984;95:261–269.
14. Longo JM, Bilbao JI, Rousseau HP, et al. Transjugular intrahepatic portosystemic shunt: evaluation with Doppler sonography. *Radiology* 1993;186:529–534.
15. Davis P, Van Thiel D, Zajkoa A, et al. Imaging in hepatic transplantation. *Semin Liver Dis* 1989;9:90–101.
16. Bolandi L, Mazzi A, Arenti V, et al. Ultrasonographic study of portal venous system in portal hypertension and after portosystemic shunt operations. *Surgery* 1984;95:261–269.

## 21

DUPLEX STUDIES OF DIALYSIS ACCESS GRAFTS

MOLLY J. ZACCARDI

The placement of dialysis access grafts for the treatment of chronic renal failure is now a commonly performed procedure in the health care system. The type of shunting performed varies a great deal, as shown in Figs. 21.1 and 21.2. These techniques are all designed to provide an arteriovenous shunt of adequate volume flow to permit dialysis. Because these have to be accessed one or more times a week by the placement of needles, it is essential that enough blood flow be available during the dialysis procedure. Multiple problems can develop that lead to failure of the shunting procedure. Many of these problems are unique to the type of shunt used. However, each of the shunt types shown in Figs. 21.1 and 21.2 can be completely evaluated by the vascular diagnostic laboratory. Our laboratory is not involved in a regular ongoing surveillance program to detect problems that may compromise shunt function. Although there have been reports suggesting that such a program can reduce the rate of total shunt occlusion, this remains a controversial subject (1,2).

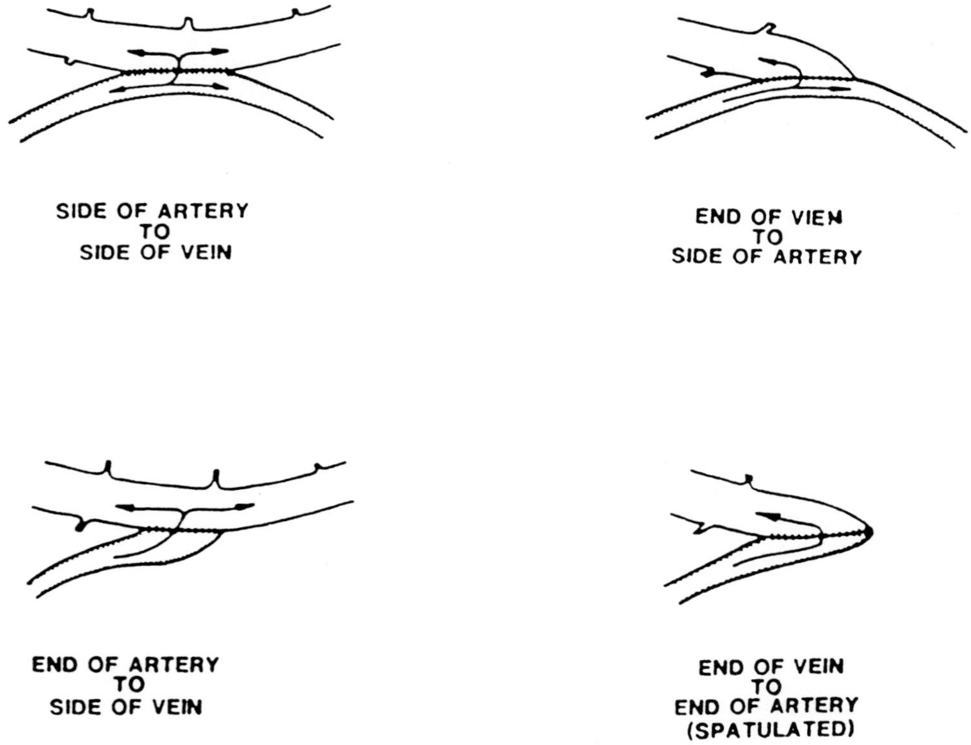

SIDE OF ARTERY
TO
SIDE OF VEIN

END OF VEIN
TO
SIDE OF ARTERY

END OF ARTERY
TO
SIDE OF VEIN

END OF VEIN
TO
END OF ARTERY
(SPATULATED)

FIGURE 21.1. The variety of arteriovenous anastomoses that can be used for renal dialysis access. It is clear from these types of anatomoses how critical it is in the course of a study of these fistulas to know exactly how the reconstruction was made. (From Guthrie CR, Wilson SE. *Vascular disorders of the upper extremity*, 2nd revised ed. Mount Kisco, NY: Futura, 1989:134, with permission).

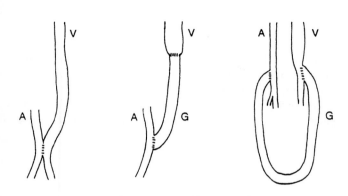

FIGURE 21.2. Examples of other types of fistulas that can be created. The fistula shown is commonly referred to as the *Brescia-Cimino fistula*. (From Tordoir JH, de Bruin HG, Hoenevald H, et al. Duplex ultrasound scanning in the assessment of arteriovenous fistulas created for hemodialysis access: comparison with digital subtraction angiography. *J Vasc Surg* 1989;10:122–128, with permission.)

UNIVERSITY OF WASHINGTON MEDICAL CENTER - VASCULAR DIAGNOSTIC SERVICE

PRE-DIALYSIS ACCESS DUPLEX EXAM   HISTORY _____

_____

DATE   _____

UH#   _____

NAME   _____

D.O.B.   _____

_____

REFERRED BY _____ PHONE _____

ADDRESS _____

DUPLEX FINDINGS   RIGHT   LEFT

SITE	SPONT	PHASIC	AUGMENT	COMPRESS	THROMBUS
RIGHT					
IJV					
BR-CEPH					
SUBCLAV					
AXILLARY					
BRACHIAL					
RADIAL					
ULNAR					
CEPHALIC					
BASILIC					

SITE	SPONT	PHASIC	AUGMENT	COMPRESS	THROMBUS
LEFT					
IJV					
BR-CEPH					
SUBCLAV					
AXILLARY					
BRACHIAL					
RADIAL					
ULNAR					
CEPHALIC					
BASILIC					

CEPHALIC SIZE   BASILIC SIZE   CEPHALIC SIZE

FOR VEIN MAP

sizes in cms

MODIFIED ALLEN'S TEST

RIGHT	Doppler signal change	LEFT
	RADIAL(Ulnar comp)	
	ULNAR(Radial comp)	

A = Augment
NC = No Change
O = Obliterate
R = Reverse

BRACHIAL ARTERY WAVEFORM   Right_____   Left_____

	R	L
TECH		
TAPE #		

PHONE/PRELIMINARY REPORT IN CHART_____

DICTATED_____

DR. SIGNATURE/DISTRIBUTION_____

FIGURE 21.3. A sample worksheet for the preoperative evaluation.

At our institution, duplex studies are requested before shunt creation for assistance in selection of appropriate sites for access construction. The patient population needing dialysis access grafts often has a long history of venous and arterial lines. Obstruction of the inflow and outflow vessels could seriously compromise the outcome of the access graft. Because of this, these vessels are evaluated before graft placement. Vein mapping of the superficial veins and evaluation of the palmar arch are also a routine part of the preoperative evaluation. Protocols describing each of these

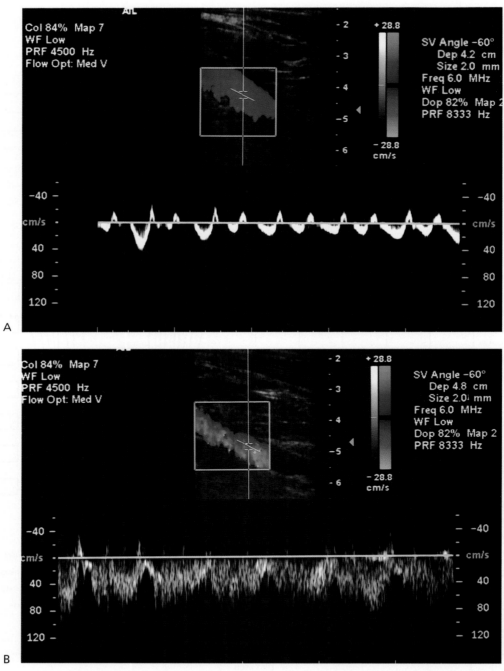

FIGURE 21.4. The differences found in the subclavian artery on the side not used for the access **(A)** as compared with that which is providing the blood to the shunt **(B)**. Note that the velocity scale is reversed so that flow in an antegrade direction is shown below the zero (0) flow line.

methods are covered in other chapters in this book (see Chapters 16, 23, and 24). A sample worksheet for the preoperative evaluation is included in Section IV (see also Fig. 21.3). This chapter will concentrate on evaluation of the existing dialysis access graft.

Ultrasound is an ideal method to provide the imaging and hemodynamic details of the dialysis access because the vessels being evaluated are superficial and are therefore easily seen. It is possible to monitor flow direction, flow velocity, the development of stenoses or occlusion, aneurysmal changes, steals, and hematomas. It is also important at this stage to evaluate both the inflow and outflow vessels. These critical components of the access system can also have lesions that affect the performance of the graft. It is necessary to understand normal flow patterns in both arteries and veins to perform these examinations successfully. A dialysis access graft directly joins the arterial and venous systems. This removes the high-resistance bed on the arterial side of the circulation, shunting the blood into the low-resistance venous system. A complete evaluation of the function of an access graft involves interrogation of the following:

- Entire length of the inflow artery
- Entire length of the outflow conduit
- Site of the arteriovenous anastomosis
- Site from which the blood is drawn for dialysis
- Circulation to the hand, if there is any question about a significant steal being present

As mentioned earlier, the performance of a shunt creates a new hemodynamic situation that is not normally found. A segment of the arterial circulation is converted into an arteriovenous shunt, removing the high-resistance arterioles from the circuit. Thus, the hemodynamic changes recorded during the examination will differ from those usually encountered. For example, the subclavian artery flow patterns seen on the side of a shunt will be entirely different than one might normally expect (Fig. 21.4).

The following paragraphs describe our methods for evaluating the dialysis access graft, followed by some abnormal examples.

EQUIPMENT

The equipment required is a color duplex ultrasound system with a mid-range to superficial range (5 to 10 MHz) transducer. As with other examinations, a printer and videotape recorder are used to document the findings. Color Doppler is valuable because it allows the examiner to detect branches of the artery and vein that may be diverting flow and reducing the chance of the graft to mature. An example of a branch vessel identified with color Doppler is shown in Fig. 21.5.

EQUIPMENT SETTINGS

The color Doppler and Doppler settings should be optimized for recording peak systolic flow velocities of at least 150 cm/sec. The B-mode setting should be optimized for superficial structures. For documentation of flow velocities, it is imperative that all recordings be made with the angle of the sound beam 60 degrees to the long axis of the vessel.

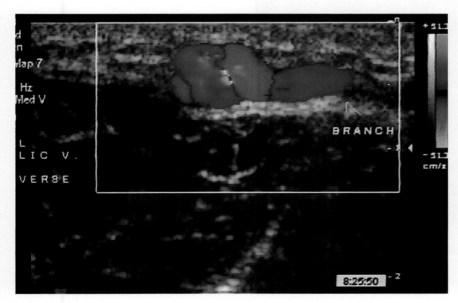

FIGURE 21.5. Cross-sectional color Doppler view of the distal radial artery showing a very large branch artery.

PATIENT PREPARATION

The time required for the examination is anywhere between 30 and 60 minutes. This examination is not done while the patient is undergoing dialysis. It is easiest to perform the examination from the side of the bed with the patient resting the arm comfortably on the bed.

EXAMINATION TECHNIQUE

Before any exam, the technologist must have information about the nature of the shunt and the problem for which the patient is being referred. This description of the examination will assume that an autogenous arteriovenous fistula at the wrist was performed. With the equipment set-

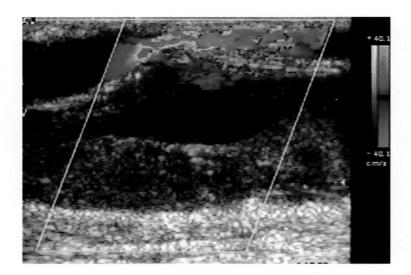

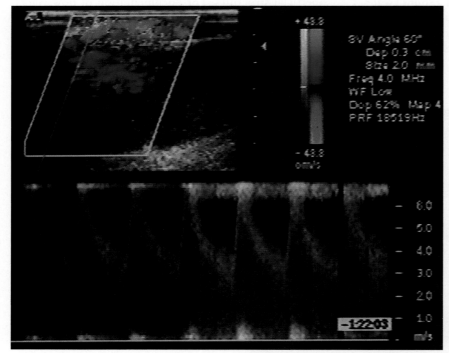

FIGURE 21.6. A very large hematoma that is compressing the access graft, creating a color Doppler bruit and velocity increase.

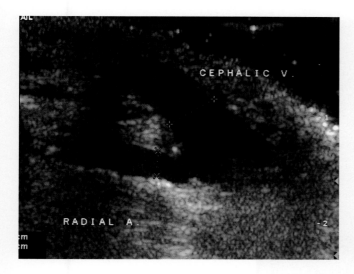

FIGURE 21.7. B-mode image of the large-diameter discrepancy at the anastomosis.

tings optimized to evaluate the subclavian and axillary artery and vein, the patency of those vessels is evaluated and documented. Using equipment settings for studies of superficial vessels, the entire brachial artery is examined in long axis, evaluating the flow velocities. This is done to document any focal velocity increase that may occur as a result of a stenosis. The radial artery is followed down the arm in the same fashion. At this point, it is important to be searching for any branches of the radial artery that may hinder the maturation process (Fig. 21.5). When this is noted, it is helpful to identify the branches on the arm with a permanent marking pen. The anastomosis of the

artery and vein is a common site for velocity increase because the vein and artery may be of different caliber (Fig. 21.6). The anastomosis is also subject to development of intimal hyperplasia and stenosis (Fig. 21.7). If a velocity increase is noted at the anastomosis site, the examiner must optimize the B mode to differentiate stenosis, caliber discrepancy, or extrinsic compression from a hematoma (Fig. 21.8). After the anastomosis has been evaluated, the cephalic vein is followed along the arm to identify any areas of stenosis or branch vessels. It is not uncommon to notice several areas of narrowing along the graft, which are presumably thrombus formation at the

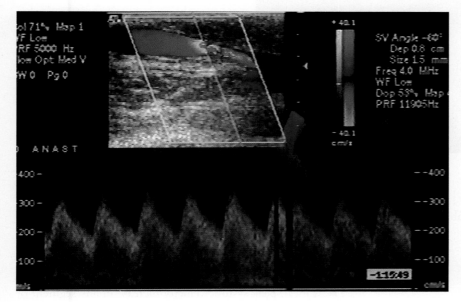

FIGURE 21.8. Color Doppler revealing a significant velocity increase at the site of an anastomosis.

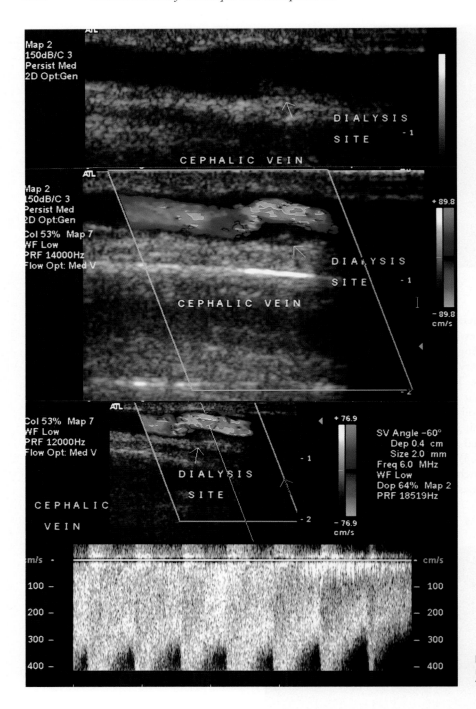

FIGURE 21.9. A high-velocity signal was recorded at the dialysis site with peak systolic velocities in excess of 400 cm/sec.

sites of needle entry during dialysis (Fig. 21.9). Evaluation continues over the entire length of the cephalic vein to the confluence to the axillary vein.

DIAGNOSTIC CRITERIA

Normal findings are described as the following:

■ Low-resistance flow pattern with peak systolic velocities ranging from 100 to 200 cm/sec throughout both the venous and arterial systems
■ Uniform flow velocities without evidence of poststenotic turbulence

Abnormal findings are described as the following:

■ A focal, peak systolic velocity increase in any segment of the graft or inflow and outflow vessels, which produces a

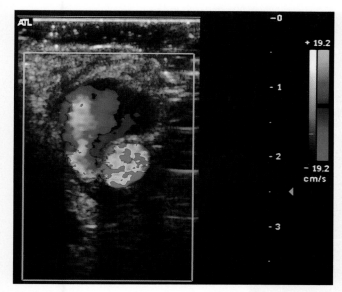

FIGURE 21.10. In cross-section , a pseudoaneurysm is easily seen originating from this Gore-Tex dialysis access graft.

poststenotic flow disturbance. A bruit may also suggest the same.

- Low-flow peak systolic velocities (less than 100 cm/sec) in the distal (venous side) segment of the graft
- Hematoma
- Extrinsic compression due to hematoma

- Large branch vessels
- Visualization of thrombus or intimal hyperplasia
- Aneurysmal dilatation
- Pseudoaneurysm (Fig. 21.10)

INTERPRETATION OF RESULTS

The criteria for establishing a hemodynamically significant stenosis on the arterial side will not be the same as described elsewhere for the grading of arterial lesions. Nonetheless, it is possible to document areas of narrowing and increased flow velocities that might be contributing factors of an access graft not functioning well. The findings that are reported are based on the focal increase in peak systolic velocity and the poststenotic turbulence. Although other methods have been used in reporting the findings, we have resorted to those described earlier as being the simplest and most useful. The reporting methods have included the resistive index, volume flow, and color flow alone (3–6). In our laboratory, the finding of poststenotic turbulence or a bruit in relationship to the site of narrowing indicates a greater than 50% diameter reduction. An example of the poststenotic flow pattern that is often seen in the presence of a stenosis is shown in Fig. 21.11. In addition to reporting sites with significant narrowing, we also report the presence of low flow produced by an area of narrowing. An example of this is shown in Fig. 21.12.

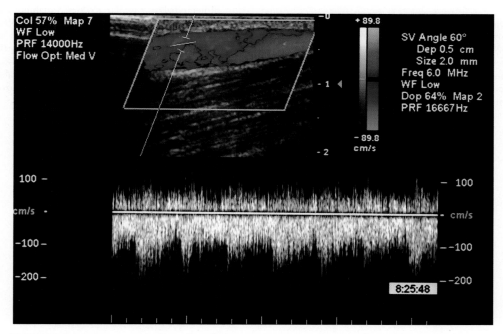

FIGURE 21.11. Poststenotic flow disturbance in the spectral display. As noted in the text, we consider these findings to be consistent with a hemodynamically significant stenosis.

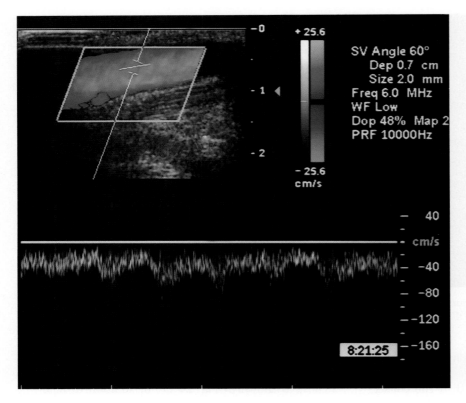

FIGURE 21.12. This case demonstrates a marked reduction in flow velocities distal to a high-grade stenosis.

REFERENCES

1. Schwab SJ, Raymond JR, Saeed M, et al. Prevention of hemodialysis fistula thrombosis: early detection of venous stenosis. *Kidney Int* 1989;36:707–711.
2. Pagano D, Green MA, Henderson MJ, et al. Surveillance policy for early detection of failing arteriovenous fistula for hemodialysis. *Nephrol Dial Transplant* 1994;9:277–279.
3. Baird DE, Omdal DG, Yuill SC, et al. Doppler analysis of hemodialysis grafts: resistive index as a predictor of stenosis. *J Ultrasound Med* 1994;13:791–796
4. Miranda CL. Ultrasound derived flow volumes in the evaluation of hemodialysis vascular accesses: variability due to measurement technique. *J Vasc Technol* 1997;21(3):155–159.
5. Middleton WD, Picus DD, Marx MV, et al. Color Doppler sonography of hemodialysis vascular access: compared with angiography. *Am J Roentgenol* 1989;152:633–639.
6. Finlay DE, Longley DG, Foshager MC, et al. Duplex and color Doppler sonography of hemodialysis arteriovenous fistulas and grafts. *Radiographics* 1993;13:983–999.

## 22

ANEURYSMAL DISEASE

MOLLY J. ZACCARDI

Aortic aneurysms involving the abdominal aorta are commonly referred for study to document exact location and size. This is done to determine whether the dilation is of sufficient size to warrant an aggressive approach for therapy. In addition, the study is often used for comparison when follow-up studies are required. With increasing interest in the application of endovascular therapy for such lesions, the role of the vascular laboratory has been extended not only to the preintervention evaluation but also to follow-up. The studies after endovascular intervention are in the evolutionary phase; thus, the final word on how these may contribute to management remains in question.

Ultrasound is uniquely qualified to evaluate aneurysmal lesions from sites that can be accessed. These include the abdomen, neck, and upper and lower extremities. It is not possible to study thoracic lesions because of the problem of air in the intervening lung. Although the study of these lesions is rather straightforward, it is important to review what can be provided to the referring physician. These include the following:

- Location
- Dimensions—lateral and anteroposterior
- Length
- Presence or absence of coexisting occlusive disease
- Single versus multiple sites (e.g., abdominal, iliac, femoral, popliteal)
- Presence or absence of laminated thrombus
- Flow patterns within and distal to lesion
- Dissection—present—and site
- Presence of coexisting lesions in the renal and superior mesenteric arteries

All this information is helpful in planning therapy. One of the key elements for the abdominal aorta is the relationship to the origin of the renal arteries. Regardless of the form of therapy (surgical or endovascular), the length of the "neck" at the proximal end is of critical importance. It is also important to understand that the ultrasound examination may be followed by computed tomography (CT) scans, which may provide additional information on size, length, and tortuosity. It is also clear that if the lesion is considered suitable for endovascular therapy, a CT scan is mandated.

Although the field is still evolving, it appears that color Doppler studies done after endovascular therapy may be useful and even better than CT scanning for the detection of endovascular leaks. This can be of critical importance because leaks may be responsible for the aneurysm to increase in size, putting the patient at continued risk.

Abdominal aortic aneurysms (AAAs) are described as being saccular, fusiform, or cylindrical (Fig. 22.1). Cylindrical is less uncommon. AAAs often have mural thrombus, which is usually on the anterior wall (1) (Fig. 22.2) and is expected to be the cause of embolization. Most are fusiform in shape, located below the renal arteries (infrarenal) and involving one or both iliac arteries. AAAs are often eccentric in shape and involve one aspect of the aortic wall more severely. Studies report an annual growth rate of AAAs measuring 3 to 5.9 cm in diameter to be 0.23 to 0.28 cm per year (2). Dissection can occur with AAAs but is less common. A dissection will have a false lumen and is documented by visualizing a flap in the transverse plane and by noting the separate flow channel documented by Doppler or color Doppler (Fig. 22.3).

A moderately dilated abdominal aorta is described as *ectatic*. It is reported as *aneurysmal* when the diameter is greater than 3 cm. Normal diameters were reported comparing measurements of aortography to ultrasound, as follows:

Type of Procedure	At 11th Rib (mm)	Above Renal Arteries (mm)	Below Renal Arteries (mm)	At Bifurcation (mm)
Aortography transverse diameter (3)	24	21	19	17
Aortography anteroposterior diameter (4)	25	22	19	15
Ultrasound (4)	23	20	18	15

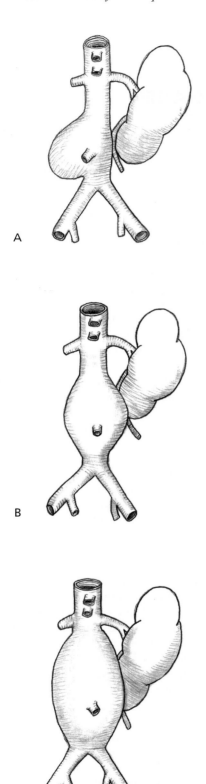

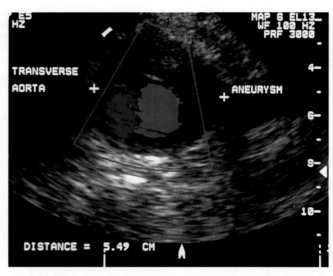

FIGURE 22.2. Mural thrombus in the abdominal aortic aneurysm is most often located on the anterior wall as depicted in this B-mode image.

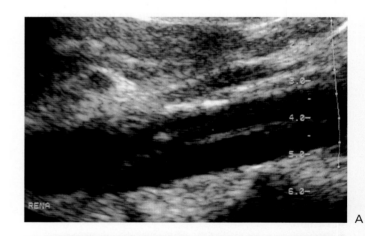

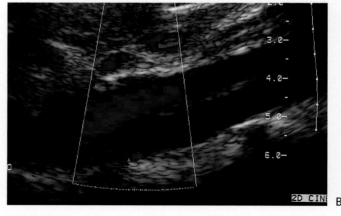

FIGURE 22.1. Three types of aortic aneurysms: **(A)** saccular, **(B)** fusiform, **(C)** cylindrical.

FIGURE 22.3. A dissection of the aorta **(A)** is documented with Doppler by separate flow channels **(B)**.

EQUIPMENT

An ultrasound system with a low-frequency transducer (2 to 4 MHz) is needed to evaluate the aortoiliac segment. A mid-range transducer (4 to 8 MHz) is ideal to rule out femoral or popliteal aneurysms.

PROCEDURE

The patient is evaluated lying supine and is not ordinarily required to fast. For every examination of an aneurysm, the following questions need to be answered: What is the aneurysm's size, shape, location (infrarenal or suprarenal), and distance from other arterial segments (neck)? Is other peripheral arterial disease present? The evaluation includes the following:

- Measure the greatest diameter of the aorta in cross-section (anteroposterior and transverse).
- Measure the length of the AAA.

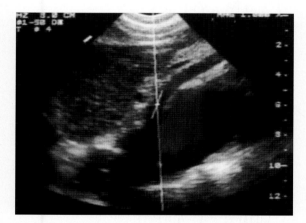

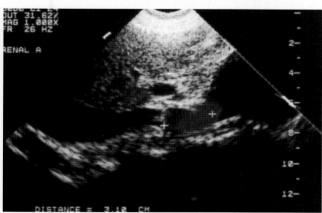

FIGURE 22.4. The length of the neck of the abdominal aortic aneurysm is measured proximally and is absent in **(A)** and present in **(B)**.

- Document the presence of a neck above and below the AAA. In other words, note the point at which a normal diameter is measured and the relationship to the renal arteries proximally and iliac bifurcation distally (Fig. 22.4).
- Describe the presence of mural thrombus.
- Image the iliac, common femoral, and popliteal arteries with B mode to rule out other aneurysms.
- Measure the ankle/brachial indices to screen for peripheral vascular disease.
- A complete arterial duplex examination is not usually performed unless requested.

An example of a worksheet used for documenting is shown in Fig. 22.5.

PITFALLS

The lateral measurements of an AAA are often less accurate because of specular reflection artifact from the vessel wall. The anteroposterior measurement is more reliable (5). A tortuous aorta is also more difficult to measure. It is recommended by some that to avoid an exaggerated reading in oblique, the best view is sagittal with an anteroposterior measurement (6). Obesity and bowel gas may hinder the ability to visualize the renal arteries and to report the proximal neck as infrarenal or suprarenal. Thoracoabdominal aneurysms cannot be evaluated by ultrasound other than describing the abdominal portion of the aneurysm.

PERIPHERAL ARTERY ANEURYSMS

Iliac artery aneurysms cannot be palpated as easily as femoral or popliteal artery aneurysms. Popliteal artery aneurysms account for 70% of the most common type of peripheral artery aneurysms. They are found to be almost entirely atherosclerotic in nature. Popliteal artery entrapment may cause dilatation but is extremely rare. Popliteal artery aneurysms are bilateral 50% of the time; 40% of these patients also have an AAA or femoral artery aneurysm.

The iliac, femoral, and popliteal arteries are considered aneurysmal if the diameter increases to 1.5 to 2 times the preaneurysmal diameter. Ultrasound is easily the most accurate and efficient method to diagnose and follow these patients. The measurements made when a peripheral artery aneurysm is detected include the diameter measurement proximal to the aneurysm. Because peripheral artery and abdominal aortic aneurysms are interrelated, the examination protocol is the same as with an AAA. The worksheet in Fig. 22.6 is an example of the data collected.

UNIVERSITY OF WASHINGTON MEDICAL CENTER - VASCULAR DIAGNOSTIC SERVICE

LOWER EXTREMITY ARTERIAL DUPLEX EXAM   HISTORY _____

_____

DATE   _____

UH#   _____

NAME   _____

D.O.B.   _____

_____

REFERRED BY _____   PHONE _____

ADDRESS _____

RISK FACTORS	
HTN	+
SMOKING	+
DIABETES	—
LIPIDS	+
CAD/PVD	

SYSTOLIC PRESSURES:	R	L
BRACHIAL ARTERY	130	130
POST TIBIAL ARTERY	150	152
ANT TIBIAL ARTERY	152	150
PERONEAL ART		
ANKLE/ARM INDEX	>1.0	>1.0

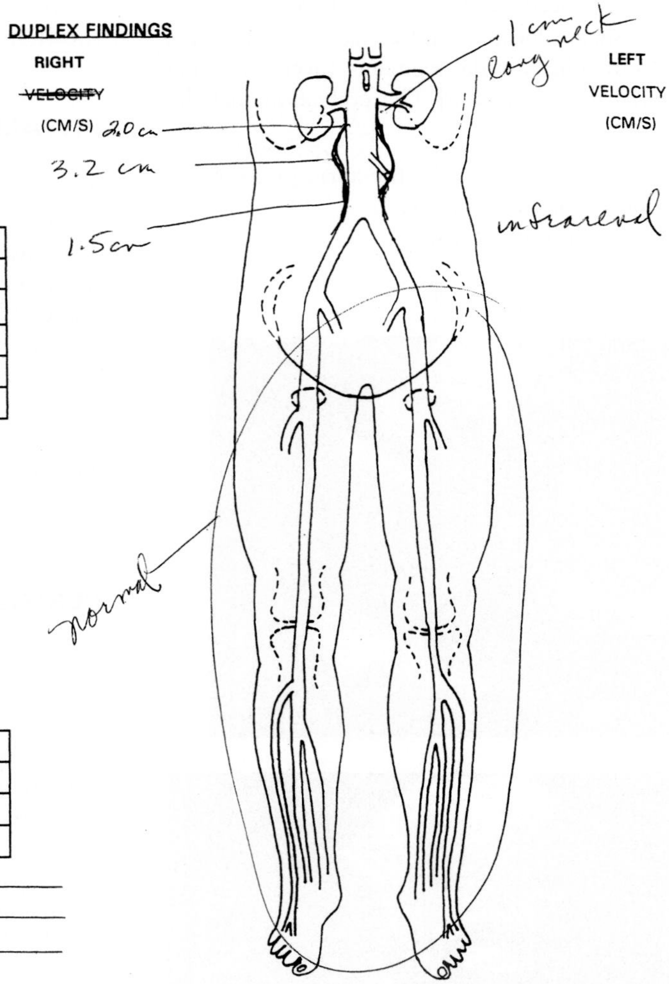

<u>DUPLEX FINDINGS</u>

RIGHT   LEFT

~~VELOCITY~~   VELOCITY

(CM/S) 2.0 cm   (CM/S)

3.2 cm

1.5 cm

1 cm neck
long neck

infrarenal

normal

	RIGHT	LEFT
<u>TECH</u>		
<u>TAPE #</u>		

PHONE/PRELIMINARY REPORT IN CHART:_____

DICTATED:_____

DR. SIGNATURE/DISTRIBUTION:_____

FIGURE 22.5. This worksheet is an example of the data collected for an abdominal aortic aneurysm examination.

UNIVERSITY OF WASHINGTON MEDICAL CENTER - VASCULAR DIAGNOSTIC SERVICE

LOWER EXTREMITY ARTERIAL DUPLEX EXAM   HISTORY _____

DATE   _____

UH#   _____

NAME   _____

D.O.B.   _____

                                  _____

                                  _____

REFERRED BY _____   PHONE _____

ADDRESS _____

RISK FACTORS	
HTN	+
SMOKING	+
DIABETES	—
LIPIDS	?
CAD/PVD	

SYSTOLIC PRESSURES:	R	L
BRACHIAL ARTERY	138	132
POST TIBIAL ARTERY	124	130
ANT TIBIAL ARTERY	0	136
PERONEAL ART	118	
ANKLE/ARM INDEX	.86	>1.0

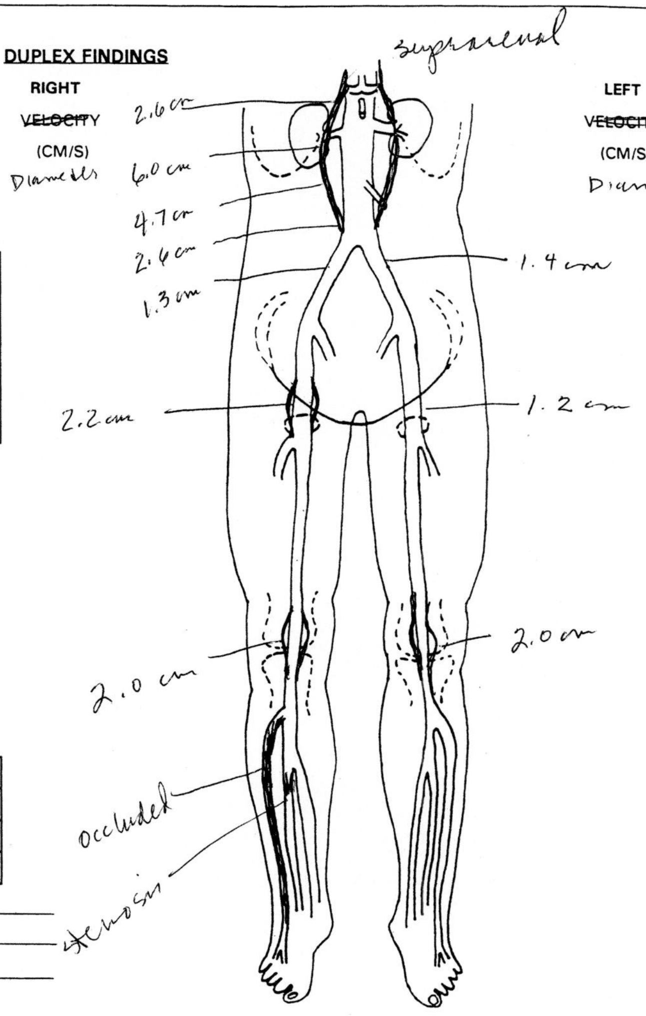

DUPLEX FINDINGS

	RIGHT	LEFT
VELOCITY (CM/S)		VELOCITY (CM/S)
Diameters		Diameter

Handwritten annotations on diagram: suprarenal, 2.6 cm, 6.0 cm, 4.7 cm, 2.4 cm, 1.3 cm, 1.4 cm, 2.2 cm, 1.2 cm, 2.0 cm, 2.0 cm, 2.0 cm, occluded, stenosis

	RIGHT	LEFT
TECH		
TAPE #		

PHONE/PRELIMINARY REPORT IN CHART: _____

DICTATED: _____

DR. SIGNATURE/DISTRIBUTION: _____

FIGURE 22.6. This worksheet is an example of the data collected for a peripheral arterial aneurysm.

REFERENCES

1. Harter LP, Gross BH, Callen PW. Ultrasonic evaluation of abdominal aortic thrombus. *J Ultrasound Med* 1982;1:315.
2. Gomes NM. Clinical and surgical aspects of abdominal aortic aneurysms. In: Raymond HW, Zweibel WJ, eds. *Seminars in ultrasound*, Vol 3. New York: Grune & Stratton, 1982:156.
3. Steinberg CR, Archer M, Steinberg L. Measurement of the abdominal aorta after intravenous aortography in health and artero-sclerotic peripheral vascular disease. *Am J Roentgenol* 1965;95:703.
4. Goldberg BB, Ostrum BJ, Isard HJ. Ultrasonic aortography. *JAMA* 1966;198:353–358.
5. Hardy DC, Lee JKT, Weyman PJ, et al. Measurement of the abdominal aortic aneurysms: plain radiographic and ultrasonic correlation. *Radiology* 1981;141:821.
6. Yucel EK, Fillmore DJ, Knox TA, et al. Interobserver reproducibility of measurement of the abdominal aorta. *Radiology* 1990;177(P):253.

## 23

DUPLEX EVALUATION OF THE RADIAL ARTERY PRIOR TO CORONARY ARTERY BYPASS GRAFT

MOLLY J. ZACCARDI

When the radial artery is to be used as a coronary artery bypass graft, the clinical vascular laboratory is asked to evaluate radial artery patency, identify possible anomalies, and document the status of the palmar arch (Fig. 23.1). The brachial artery normally bifurcates at the elbow, but it has been reported that 9% to 22% of the population may have a bifurcation several centimeters above the elbow or other aberrant anatomy (1). It is also important to document the presence of calcification of the arterial wall. A calcified radial artery may not be suitable for use as a graft. This finding is not uncommon in this patient population and age group (2). Finally, it would not be prudent to sacrifice this artery if the palmar arch were incomplete. This has been described in 11% to 20% of the population (3–5).

EQUIPMENT

A duplex ultrasound scanner with a mid to superficial range transducer (range, 4 to 10 MHz) is recommended to visualize the radial artery. Data are recorded on a videotape and a printer to provide hard-copy documentation. A photoplethysmograph is used to document the status of the palmar arch. All evaluations should include measurement of the arm blood pressure as well as interrogation of the arterial inflow with duplex scanning.

PATIENT PREPARATION

The only preparation necessary for this examination is to determine which is the dominant hand. If the radial artery

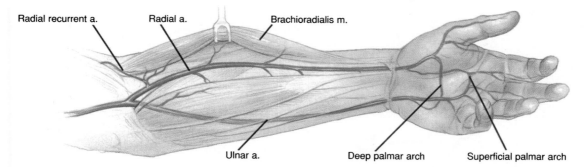

FIGURE 23.1. Normal arterial supply to the hand. The superficial and deep palmar arch normally found can provide circulation to the opposite side of the hand when either the radial or ulnar artery is occluded. (From Urken M. Free flaps: radial forearm. In: Urken M, Cheney M, Sullivan M, et al., eds. *Atlas of regional and free flaps for head and neck reconstruction.* New York: Raven, 1995:155, with permission.)

to the nondominant hand is adequate by our test criteria, a bilateral examination may not be necessary.

EXAMINATION TECHNIQUE

With the patient in the supine position, double-stick tape is placed on the thumb of the nondominant hand, and the photocell of the photoplethysmograph is attached. A strip chart recorder (AC coupled) documents the amplitude and shape of the waveform recorded from the thumb. The radial artery is then digitally compressed to document the effect on the waveform recorded from the thumb (Fig 23.2).

The waveform response leads to one of three interpretations. If there is no change in the amplitude of the digit pulse, one can assume that the palmar arch is intact. If it decreases but is still detectable, it indicates that the arch may be intact but not adequate to maintain the normal pulsatility with acute occlusion of the radial artery. Presumably, this situation would improve with time. If, however, the pulse disappears, one can assume the arch is functionally incomplete. These three possibilities are illustrated in Fig. 23.3.

The palmar arch is noted to be incomplete if the waveform obliterates. An incomplete palmar arch indicates that the radial artery cannot be harvested without sacrificing blood flow to the hand. At this point, we evaluate the dominant hand and report our findings when the duplex evaluation has been completed. If the palmar arch is documented to be complete, arm blood pressures are then taken from the upper arm as well as the forearm (radial and ulnar arteries). A 12-cm cuff is used for the upper arm and a 10-cm cuff for the forearm. All pressures recorded should be within 10 mm Hg of each other.

If the palmar arch is complete and the arm pressures are in the normal range, we proceed to perform a duplex scan of the radial artery. The purposes of this portion of the examination are to (a) measure the diameter of the radial artery, (b) document calcification of the radial artery, and (c) note any anatomic variants that the surgeon should be aware of before harvesting the artery. The transducer is placed longitudinally to the radial artery at the wrist. A Doppler velocity waveform (using a 60-degree angle of insonance) is recorded to document patency. The transducer is rotated 90 degrees to provide a transverse view of the artery. This permits a measurement of the diameter. It is also important to document the presence of calcium in the wall of the artery (Fig. 23.4). The scan is continued along the entire length of the radial artery. The screening should also include a statement about the uniformity of the dimensions as well as the distribution of the calcification. If the brachial artery has an abnormally located bifurcation, this is also reported.

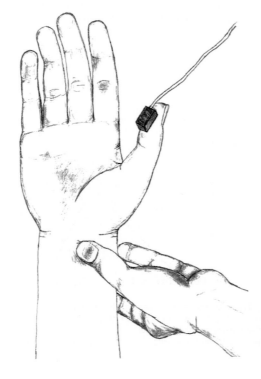

FIGURE 23.2. Radial artery compression is performed while monitoring the flow pattern in the thumb. This is a method of documenting the Allen's test, which can assess the completeness of the palmar arch.

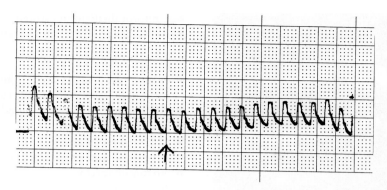

No Change

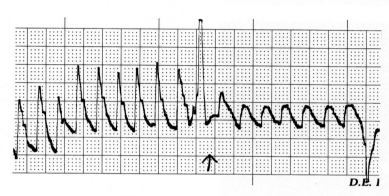

Decrease

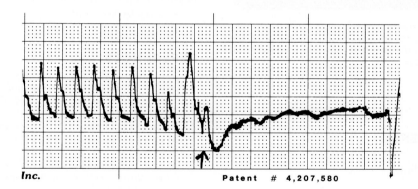

Obliterate

FIGURE 23.3. The types of changes in the pulsatility recorded from the thumb when the radial artery is digitally occluded. See text for explanation.

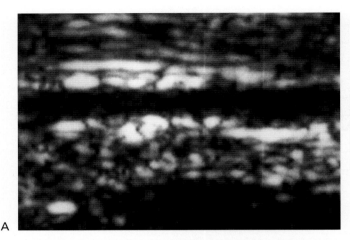

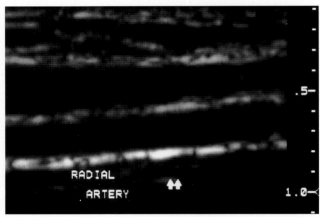

FIGURE 23.4. A: In the upper half of this illustration, the bright echoes seen are secondary to calcification of the media of the radial artery. **B:** A normal radial artery is shown in the lower half to emphasize the differences.

DIAGNOSTIC CRITERIA

Normal criteria are as follows:

- Complete palmar arch documented by photoplethysmography
- Symmetric arm systolic pressures bilaterally
- No evidence of stenosis in the radial artery
- No evidence of calcification in the radial artery

- Uniform diameter measurements in the radial artery
- No evidence of anatomic variants

Abnormal criteria are as follows:

- Incomplete palmar arch (photoplethysmograph waveform obliterates with radial artery compression)
- Asymmetric arm systolic blood pressures
- Radial artery stenosis
- Calcified radial artery
- Irregular diameter measurements of the radial artery
- Anatomic variant

The significance of performing a radial artery duplex evaluation before coronary artery bypass graft is summarized in a review of patients at the University of Washington Medical Center over a 24-month period. We evaluated 89 patients (145 limbs). This group was composed of 68 men and 21 women aged 24 to 79 years. The abnormal findings are as follows:

- Twelve patients with an incomplete Palmar arch
- Three patients with subclavian artery stenosis or occlusion
- Nine patients with calcified radial arteries
- Fourteen anomalies (tortuous radial artery, radial artery dominant, high radial artery bifurcation)

Because of the significant number of patients with abnormal findings, the cardiac surgery team continues to request duplex assessment of the radial artery before coronary artery bypass graft.

REFERENCES

1. Uglietta JP, Kadir S. Arteriographic study of variant arterial anatomy of the upper extremities. *Cardiovasc Intervent Radiol* 1989;12(3):145–148.
2. Thomson PJ, Musgrove BT. Preoperative vascular assessment: an aid to radial forearm surgery. *Br J Oral Madillofac Surg* 1997;35 (6):419–423.
3. Doscher W, Viswanathan B, Stein T, et al. Physiological anatomy of the palmar circulation in 200 normal hands. *J Cardiovasc Surg* (Torino) 1985;26(2):171–174.
4. Ozkus K, Pestelmaci T, Soyluoglu AI, et al. Variations of the superficial palmar arch. *Folia Morphol* (Warsz) 1998;57(3):251–255.
5. Ikeda A, Ugawa A, Kazihara Y, et al. Arterial patterns in the hand based on a three dimensional analysis of 220 cadaver hands. *J Hand Surg* (Am) 1988;13(4):501–509.

## 24

PREOPERATIVE VEIN MAPPING

KAREN A. GATES

For a variety of bypass procedures, the use of autologous vein remains the conduit of choice. This is because the long-term patency and durability are much better than can be achieved for prosthetic devices, particularly when used below the knee. A great deal is known about the long-term results of vein grafting largely because of the surveillance programs that are in place. The issue of graft surveillance is covered in Chapter 18. The most commonly used vein for bypass grafting is the greater saphenous vein, which has excellent length and dimensional features, making it ideal for even the longest grafts that need to be placed. However, on occasion, the greater saphenous vein has been previously harvested for lower extremity or coronary bypass purposes. It may also have been removed because it was varicose. In these circumstances, one may need to look for alternative vein from the lesser saphenous or the veins of the arm.

The advantage of preoperative vein mapping has now become obvious in that we can document length, diameter, branching, and anomalies before the procedure itself. In addition, we have discovered much to our surprise that a greater saphenous vein that had been "removed" was in fact present, or there was an accessory greater saphenous that was perfectly adequate for bypass purposes. Obviously, the greater saphenous vein is the first choice for most surgeons, but we are increasingly faced with the use of alternate veins. It is for this reason that we also examine the upper extremities for suitable veins. We prefer the cephalic and basilic veins of the upper extremities to the lesser saphenous vein of the calf because the upper extremity veins are often of larger diameter and length. On occasion, we may have to use more than one vein, performing a venovenal anastomosis at the time of operation.

Preoperative marking of the veins, along with a written report as to size, length, and branching, is essential. The marking of the venous segments permits the surgeon to cut down on the vein directly without having to create flaps, which on occasion can lead to skin necrosis. In addition, healing of the incision is promoted when unnecessary dissection is avoided (1–9).

The most advantageous practice is to order a vein mapping procedure at the time the patient undergoes a duplex scan of the peripheral arterial system. This, of course, depends on the surgeon knowing with some certainty that a bypass procedure may be necessary. If adequate conduit is found on this preliminary examination, the patient will return preoperatively to have the vein marked on the skin. If evaluation of the vein is not performed during the initial visit, we have the patient come back to be scanned and marked on the day before the operation. This procedure has worked very well.

The vessel most commonly evaluated during a preoperative vein mapping procedure is the greater saphenous vein. The other vessels evaluated are the lesser saphenous, basilic, and cephalic veins (Fig. 24.1). Communication with the ordering physician is imperative to obtain the information necessary for operative planning. The information that should be obtained from the ordering physician includes the type of bypass procedure being considered (e.g., femorodistal bypass graft, femoropopliteal bypass graft, segmental vein patch), which assists the technologists in knowing the length of vein necessary for the operative procedure; the patient's history of previous vein ligations; and if adequate vein is found, whether the vein needs to be marked on the leg during this examination or whether the patient will be returning at a later date for surgery. A vein map procedure is done from several days to a week in advance of surgery, in which case it is helpful to send the patient home with a marking pen to reinforce the line on the skin.

Vein mapping studies are performed using a duplex ultrasound machine equipped with a medium- to high-frequency transducer. In our laboratory, we often use an intraoperative probe because of its high frequency, excellent near-field resolution, and ease of handling. Other equipment that should be readily available includes an indelible pen to mark the skin, measuring tape to measure the length of adequate vein, a tourniquet to maximize venous distention, and extra pillows to help support the extremity. There are pens being marketed for the sole purpose of vein mapping; however, we use standard black permanent markers. There are several techniques in use in our laboratory for making the actual mark on the skin, keeping in mind that most pens will not write through ultrasound gel. Using a

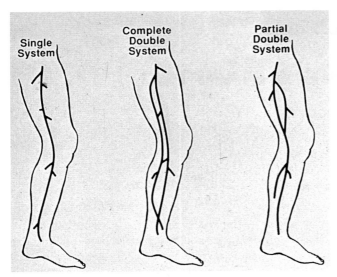

FIGURE 24.1. Some of the common variants of the greater saphenous vein. At the time of study, each of the findings is marked on the skin.

When evaluating the upper extremity veins (cephalic and basilic), the head should be elevated with the arm in a dependent position (Fig. 24.2). The arm should be slightly flexed at the elbow, again to optimize comfort and relaxation of the limb. Placing a pillow under the forearm may be helpful. When scanning the cephalic vein, the arm may rest in its normal position at the patient's side; however, when evaluating the basilic vein, the arm needs to be externally rotated.

Initial evaluation of the venous segment under interrogation should be done to prove patency. When a Doppler signal is obtained by the presence of spontaneous flow or augmentation, it is important to test for reflux by proximal compression. The presence of intraluminal defects must also be assessed using transverse compression maneuvers. Anatomic variants, structural abnormalities, wall thickening, varicosities, and valvular incompetence must be looked for and, when found, noted and transmitted to the surgeon.

After patency has been determined, diameter measurements are performed. Starting at the proximal aspect of the vein, diameter measurements are obtained from the trans-

minimal amount of gel is helpful, as is using a washcloth or a spoon to wipe the limb while holding the probe in place. Another technique is to use a straw to make a mark on the skin where the map will be drawn. The straw needs to be pressed into the skin hard enough to leave an imprint, but not so hard as to cause the patient discomfort.

It is important that the extremity under investigation be relaxed and comfortable, while at the same time allowing for the easiest access for the technologist to scan and mark the limb. The patient should be warm, and often it is necessary to cover the limb with a blanket for 10 to 15 minutes before beginning the evaluation in order to dilate the veins maximally.

When evaluating the greater saphenous vein, the patient is in reverse Trendelenburg's position with the head elevated about 30 degrees and the leg externally rotated with the knee slightly flexed, remembering to make the effort to keep the patient comfortable while allowing for easy access to the medial aspect of the leg.

For evaluation of the lesser saphenous vein, the patient is again placed in reverse Trendelenburg's position, lying either prone or on the contralateral side with the leg dependent and slightly flexed. The posterior aspect of the calf should be easily accessible to the technologist, and again the leg should be in a relaxed position. Extra pillows are especially helpful when evaluating this particular venous segment. It is important to note the point of entry of the lesser saphenous into the deep system. It is known that this can be extremely variable and important if this vein is to be harvested.

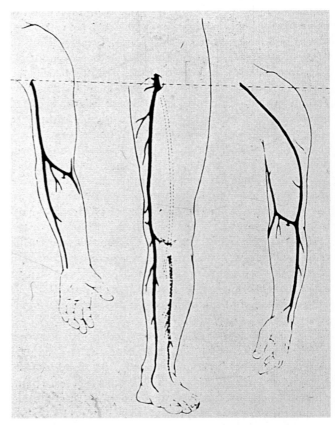

FIGURE 24.2. This depicts the major anatomic distribution of the cephalic and basilic veins that might be used for peripheral bypass grafting.

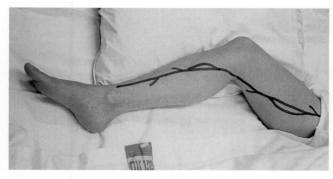

FIGURE 24.3. The type of vein marking that is used and preserved up to the time of operation. This facilitates the harvest of the vein without the need for extensive dissection and creation of large skin flaps.

verse scan at specified points along the length of the vein. It is important to maintain very light contact on the skin to avoid compressing the walls of the vein. It is our experience that a vein measuring 2 to 3 mm in transverse scan is acceptable for use as a bypass conduit. If the vein diameter is found to be borderline (less than or equal to 2 mm), it is necessary to apply a tourniquet to the more proximal limb to maximize venous distention. Obviously, if this is found, it could be important in planning the procedure. On occasion, one needs to use the vein from the opposite leg.

The final step in vein mapping is marking the vein location on the patient's skin. In long axis, or transverse scan, the vein is insonated, and a mark is made on the skin to identify its location (Fig. 24.3).

Depending on the technique the technologist uses, diameter measurements may be somewhat variable. It is important to develop a technique that is comfortable and accurate. There are also some gray areas in regard to veins being evaluated for bypass purposes, including wall thick-

ening and sclerosis. These have not been adequately defined, but they are important potential problems that need to be transmitted to the surgeon so that there are no surprises at the time of operation.

Communication with the requesting surgeon is of paramount importance before, after, and often during this examination. The vein location should be marked directly onto the skin, and vein diameters should be documented along with a description when necessary of the vein anatomy (i.e. branches, duplicate systems), with a copy of a report being sent directly to the surgeon. Verbal communication along with documentation in the medical record is done routinely.

REFERENCES

1. Cousens KA, Altemus A, Musson A, et al. Utility of preoperative vein mapping. *J Vasc Technol* 1997;21:231.
2. Kupinski AM, Leather R, Chang BB, et al. Preoperative vein mapping of the saphenous vein. In: Bernstein EF, ed. 4th ed. St. Louis: CV Mosby, 1993:897–901.
3. Salles-Cunha SX, Andros G, Harris RW, et al. Preoperative noninvasive assessment of arm veins to be used as bypass grafts in the lower extremities. *J Vasc Surg* 1986;3:813–816.
4. Chang BB, Paty PSK, Shah DM. The lesser saphenous vein: an under appreciated vein. *J Vasc Surg* 1992;15:152–157.
5. Head HD, Brown M. Preoperative vein mapping for coronary artery bypass operations. *Ann Thorac Surg* 1995;59:144–148.
6. Veith FJ, Moss CM, Sprayregen S, et al. Preoperative saphenous venography in arterial reconstructive surgery of the lower extremity. *Surgery* 1979;85(3):253–256.
7. Leopold PW, Shandall AA, Corson JD, et al. Initial experience comparing B-mode imaging and venography of the saphenous vein before in-situ bypass. *Am J Surg* 1986;152:206–210.
8. Seeger JM, Schmidt JH, Flynn TC. Preoperative saphenous and cephalic vein mapping as an adjunct to reconstructive arterial surgery. *Ann Surg* 1987;205:733–739.
9. Leopold PW, Shandall A, Kupinski AM, et al. Role of B-mode venous mapping in infrainguinal in situ vein-arterial bypasses. *Br J Surg* 1989;76:305–307.

## 25

DUPLEX EVALUATION PRIOR TO TRANSVERSE RECTUS ABDOMINIS MYOCUTANEOUS FLAP BREAST RECONSTRUCTION

MOLLY J. ZACCARDI

Transverse rectus abdominis myocutaneous flap (also called TRAM flap) is a surgery performed to reconstruct the breast following mastectomy. In 1993, Cramer and colleagues developed a noninvasive vascular duplex examination to locate and evaluate the vessels that directly and indirectly supply the rectus abdominis muscle, which is used for breast reconstruction (1). Those vessels providing blood to this muscle include the common femoral artery, inferior epigastric artery, perforating

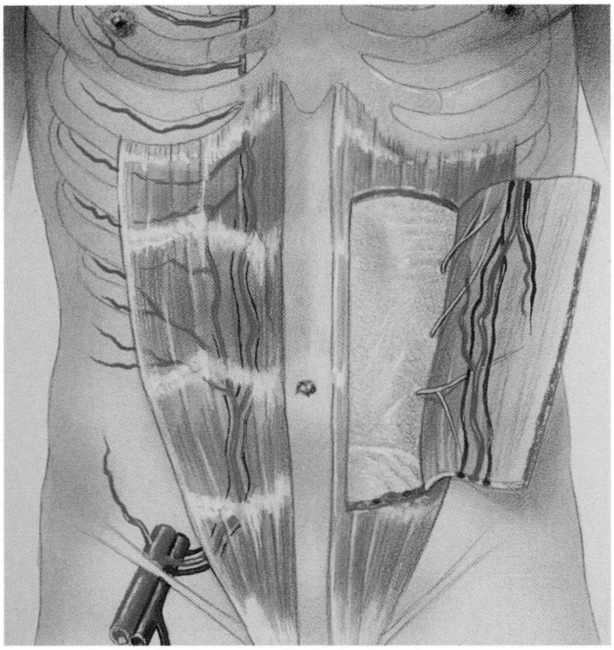

FIGURE 25.1. Origin of the inferior epigastric artery from the external iliac artery. It courses up the posterior aspect of the rectus abdominis muscle to anastomose with the superior epigastric artery. Perforating branches of these arteries are mapped by their location in the zones shown in Fig. 25.2. (From Urken M, Cheney M, Sullivan M, et al. *Atlas of regional and free flaps for head and neck reconstruction*. New York: Raven, 1995, with permission.)

arteries of the epigastric artery, and internal mammary arteries. The location of the perforating arteries is marked on the skin to allow the surgeon to incorporate the best-perfused segments of muscle into the graft. Patients who have epigastric artery perforators that have been damaged by radiation, previous abdominal surgery, or atherosclerosis, or who have variant anatomy may fare better with a different type of flap procedure. The protocol employed is the subject of this discussion. The pertinent anatomy of the rectus abdominis muscle and perforating arteries is shown in Fig. 25.1.

PATIENT PREPARATION

The examination requires a great deal of patience because the perforating arteries are small. For this reason, the patient is scheduled for a 1.5- to 2-hour time period. There is no preparation for the patient other than the time allowance. If possible, the examination is done close to the date of surgery to ensure that the skin markings delineating the perforating arteries will remain clear. It may be necessary to have the patient reinforce the markings with permanent ink if they become faint.

EQUIPMENT

The equipment necessary for this examination is an ultrasound system with color Doppler. A transducer range from 5 to 10 MHz is adequate. The location of the perforating arteries is documented using a permanent marking pen, straw, and ruler. The examination is recorded on a standard videotape, and a printer is used to provide hard-copy prints of the spectral patterns from each vessel.

EXAMINATION TECHNIQUE

The patient is asked to lie supine with the abdomen exposed. With a ruler and marking pen, a grid is drawn on the patient's

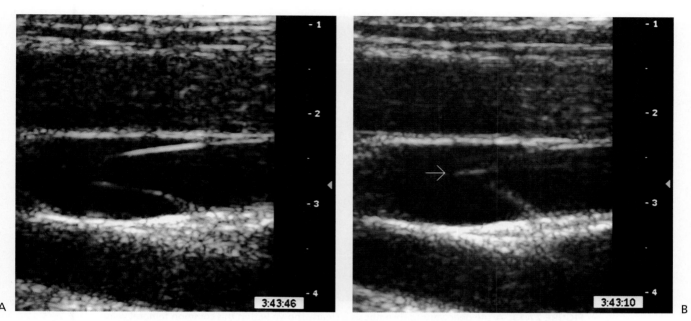

FIGURE 27.11. A: The valves shown here are within the superficial femoral vein. **B:** With proximal compression or Valsalva's maneuver, the valves should normally close, as is shown here.

penetration, the color Doppler criterion depends on symmetry with the asymptomatic side.

- If the vein segment is poorly visualized for any reason, we report findings suggested by the flow patterns but note that partial obstruction cannot be ruled out.

Abnormal Examination Criteria

B Mode

- Incomplete collapse of vein walls with compression of the transducer (Fig. 27.13)

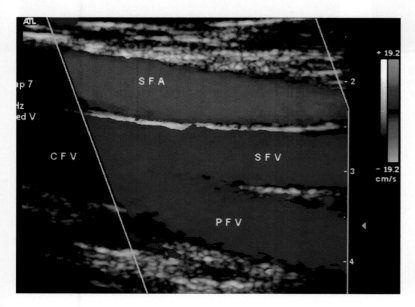

FIGURE 27.12. Color filling is shown within the profunda femoris (*PFV*) and superficial femoral veins (*SFV*) at their confluence.

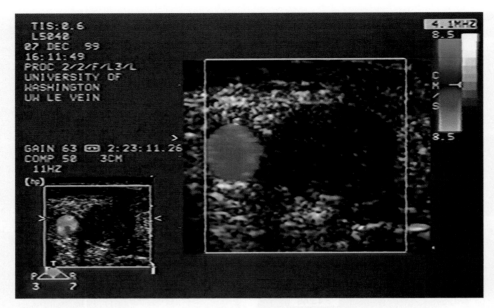

FIGURE 27.13. Acute deep venous thrombosis is clearly shown within this common femoral vein.

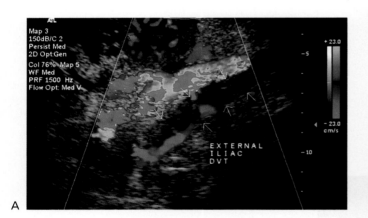

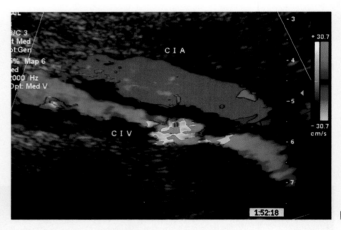

A

B

FIGURE 27.14. A: Partial color filling is seen here with external iliac DVT. **B:** Color aliasing is displayed here at the site of extrinsic compression of the common iliac vein. In this case, the patient was found by computed tomography to have lymphadenopathy at this location compressing on the iliac vein.

■ Echogenic material visible in the vein or attached to the vein wall

Doppler Spectral Analysis

■ Absent or decreased venous Doppler flow is present in comparison to the opposite side.

■ Continuous venous flow without respiratory variation suggests proximal obstruction. It is important to remember that obstruction may be due to proximal iliac thrombosis (Fig. 27.14) or to iliac vein extrinsic compression. With extrinsic compression, there is typically high-velocity continuous Doppler flow noted at the area of compression (Fig. 27.15).

■ Pulsatile venous flow in both lower extremities and throughout the inferior vena cava and iliac veins suggests increased central venous pressure.

■ No augmentation or decreased augmentation with distal compression maneuvers may indicate venous obstruction between the transducer and the level of distal compression. However, this can be misinterpreted if the patient's knee is locked. Make sure the patient's leg is in a relaxed position.

Color Doppler

■ With appropriate gain settings, the vein will have incomplete color filling or absent color filling in the presence of DVT.

PITFALLS OF THE EXAMINATION

Lower extremity venous duplex scanning does have pitfalls. As mentioned, the distal superficial femoral vein at the level of the adductor canal can be difficult to evaluate because of its depth and can produce false-positive examination results. Augmentations can be misinterpreted if not performed correctly. Also, a duplicate venous segment may result in false-negative examination results.

Ultrasonic duplex scanning, when used appropriately, appears to answer many of the needs for screening of DVT. The development of color Doppler and a wider range of transducers has contributed to the ability of skilled technologists to assess the entire venous system from the calf to the inferior vena cava.

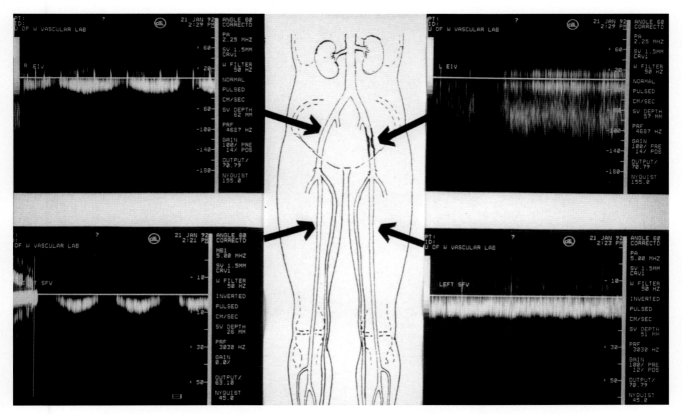

FIGURE 27.15. Doppler velocity patterns shown in left leg are continuous and of the type seen with extrinsic compression of the external iliac vein.

REFERENCES

1. Homans J. Diseases of the veins. *N Eng J Med* 1944;231:51–60.
2. Haeger K. Problems of acute venous thrombosis. I. The interpretation of symptoms and signs. *Angiology* 1969;20:219–223.
3. Bauer G. Venographic study of thrombo-embolic problems. *Acta Chir Scand Suppl* 1940;61:1–75.
4. Bauer G. Diseases and management of peripheral venous diseases. *Am J Med Sci* 1957;23:713–723.
5. Killewich LA, Bedford GR, Beach KW, et al. Diagnosis of deep venous thrombosis: a prospective study comparing duplex scanning to contrast venography. *Circulation* 1989;79:810–814.
6. Markel A, Manzo RA, Bergelin R, et al. Acute deep vein thrombosis: diagnosis, localization, risk factors. *J Vasc Med Biol* 1992;3:432–439.
7. Markel A, Weich Y, Gaitini D. Doppler ultrasound in the diagnosis of venous thrombosis. *Angiology* 1995;46:65–73.
8. Meissner MH, Caps MT, Bergelin RO, et al. Early outcome after isolated calf vein thrombosis. *J Vasc Surg* 1997;26:749–756.
9. Passman MA, Moneta GL, Taylor LM Jr, et al. Pulmonary embolism is associated with the combination of isolated calf vein thrombosis and respiratory symptoms. *J Vasc Surg* 1997;25:39–45.
10. Kahn SR, Joseph L, Abenhaim L, et al. Clinical prediction of deep vein thrombosis in patients with leg symptoms. *Thromb Haemost* 1999;81:353–357.
11. Anderson DR, Wells PS, Stiell I, et al. Thrombosis in the emergency department: use of a clinical diagnosis model to safely avoid the need for urgent radiological investigation. *Arch Intern Med* 1999;159:477–482.
12. Killewich LA, Bedford GR, Beach KW, et al. Spontaneous lysis of deep venous thrombosis: rate and outcome. *J Vasc Surg* 1989;9:89–97.
13. Meissner MH, Caps MT, Bergelin RO, et al. Propagation, rethrombosis and new thrombus formation after acute deep venous thrombosis. *J Vasc Surg* 1995;22:558–567.
14. Caps MT, Meissner MT, Tullis MJ, et al. Venous thrombus stability during acute phase of therapy. *Vasc Med* 1999;4:(1)15–23.
15. Wells PS, Lensing AWA, Davidson BL, et al. Accuracy of ultrasound for the diagnosis of deep venous thrombosis in asymptomatic patients after orthopedic surgery: a meta-analysis. *Ann Intern Med* 1995;122:47–53.

## 28

DUPLEX EVALUATION OF CHRONIC VENOUS DISEASE

RICHARD MANZO

Although a great deal of time is spent ruling in or out the problem of acute deep venous thrombosis (DVT), little attention has been given to the patient who has chronic venous insufficiency. The reasons for this are not entirely clear but relate in part to the idea that the observed changes are of little importance in understanding the pathophysiology of the disorder or how to manage it. The two major categories of patients seen are those who present with varicose veins (primary or secondary) and those who present with symptoms or signs suggestive of the postthrombotic syndrome (1,2). The evaluation process and its interpretation have become of increasing importance.

The patient with varicose veins needs an evaluation to assist in determining the etiology and how the varicosities should be managed. The two major categories of problems are referred to as primary and secondary. By definition, the patient with *primary varicose veins* does not have involvement of the deep venous system. This can be effectively determined by ultrasonic duplex scanning, which shows a patent and competent deep system from the level of the iliac veins to below the knee. The patient with *secondary varicose veins* has them due to damage to the deep venous system, usually due to DVT. This problem can be settled by a careful ultrasonic duplex scan establishing that certain venous segments in the deep system are chronically occluded and/or that the valves are incompetent (3–7).

For a complete duplex study to be done, it is necessary to be able to study the entire venous system of the leg. Although some have neglected the veins of the calf, they must be included in the evaluation (8). Most venous valves are found in the calf. This is undoubtedly a result of the need for protection of the lower limb from the high-pressure swings that occur secondary to the effects of gravity and the forces generated by the calf muscle pump (9).

As will be noted, the two major elements in the study of the venous system revolve around documentation of patency and venous valvular competence (1). *Patency* is simply a matter of noting whether flow is present and determining whether it has a normal pattern (10). *Valvular competence* is determined by noting whether reverse flow occurs under circumstances in which only unidirectional flow should be occurring (5). As will be noted, there are two methods of documenting

reverse flow. Although we prefer the standing method, it is permissible to use a combination of Valsalva's maneuver and limb compression in some circumstances (3,11,12).

It is also clear that thrombus stability is an important issue. We now know that spontaneous lysis can and does occur and affects both long-term patency and venous valvular function. It is also important that the testing be done to detect recurrent DVT when this occurs. The protocol is to perform a follow-up scan at the point at which the venous involvement has stabilized. This is usually at the end of the first 3 months. As a general rule, we recommend that repeat testing be done when the anticoagulation is completed. At this time, the repeat duplex scan serves as the baseline for comparison when and if future problems develop.

TEST DESCRIPTION

The ultrasonic venous duplex examination for chronic venous insufficiency of the lower extremities involves the use of both B-mode imaging and spectral Doppler analysis. The imaging permits examination of specific sites from which the flow velocity data can also be collected and evaluated. It is important to study all sites at which DVT can or has occurred. The purpose of the examination is to evaluate the deep, superficial, and perforating venous systems for evidence of chronic occlusion, chronic partial residual occlusion, or valvular incompetence. The venous system is examined from the level of the inferior vena cava distally to include the common femoral, profunda femoris, superficial femoral, popliteal, gastrocnemial, soleal, tibial, peroneal, greater and lesser saphenous, and perforating veins. The screening examination is done with the patient in the reverse Trendelenburg's position, with the evaluation of valvular competence done in the upright position. As will be noted, however, valvular function can also be tested with the patient supine, but the valve closure times will be different.

EQUIPMENT

At least two imaging pulsed wave transducers are necessary for a complete examination. A 5- to 7.5-MHz or a 7- to 4-

MHz linear transducer can be used for the lower extremities from just below the inguinal ligament in the groin down through the thigh and calf. A 2- to 3.5-MHz phased array transducer can be used for the inferior vena cava and iliac venous segments. A videotape recorder is used to record and document studies. A thermal printer for "black-and-white" hard-copy documentation of the examination at specific anatomic sites is also needed. A color printer is also used for presenting color Doppler data that are collected.

EQUIPMENT SETTINGS
B-Mode Imaging

Imaging requires a continual adjustment of controls to give optimal results throughout the examination. Overall power must be increased for deeper vessels and decreased for superficial vessels. The gray scale and dynamic range must be continuously adjusted throughout the examination. The dynamic range should be increased to image thrombus in the setting of an acute DVT; this helps to bring out the subtle echoes that may be present. In the setting of chronic residual DVT, increasing the contrast of the image may help to delineate the vein wall from the residual DVT.

Doppler Settings

Venous duplex imaging requires the Doppler and color Doppler parameter setting to be set low. The wall filter should be set at the lowest setting to avoid cutting off low-velocity flow. Increasing the power and gain maximizes the Doppler flow signal with increasing depth through tissue. Overcompensation of the overall gain of the Doppler settings produces a mirror-like image of flow signals in the spectral analysis above and below the zero baseline, owing to the increased harmonics of the Doppler signal produced; decreasing the gain will correct it. Doppler and color Doppler (mean velocities) settings should be set to optimize peak velocities in the range of 50 to 100 cm/sec. Documentation of valvular incompetence and its sites is one of the major goals of the examination. Determine which way antegrade flow (outflow) will be, either below or above the zero baseline, and be consistent. We have determined at our institution that greater than 2 seconds of reverse flow is considered evidence of incompetent venous valves when a Valsalva's maneuver and manual compression maneuvers have been used. The reflux time that is abnormal when the standing cuff inflation and deflation method is used is more than 0.5 second.

PATIENT PREPARATION

Patients are not asked to fast overnight, but in some cases, examination of the inferior vena cava and iliac veins might

be difficult because of bowel gas. Before each examination, a brief history is taken and recorded along with the duplex findings. The patient is also examined to assess the status of the skin and the presence, location, and size of ulcers.

PATIENT POSITION

Begin with the patient supine and in reverse Trendelenburg's position with the leg to be examined externally rotated and with the knee bent (Fig. 28.1). The external iliac, common femoral, profunda femoris, and superficial femoral veins can easily be examined with the leg in this position. However, it is best to examine the popliteal vein with the patient in the prone position and with the calf supported on pillows (Fig. 28.2). If the patient is unable to assume the prone position, the popliteal vein may be exam-

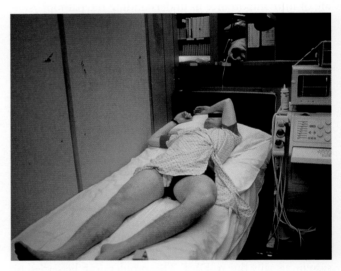

FIGURE 28.1. Position that is used for the screening examination. The patient is in minus 10 degrees Trendelenburg's position, with the leg externally rotated and the knee slightly flexed.

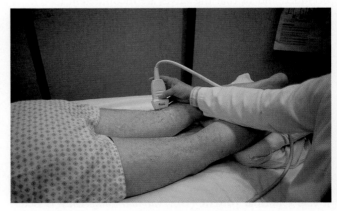

FIGURE 28.2. The distal superficial femoral and popliteal vein are best studied with the patient in a prone position with the knee slightly flexed and resting on a pillow.

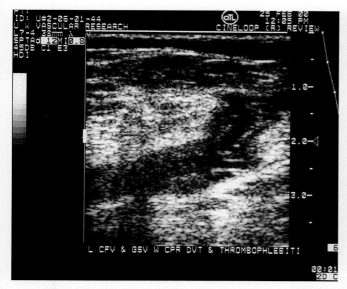

FIGURE 28.3. This is a longitudinal scan of a common femoral–proximal superficial femoral vein with considerable intraluminal irregularities (echoes) signifying the previous episode of deep venous thrombosis 1 year ago.

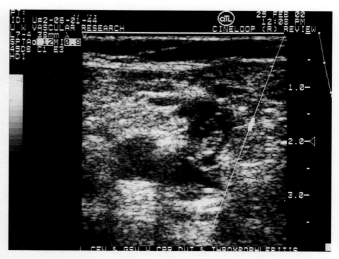

FIGURE 28.4. Cross-sectional view of the common femoral vein shown in Fig. 28.3. The extensive intraluminal echoes are obvious.

ined by turning the patient on the side (lateral decubitus), or in the supine position by rotating the knee externally.

EXAMINATION PROCEDURE SEQUENCE

Place the transducer in the groin to image the external iliac, common femoral, greater saphenous, profunda femoris, and proximal superficial femoral veins. The transducer is placed just below the inguinal ligament medial to the common femoral artery, which is easily seen in long axis (Figs. 28.3 and 28.4). By moving distally a few centimeters, the junction of the superficial femoral–profunda femoris bifurcation can be seen. With the veins seen in longitudinal view, it is important to determine the venous flow characteristics. Venous flow in the veins of the abdomen, thigh, and popliteal vein is normally phasic with respiration. However, the flow patterns in the tibial and peroneal veins may not be spontaneous, particularly if the patient is vasoconstricted. When this occurs, it may be necessary to use foot compression to augment flow to document patency. When the veins are visualized with the sample volume in the center of the vein, valvular competence can be determined by using Valsalva's maneuver for the upper thigh segments and limb compression for the veins below the knee (Fig. 28.5). When this method is used for documenting valve competency, the time normally required for valve closure is 2 seconds or less. As will be covered later, this is longer than occurs when the patient is studied in the upright position.

In the groin, the probe is angled medially to visualize the greater saphenous vein at the saphenofemoral junction. The greater saphenous vein is examined both for patency and valvular competence. If the greater saphenous vein is found to be incompetent in the upper thigh, it should be studied in its entire length. With the veins seen in a transverse view, the segment is tested for compressibility to document the presence or absence of intraluminal material, such as acute and chronic thrombi. Because compression of the superficial femoral vein in the adductor canal may be difficult, patency may have to be documented by flow parameters. It is also important to look for reduplication of the superficial femoral and popliteal veins.

The popliteal vein is located lateral and superficial to the popliteal artery. It is easily compressed normally. The popliteal vein may also be duplicated (bifid). The lesser saphenous vein is usually seen at the middle to proximal popliteal fossa. Its anatomy is quite variable in terms of the point where it enters the deep venous system. This information can be of great importance when a vein stripping procedure is being contemplated. The gastrocnemius vein branches come off very close to the lesser saphenous vein, where it enters the popliteal fossa to connect with the popliteal vein.

The transducer at the ankle is placed posterior to the medial malleolus to image the posterior tibial veins in long axis (Fig. 28.6). The veins are paired on either side of the artery. The posterior tibial artery is a useful landmark because flow in these small vessels is not always spontaneous and, in the case of chronic DVT, may be very difficult to visualize. The peroneal veins can be examined from the medial approach, deeper but parallel to the posterior tibial veins. The soleal plexus of veins is located in the soleus muscle and connects with the posterior tibial veins (PTVs) and peroneal veins, usually at diagonal angles.

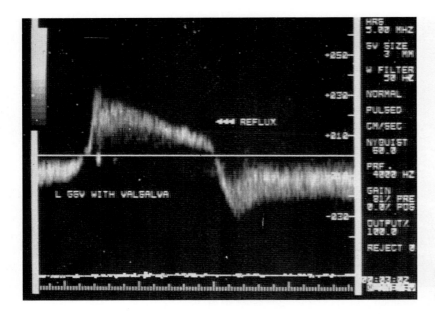

FIGURE 28.5. Bidirectional flow occurring in response to a Valsalva's maneuver. This is a good example of reflux through incompetent valves.

Subfascial endoscopic perforator surgery has become popular in recent years. Examining the location and size of the perforating veins is essential in planning the operation. The major medial lower leg perforators are found 10 to 15 cm proximal from the medial malleolus. These are referred to as the Cockett I, II, and III perforators (Fig. 28.7). Using B-mode imaging, these perforators can be seen to penetrate the deep fascia and connect with the posterior arch vein. The perforating veins along the medial lower leg are the most important in planning the procedure (Fig. 28.8) (13).

If surgery is planned, the location of the perforating veins is marked. It is also important to relate to the surgeon the status of the deep system as well as the greater and lesser saphenous veins. These findings will dictate whether additional surgical options will need to be considered.

If an ulcer is present, it is important to determine its relationship to underlying perforating veins. A surgical lubricant and transparent dressing should be used to cover the ulcer. A latex cover for the transducer should be used as well (14–19).

To examine the inferior vena cava and iliac veins, a low-frequency transducer is used. The transducer is placed below the xiphoid process to visualize the inferior vena cava in long axis. Flow should be spontaneous and phasic (pulsatile). No augmentation is necessary at this level. Rotate the transducer to evaluate compression of the inferior vena cava in cross-section by moving toward the umbilicus. Evaluate with compression of vein walls. If a patient has a history of recurrent chronic DVT and pulmonary emboli, an inferior vena cava filter placement procedure may have been

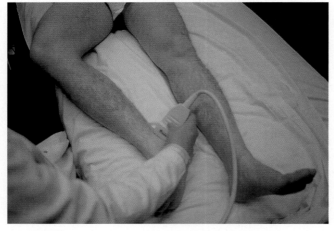

FIGURE 28.6. Position of the leg and the transducer when one is examining the posterior tibial and peroneal veins.

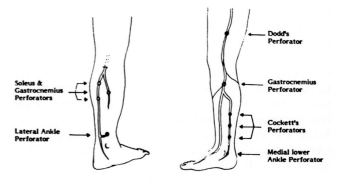

FIGURE 28.7. Location of the perforators on the medial and lateral side of the leg. All of these sites are accessible to ultrasonic scanning.

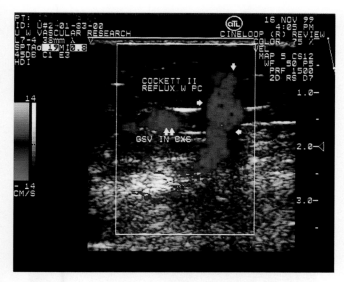

FIGURE 28.8. Color Doppler picture illustrating marked reflux out *(red)* through a very large Cockett 2 perforator.

Standing Cuff Examination

The standing cuff examination is done after the screening examination is completed to evaluate for the presence of chronic occlusive or partial DVT. A two-step stand with a frame for support is used. While the patient is facing the examiner, the leg examined is suspended, and weight is placed on the contralateral leg. A 24-cm pneumatic cuff is used on the thigh and inflated to 80 mm Hg (Fig. 28.10). A 12-cm cuff is used on the calf and inflated to 100 mm Hg (Fig. 28.11). A 7- or 10-cm cuff is used on the foot and inflated to 120 mm Hg (Fig. 28.12). The transducer is placed proximal to the cuff and is kept in close proximity to isolate specific valves of interest. An automatic rapid cuff inflator (Hokanson, Bellevue, WA) is used for a controlled inflation and deflation. The cuff is rapidly inflated and held at the described pressures for 3 seconds. The time for deflation is 0.3 second, which will result in a reverse transvalvular velocity of more than 30 cm/sec. When the veins of the lower extremity are normal, the time for valve closure is 0.5 second or less (Fig. 28.13). A reflux time greater than 0.5

done. It is important to visualize the location of the filter relative to the renal veins (Fig. 28.9). Doppler velocity signals should be taken proximal to, in, and distal to the filter. It may be possible to visualize thrombus within the filter.

At the umbilicus, the transducer is rocked to the right and left to evaluate the common iliac veins. The thigh is compressed to augment the flow to the iliac veins. With the transducer medial to the iliac crest, it can be angled medially to image the confluence of the iliac veins (common, internal, and external). The flow characteristics of the distal common and external iliac veins are evaluated by augmentation of flow with distal compression maneuvers. Once again, observe the B-mode image for evidence of chronic residual obstruction or partial obstruction.

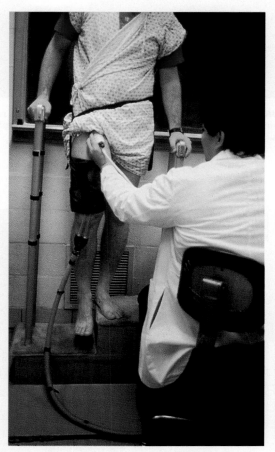

FIGURE 28.10. Stand used for the standing cuff deflation test. The transducer is placed just above the cuff to document the forward–reverse flows that might accompany the sudden deflation of the cuff. The cuff is deflated very rapidly (less than 0.3 second).

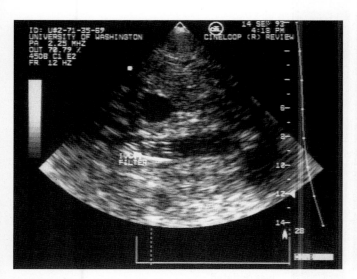

FIGURE 28.9. This longitudinal view of the inferior vena cava shows a Greenfield filter in place.

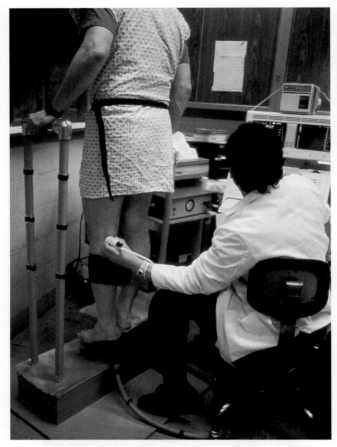

FIGURE 28.11. In this position, with the cuff on the calf, reflux is being tested for the distal superficial femoral and popliteal veins.

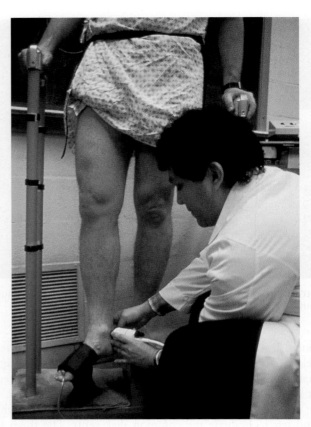

FIGURE 28.12. With the cuff on the foot, it is possible to document the status of forward–reverse flow in the posterior tibial and peroneal veins.

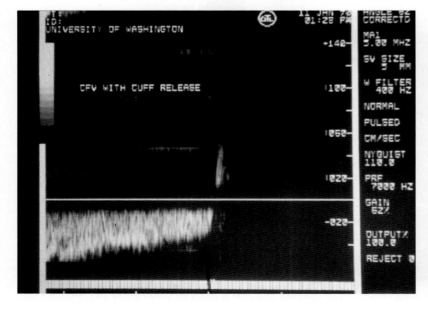

FIGURE 28.13. Example of a normal valve closure that occurred in less than 0.5 second when the cuff was deflated.

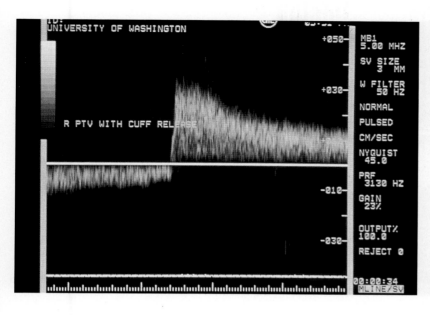

FIGURE 28.14. Marked reflux after sudden cuff deflation.

second is usually indicative of venous valvular incompetence (Fig. 28.14).

This method employs pressures within the physiologic range and allows for reproducible results. This upright position is the method of choice. Because not all patients are able to stand for the test, it is possible to use reverse Trendelenburg's position. In this position, Valsalva's maneuver is used to test the competency of the proximal venous segments, with compression of the lower thigh for the valves below the knee. Valve closure time when this position is used is 2 seconds or less.

DIAGNOSTIC CRITERIA: DUPLEX EVALUATION OF LOWER EXTREMITY CHRONIC VENOUS DISEASE

Doppler Flow Pattern

Doppler flow signals may be classified as phasic with respiration (normal) or continuous. Normal Doppler signals can be detected with chronic partial occlusion. This will depend as well on the status of the venous collateral circulation. Continuous flow is generally seen in the presence of acute DVT or when collateral venous flow is not adequate.

Diminished continuous venous signals may indicate chronic partial residual DVT proximal to the venous segment that is being studied as well as the specific segment that is being interrogated. The extent of the diminished continuous signal depends on several factors, which again include the number of venous segments involved, overall thrombus load (usually extensive), and inadequate collateral flow. Severe extrinsic compression of the iliac venous segments can also cause diminished continuous flow. Contin-

uous venous flow with normal velocities (Fig. 28.15) can and does occur with proximal partial obstruction or with partial obstruction at the segmental site of examination (usually moderate). The absence of venous Doppler flow signals and of color Doppler flow signals is indicative of chronic residual occlusion (in the absence of the sudden onset of symptoms of pain, edema, chest pain, etc.), provided that Doppler and color Doppler parameters are correctly set low. If there is a question about a Doppler signal obtained at any venous segment level, it is always compared with the same sites in the contralateral leg.

B-Mode Image

B-mode imaging findings in chronic venous insufficiency vary a great deal. Venous segments can and will sometimes appear completely normal. Complete recanalization with restoration of patency is relatively common. Minimal or isolated valvular incompetence may be the only evidence of a previous episode of DVT. The rate of recanalization is a significant determinant of the outcome after an episode of acute DVT.

When either partial or complete obstruction is the outcome, it can be detected by a combination of B-mode and Doppler testing. The normal response to probe pressure on the leg over a patent venous segment is complete compressibility of the vein walls. Incompressibility or partial compressibility of vein walls with transducer pressure is seen with partial or complete occlusion.

The consistency of the echogenic material within the vein also varies considerably. It depends on the age of the DVT and the efficiency of the fibrinolytic system in resolving a DVT event. The longer a chronic occlusive or partial

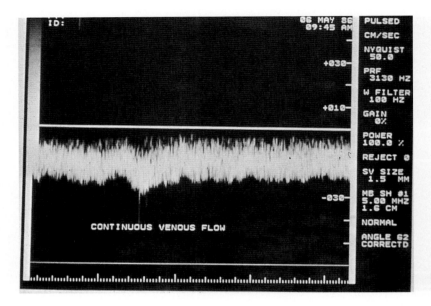

FIGURE 28.15. Continuous venous flow with no changes with respiration.

residual obstruction exists within a venous segment, the brighter and stronger the echoes within the lumen appear on B-mode image. This is because of the strong echogenic nature of fibrous material of the residual DVT. At times, the echogenic material will appear as fibrin strands within the vein, vein walls will compress with probe pressure, and color flow will be noted through the mural thrombus (Fig. 28.16) within the venous segment of interest (20–22).

Color Doppler

Color Doppler imaging greatly expedites the venous duplex examination. This is most apparent in the calf. Using color as a roadmap to visualize the small, complex, and numerous vessels, including perforators of the calf, is remarkable. Minimal or incomplete color filling of venous segments will be noted with chronic partial residual obstruction in any

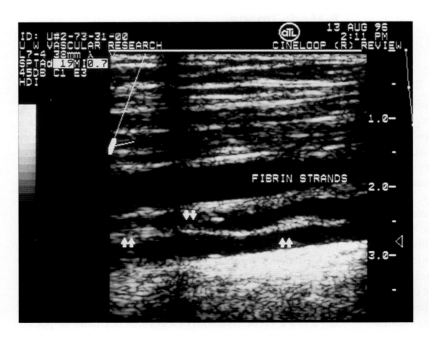

FIGURE 28.16. This shows the presence of fibrous strands in the vein after partial recanalization had taken place.

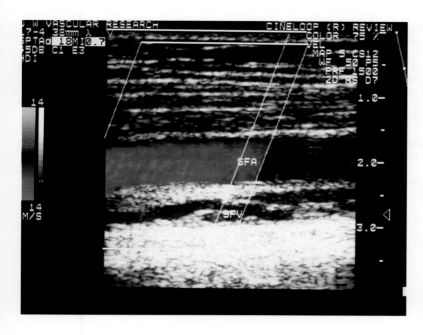

FIGURE 28.17. The femoral artery is illustrated in *red* with the recanalized, very shrunken vein visible immediately below.

segment of the lower extremity. Absence of color filling in any venous segment studied will be noted with chronic occlusive obstruction (Fig. 28.17). However, this is possible provided that the color Doppler imaging parameters of the duplex ultrasound equipment are correctly set low and are sensitive to a venous low-flow state.

Color Doppler imaging can be used to detect reflux but is not recommended as the sole criterion for the diagnosis of valvular incompetence. A change in color through a venous segment may not necessarily equate to reflux or valvular incompetence. Keep in mind that the color change is relative to the direction of flow, which is relative to the transducer.

GENERAL LIMITATIONS (PITFALLS)

All diagnostic modalities have limitations. Duplex ultrasound in this area has its share. Obesity will limit the capacity to image and obtain Doppler signals of the deep venous system, specifically the abdomen (inferior vena cava and iliac segments). Edema may limit the ability to visualize and obtain signals in the lower extremities. When edema is extreme and combined with chronic obstruction, obtaining good visualization of the B-mode image and Doppler signals can be very difficult. Complex varicose veins are frequently seen with chronic venous duplex imaging. Persistent fibrous echogenic chronic obstruction and partial residual obstruction (DVT) limit the ability to image and obtain Doppler information from specific involved venous segments. Over time, if the obstruction is extensive and is accompanied by valvular incompetence, the B-mode image may degrade. Fortunately, most thrombi eventually recanalize.

Venous duplex imaging is a highly operator-dependent examination. The learning curve can be long and requires patience. Initially, emphasis should be on developing a careful and thorough scanning technique. Quicker examination times will come with familiarity and confidence in the ability to operate the equipment and to recognize the changes associated with chronic venous insufficiency and the postthrombotic syndrome.

REFERENCES

1. Johnson BF, Manzo RA, Bergelin RO, et al. Relationship between changes in the deep venous system and the development of the postthrombotic syndrome after an acute episode of lower limb deep vein thrombosis: a one- to six-year follow-up. *J Vasc Surg* 1995;21:307–313.
2. Killewich LA, Martin R, Cramer M, et al. Pathophysiology of venous claudication. *J Vasc Surg* 1984;1:507–511.
3. Van Bemmelen PS, Bedford G, Strandness DE Jr. Quantitative segmental evaluation of venous valvular reflux with ultrasonic duplex scanning. *J Vasc Surg* 1989;10:425–431.
4. Van Bemmelen PS, Bedford G, Beach K, et al. Status of the valves in the superficial and deep venous system in chronic venous disease. *Surg* 1991;109:730–734.
5. Van Bemmelen PS, Beach KW, Bedford G, et al. The mechanism of venous valve closure: its relationship to the velocity of reverse flow. *Arch Surg* 1990;125:617–619.
6. Labropoulos N, Volteas N, Leon M, et al. The role of venous outflow obstruction in patients with chronic venous dysfunction. *Arch Surg* 1997;132:46–51.
7. Strandness DE Jr, Langlois YE, Cramer ME, et al. Long-term sequelae of acute venous thrombosis. *JAMA* 1983;250:1289–1292.
8. Meissner MH, Caps MT, Bergelin RO, et al. Early outcome after isolated calf vein thrombosis. *J Vasc Surg* 1997;26:749–756.
9. Strandness DE Jr. Hemodynamics of the normal arterial and venous system. In: Strandness DE Jr, ed. *Duplex scanning in vascular disorders,* 2nd ed. New York: Raven, 1993:45–79.

10. Moneta GL, Bedford G, Beach K, et al. Duplex ultrasound assessment of venous diameters, peak velocities and flow patterns. *J Vasc Surg* 1988;8:286–291.
11. Markel A, Meissner MH, Manzo RA, et al. A comparison of the cuff deflation method with Valsalva's maneuver and limb compression in detecting venous valvular reflux. *Arch Surg* 1994;129:701–705.
12. Meissner MH, Manzo RA, Bergelin RO, et al. Deep venous insufficiency: the relationship between lysis and subsequent reflux. *J Vasc Surg* 1993;18:596–608.
13. Mozes G, Gloviczki P, Menawat SS, et al. Surgical anatomy for endoscopic subfascial division of perforating veins. *J Vasc Surg* 1996;24:800–808.
14. Hanrahan LM, Araki CT, Rodriguez AA, et al. Distribution of valvular incompetence in patients with venous stasis ulceration. *J Vasc Surg* 1991;13:805–812.
15. Labropoulos N, Delis K, Nicolaides N, et al. The role of the distribution and anatomic extent of reflux in the development of signs and symptoms in chronic venous insufficiency. *J Vasc Surg* 1996;23:504–510.
16. Labropoulos N, Giannoukas AD, Delis K, et al. Where does venous reflux start? *J Vasc Surg* 1997;26:736–742.
17. Labropoulos N, Delis K, Mansour MA, et al. Prevalence and clinical significance of posterolateral thigh perforator vein incompetence. *J Vasc Surg* 1997;26:743–748.
18. Quigley S, Raptis M, Cashman M, et al. Duplex ultrasound mapping of sites of deep to superficial incompetence in primary varicose veins. *Aust N Z J Surg* 1992;62:276–278.
19. Delis KT, Ibegbuna V, Nicolaides AN, et al. Prevalence and distribution of incompetent perforating veins in chronic venous insufficiency. *J Vasc Surg* 1998;28:815–825.
20. Meissner MH, Caps MT, Zierler BK, et al. Determinants of chronic venous disease after acute venous thrombosis. *J Vasc Surg* 1998;28:826–833.
21. Meissner MH, Caps MT, Bergelin RO, et al. Propagation, rethrombosis, and new thrombus formation after acute deep venous thrombosis. *J Vasc Surg* 1995;22:558–567.
22. Meissner M. The effect of recanalization of venous thrombi on valve function. *Vasc Med Rev* 1995;6:143–152.

## 29

DUPLEX EVALUATION OF THE UPPER EXTREMITY

BRIDGET A. MRAZ

Thrombotic occlusion of the major veins of the upper extremity and thorax was once a relatively unusual complication. However, with the increased use of central venous catheters, it has now become a very common disorder in nearly all hospitals. Up to 80% of these cases develop in response to an easily identified problem, such as a central venous catheter (1,2). The remaining cases are often classified as "effort" thrombosis or Paget-Schroetter syndrome (3–6). It is also important to remember that some cases involve obstruction or compression of the great central veins, such as occurs with the superior vena cava syndrome. In addition, more requests are now made for screening the subclavian and central veins for documentation of patency and suitability for catheter placement.

The anatomy of the upper extremity venous system that is of particular interest to the vascular diagnostic laboratory centers on the thoracic inlet (the axillary and subclavian veins), the jugular vein in the neck, and the major draining veins within the thorax. Although venous thrombosis can also involve the deep veins outside the thorax, it is very unusual for this to occur unless there is some underlying and very serious coagulopathy. The deep veins of the upper extremities include the innominate (brachiocephalic), internal jugular, subclavian, axillary, brachial, radial, and ulnar veins. Two superficial veins in the upper extremities, the basilic and cephalic veins, are also important to include in a basic upper extremity venous duplex examination to rule out superficial thrombophlebitis.

Effort thrombosis is a relatively uncommon vascular event, affecting 1% to 2% of all cases of upper extremity deep venous thrombosis (DVT). It occurs more commonly in men and more often affects the right arm. To illustrate the type of presentation and how it is evaluated, the following case will bring out the salient features. This 19-year-old competitive swimmer had subclavian vein thrombosis after a pool collision with another freestyle swimmer traveling in the opposite direction. She was initially referred to the Vascular Diagnostic Service from the Sports Medicine clinic to rule out acute upper extremity DVT. The subclavian and

proximal axillary veins were totally occluded—they had no Doppler flow and were dilated with echogenic material within the lumen of the vessels. The patient underwent catheter-directed thrombolysis for a 24-hour period, after which time the thrombus was completely lysed as confirmed by repeat ultrasound studies. A postlysis venogram revealed an underlying 70% stenosis of the subclavian vein. A transluminal angioplasty was done to open the stenotic area. Provocative maneuvers under fluoroscopy demonstrated occlusion of the subclavian vein with abduction of the arm. The vein was subsequently decompressed by first rib resection. A follow-up duplex evaluation revealed nonocclusive wall thickening but no scarring of the vein. After 2 weeks, heparin therapy was discontinued, and the patient returned to full-time competitive swimming at the collegiate level.

Cases of this type are screened with duplex scanning to document both the site and extent of the occlusive process. In some cases, particularly with Paget-Schroetter syndrome, catheter-directed thrombolysis is carried out to determine the underlying cause of the problem.

As with the lower extremities, the technologist will image and evaluate flow characteristics in the deep veins of the upper extremity to rule out DVT. The patency of the superficial veins is also important to know preoperatively when dialysis access is planned or the veins are being proposed for use in lower limb arterial bypass grafting.

For the upper extremities, a 5- to 7.5-MHz transducer is best for most patients. However, for large patients, a curved linear transducer may be helpful when evaluating the innominate, subclavian, and axillary veins. For very superficial basilic and cephalic veins, a high-frequency transducer (even an intraoperative scanhead) will give the best detail for diameter measurements.

No patient preparation is required for examining the upper extremities. The examiner should allow 30 minutes for the examination (60 minutes if also mapping the superficial veins). Examine the patient from the head of the bed, with the patient lying supine and the head of the bed flat.

If only examining one arm, it may be easiest to scan from that side of the bed in order to adjust the patient's arm position.

EXAMINATION PROCEDURE

The transducer is lightly placed on the neck to visualize the internal jugular vein in a longitudinal plane (Fig. 29.1). The effect of body position on the diameter of the vein is shown in Fig. 29.2. However, it must be remembered that a vein with an acute thrombus may be larger than normal (Fig. 29.3). If the vein appears to be patent, a Doppler signal is recorded with the angle of the incident sound beam 60 degrees or less to the long axis of the vein. The flow pattern should be spontaneous, phasic, and pulsatile but should have a different relationship to the respiratory cycle, as seen in the veins of the lower leg. Rotate the transducer to the cross-sectional view of the internal jugular vein and compress the vein throughout its length to rule out partial obstruction.

Visualize the internal jugular vein as it drains into the brachiocephalic vein. Angle the probe medial and caudal. Record the Doppler signal from the innominate vein, and document the flow pattern. Color Doppler filling may be helpful in identifying the correct vessels.

At the level of the innominate vein, angle the probe laterally to view the origin of the subclavian vein. Document the flow pattern, and note any collateral flow channels.

Place the transducer inferior to the clavicle to visualize the distal subclavian and axillary veins in long axis, and record the Doppler signal. Evaluate for compression in

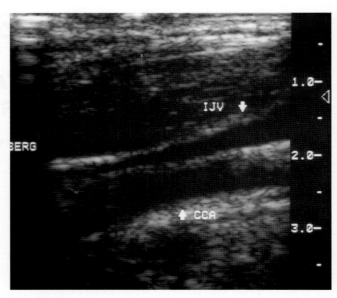

FIGURE 29.2. With the patient in reverse Trendelenburg's position, the internal jugular vein *(IJV)* is seen.

cross-section. If unable to compress the subclavian vein, ask the patient to sniff quickly through the nose. This may decrease the pressure within the vein and allow the vein walls to collapse. Also, evaluate the vein for color filling. Rotate the transducer to visualize the brachial vein longitudinally (Fig. 29.4), and record the Doppler signal. Continue compression of the brachial vein to the level of the elbow. Flow signals should also be recorded here in the longitudinal plane of the vein.

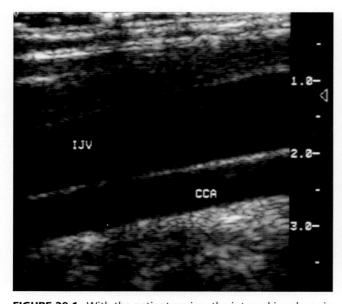

FIGURE 29.1. With the patient supine, the internal jugular vein *(IJV)* is easily seen adjacent to the common carotid artery *(CCA).*

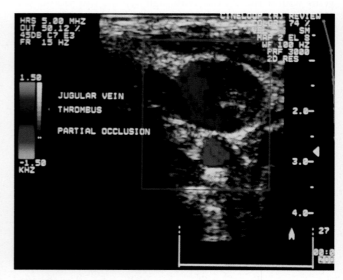

FIGURE 29.3. This cross-sectional view of the neck shows the presence of a large thrombus in the internal jugular vein, which is partially occlusive. Its large size relative to the common carotid artery *(red)* is obvious.

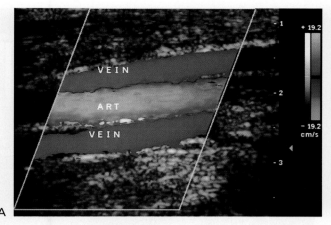
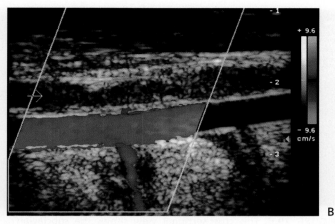

FIGURE 29.4. A: With the arm at the patient's side in a relaxed position, the brachial veins are identified in long axis. **B:** Brachial vein deep venous thrombosis.

DIAGNOSTIC CRITERIA

The diagnostic criteria are similar to those of the lower extremities. The main difference is the normal pulsatility in the spectral waveform with the upper extremities, especially the internal jugular, innominate, and subclavian veins, owing to their proximity to the heart.

Normal Examination Criteria

B-Mode Image

- Vein walls collapse completely distal to the clavicle with transducer pressure.
- Interior of vein appears anechoic.

Doppler Spectral Analysis

- Spontaneous
- Phasic and pulsatile (Fig. 29.5)
- Augments with distal compression

Color Doppler

- Complete color Doppler filling

Abnormal Examination Criteria

B-Mode Image

- Incomplete collapse of vein walls distal to the clavicle with compression of the transducer

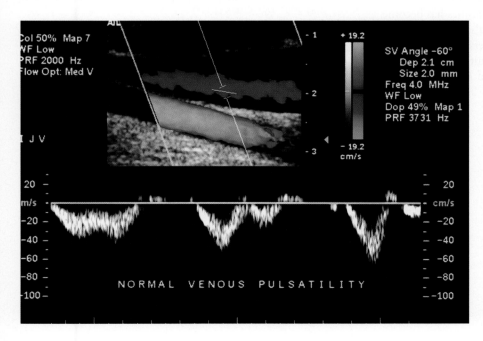

FIGURE 29.5. Normal venous pulsatility obtained from the internal jugular vein.

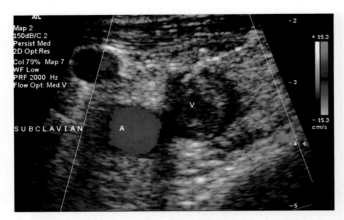

FIGURE 29.6. This cross-sectional view shows the subclavian vein with occlusive thrombus.

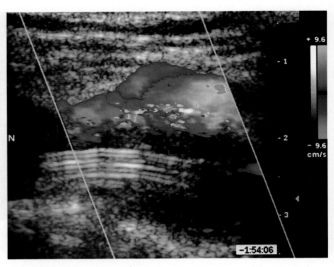

FIGURE 29.7. Longitudinal view of the subclavian vein with occlusive thrombus surrounding venous catheter. Subclavian artery is shown adjacent.

- Echogenic material visible within the vein or attached to the vein wall (Fig. 29.6)

Doppler Spectral Analysis

- Absent or decreased in comparison to the contralateral side
- Continuous or decreased pulsatility, suggestive of a proximal obstruction
- No augmentation or decreased augmentation with distal compression maneuvers. This may indicate a distal obstruction.

Color Doppler

- Incomplete color filling or absent color filling
- Venous thrombosis in the upper extremities has become a relatively common problem in hospitals with the increased use of upper extremity venous catheters (Fig. 29.7).
- Duplex scanning of the upper extremities can prove beneficial in the diagnosis of DVT and superficial thrombophlebitis and in the documentation of patency and adequacy for catheter placement.

REFERENCES

1. Prandoni P, Bernardi E. Upper extremity deep vein thrombosis. *Curr Opin Pulm Med* 1999;5:222–226.
2. Prandoni P, Polistena P, Bernardi E, et al. Upper-extremity deep vein thrombosis: risk factors, diagnosis, and complication. *Arch Intern Med* 1997;157:57–62.
3. Machleder H. Vaso-occlusive disorders of the upper extremity. *Curr Probl Surg* 1988;25:1–67.
4. Viera AJ. Primary upper-extremity deep venous thrombosis. *Milit Med* 1997;162:829–831.
5. Sayinalp N, Ozcebe OI, Kirazli S, et al. Paget-Schroetter syndrome associated with FV:Q506 and prothrombin 20210A: a case report. *Angiology* 1999;50:689–692.
6. Nair KP, Poulose KP, Sudheer VM. Paget-Schroetter's syndrome. *J Assoc Physicians India* 1990;38:951–952.

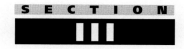

EXAM WORK SHEETS

EXAM WORK SHEETS

Carotid Artery Duplex Exam
Pre Fibula Flap Vascular Evaluation
Thoracic Outlet Arterial Compression Exam
Lower Extremity Arterial Exercise Exam
Renal Artery Duplex Exam
Lower Extremity Arterial Duplex Exam
Lower Extremity Venous Duplex Exam
Mesenteric Artery Duplex Exam

Upper Extremity Venous Duplex Exam
Pre-Dialysis Access Duplex Exam
Transcranial Doppler Exam
Upper Extremity Arterial Duplex Exam
Tram Flap Perforator Duplex Exam
Abdominal Venous Duplex Exam
TCD Monitoring-Carotid Endarterectomy

UNIVERSITY OF WASHINGTON MEDICAL CENTER - VASCULAR DIAGNOSTIC SERVICE

CAROTID ARTERY DUPLEX EXAM   HISTORY _____

_____

DATE   _____

UH#   _____

NAME   _____

D.O.B.   _____

_____

REFERRED BY _____   PHONE _____

ADDRESS _____

<u>DUPLEX FINDINGS</u>

BRUITS	RIGHT	LEFT	BLOOD PRESS.	RIGHT	LEFT	RISK FACTORS	
NONE			DOPPLER			HTN	
CARDIAC			STETH	/	/	SMOKING	
SUBCL						DIABETES	
CAR-LO						LIPIDS	
CAR-HI						CAD/PVD	

RIGHT   **LEFT**

PSV	EDV	FLOW SEP	SPECT BROAD	TORT	PLAQUE	SPECT CLASS		PSV	EDV	FLOW SEP	SPECT BROAD	TORT	PLAQUE	SPECT CLASS
							CCAo							
							CCAm							
							CCAd							
							ICAp							
							ICAm							
							ICAd							
							ECA							

ICA/CCA RATIO [   ]   [   ]

SUBCLAVIAN ART		VERTEBRAL ART	
SYST VEL		SYST VEL	
WAVEFORM		ANTEGRADE	
TURBULENCE		RETROGRADE	
TORTUOSITY		TORTUOSITY	
PLAQUE		NOT LOCATED	
Normal	< 50%	Normal	Stenotic
< 50%	Occluded	Steal	Occluded

SUBCLAVIAN ART		VERTEBRAL ART	
SYST VEL		SYST VEL	
WAVEFORM		ANTEGRADE	
TURBULENCE		RETROGRADE	
TORTUOSITY		TORTUOSITY	
PLAQUE		NOT LOCATED	
Normal	< 50%	Normal	Stenotic
< 50%	Occluded	Steal	Occluded

	RIGHT	LEFT
TECH:		
TAPE #:		

PHONE/PRELIMINARY REPORT IN CHART _____

DICTATED _____

DR. SIGNATURE/DISTRIBUTION _____

PRE FIBULA FLAP VASCULAR EVALUATION

HISTORY _____

DATE

UH#

NAME

D.O.B.

REFERRED BY _____   PHONE _____

ADDRESS _____

DUPLEX FINDINGS

SYSTOLIC PRESSURES:	R	L
BRACHIAL ARTERY		
POST TIBIAL ARTERY		
ANT TIBIAL ARTERY		
PERONEAL ART		
ANKLE/ARM INDEX		

PERONEAL ARTERIES

DIAMETER MEASUREMENTS		
	R	L
PROXIMAL		
MIDDLE		
DISTAL		

PERONEAL ARTERIES

	R	L
CALCIFICATION		
VISUALIZED		
ANATOMICAL		
VARIANTS		

DUPLEX OF PERONEAL VEINS

COMPRESSION (Y/N)		
	R	L
PROXIMAL		
MIDDLE		
DISTAL		

PERONEAL ARTERIES

VELOCITY MEASUREMENTS		
	R	L
PROXIMAL		
MIDDLE		
DISTAL		

PERONEAL ARTERIES

WAVEFORM ANALYSIS		
	R	L
PROXIMAL		
MIDDLE		
DISTAL		

RIGHT		RIGHT
# PERFORATORS:		
DISTANCE FROM		
MALLEOLUS (cm)		

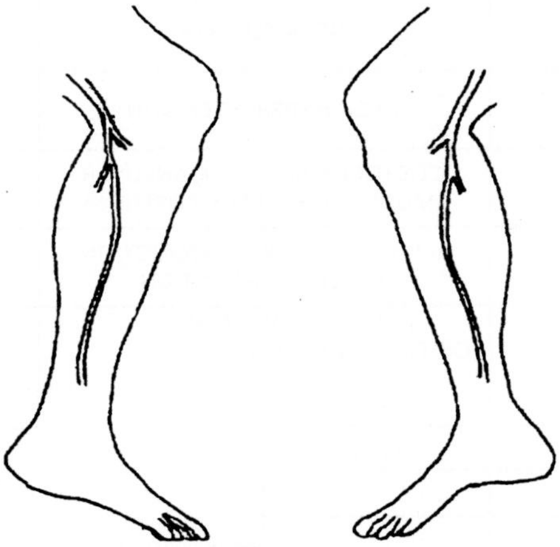

LEFT	LEFT
# PERFORATORS:	
DISTANCE FROM	
MALLEOLUS (cm)	

	R	L
TAPE #		
TECH		

PHONE/PRELIMINARY REPORT IN CHART: _____

DICTATED: _____

DR. SIGNATURE/DISTRIBUTION: _____

UNIVERSITY OF WASHINGTON MEDICAL CENTER - VASCULAR DIAGNOSTIC SERVICE

THORACIC OUTLET ARTERIAL COMPRESSION EXAM HISTORY_____

_____

DATE _____

UH# _____

NAME _____

D.O.B. _____

REFERRED BY_____ PHONE_____

ADDRESS_____

RIGHT		PATIENT POSITION	LEFT	
SYMPTOMS	DOPPLER/PPG RESPONSE		DOPPLER/PPG RESPONSE	SYMPTOMS
		SEATED		
		HYPERABDUCTION/EXTENSION BOTH ARMS		
		HYPERABDUCTION/EXTENSION LEFT ARM		
		HYPERABDUCTION/EXTENSION RIGHT ARM		
		ADSON MANEUVER HEAD TO LEFT		
		ADSON MANEUVER HEAD TO RIGHT		
		NECK FLEXION		
		NECK HYPEREXTENSION		
		COSTOCLAVICULAR MANEUVER (MODIFIED MILITARY POSITION)		
		AER POSITION 90* ABDUCTION- EXTERNAL ROTATION		
		OTHER SYMPTOMATIC POSITION -- DESCRIBE:		

	RIGHT	LEFT
TECH		
TAPE #		

PHONE/PRELIMINARY REPORT IN CHART: _____

DICTATED: _____

DR. SIGNATURE/DISTRIBUTION: _____

LOWER EXTREMITY ARTERIAL EXERCISE EXAM HISTORY _____

_____

DATE   _____

UH#   _____

NAME   _____

D.O.B.   _____

_____

REFERRED BY _____   PHONE _____

ADDRESS _____

SYSTOLIC PRESSURES	RIGHT	LEFT
BRACHIAL ARTERY		
POSTERIOR TIBIAL ARTERY		
ANTERIOR TIBIAL ARTERY		
PERONEAL ARTERY		
ANKLE/ARM INDEX		

RISK FACTORS	
HTN	
SMOKING	
DIABETES	
LIPIDS	
CAD/PVD	

EXERCISE TREADMILL: Speed _____ mph Grade _____ %

TIME	SYMPTOMS WITH EXERCISE
:	
:	
:	
:	
:	
TOTAL WALK TIME: _____ MIN. _____ SEC.	
STOPPED DUE TO:	

POST EXERCISE PRESSURES

RT _____	TIME	LT _____	ARM
	1 MIN		
	2 MIN		
	4 MIN		
	6 MIN		
	8 MIN		
	10 MIN		
	12 MIN		

	RIGHT	LEFT
TECH		
TAPE #		

PHONE/PRELIMINARY REPORT IN CHART _____

DICTATED _____

DR. SIGNATURE/DISTRIBUTION _____

RENAL ARTERY DUPLEX EXAM

HISTORY _____

_____

DATE   _____

UH#   _____

NAME   _____

D.O.B.   _____

_____

REFERRED BY _____ PHONE _____

ADDRESS _____

DUPLEX FINDINGS

SYSTOLIC PRESSURES	R	L
BRACHIAL ARTERY		
POST TIBIAL ARTERY		
ANT TIBIAL ARTERY		
ANKLE/ARM INDEX		
STETHOSCOPE B/P	/	/

RISK FACTORS	
HYPERTENSION	
SMOKING	
DIABETES	
LIPIDS	
CAD/PVD/AAA	

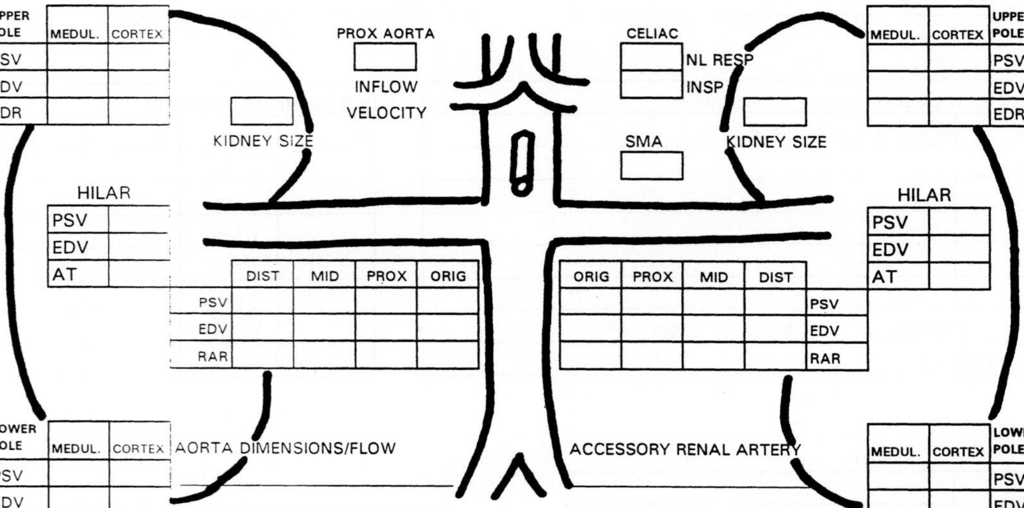

UPPER POLE

	MEDUL.	CORTEX
PSV		
EDV		
EDR		

PROX AORTA

INFLOW
VELOCITY

KIDNEY SIZE

CELIAC
NL RESP
INSP

SMA

KIDNEY SIZE

UPPER POLE

MEDUL.	CORTEX	
		PSV
		EDV
		EDR

HILAR

PSV	
EDV	
AT	

	DIST	MID	PROX	ORIG
PSV				
EDV				
RAR				

ORIG	PROX	MID	DIST	
				PSV
				EDV
				RAR

HILAR

PSV	
EDV	
AT	

LOWER POLE

	MEDUL.	CORTEX
PSV		
EDV		
EDR		

AORTA DIMENSIONS/FLOW

_____

_____

_____

ACCESSORY RENAL ARTERY

_____

_____

_____

LOWER POLE

MEDUL.	CORTEX	
		PSV
		EDV
		EDR

RENAL VEIN PATENT _____

RENAL VEIN PATENT

TECH		
	RIGHT	LEFT
TAPE #		

PHONE/PRELIMINARY REPORT IN CHART _____

DICTATED _____

DR. SIGNATURE/DISTRIBUTION _____

LOWER EXTREMITY ARTERIAL DUPLEX EXAM   HISTORY _____

_____

DATE   _____

UH#   _____

NAME   _____

D.O.B.   _____

_____

REFERRED BY _____   PHONE _____

ADDRESS _____

RISK FACTORS	
HTN	
SMOKING	
DIABETES	
LIPIDS	
CAD/PVD	

DUPLEX FINDINGS

	RIGHT		LEFT	
	VELOCITY		VELOCITY	
	(CM/S)		(CM/S)	

SYSTOLIC PRESSURES:	R	L
BRACHIAL ARTERY		
POST TIBIAL ARTERY		
ANT TIBIAL ARTERY		
PERONEAL ART		
ANKLE/ARM INDEX		

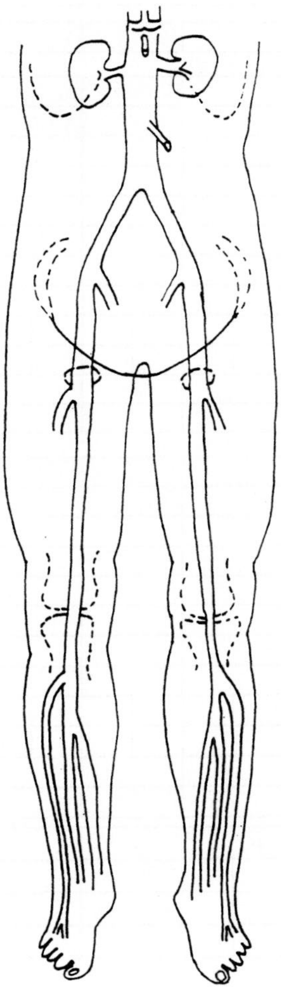

	RIGHT	LEFT
TECH		
TAPE #		

PHONE/PRELIMINARY REPORT IN CHART: _____

DICTATED: _____

DR. SIGNATURE/DISTRIBUTION: _____

UNIVERSITY OF WASHINGTON MEDICAL CENTER - VASCULAR DIAGNOSTIC SERVICE

LOWER EXTREMITY VENOUS DUPLEX EXAM   HISTORY _____

DATE

UH#

NAME

D.O.B.

REFERRED BY _____   PHONE _____

ADDRESS _____

DUPLEX FINDINGS

SITE	SPONT	PHASIC	AUGMENT	REFLUX	COMPRESS	THROMBUS
IVC			░░░	░░░		
RIGHT						
CIV			░░░	░░░		
EIV			░░░	░░░		
CFV						
Prof						
SFVp						
SFVm						
SFVd						
Pop						
PTV						
PER						
GrSp						
GrSm						
LEFT						
CIV			░░░	░░░		
EIV			░░░	░░░		
CFV						
Prof						
SFVp						
SFVm						
SFVd						
Pop						
PTV						
PER						
GrSp						
GrSm						

RIGHT   LEFT

GSV DIAM   GSV DIAM

LSV DIAM

sizes in cm

	R			L	
TECH					
TAPE #					

PHONE/PRELIMINARY REPORT IN CHART _____

DICTATED _____

DR. SIGNATURE/DISTRIBUTION _____

UNIVERSITY OF WASHINGTON MEDICAL CENTER - VASCULAR DIAGNOSTIC SERVICE

MESENTERIC ARTERY DUPLEX EXAM   HISTORY _____

DATE

UH#

NAME

D.O.B.

REFERRED BY _____   PHONE _____

ADDRESS _____

SYSTOLIC PRESSURES	RIGHT	LEFT
BRACHIAL ARTERY		
POST TIBIAL ARTERY		
ANT TIBIAL ARTERY		
ANKLE/ARM INDEX		

ABDOMINAL BRUIT: _____

WITH DEEP INSP: _____

POST-PRANDIAL: After _____ oz. Ensure Plus

SITE MONITORED:

MINUTE	SYSTOLIC VELOCITY	REVERSE FLOW	DIASTOLIC VELOCITY
5			
10			
15			
20			

DUPLEX FINDINGS

FASTING:	SYSTOLIC VELOCITY	REVERSE FLOW	DIASTOLIC VELOCITY
Ao			
SMA Orig			
SMA Prox			
SMA Dist			
Celiac Orig			
Celiac Mid			
Hepatic Orig			
Splenic Orig			
IMA Orig			

Celiac Axis Compression:

Deep Insp		

TECH		
	CELIAC	
TAPE #	SMA	
	IMA	

PHONE/PRELIMINARY REPORT IN CHART: _____

DICTATED: _____

DR. SIGNATURE/DISTRIBUTION: _____

393

UPPER EXTREMITY VENOUS DUPLEX EXAM HISTORY _____

_____

DATE _____

UH# _____

NAME _____

D.O.B. _____

_____

REFERRED BY _____ PHONE _____

ADDRESS _____

DUPLEX FINDINGS   RIGHT   LEFT

SITE	SPONT	PHASIC	AUGMENT	COMPRESS	THROMBUS
RIGHT					
IJV					
BR-CEPH					
SUBCLAV					
AXILLARY					
BRACHIAL					
RADIAL					
ULNAR					
CEPHALIC					
BASILIC					

SITE	SPONT	PHASIC	AUGMENT	COMPRESS	THROMBUS
LEFT					
IJV					
BR-CEPH					
SUBCLAV					
AXILLARY					
BRACHIAL					
RADIAL					
ULNAR					
CEPHALIC					
BASILIC					

CEPHALIC SIZE   BASILIC SIZE   CEPHALIC SIZE

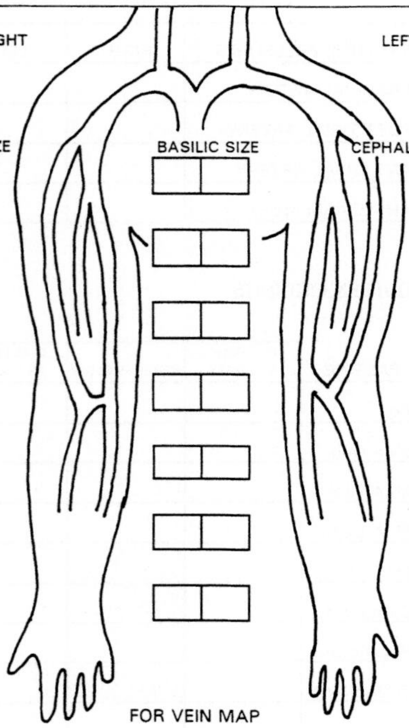

FOR VEIN MAP

sizes in cms

	RIGHT	LEFT
TECH		
TAPE #		

PHONE/PRELIMINARY REPORT IN CHART _____

DICTATED _____

DR. SIGNATURE/DISTRIBUTION _____

UNIVERSITY OF WASHINGTON MEDICAL CENTER - VASCULAR DIAGNOSTIC SERVICE

PRE-DIALYSIS ACCESS DUPLEX EXAM

HISTORY _____

_____

DATE

_____

UH#

_____

NAME

_____

D.O.B.

_____

_____

REFERRED BY _____ PHONE _____

ADDRESS _____

DUPLEX FINDINGS

RIGHT   LEFT

SITE	SPONT	PHASIC	AUGMENT	COMPRESS	THROMBUS
RIGHT					
IJV					
BR-CEPH					
SUBCLAV					
AXILLARY					
BRACHIAL					
RADIAL					
ULNAR					
CEPHALIC					
BASILIC					

SITE	SPONT	PHASIC	AUGMENT	COMPRESS	THROMBUS
LEFT					
IJV					
BR-CEPH					
SUBCLAV					
AXILLARY					
BRACHIAL					
RADIAL					
ULNAR					
CEPHALIC					
BASILIC					

CEPHALIC SIZE   BASILIC SIZE   CEPHALIC SIZE

FOR VEIN MAP
sizes in cms

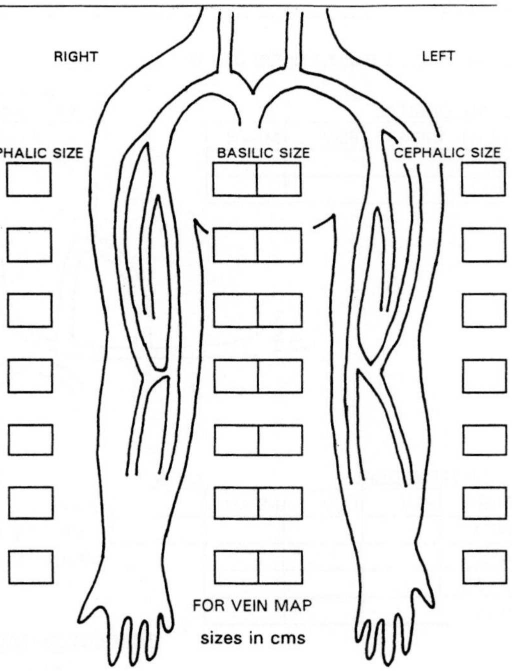

MODIFIED ALLEN'S TEST

RIGHT	Doppler signal change	LEFT
	RADIAL(Ulnar comp)	
	ULNAR(Radial comp)	

A = Augment
NC = No Change
O = Obliterate
R = Reverse

BRACHIAL ARTERY WAVEFORM		Right_____	Left_____

	R	L	
TECH			
TAPE #			

PHONE/PRELIMINARY REPORT IN CHART_____

DICTATED_____

DR. SIGNATURE/DISTRIBUTION_____

TRANSCRANIAL DOPPLER EXAM HISTORY _____

_____

DATE   _____

UH#   _____

NAME   _____

D.O.B.   _____

_____

REFERRED BY _____   PHONE _____

ADDRESS _____

EXTRA-CRANIAL DUPLEX FINDINGS: R = _____   L = _____

TRANSORBITAL

RIGHT	PSV	EDV	MEAN
ICA			
OPHTH			

All velocities in cm/sec

TRANSORBITAL

LEFT	PSV	EDV	MEAN
ICA			
OPHTH			

TRANSTEMPORAL   DICA

RIGHT	PSV	EDV	MEAN	
MCA				PSV
ACA				EDV
BIFUR				MEAN
PCA				

DICA   TRANSTEMPORAL

	LEFT	PSV	EDV	MEAN
PSV	MCA			
EDV	ACA			
MEAN	BIFUR			
	PCA			

TRANSOCCIPITAL

	PSV	EDV	MEAN
LEFT VERT			
RIGHT VERT			
BASILAR ARTERY			

MCA/ICA velocity ratio _____

MCA pulsatility index _____

MCA/ICA velocity ratio _____

MCA pulsatility index _____

	RIGHT	LEFT
TECH		
TAPE #		

PHONE/PRELIMINARY REPORT IN CHART: _____

DICTATED: _____

DR. SIGNATURE/DISTRIBUTION: _____

UNIVERSITY OF WASHINGTON MEDICAL CENTER -- VASCULAR DIAGNOSTIC SERVICE

UPPER EXTREMITY ARTERIAL DUPLEX EXAM HISTORY _____

DATE

UH#

NAME

D.O.B.

REFERRED BY _____ PHONE _____

ADDRESS _____

RIGHT	SYSTOLIC PRESSURES	LEFT
	BRACHIAL	
	RADIAL	
	ULNAR	

RIGHT	DUPLEX FINDINGS	LEFT
	INNOMINATE	
	P SUBCLAVIAN P	
	M M	
	D D	
	P AXILLARY P	
	D D	
	P BRACHIAL P	
	D D	
	P RADIAL P	
	D D	
	WITH ULNAR COMPRESSION	
	P ULNAR P	
	D D	
	WITH RADIAL COMPRESSION	

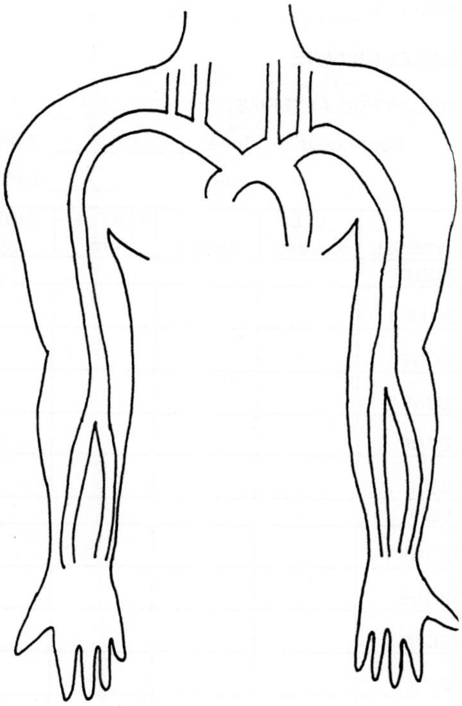

NOTE:

A = Augment   O = Obliterate

NC = No Change   R = Reverse

RIGHT	LEFT		
		TECH	
			PHONE/PRELIMINARY REPORT IN CHART_____
		TAPE #	DICTATED_____
			DR. SIGNATURE/DISTRIBUTION_____

TRAM FLAP PERFORATOR DUPLEX EXAM   HISTORY _____

_____

DATE   _____

UH#   _____

NAME   _____

D.O.B.   _____

_____

REFERRED BY _____   PHONE _____

ADDRESS _____

<u>DUPLEX FINDINGS</u>

EPIGASTRIC ARTERIES:

    Continuous to Zone _____ Right

                Zone _____ Left

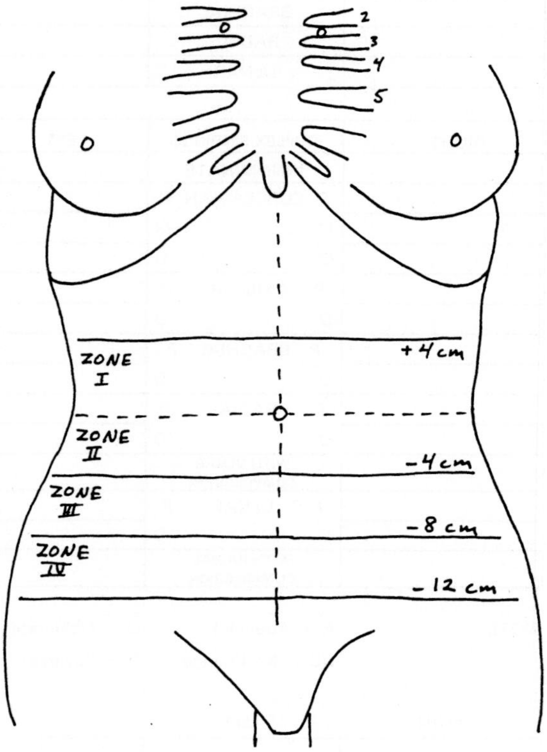

VESSEL	VEL cm/sec	ANGLE	VERT +/- cm	HORIZ cms
RIGHT				
ZONE I				
ZONE				
ZONE				
ZONE				
ZONE IV				
LEFT				
ZONE I				
ZONE				
ZONE				
ZONE				
ZONE IV				

IMA RT		
IMA LT		

# PERFORATORS:	R_____	L_____

<u>TECH</u>	
<u>TAPE #</u>	

PHONE/PRELIMINARY REPORT IN CHART_____

DICTATION_____

DR. SIGNATURE/DISTRIBUTION_____

ABDOMINAL VENOUS DUPLEX EXAM   HISTORY _____

_____

DATE   _____

UH#   _____

NAME   _____

D.O.B.   _____

_____

REFERRED BY _____   PHONE _____

ADDRESS _____

DUPLEX FINDINGS

HEPATIC VEIN	
VELOCITY	
DIRECTION	
THROMBUS	
PHAS/PULSE	

IVC	
SIZE	
VELOCITY	
THROMBUS	
PHAS/PULSE	

SMV	
VELOCITY	
DIRECTION	
SIZE	
THROMBUS	

RIGHT RENAL VEIN	
VELOCITY	
DIRECTION	
SIZE	
THROMBUS	

MAIN PORTAL VEIN	
VELOCITY	
DIRECTION	
SIZE	
THROMBUS	

RIGHT PORTAL VEIN	
VELOCITY	
DIRECTION	
SIZE	
THROMBUS	

LEFT PORTAL VEIN	
VELOCITY	
DIRECTION	
SIZE	
THROMBUS	

SPLENIC VEIN	
VELOCITY	
DIRECTION	
SIZE	
THROMBUS	

LEFT RENAL VEIN	
VELOCITY	
DIRECTION	
SIZE	
THROMBUS	

ASCITES   HEPATOMEGALY   SPLENOMEGALY

	PORTAL VEIN	HEPATIC VEIN
TECH		
TAPE #		

PHONE/PRELIMINARY REPORT IN CHART _____

DICTATED _____

DR. SIGNATURE/DISTRIBUTION _____

UNIVERSITY OF WASHINGTON MEDICAL CENTER

TCD MONITORING - CAROTID ENDARTERECTOMY

Date
UH#
Name
D.O.B.

Pre-Op Findings - Angio/Duplex:	
Left Carotid	______
Right Carotid	______
Other	______
Symptoms	______
	______
	______

Type of Surgery ______
Surgeons: ______
Baseline Exam Date: ______
Baseline Exam Findings: ______
______
Vessel Monitored ______
Vessel Depth ______

	MV	PI	Air Emboli	Paticul. Emboli	
Pre-Anesthesia					
Post-Anesthesia					40%=
Prior to Clamp					40%=
Imm. Post Clamp					%Baseline=
5 min Post Clamp					%Baseline=

Shunt Used?__________ Stump Pressure___________
Duration of Shunt_______

	MV	PI	Air Emboli	Paticul. Emboli	
During CEA					%Baseline=
Imm. Post Clamp					%Baseline=
5 min Post Clamp					%Baseline=

Total Air Emboli________ Total Particulate Emboli______ Total Emboli______

	MV	PI	Air Emboli	Paticul. Emboli
Recovery Room				
____Hours After				

Comments: ______
______
______
______

		Right	Left
Tech			
Tape#			

VASCULAR DIAGNOSTIC SERVICE

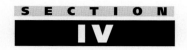

EXAMPLES OF REPORTS

EXAMPLES OF REPORTS

Lower Extremity Arterial Duplex Exam
Upper Extremity Arterial Duplex Exam
Pre-Dialysis Access Duplex Exam
Carotid Artery Duplex Exam
TCD Monitoring-Carotid Endarterectomy
Thoracic Outlet Arterial Compression Exam
Transcranial Doppler Exam
Renal Artery Duplex Exam
Carotid Artery Duplex Exam

Abdominal Venous Duplex Exam
Tram Flap Perforator Duplex Exam
Pre Fibula Flap Vascular Evaluation
Mesenteric Artery Duplex Exam
Dialysis Access Graft Duplex Study
Lower Extremity Venous Duplex Exam
Upper Extremity Venous Duplex Exam
Lower Extremity Arterial Exercise Exam

UNIVERSITY OF WASHINGTON MEDICAL CENTER - VASCULAR DIAGNOSTIC SERVICE

LOWER EXTREMITY ARTERIAL DUPLEX EXAM

HISTORY 83 year old female w/ nonhealing wound of Ⓛ mid anterior tibial region. This is possible osteomyelitis vs. extremity ischemia.

DATE

UH#

NAME

D.O.B.

REFERRED BY

PHONE

ADDRESS

RISK FACTORS	
HTN	⊕ oral meds (2)
SMOKING	⊕ 20+ yr. x 1 pack /day
DIABETES	⊖
LIPIDS	⊕ oral meds (1)
CAD/PVD	Ø CVA ; MI x 1

SYSTOLIC PRESSURES:	R	L
BRACHIAL ARTERY	110	104
POST TIBIAL ARTERY	80	50
ANT TIBIAL ARTERY	74	66
PERONEAL ART		
ANKLE/ARM INDEX	0.72	0.60

DUPLEX FINDINGS

RIGHT VELOCITY (CM/S) — LEFT VELOCITY (CM/S)

80 (Aorta P)
AAA
102 (Aorta M - AAA)
97-115 (Aorta D)
115
200
180
160
160
194
180
131
85
120
161
100
120
120
150
80
110
140
140
110
120
180
100
80
* Arterio-Venous Fistula from branch of PFA to the CFV
PSV= 550 cm/s
EDV= 312 cm/s
* Pulsatile CFV
* Decreased resistance flow CFA
50
ATA
70
50
PTA
40
ATA
40
30
PER

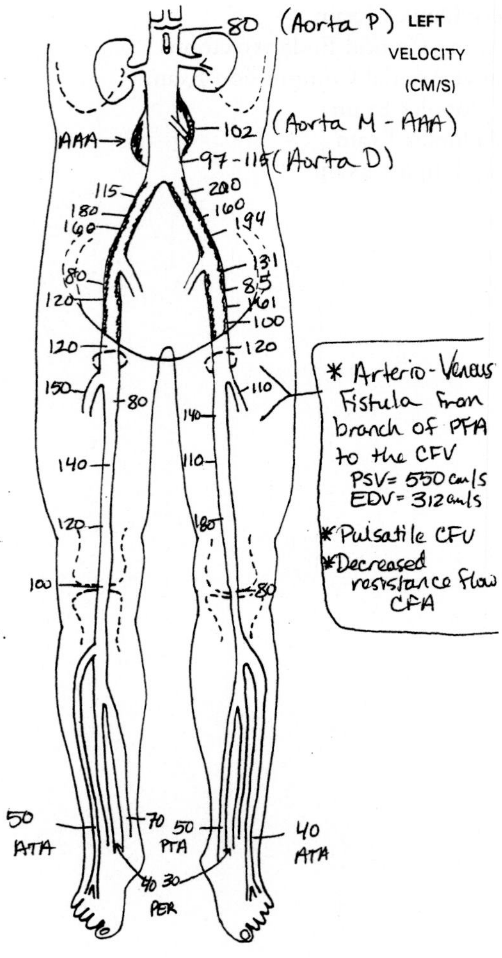

Abdominal Aortic Aneurysm: (Diameter)

Prox: 1.5 cm

Mid-AAA: 6.3 cm x 6.2 cm x 6.0 cm length

Dist: 2.15 cm

Intramural, nonocclusive thrombus in AAA.

	RIGHT	LEFT
TECH Ko		
TAPE #		

PHONE/PRELIMINARY REPORT IN CHART:

DICTATED:

DR. SIGNATURE/DISTRIBUTION:

UWMC/VASCULAR DIAGNOSTIC SERVICES

1654138 27-Oct-2000 1025
AORTA-ILIAC ART. DUPLEX
Requester:
Attending:
Preauth/Referral:

1654139 27-Oct-2000 1125
LEA DUPLEX LTD/UNILAT
Preauth/Referral:

Diagnosis:
Clinical History:

Vascular Diagnostic Service

This is an 83-year-old woman who presents with a nonhealing wound of the left anterior tibial region. This is possible osteomyelitis versus extremity ischemia. We are asked to evaluate for lower extremity arterial perfusion.

Lower Extremity Arterial Duplex Exam

Resting Systolic Pressures	Right	Left
Brachial artery	110	104
Posterior tibial artery	80	50
Anterior tibial artery	74	66
Ankle/arm index	0.72	0.60

By duplex exam, there is an abdominal aortic aneurysm identified in the mid- and distal aorta, measuring approximately 6.3 × 6.2 × 6.0 cm in length. Unable to visualize the origin of the right and left renal arteries secondary to abdominal gas. Intramural, nonocclusive thrombus is visualized within the abdominal aortic aneurysm.

There are mild to moderate diffuse and focal velocity elevations noted throughout the right and left common and external iliac arteries.

On the left, there is a fistula identified between the left branch of the profunda femoris artery and the common femoral vein. Decreased resistance to flow is noted throughout the left proximal femoral arteries. High, turbulent, and pulsatile venous flow signals are obtained within the left proximal femoral veins. There are mild to moderate diffuse and focal velocity elevations noted throughout the common femoral, proximal profunda femoris, superficial femoral, popliteal, distal posterior tibial, and distal peroneal arteries, upon somewhat limited evaluation. The left anterior tibial artery is seen to be open with monophasic flow at the level of the mid-calf, with no Doppler flow obtainable in its distal segment.

On the right, the common femoral, proximal profunda femoris, and superficial femoral arteries have no evidence of significant velocity elevation. Bitriphasic Doppler flow signals are obtained.

Impression

1. There is an abdominal aortic aneurysm identified, measuring 6.3 cm in diameter, with intramural nonocclusive thrombus visualized, as described above.
2. Moderately abnormal right and left ankle/arm indices.
3. Arteriovenous fistula from the left profunda femoris artery branch to the common femoral vein.
4. Diffuse and focal 50% stenoses throughout the right and left iliac arteries and the left femoral, popliteal, and tibial arteries, upon somewhat limited evaluation (described in detail above).
5. Right proximal femoral arteries have no significant stenosis.

Vascular technologist: Kari A. Olmsted, BS/RVT

Vascular Diagnostic Service Report

I have personally reviewed these images, and I agree with the report above (or as edited if so indicated below).

Attending Physician: R. Eugene Zierler, MD
/signed by/ R. Eugene Zierler, MD

UNIVERSITY OF WASHINGTON MEDICAL CENTER -- VASCULAR DIAGNOSTIC SERVICE

UPPER EXTREMITY ARTERIAL DUPLEX EXAM HISTORY ___21 year old male w/ endocarditis and possible thromboembolization to the (L) brachial artery. Pt. presents with absent (L) brachial pulse and decreased (L) radial pulse. Painful (L) upper extremity.___

DATE

UH#

NAME

D.O.B.

REFERRED BY

ADDRESS ____   ____ PHONE _____

RIGHT	SYSTOLIC PRESSURES	LEFT
	BRACHIAL	
	RADIAL	
	ULNAR	

RIGHT	DUPLEX FINDINGS		LEFT
	INNOMINATE		Normal
	P SUBCLAVIAN	P	Triphasic
	M	M	"
	D	D	"
	P AXILLARY	P	Triphasic
	D	D	"
	P BRACHIAL	P	Triphasic, ↓PSV resistive
	D	D	Occluded
	P RADIAL	P	Occluded
	D	D	Biphasic
	WITH ULNAR COMPRESSION		
	P ULNAR	P	Occluded
	D	D	Biphasic
	WITH RADIAL COMPRESSION		

NOTE: A = Augment   O = Obliterate

NC = No Change   R = Reverse

120
70
80

Large Collateral arteries; Good flow distally

RIGHT	LEFT	
		TECH
		Ko
		TAPE #

PHONE/PRELIMINARY REPORT IN CHART_____

DICTATED_____

DR. SIGNATURE/DISTRIBUTION_____

UWMC/VASCULAR DIAGNOSTIC SERVICES

1667985 27-Nov-2000 1000
UEA DUPLEX LTD
Requester:
Attending:
Preauth/Referral:

1667986 27-Nov-2000 1100
UEV DUPLEX LTD
Preauth/Referral:

Diagnosis:
Clinical History:

Vascular Diagnostic Service

This is a 21-year-old man with endocarditis and possible thromboembolization to the left brachial artery. He has absent left brachial pulse and decreased left radial pulse. We are asked to evaluate for arterial thrombosis.

Left Upper Extremity Arterial/Venous Duplex Exam

By duplex exam, triphasic Doppler flow signals are obtained within the axillary and proximal to mid-brachial arteries. The left distal brachial artery from approximately 2.0 cm above the brachial bifurcation is seen to be Doppler silent distally. No Doppler flow signals are obtainable from this level distally through the brachial bifurcation, origin of radial artery, and proximal ulnar artery. Multiple collateral arteries are identified proximal and distal to the level of the occlusion. The radial artery flow is reconstituted essentially at its origin via large collateral branches. The ulnar artery remains thrombosed proximally, and flow is reconstituted at approximately mid-forearm via large collateral branches. Flow signals within the radial and ulnar arteries at the wrist demonstrate decreased flow velocity. However, flow signals suggest good collateral flow/compensation. The radial and ulnar arteries are open at the wrist. Unable to completely rule out nonocclusive thrombus at this level.

Flow signals and vein wall compression are within normal limits throughout the axillary, brachial, basilic, radial, ulnar, and cephalic veins.

Impression

1. There is complete occlusion/thrombosis of the left distal brachial artery from approximately 2.0 cm above the brachial bifurcation and distal, with multiple collateral branches identified.
2. The radial artery is reconstituted essentially at its origin. The ulnar artery is reconstituted in the mid-forearm. Flow signals within the radial and ulnar arteries at the wrist suggest good collateral flow/compensation.
3. No other evidence of thrombosis or obstruction in the arteries of the left upper extremity.
4. No evidence of deep or superficial venous thrombosis in the left upper extremity.

Vascular technologist: Kari A. Olmsted, BS/RVT

Vascular Diagnostic Service Report

I have personally reviewed these images, and I agree with the report above (or as edited if so indicated below).

Attending Physician: Eugene Strandness, MD 356410
/signed by/ Eugene Strandness, MD 356410

UNIVERSITY OF WASHINGTON MEDICAL CENTER - VASCULAR DIAGNOSTIC SERVICE

PRE-DIALYSIS ACCESS DUPLEX EXAM

HISTORY _50 year-old male who is in need of dialysis access. No history of upper extremity DVT, or Prior central venous access._

DATE

UH#

NAME

D.O.B.

REFERRED BY _____ ONE _____

ADDRESS _____

DUPLEX FINDINGS

RIGHT   LEFT

SITE	SPONT	PHASIC	AUGMENT	COMPRESS	THROMBUS
RIGHT					
IJV	Nl			→	Ø
BR-CEPH	Nl			→	Ø
SUBCLAV	Nl			→	Ø
AXILLARY	Nl			→	Ø
BRACHIAL	Nl			→	Ø
RADIAL	Nl			→	Ø
ULNAR	Nl			→	Ø
CEPHALIC	Nl			→	Ø
BASILIC	Nl			→	Ø

SITE	SPONT	PHASIC	AUGMENT	COMPRESS	THROMBUS
LEFT					
IJV	Nl			→	Ø
BR-CEPH	Nl			→	Ø
SUBCLAV	Nl			→	Ø
AXILLARY	Nl			→	Ø
BRACHIAL	Nl			→	Ø
RADIAL	Nl			→	Ø
ULNAR	Nl			→	Ø
CEPHALIC	Nl			→	Ø
BASILIC	Nl			→	Ø

CEPHALIC SIZE (RIGHT): .59, .46, .47, .60, .51, .42, .40

BASILIC SIZE: .59 | 1.05, .47 | .72, .51 | .71, .30 | .48, .27 | .22, .30 | .22, .30 | .24

CEPHALIC SIZE (LEFT): .50, .52, .54, .55, .48, .43, .45

FOR VEIN MAP
sizes in cms

MODIFIED ALLEN'S TEST

RIGHT	Doppler signal change	LEFT
A	RADIAL(Ulnar comp)	A
A	ULNAR(Radial comp)	A

A = Augment
NC = No Change
O = Obliterate
R = Reverse

BRACHIAL ARTERY WAVEFORM   Right _Triphasic_   Left _Triphasic_

	R	L
TECH Ko		
TAPE #		

PHONE/PRELIMINARY REPORT IN CHART _____

DICTATED _____

DR. SIGNATURE/DISTRIBUTION _____

UWMC/VASCULAR DIAGNOSTIC SERVICES

1608269 19-Jul-2000 1410
UEA DUPLEX LTD/SPECIAL BILLING
Requester: Req ID: UPIN# RES000
Attending: Att ID: UPIN# RES000
Preauth/Referral:

1608271 19-Jul-2000 1610 Requester:
UE VEIN MAPPING BILAT/SPECIAL BILLING
Preauth/Referral: aaa va, pre dag 2121035

1608270 19-Jul-2000 1510 Requester:
UE VENOUS DUPLEX BILAT/SPECIAL BILLING
Preauth/Referral: aaa va, pre dag 2121035

Diagnosis:
Clinical History:

Vascular Diagnostic Service

This is a 50-year-old man who is in need of dialysis access. We are asked to evaluate preoperatively.

Predialysis Access Duplex Exam

On the right, flow signals and vein wall compression are within normal limits throughout the subclavian, axillary, brachial, radial, and ulnar veins. Flow through the subclavian, axillary, brachial, radial, and ulnar arteries is triphasic, with normal velocities. On the left, flow signals and vein wall compression are within normal limits throughout the subclavian, axillary, brachial, radial, and ulnar veins. Flow through the subclavian, axillary, brachial, radial, and ulnar arteries is triphasic, with normal velocities.

Modified Allen Test

On the right and left, radial artery Doppler flow demonstrates a normal response with ulnar artery compression. On the right and left, ulnar artery Doppler flow demonstrates a normal response with radial artery compression.

Cephalic/Basilic Vein Diameters

Right	Cephalic (cm)	Basilic (cm)
Proximal Upper Arm	0.59	0.59
Mid-upper arm	0.46	0.47
Distal upper arm	0.47	0.51
Proximal lower arm	0.60	0.30
Mid-lower arm	0.51	0.27
Distal lower arm	0.42	0.30

Left	Cephalic (cm)	Basilic (cm)
Proximal upper arm	0.50	1.05
Mid-upper arm	0.52	0.72
Distal upper arm	0.54	0.71
Proximal lower arm	0.55	0.48
Mid-lower arm	0.48	0.22
Distal lower arm	0.43	0.22

Impression

1. No evidence of venous thrombosis or obstruction in right or left upper extremity.
2. No evidence of significant arterial disease in right or left upper extremity.
3. Complete right and left palmar arches.
4. Right and left cephalic and basilic veins appear normal (sizes listed above).

Vascular technologist: Kari A. Olmsted, BS/RVT

Vascular Diagnostic Service Report

I have personally reviewed these images, and I agree with the report above (or as edited if so indicated below).

Attending Physician: R. Eugene Zierler, MD
/signed by/ R. Eugene Zierler, MD

UNIVERSITY OF WASHINGTON MEDICAL CENTER - VASCULAR DIAGNOSTIC SERVICE

CAROTID ARTERY DUPLEX EXAM

HISTORY _____
Bruit in Ⓡ neck
Ⓡ eye vision loss × 2 min.
Ⓡ Hand weakness)

DATE

UH#

NAME

D.O.B.

REFERRED BY _____ PHONE _____

ADDRESS _____

DUPLEX FINDINGS

BRUITS	RIGHT	LEFT	BLOOD PRESS.	RIGHT	LEFT	RISK FACTORS	
NONE		X	DOPPLER			HTN	+
CARDIAC			STETH	132/84	/	SMOKING	+
SUBCL						DIABETES	0
CAR-LO						LIPIDS	0
CAR-HI	X					CAD/PVD	CAD

RIGHT / **LEFT**

PSV	EDV	FLOW SEP	SPECT BROAD	TORT	PLAQUE	SPECT CLASS		PSV	EDV	FLOW SEP	SPECT BROAD	TORT	PLAQUE	SPECT CLASS
							CCAo							
80							CCAm	80						
							CCAd							
104	45			++		C	ICAp	417	161				non calc. D+	>80
							ICAm							
							ICAd							
80							ECA	180						

NA	ICA/CCA RATIO	NA

SUBCLAVIAN ART		VERTEBRAL ART	
SYST VEL	120	SYST VEL	80
WAVEFORM		ANTEGRADE	
TURBULENCE		RETROGRADE	
TORTUOSITY		TORTUOSITY	
PLAQUE		NOT LOCATED	
(Normal) < 50%		(Normal) Stenotic	
< 50% Occluded		Steal Occluded	

SUBCLAVIAN ART		VERTEBRAL ART	
SYST VEL	126	SYST VEL	80
WAVEFORM		ANTEGRADE	
TURBULENCE		RETROGRADE	
TORTUOSITY		TORTUOSITY	
PLAQUE		NOT LOCATED	
(Normal) < 50%		(Normal) Stenotic	
< 50% Occluded		Steal Occluded	

	RIGHT	LEFT	
TECH:			PHONE/PRELIMINARY REPORT IN CHART _____
TAPE #:			DICTATED _____
			DR. SIGNATURE/DISTRIBUTION _____

UWMC/VASCULAR DIAGNOSTIC SERVICES

1444552 1-Sep-1999 0850
CAROTID/VERTEBRAL DUPLEX
Requester:
Attending:
Preauth/Referral:

Diagnosis:
Clinical History:

Vascular Diagnostic Service

This is a 64-year-old woman with a carotid bruit in the right neck and a history of TIA's. She is to be evaluated for possible carotid artery disease.

Carotid Duplex Exam

On the left, increased velocities are noted at the origin of the internal carotid artery (focal lesion). The peak systolic velocity is noted to be 417 cm/sec, and the end diastolic velocity is 161 cm/sec. This indicates an 80%–99% diameter reduction. The bifurcation is at midneck, approximately 4.5 cm from the angle of the jaw. Increased flow rate in the external carotid artery may be due to increased flow (compensatory) rather than stenosis. The subclavian and vertebral arteries on this side are within normal limits. On the right, moderate spectral broadening with no velocity increase is noted in the internal carotid artery, consistent with a 16%–49% diameter reduction. The external carotid, subclavian, and vertebral arteries on this side are within normal limits.

Impression

1. 80%–99% diameter reduction of the left internal carotid artery.
2. 16%–49% diameter reduction of the right internal carotid artery.

Vascular technologist: Molly Zaccardi, BA/RVT

Vascular Diagnostic Service Report

I have personally reviewed these images, and I agree with the report above (or as edited if so indicated below).

Attending Physician: R. Eugene Zierler, MD
/signed by/ R. Eugene Zierler, MD

UNIVERSITY OF WASHINGTON MEDICAL CENTER

TCD MONITORING - CAROTID ENDARTERECTOMY

Date
UH#
Name
D.O.B.

Pre-Op Findings - Angio/Duplex:	
Left Carotid	C
Right Carotid	D+
Other	(L) vertebral "damped"
Symptoms	CVA's

Type of Surgery (R) CEA
Surgeons: Zierler, Gibson
Baseline Exam Date:
Baseline Exam Findings: 5-4-99 posterior to anterior collateralization on the (R) (R) MCA MV - 17 cms/sec
Vessel Monitored (R) MCA
Vessel Depth 45

	MV	PI	Air Emboli	Paticul. Emboli	
Pre-Anesthesia	39				40% = 15.6
Post-Anesthesia	25				40%=
Prior to Clamp					40%= ·
Imm. Post Clamp	5-8				%Baseline= 15-21 %
5 min Post Clamp					%Baseline=

Shunt Used? Yes 22 cms/sec Stump Pressure__________
Duration of Shunt______

	MV	PI	Air Emboli	Paticul. Emboli	
During CEA	22				%Baseline=
Imm. Post Clamp	35		3		%Baseline=
5 min Post Clamp					%Baseline=

Total Air Emboli_______ Total Particulate Emboli______ Total Emboli______

	MV	PI	Air Emboli	Paticul. Emboli
Recovery Room	42			
____Hours After				

Comments: multiple small "air emboli" with shunt

		Right	~~Left~~
Tech	WS	NL	
Tape#	∅		

VASCULAR DIAGNOSTIC SERVICE

UWMC/VASCULAR DIAGNOSTIC SERVICES

1390681 5-May-1999 1045
TCD LTD.
Requester:
Attending:
Preauth/Referral:

1392144 5-May-1999 1055
PORTABLE FEE
Preauth/Referral:

Diagnosis:
Clinical History:

Vascular Diagnostic Service

This is a 79-year-old man undergoing a right carotid endarterectomy.

Intraoperative Transcranial Doppler Exam

The right middle cerebral artery was monitored continously during the procedure:

	Mean Velocity (cm/sec)	Pulsative Index	Particulate Emboli	Air Emboli
Preanesthesia	39			
Postanesthesia	25			
Postclamp	5–8 (15%–21% baseline)			
With shunt	22			
During carotid endarterectomy	22			Multiple small
S/P shunt removal	35			3
End of procedure	35			
Recovery room	42			

Impression

1. Satisfactory right middle cerebral artery velocities/pulsatilities were maintained throughout the procedure.
2. Right middle cerebral artery velocities/pulsatilities remained normal postoperatively in the recovery room.

Vascular technologist: Watson B. Smith, RDMS/RVT

Vascular Diagnostic Service Report

I have personally reviewed these images and I agree with the report above (or as edited if so indicated below).

Attending Physician: Eugene Strandness, MD 356410
/signed by/ Eugene Strandness, MD 356410

UNIVERSITY OF WASHINGTON MEDICAL CENTER - VASCULAR DIAGNOSTIC SERVICE

THORACIC OUTLET ARTERIAL COMPRESSION EXAM

HISTORY _____

44 y/o male w/ Ⓛ UE pain
w/ position changes

he is s/p tumor surgery
Ⓛ clavicular area

DATE

UH#

NAME

D.O.B.

REFERRED BY _____ PHONE _____

ADDRESS _____

RIGHT				LEFT	
SYMPTOMS	DOPPLER/PPG RESPONSE	PATIENT POSITION		DOPPLER/PPG RESPONSE	SYMPTOMS
∅	NL	SEATED			
		HYPERABDUCTION/EXTENSION BOTH ARMS		NL	
		HYPERABDUCTION/EXTENSION LEFT ARM		diminished	↑ pain
		HYPERABDUCTION/EXTENSION RIGHT ARM		NL	
		ADSON MANEUVER HEAD TO LEFT		NL	
		ADSON MANEUVER HEAD TO RIGHT		NL	
		NECK FLEXION		NL	
		NECK HYPEREXTENSION		NL	
		COSTOCLAVICULAR MANEUVER (MODIFIED MILITARY POSITION)		NL	
		AER POSITION 90* ABDUCTION- EXTERNAL ROTATION		diminished	↑ pain
↓	↓	OTHER SYMPTOMATIC POSITION -- DESCRIBE:			

	RIGHT	LEFT	
TECH			
			PHONE/PRELIMINARY REPORT IN CHART: _____
TAPE #			DICTATED: _____
			DR. SIGNATURE/DISTRIBUTION: _____

UWMC/VASCULAR DIAGNOSTIC SERVICES

1263394 13-Jul-1998 1200
THORACIC OUTLET EVAL.
Requester:
Attending: Diagnosis:
Preauth/Referral: Clinical History:

Vascular Diagnostic Service

This is a 44-year-old man with left upper extremity pain/tingling S/P tumor surgery in the left clavicular area. His symptoms are exacerbated by positional changes.

Thoracic Outlet Arterial Duplex Exam

Segmental Pressures	Right	Left
Brachial artery	128	122
Radial artery	128	118
Ulnar artery	120	126

By duplex exam, left subclavian, axillary, brachial, radial, and ulnar arteries are patent with normal Doppler waveforms and velocities. No abnormalities are seen on Bmode image.

Modified Allen Test

On the right and left, radial artery Doppler flow augments with ulnar artery compression.
On the right and left, ulnar artery Doppler flow augments with radial artery compression.

Waveform Evaluation Exam

Normal photoplethysmographic waveforms are detectable in the second, third, fourth, and fifth fingers.

Positional Exam

Doppler flow signals in the left brachial artery were monitored in the following positions:

Hyperabduction/extension of the left arm
Hyperabduction/extension of the right arm
The Adson maneuver, head to the right
Neck flexion
Neck hyperextension

The costoclavicular maneuver
A 90-degree abduction/external rotation of both arms
simultaneously
Passive left upper extremity abduction to approximately
70–90 degrees

Doppler flow diminished and then became undetectable in the left brachial artery with hyperabduction/extension of the left upper extremity, 90-degree abduction/external rotation of the left upper extremity, and passive abduction to approximately 70–90 degrees. The subclavian and axillary arteries were evaluated with duplex ultrasound while the brachial artery was monitored with continuous wave Doppler to localize the level of obstruction. The subclavian artery flow became undetectable at approximately the level of the clavicle in those three positions. The vessel could not be imaged proximal to the clavicle.

Impression

1. Duplex, Doppler, and PPG exams find no evidence of fixed arterial lesions in left upper extremity or digit arteries.
2. Positional exam finds complete arterial obstruction of the left subclavian artery at approximately the level of the clavicle with hyperabduction/extension of the left upper extremity with 90-degree abduction/external rotation and with passive abduction at approximately 70–90 degrees.

Vascular technologist: Watson B. Smith, RDMS/RVT

Vascular Diagnostic Service Report

I have personally reviewed these images, and I agree with the report above (or as edited if so indicated below).

Attending Physician: R. Eugene Zierler, MD
/signed by/ R. Eugene Zierler, MD

TRANSCRANIAL DOPPLER EXAM

HISTORY _____

_____ 28 F _____

DATE _____ Vasculitis per angio _____

UH# _____ recent transient numbness _____

NAME _____ (R) hand and face _____

D.O.B. _____

_____

REFERRED BY _____ PHONE _____

ADDRESS _____

EXTRA-CRANIAL DUPLEX FINDINGS: MCA/ICA "99% occlusion   MCA stenosis

R = _per angio_   L = _per angio_

TRANSORBITAL

RIGHT	PSV	EDV	MEAN
ICA			
OPHTH			

All velocities in cm/sec

TRANSORBITAL

LEFT	PSV	EDV	MEAN
ICA			
OPHTH			

22   326   140

72

TRANSTEMPORAL   DICA

RIGHT	PSV	EDV	MEAN	
MCA	31	.17	22	PSV
ACA	?			EDV
BIFUR				MEAN
PCA			72	

DICA   TRANSTEMPORAL

	LEFT	PSV	EDV	MEAN
PSV	MCA			326
EDV	ACA			130
MEAN	BIFUR			
	PCA			102

D MCA   140

TRANSOCCIPITAL

	PSV	EDV	MEAN
LEFT VERT			
RIGHT VERT			
BASILAR ARTERY			72

MCA/ICA velocity ratio _____
MCA pulsatility index _.63_

MCA/ICA velocity ratio _7.2_
MCA pulsatility index _.43_

	RIGHT	LEFT	
TECH WS	collat	STEN	
TAPE # ∅			

PHONE/PRELIMINARY REPORT IN CHART: _____

DICTATED: _____

DR. SIGNATURE/DISTRIBUTION: _____

UWMC/VASCULAR DIAGNOSTIC SERVICES

1010738 8-Oct-1996 1400
TRANSCRANIAL DOPPLER
Requester:
Attending:
Preauth/Referral:

Diagnosis:
Clinical History:

Vascular Diagnostic Service

This is a 28-year-old woman with vasculitis. She experienced a recent episode of transient numbness of right hand and face.

Transcranial Duplex Exam

Elevated flow velocities are found proximally in the left middle cerebral artery (mean velocity = 326 cm/sec; ICA/CCA ratio = 7.2; pulsatility index = 0.43). Mildly elevated flow is also found at the left carotid siphon and in the left posterior cerebral artery. Normal waveforms and velocities are found in the left anterior cerebral artery.

On the right side, middle cerebral artery velocities/pulsatilities are abnormally low (mean velocity = 18 cm/sec; pulsatility index = 0.45). The right anterior cerebral artery can not be identified. Elevated flow is found in the posterior cerebral artery.

Basilar artery velocities are mildly elevated (72 cm/sec).

Impression

1. The moderate-severe left middle cerebral artery stenosis identified on previous duplex exam 07/30/96 appears to be progressive and is now severe by velocity, hemispheric index, and pulsatility index.
2. Elevated flow velocities found in the left carotid siphon are consistent with mild stenosis.
3. There are elevated flow velocities in the left posterior cerebral artery, which may represent collateral flow or mild stenosis.
4. There is no significant change in right side findings, with posterior to anterior collateralization and abnormally low right middle cerebral artery velocities/pulsatilities.
5. The right anterior cerebral artery can not be identified. The left anterior cerebral artery appears to be normal.
6. Basilar artery waveforms/velocities are mildly elevated, which may be secondary to collateral flow.

Vascular technologist: Watson B. Smith, RDMS/RVT

Vascular Diagnostic Service Report

I have personally reviewed these images, and I agree with the report above (or as edited if so indicated below).

Attending Physician: R. Eugene Zierler, MD
/signed by/ R. Eugene Zierler, MD

UNIVERSITY OF WASHINGTON MEDICAL CENTER - VASCULAR DIAGNOSTIC SERVICE

RENAL ARTERY DUPLEX EXAM

HISTORY _____

52 yr old woman s/p liver
tx. w/ CT report
Small (R) kidney and
↑ htn.

DATE

UH#

NAME

D.O.B.

_____
_____

REFERRED BY _____ PHONE _____

ADDRESS _____

DUPLEX FINDINGS

SYSTOLIC PRESSURES	R	L
BRACHIAL ARTERY		
POST TIBIAL ARTERY		
ANT TIBIAL ARTERY		
ANKLE/ARM INDEX		
STETHOSCOPE B/P	156/88	/

RISK FACTORS			
HYPERTENSION	+		
SMOKING	0		
DIABETES	0		
LIPIDS	0		
CAD/PVD/AAA	0	0	0

UPPER POLE

	MEDULA	CORTEX
PSV	25	18
EDV	9	8
EDR	.36	.44

PROX AORTA
| 69 |
INFLOW
VELOCITY

7.8cm
KIDNEY SIZE

CELIAC
| 190 | NL RESP
INSP

SMA
| 90 |

9.3cm
KIDNEY SIZE

UPPER POLE

MEDULA	CORTEX	
33	16	PSV
10	9	EDV
.30	.56	EDR

HILAR

PSV	
EDV	
AT	

	DIST	MID	PROX	ORIG
PSV	60	92	377	320
EDV				
RAR				

ORIG	PROX	MID	DIST	
93	87	77	41	PSV
				EDV
				RAR

HILAR

PSV	
EDV	
AT	

LOWER POLE

	MEDULA	CORTEX
PSV	25	12
EDV	12	4
EDR	.48	.33

AORTA DIMENSIONS/FLOW
_____

RAR = 5.4

ACCESSORY RENAL ARTERY
_____
_____
_____

LOWER POLE

MEDULA	CORTEX	
17	18	PSV
9	5	EDV
.53	.28	EDR

RENAL VEIN PATENT _____

_____ RENAL VEIN PATENT

TECH	RIGHT	LEFT
TAPE #		

PHONE/PRELIMINARY REPORT IN CHART_____

DICTATED_____

DR. SIGNATURE/DISTRIBUTION_____

UWMC VASCULAR DIAGNOSTIC SERVICES

1651322 24-Oct-2000 0900
RENAL ARTERY DUPLEX
Requester:
Attending:
Preauth/Referral:

Diagnosis:
Clinical History:

Vascular Diagnostic Service

This is a 52-year-old woman S/P liver transplant in 1997. Ultrasound reports a small right kidney of 8 cm in length and a left kidney of 10 cm in length. She recently has increased creatinine and is known to have protein C deficiency. She has a history of paradoxical emboli and CVA.

Renal Artery Duplex Exam

On the right, increased velocities in the origin and proximal segment of the main renal artery are consistent with a more than 60% diameter reduction. The renal/aortic ratio is 5.4. On the left, flow velocities are within normal limits throughout the main renal artery.

Flow in both kidneys demonstrates low resistance. The peak systolic velocity in the cortex of the right kidney ranges from 10 to 18 cm/sec, and the peak systolic velocity in the cortex of the left kidney is also low, ranges from 16 to 17 cm/sec.

The right kidney measures 7.8 cm in length, and the left kidney measures 9.3 cm in length.

Impression

1. Greater than 60% diameter reduction of the proximal right main renal artery.
2. Low resistance, low flow in both kidneys.
3. Small right kidney.

Vascular technologist: Molly Zaccardi, BA/RVT

Vascular Diagnostic Service Report

I have personally reviewed these images, and I agree with the report above (or as edited if so indicated below).

Attending Physician: R. Eugene Zierler, MD
/signed by/ R. Eugene Zierler, MD

CAROTID ARTERY DUPLEX EXAM

HISTORY _____

DATE

UH#

NAME

D.O.B.

68 y/o man w/ new onset of (L) hemiparesis

REFERRED BY _____ PHONE _____

ADDRESS _____

DUPLEX FINDINGS

BRUITS	RIGHT	LEFT	BLOOD PRESS.	RIGHT	LEFT	RISK FACTORS	
NONE			DOPPLER			HTN	+
CARDIAC			STETH	160/88	/	SMOKING	+
SUBCL						DIABETES	0
CAR-LO						LIPIDS	0
CAR-HI						CAD/PVD	0 / 0

RIGHT / **LEFT**

PSV	EDV	FLOW SEP	SPECT BROAD	TORT	PLAQUE	SPECT CLASS		PSV	EDV	FLOW SEP	SPECT BROAD	TORT	PLAQUE	SPECT CLASS
							CCAo							
73							CCAm	67						
70							CCAd	80						
149						<70	ICAp	45			++			C
120							ICAm	40						
60							ICAd	40						
120							ECA	80						

2.0	ICA/CCA RATIO	NA

SUBCLAVIAN ART		VERTEBRAL ART	
SYST VEL		SYST VEL	45
WAVEFORM		ANTEGRADE	
TURBULENCE		RETROGRADE	
TORTUOSITY		TORTUOSITY	
PLAQUE		NOT LOCATED	
(Normal)	< 50%	(Normal)	Stenotic
< 50%	Occluded	Steal	Occluded

SUBCLAVIAN ART		VERTEBRAL ART	
SYST VEL	140	SYST VEL	30
WAVEFORM		ANTEGRADE	
TURBULENCE		RETROGRADE	
TORTUOSITY		TORTUOSITY	
PLAQUE		NOT LOCATED	
(Normal)	< 50%	(Normal)	Stenotic
< 50%	Occluded	Steal	Occluded

	RIGHT	LEFT	
TECH:			PHONE/PRELIMINARY REPORT IN CHART _____
TAPE #:			DICTATED _____
			DR. SIGNATURE/DISTRIBUTION _____

UWMC/VASCULAR DIAGNOSTIC SERVICES

1666301 20-Nov-2000 1530
CAROTID/VERTEBRAL DUPLEX
Requester:
Attending:
Preauth/Referral:

Diagnosis:
Clinical History:

Vascular Diagnostic Service

This is a 68-year-old man with new onset of left hemiparesis.

Carotid Duplex Exam

On the right, increased velocities in the internal carotid artery are consistent with a 50%–79% diameter reduction. The peak systolic velocity is 149 cm/sec, and end diastolic velocity 25 cm/sec. The ICA/CCA velocity ratio is 2.0, which suggests this is a less than 70% diameter reduction.

On the left, moderate flow disturbances are noted in the internal carotid artery, with no evidence of velocity increase, consistent with 16%–49% diameter reduction.

Bilaterally, the subclavian, vertebral, and external carotid arteries are within normal limits.

Impression

1. Less than 70% diameter reduction of the right internal carotid artery.
2. 16%–49% diameter reduction of the left internal carotid artery.

Vascular technologist: Molly Zaccardi, BA/RVT

Vascular Diagnostic Service Report

I have personally reviewed these images, and I agree with the report above (or as edited if so indicated below).

Attending Physician: R. Eugene Zierler, MD
/signed by/ R. Eugene Zierler, MD

UNIVERSITY OF WASHINGTON MEDICAL CENTER - VASCULAR DIAGNOSTIC SERVICE

ABDOMINAL VENOUS DUPLEX EXAM HISTORY _57 YEAR OLD FEMALE WHO PRESENTS_
WITH RIGHT UPPER QUADRANT PAIN,
DATE _____ _ABDOMINAL SPASM AND DECREASED_
UH# _____ _APPETITE FOLLOWING NISSEN_
NAME _____ _FUNDOPLICATION._
D.O.B. _____ _____

REFERRED BY _____ PHONE _____
ADDRESS _____

DUPLEX FINDINGS

HEPATIC VEIN	
VELOCITY	25 cm/s
DIRECTION	NL
THROMBUS	
PHAS/PULSE	+

IVC	
SIZE	
VELOCITY	75 cm/s
THROMBUS	—
PHAS/PULSE	+

SMV	
VELOCITY	∅
DIRECTION	∅
SIZE	
THROMBUS	+

RIGHT RENAL VEIN	
VELOCITY	30 cm/s
DIRECTION	NL
SIZE	
THROMBUS	—

MAIN PORTAL VEIN	
VELOCITY	∅
DIRECTION	∅
SIZE	2.1 cm
THROMBUS	+

RIGHT PORTAL VEIN	
VELOCITY	∅
DIRECTION	∅
SIZE	
THROMBUS	+

LEFT PORTAL VEIN	
VELOCITY	∅
DIRECTION	∅
SIZE	
THROMBUS	+

SPLENIC VEIN	
VELOCITY	∅
DIRECTION	∅
SIZE	
THROMBUS	+

LEFT RENAL VEIN	
VELOCITY	30 cm/s
DIRECTION	NL
SIZE	
THROMBUS	—

ASCITES	HEPATOMEGALY	SPLENOMEGALY
—	—	—

	PORTAL VEIN	HEPATIC VEIN
TECH		
TAPE #		

PHONE/PRELIMINARY REPORT IN CHART _____
DICTATED _____
DR. SIGNATURE/DISTRIBUTION _____

UWMC/VASCULAR DIAGNOSTIC SERVICES

1643679 9-Oct-2000 1245
PORTAL VEIN DUPLEX
Requester:
Attending:
Preauth/Referral:

Diagnosis:
Clinical History:

Vascular Diagnostic Service

This is a 57-year-old woman who presents with possible portal vein thrombosis.

Portal Vein Duplex Exam

The IVC was open. Hepatic veins were also open.

The main portal vein, right and left portal veins, and superior mesenteric veins had no Doppler flow, with echogenic material noted within the lumen of the vessel. Thrombus appeared to involve approximately 1.5 cm of the splenic vein at the confluence with the superior mesenteric vein. The remainder of the splenic vein appeared to be open, with reversed flow (towards the spleen) supplied by a collateral.

Impression

1. Portal, superior mesenteric, and partial splenic vein thrombosis. Only the very proximal splenic vein appears to be thrombosed at this time (near the confluence with the SMV). The remainder of the splenic vein appears to be open, with reversed Doppler flow (toward the spleen) supplied by a collateral.

Vascular technologist: Bridget Mraz, BS/RDMS/RVT

Vascular Diagnostic Service Report

I have personally reviewed these images, and I agree with the report above (or as edited if so indicated below).

Attending Physician: Eugene Strandness, MD 356410
/signed by/ Eugene Strandness, MD 356410

TRAM FLAP PERFORATOR DUPLEX EXAM

HISTORY _____

54 y/o woman
s/p ⒷB mastectomy

DATE

UH#

NAME

D.O.B.

REFERRED BY _____ PHONE _____

ADDRESS _____

DUPLEX FINDINGS

VESSEL	VEL cm/sec	ANGLE	VERT +/- cm	HORIZ cm
RIGHT				
ZONE I	40	36	+2	5.5
	51	30	+3	5.0
ZONE II	14	14	0	7
	32	12	-2.5	4.5
ZONE III	17	40	-5	5.0
	34	46	-6	4.5
ZONE IV	15	60	-8	5.5
LEFT				
ZONE I	28	40	+2	3.0
	19		+3.5	5.0
ZONE II	25	40	-.5	1.5
	32	40	-.5	3.5
	19		-1.5	4.5
ZONE III	50	46	-5	1.5
	22	24	-5	3.5
ZONE IV	14	46	-8.5	3.0
	18	10	-8	4.0

IMA RT	79	60
IMA LT	92	60

# PERFORATORS	R _____	L _____

EPIGASTRIC ARTERIES:

Continuous to Zone _____ Right

Zone _____ Left

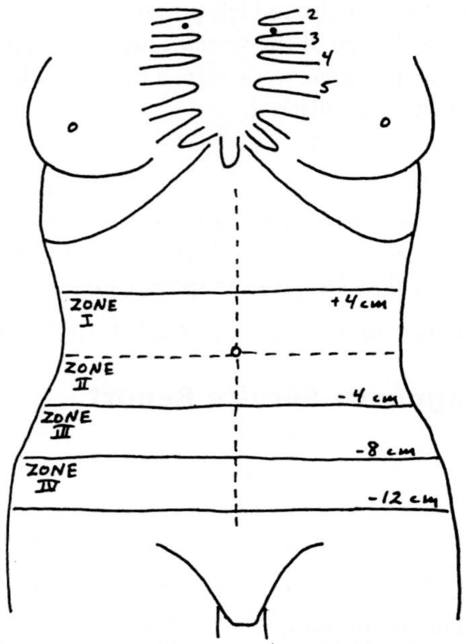

ZONE I +4 cm
ZONE II -4 cm
ZONE III -8 cm
ZONE IV -12 cm

TECH	RIGHT	LEFT
TAPE #		

PHONE/PRELIMINARY REPORT IN CHART _____

DICTATION _____

DR. SIGNATURE/DISTRIBUTION _____

UWMC/VASCULAR DIAGNOSTIC SERVICES

1400530 26-May-1999 1020
TRAM FLAP DUPLEX
Requester:
Attending:
Preauth/Referral:

Diagnosis:
Clinical History:

Vascular Diagnostic Service

This is a 54-year-old woman with a history of breast cancer, preoperative for mastectomy, and transverse rectus abdominis myocutaneous (TRAM) flap.

TRAM Flap Duplex Exam

By duplex, the right and left inferior epigastric arteries are seen to be patent from the origins of the external iliac arteries to the level of the umbilicus.

The total of 16 epigastric perforators were identified and marked on the skin.

Peak Systolic Velocities

Right	Velocity (cm/sec)	Vertical (cm)	Horizontal (cm)
Zone I	40	+2.0	5.5
	51	+3.0	5.0
Zone II	14	0	7.0
	32	−2.5	4.5
Zone III	17	−5.0	5.0
	34	−6.0	4.5
Zone IV	15	−8.0	5.5

Left	Velocity (cm/sec)	Vertical (cm)	Horizontal (cm)
Zone I	28	+2.0	3.0
	19	+3.5	5.0
Zone II	25	−0.5	1.5
	32	−0.5	3.5
	19	−1.5	4.5
Zone III	50	−5.0	1.5
	22	−5.0	3.5
Zone IV	14	8.5	3.0
	18	8.0	4.0

Peak systolic velocities in the internal mammary artery are 79 cm/sec on the right and 92 cm/sec on the left.

Impression

1. The right and left inferior epigastric arteries are seen to be patent from origin to umbilicus.
2. A total of 16 epigastric perforators were seen and marked as above.
3. The internal mammary artery peak systolic velocities are 70 cm/sec on the right and 92 cm/sec on the left.

Vascular technologist: Molly Zaccardi, BA/RVT

Vascular Diagnostic Service Report

I have personally reviewed these images, and I agree with the report above (or as edited if so indicated below).

Attending Physician: Eugene Strandness, MD 356410
/signed by/ Eugene Strandness, MD 356410

PRE FIBULA FLAP VASCULAR EVALUATION

HISTORY _____
56 y/o man
preop for Fib Flap

DATE

UH#

NAME

D.O.B.

REFERRED BY _____ PHONE _____

ADDRESS _____

DUPLEX FINDINGS

SYSTOLIC PRESSURES:	R	L
BRACHIAL ARTERY	140	140
POST TIBIAL ARTERY	126	140
ANT TIBIAL ARTERY	124	120
PERONEAL ART	120	120
ANKLE/ARM INDEX	.90	1.0

PERONEAL ARTERIES DIAMETER MEASUREMENTS	R	L
PROXIMAL	.26	.31
MIDDLE	.31	.28
DISTAL	.21	.24

PERONEAL ARTERIES	R	L
CALCIFICATION VISUALIZED	Y	Y
ANATOMICAL VARIANTS	N	N

DUPLEX OF PERONEAL VEINS COMPRESSION (Y/N)	R	L
PROXIMAL	Y	Y
MIDDLE	Y	Y
DISTAL	Y	Y

PERONEAL ARTERIES VELOCITY MEASUREMENTS	R	L
PROXIMAL	40	40
MIDDLE	40	30
DISTAL	25	20

PERONEAL ARTERIES WAVEFORM ANALYSIS	R	L
PROXIMAL	tri	tri
MIDDLE	↓	↓
DISTAL	↓	↓

RIGHT		RIGHT
# PERFORATORS: 5		
DISTANCE FROM MALLEOLUS (cm)		
28		
24		
22.5		
18.5		
12		

>50% red Common fem + Superficial fem. arteries on R

LEFT	LEFT
# PERFORATORS: 4	
DISTANCE FROM MALLEOLUS (cm)	
27	
22.5	
18.5	
14	

50% diam. red Com. fem artery on L

	R	L	PHONE/PRELIMINARY REPORT IN CHART: _____
TAPE #			DICTATED: _____
TECH			DR. SIGNATURE/DISTRIBUTION: _____

UWMC/VASCULAR DIAGNOSTIC SERVICES

1665545 20-Nov-2000 1300
LEA DUPLEX LTD/UNILAT
Requester:
Attending:
Preauth/Referral:

1665546 20-Nov-2000 1400
LEV DUPLEX LTD
Preauth/Referral:

Diagnosis:
Clinical History:

Vascular Diagnostic Service

This is a 56-year-old man preoperative for fibula flap surgery. He is to be evaluated for arterial and venous patency of the lower legs.

Pre–Fibula Flap Evaluation

Resting Systolic Pressures	Right	Left
Brachial artery	140	Not taken
Posterior tibial artery	126	140
Anterior tibial artery	124	126
Ankle/arm index	0.90	1.0

Duplex of Lower Extremity Arteries

Right Lower Extremity

- A 50% diameter reduction of the common and proximal superficial femoral arteries.
- Popliteal, anteroposterior tibial, and peroneal arteries are within normal limits.

  No evidence of anatomic variance.

Left Lower Extremity

- A 50% diameter reduction of the common femoral artery.
- Profunda femoris, superficial femoral, popliteal, posteroanterior tibial, and peroneal arteries are patent

Duplex of Peroneal Perforators

Five peroneal perforators were seen in the right leg, and 4 peroneal perforators were seen in the left leg (left perforators larger than right perforators).

Peroneal Artery Diameters (cm)	Right	Left
Proximal	0.26	0.31
Middle	0.31	0.28
Distal	0.21	0.24

Deep Veins

Duplex reveals the bilateral femoral, popliteal, and all three pairs of tibial veins to be widely patent, with normal flow patterns and vein wall compression.

The abdominal veins and arteries were not evaluated.

Impression

1. Abnormal right ankle/arm index.
2. A 50% diameter reduction of the femoral arteries, bilaterally.
3. Peroneal perforators were marked on both legs.
4. Deep veins in both legs were found to be within normal limits.

Vascular technologist: Molly Zaccardi, BA/RVT

Vascular Diagnostic Service Report

I have personally reviewed these images, and I agree with the report above (or as edited if so indicated below).

Attending Physician: R. Eugene Zierler, MD
/signed by/ R. Eugene Zierler, MD

UNIVERSITY OF WASHINGTON MEDICAL CENTER - VASCULAR DIAGNOSTIC SERVICE

MESENTERIC ARTERY DUPLEX EXAM   HISTORY _____

68 y/o male S/P PTA
and Stent placement
for SMA stenosis

DATE

UH#

NAME

D.O.B.

REFERRED BY _____   PHONE _____

ADDRESS _____

SYSTOLIC PRESSURES	RIGHT	LEFT
BRACHIAL ARTERY		
POST TIBIAL ARTERY		
ANT TIBIAL ARTERY		
ANKLE/ARM INDEX		

ABDOMINAL BRUIT: _____

WITH DEEP INSP: _____

POST-PRANDIAL: After _____ oz. Ensure Plus

SITE MONITORED:

MINUTE	SYSTOLIC VELOCITY	REVERSE FLOW	DIASTOLIC VELOCITY
5			
10		*not done*	
15			
20			

DUPLEX FINDINGS

FASTING:	SYSTOLIC VELOCITY	REVERSE FLOW	DIASTOLIC VELOCITY
Ao			
SMA Orig	555	0	5
SMA Prox	600	0	5
SMA Dist	228	0	post stenotic
Celiac Orig	241		15
Celiac Mid	190		
Hepatic Orig	127		40
Splenic Orig	148		68
IMA Orig			

Celiac Axis Compression:

Deep Insp	255		18

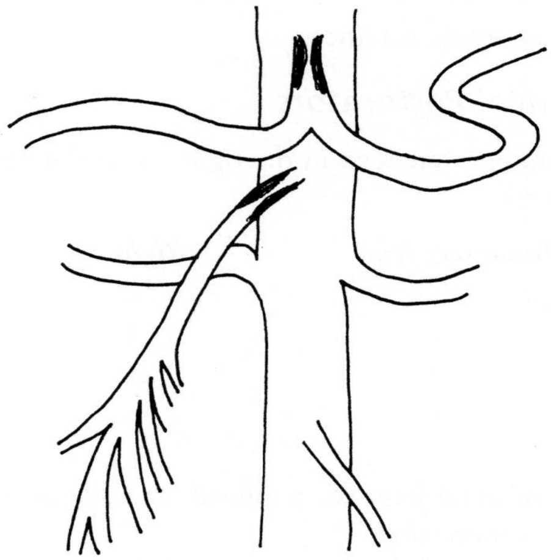

TECH	
	CELIAC
TAPE #	SMA
	IMA

PHONE/PRELIMINARY REPORT IN CHART: _____

DICTATED: _____

DR. SIGNATURE/DISTRIBUTION: _____

UWMC/VASCULAR DIAGNOSTIC SERVICES

1643646 10-Oct-2000 0830
MESENTERIC ARTERY DUPLEX
Requester:
Attending:
Preauth/Referral:

Diagnosis:
Clinical History:

Vascular Diagnostic Service

This is a 68-year-old man S/P angioplasty and stent placement for SMA stenosis.

Mesenteric Artery Duplex Exam

The abdominal aorta was noted to be within normal limits in the proximal segment. Significant velocity increase was noted in the proximal celiac axis, with peak systolic velocity of 360 cm/sec. Monophasic flow present distally in the splenic artery.

Significant velocity increase was also noted in the proximal superior mesenteric artery, with peak systolic velocity of 555 cm/sec, with turbulent flow noted distally. The distal superior mesenteric artery had a peak systolic velocity of 170 cm/sec. The SMA stent was not well visualized because of extreme bowel gas.

Impression

1. No significant change at this time from exam on 09/06/00.
2. Greater than 70% stenosis in the proximal celiac axis.
3. Greater than 70% stenosis in the proximal superior mesenteric artery, with turbulent flow noted distally.

Vascular technologist: Bridget Mraz, BS/RDMS/RVT

Vascular Diagnostic Service Report

I have personally reviewed these images, and I agree with the report above (or as edited if so indicated below).

Attending Physician: Eugene Strandness, MD 356410
/signed by/ Eugene Strandness, MD 356410

DIALYSIS ACCESS GRAFT DUPLEX STUDY HISTORY _____

93 y/o male
_w/ (L) UE_
Cadaveric dialysis
access graft

DATE

UH#

NAME

D.O.B.

REFERRED BY _____   PHONE _____

ADDRESS _____

TYPE OF GRAFT: LOCATION: DATE CREATED: _____

_____ A-V fistula   _____ Right X Left

_____ Gortex straight   _____ Forearm   DATE FIRST DIALYSIS: _____

_____ Gortex loop   X Upper arm

X Other (vein, etc.)   _____ Groin

VENOUS PRESSURES DURING LAST DIALYSIS:

Highest: _____   Lowest: _____   Mean: _____   DATE LAST DIALYSIS: _____

DUPLEX FINDINGS	Systolic	Diastolic	Mean flow
Inflow Artery	214 cm/s	50 cm/s	_____ cm/s
(_axillary_) NAME			
Art. Anast.	300 cm/s	100 cm/s	_____ cm/s
Prox. graft	60 cm/s	35 cm/s	_____ cm/s
Mid graft	57 cm/s	30 cm/s	_____ cm/s
Dist graft	114 cm/s	70 cm/s	_____ cm/s
Ven. Anast.	629 cm/s	400 cm/s	_____ cm/s
Outflow Vein	60 cm/s	40 cm/s	_____ cm/s
(_____) NAME			
Brachial Vein	40 cm/s	20 cm/s	_____ cm/s
Axillary Vein	60 cm/s	40 cm/s	_____ cm/s
Subclavian Vein	___ cm/s	___ cm/s	_____ cm/s

VOLUME FLOW: Mean flow _____ cm/s X graft diameter _____ mm X 60 = _____ ml/min
(From a straight, non-stenotic segment)

	ART	VEN	COMMENTS: _____
TECH			
TAPE #			

UWMC/VASCULAR DIAGNOSTIC SERVICES

1487397 2-Dec-1999 0905
DIALYSIS ACCESS DUPLEX

Requester:	Req ID:
Attending:	Att ID:
Preauth/Referral:	

Diagnosis:
Clinical History:

Vascular Diagnostic Service

This is a 93-year-old man with left upper arm cadaveric dialysis access graft. We are asked to rule out stenosis.

Dialysis Access Graft Duplex Exam

The left upper extremity cadaveric dialysis access graft is patent, with a midgraft velocity of 57 cm/sec.

The arterial anstomosis measured 0.83 cm in diameter.

At the venous anastomosis, a velocity increase was noted from 114 cm/sec to 629 cm/sec, with poststenotic flow suggestive of high-grade stenosis.

The left axillary and proximal to mid-brachial arteries had low-resistance Doppler flow. However, the distal brachial, proximal to mid-ulnar, and radial arteries have reversed flow throughout diastole. At the wrist, the radial and ulnar arteries have monophasic Doppler flow. The radial and ulnar arteries were quite calcified and relatively small in caliber.

The left axillary, brachial, radial, and ulnar veins are patent.

Impression

1. Patent left upper extremity cadaveric dialysis access graft, with a midgraft velocity of 57 cm/sec.
2. High-grade stenosis at the venous anastomosis.
3. Steal phenomenon was noted in the distal left brachial, ulnar, and radial arteries.
4. Patent left axillary, brachial, radial, and ulnar veins.

Vascular technologist: Bridget Mraz, BS/RDMS/RVT

Vascular Diagnostic Service Report

I have personally reviewed these images, and I agree with the report above (or as edited if so indicated below).

Attending Physician: Eugene Strandness, MD 356410
/signed by/ Eugene Strandness, MD 356410

LOWER EXTREMITY VENOUS DUPLEX EXAM

HISTORY _67 YEAR OLD FEMALE S/P LEFT KNEE SURGERY WHO PRESENTS WITH NEW ONSET LEFT CALF TENDERNESS AND SWELLING._

DATE

UH#

NAME

D.O.B.

REFERRED BY _____ PHONE _____

ADDRESS _____

DUPLEX FINDINGS

SITE	SPONT	PHASIC	AUGMENT	REFLUX	COMPRESS	THROMBUS
IVC	+	+			+	−

RIGHT

SITE	SPONT	PHASIC	AUGMENT	REFLUX	COMPRESS	THROMBUS
CIV	+	+			+	−
EIV	+	+			+	−
CFV	+	+	+	−	+	−
Prof	+	+	+	−	+	−
SFVp	+	+	+	−	+	−
SFVm	+	+	+	−	+	−
SFVd	+	+	+	−	+	−
Pop	+	+	+	−	+	−
PTV	+	+	+	+	+	+	−	−	+	+	−	−
PER	+	+	+	+	+	+	−	−	+	+	−	−
GrSp	+	+	+	−	+	−
GrSm	+	+	+	−	+	−

LEFT

SITE	SPONT	PHASIC	AUGMENT	REFLUX	COMPRESS	THROMBUS
CIV	+	+			+	−
EIV	+	+			+	−
CFV	+	+	↓		+	−
Prof	+	+	+		+	−
SFVp	+	+	↓		+	−
SFVm	−	−	−		−	+
SFVd	−	−	−		−	+
Pop	−	−	−		−	+
PTV	−	−	−	−	−	−			−	−	+	+
PER	−	−	−	−	−	−			−	−	+	+
GrSp	+	+	+	−	+	−
GrSm	+	+	+	−	+	−

RIGHT

GSV DIAM

LSV DIAM

LEFT

GSV DIAM

sizes in cm

	R			L	
TECH					
TAPE #					

PHONE/PRELIMINARY REPORT IN CHART _____

DICTATED _____

DR. SIGNATURE/DISTRIBUTION _____

UWMC/VASCULAR DIAGNOSTIC SERVICES

1137800 1-Sep-1997 0955
CHEST 1VIEW
Requester:
Attending:
Preauth/Referral:

Diagnosis:
Clinical History:

Addended Report, Revised Report

Vascular Diagnostic Service

This is a 67-year-old woman S/P left knee surgery who presents with new onset of left calf tenderness and swelling.

Bilateral Lower Extremity Venous Duplex Exam

By duplex exam, the IVC is patent, with normal flow characteristics and vein wall compressibility. Flow patterns in the right and left common and external iliac, common femoral, and right superficial femoral, proximal profunda femoris, popliteal, paired posterior tibial, anterior tibial, and peroneal veins are within normal limits (spontaneous, phasic, brisk augmentation, no reflux). Vein wall compressibility is within normal limits throughout.

On the left, no Doppler flow is obtainable from the mid- to distal superficial femoral, popliteal, posterior tibial, or peroneal veins. Vein walls are incompressible throughout.

The right and left greater saphenous veins are patent at the confluence with the common femoral veins.

Impression

1. Deep vein thrombosis in the left mid- to distal superficial femoral, popliteal, posterior tibial, and peroneal veins.
2. No evidence of deep vein thrombosis throughout the right lower extremity.

Vascular technologist: Bridget Mraz, BS/RDMS/RVT

Vascular Diagnostic Service Report

I have personally reviewed these images, and I agree with the report above (or as edited if so indicated below).

Attending Physician: R. Eugene Zierler, MD
/signed by/ R. Eugene Zierler, MD

UPPER EXTREMITY VENOUS DUPLEX EXAM HISTORY _45 YEAR OLD FEMALE WITH_
HISTORY OF BREAST CANCER AND
DATE _____ _CHEMOTHERAPY. PATIENT HAS RIGHT_
UH# _____ _SUBCLAVIAN VENOUS LINE AND NOW_
NAME _____ _PRESENTS WITH NEW ONSET OF_
D.O.B. _____ _RIGHT UPPER EXTREMITY SWELLING._

REFERRED BY _____ PHONE _____

ADDRESS _____

DUPLEX FINDINGS   RIGHT   LEFT

SITE	SPONT	PHASIC	AUGMENT	COMPRESS	THROMBUS
RIGHT					
IJV	+	+		+	−
BR-CEPH	+	+	−	+	−
SUBCLAV	−	−	−	−	+
AXILLARY	−	−	−	−	+
BRACHIAL	−	−	−	−	+
RADIAL	−	−	+	+	−
ULNAR	−	−	+	+	−
CEPHALIC	−	−	−	−	+
BASILIC	−	−	−	−	+

SITE	SPONT	PHASIC	AUGMENT	COMPRESS	THROMBUS
LEFT					
IJV	+	+		+	−
BR-CEPH	+	+	+	+	−
SUBCLAV	+	+	+	+	−
AXILLARY	+	+	+	+	−
BRACHIAL	+	+	+	+	−
RADIAL	+	+	+	+	−
ULNAR	+	+	+	+	−
CEPHALIC	+	+	+	+	−
BASILIC	+	+	+	+	−

CEPHALIC SIZE □   BASILIC SIZE □ □   CEPHALIC SIZE □

□   □ □   □

□   □ □   □

□   □ □   □

□   □ □   □

□   □ □   □

FOR VEIN MAP

sizes in cms

	RIGHT	LEFT
TECH		
TAPE #		

PHONE/PRELIMINARY REPORT IN CHART_____

DICTATED_____

DR. SIGNATURE/DISTRIBUTION_____

UWMC/VASCULAR DIAGNOSTIC SERVICES

1137800 1-Sep-1997 0955
CHEST 1VIEW
Requester:
Attending:
Preauth/Referral:

Diagnosis:
Clinical History:

Addended Report, Revised Report

Vascular Diagnostic Service

This is a 45-year-old woman with a history of breast cancer and chemotherapy. The patient has a right subclavian venous line and now presents with new onset of right upper extremity swelling.

Bilateral Upper Extremity Venous Duplex Exam

On the right, flow signals and vein wall compression were within normal limits throughout the internal jugular and brachiocephalic veins. No Doppler flow was obtainable from the subclavian, axillary, and brachial veins. Vein walls were incompressible throughout. The basilic vein had no Doppler flow and was incompressible with scanhead pressure throughout the upper arm. The cephalic vein had minimal Doppler flow and was partially compressible in the upper arm. The remainder of the right cephalic vein was within normal limits. Vein wall compressibility was within normal limits.

On the left, flow signals and vein wall compression were within normal limits throughout the internal jugular, brachiocephalic, subclavian, axillary, and brachial veins.

Impression

1. Deep vein thrombosis in the right subclavian, axillary, and brachial veins.
2. Superficial thrombophlebitis in the right cephalic and basilic veins.
3. No evidence of deep vein thrombosis throughout the left upper extremity.

Vascular technologist: Bridget Mraz, BS/RDMS/RVT

Vascular Diagnostic Service Report

I have personally reviewed these images, and I agree with the report above (or as edited if so indicated below).

Attending Physician: R. Eugene Zierler, MD
/signed by/ R. Eugene Zierler, MD

LOWER EXTREMITY ARTERIAL EXERCISE EXAM   HISTORY _59 year old Female with_
(R) hip and buttock claudication
DATE _symptoms after walking 1-2_
UH# _blocks at an incline (symptoms_
NAME _occur at 4-5 blocks of flat terrain)_
D.O.B. _with 5 minute recovery time._

REFERRED BY   PHONE _____

ADDRESS ___| _____

Resting

SYSTOLIC PRESSURES	RIGHT	LEFT
BRACHIAL ARTERY	148	142
POSTERIOR TIBIAL ARTERY	152	150
ANTERIOR TIBIAL ARTERY	138	142
PERONEAL ARTERY		
ANKLE/ARM INDEX	>1.0	>1.0

RISK FACTORS	
HTN	⊕ 2 meds
SMOKING	⊕ 1 ppd x 10 years
DIABETES	⊖
LIPIDS	⊖
CAD/PVD	⊖

EXERCISE TREADMILL: Speed 2.0 mph Grade 12 %	
TIME	SYMPTOMS WITH EXERCISE
2:00	(R) thigh tightness
2:30	(R) buttock tightness
3:30	(R) buttock, hip pain, thigh tightness
5:00	(R) buttock, hip + thigh pain + cramping

TOTAL WALK TIME: 5 MIN. 00 SEC.
STOPPED DUE TO: Patient discomfort + test completion

POST EXERCISE PRESSURES				
RT 58	TIME	LT 126	150 ARM
74	1 MIN	138	
102	2 MIN	146	
136	4 MIN	152	
148	6 MIN		
150	8 MIN		
	10 MIN		
	12 MIN		

	RIGHT	LEFT
TECH KO		
TAPE #		

PHONE/PRELIMINARY REPORT IN CHART_____

DICTATED_____

DR. SIGNATURE/DISTRIBUTION_____

UWMC/VASCULAR DIAGNOSTIC SERVICES

1137800 1-Sep-1997 0955
CHEST 1VIEW
Requester:
Attending:
Preauth/Referral:

Diagnosis:
Clinical History:

Addended Report, Revised Report

Vascular Diagnostic Service

This is a 59-year-old woman with right hip and buttock claudication symptoms after walking 1–2 blocks at an incline (symptoms occur at 4–5 blocks of flat terrain walking), with a 5-minute recovery time. We are asked to evaluate for arterial insufficiency.

Lower Extremity Arterial Duplex Exam

Resting Systolic Pressures	*Right*	*Left*
Brachial artery	148	142
Posterior tibial artery	152	150
Anterior tibial artery	138	142
Ankle/arm index	>1	>1

Exercise Treadmill Test

The patient walked on a treadmill set at 2 mph with 12% grade for the full 5-minute protocol.

Postexercise Pressures

Time	*Right*	*Left*	*Brachial*
Immediate	58	126	150
1 min	74	138	
2 min	102	146	
4 min	136	152	
6 min	148		
8 min	150		

By duplex exam, the abdominal aorta is seen to be of even diameter.

Flow signals are within normal limits for velocity and waveform contour.

On the right, flow through the common iliac artery is triphasic, with normal flow velocities. The external iliac artery demonstrates diffuse, significant velocity elevations (maximum peak systolic velocity = 360 cm/sec, increased from 156 cm/sec in the common iliac artery). Turbulence, spectral broadening, and subtle waveform changes are noted in the distal external iliac artery. Flow through the common femoral and proximal profunda femoris arteries is turbulent, with no evidence of velocity increase. Flow through the superficial femoral and popliteal arteries is bi-triphasic, with no other evidence of focal or diffuse velocity elevations. Doppler flow signals within the distal posterior tibial, anterior tibial, and peroneal arteries are essentially biphasic.

On the left, the proximal common iliac artery demonstrates focal significant velocity elevations (maximum peak systolic velocity = 298 cm/sec, increased from 85 cm/sec in the distal abdominal aorta). Turbulence, spectral broadening, and waveform changes are noted within the mid and distal common iliac artery. Flow through the external iliac, common femoral, proximal profunda femoris, superficial femoral, and popliteal arteries is bi-triphasic, with no other evidence of focal or diffuse velocity elevations. Doppler flow signals within the distal posterior tibial, anterior tibial, and peroneal arteries are essentially bi-triphasic.

Impression

1. Normal right and left resting ankle/arm indices.
2. Abnormal postexercise test pressures on the right, which return to within normal limits after 6 minutes. Essentially normal postexercise test pressures on the left (pressures return to within normal limits within 2 min postexercise).
3. Diffuse greater than or equal to 50% diameter reduction throughout the right external iliac artery.
4. Focal greater than 50% diameter reduction of the left proximal common iliac artery.
5. No other evidence of significant arterial disease in the right or left lower extremity, as described above.

Vascular technologist: Kari A. Olmsted, BS/RVT

Vascular Diagnostic Service Report

I have personally reviewed these images, and I agree with the report above (or as edited if so indicated below).

Attending Physician: Service Support, MD

Appendix

PHYSICS AND INSTRUMENTATION FOR ULTRASONIC DUPLEX SCANNING

KIRK W. BEACH

Ultrasonic duplex scanning, the combination of two-dimensional (2D) ultrasound B-mode imaging and single-gate pulse Doppler blood velocimetry with spectral waveform analysis, is the most successful and widely used method available for the examination and classification of vascular occlusive disease. This discussion focuses on the physics and instrumentation behind these ultrasound methods for the examination of blood vessels.

ULTRASOUND PROPAGATION THROUGH TISSUE

Linear Mechanics of Longitudinal Waves

The physical principles of sound and ultrasound transmission can be derived from Newton's equations using a model of balls (representing molecules) and springs (representing chemical bonds) (Fig. 1).

$$\text{Force} = \text{mass} \times \text{acceleration, } and$$
$$\text{Force} = \text{stiffness} \times \text{compression}$$

When these equations are applied to molecules in a material, setting the compression force equal to the acceleration force:

$$\text{Molecular force} = \text{density} \times \text{molecular acceleration}$$
$$= \text{stiffness} \times (\text{compression change with distance})$$

Ultrasound wave mechanics are derived from this equation. If u is the distance of each molecule from its resting position, y is distance along the direction that the wave is traveling and, t is time, the equation becomes:

$$\text{Molecular force} = \text{density} \times d^2u/dt^2 = \text{stiffness} \times d^2u/dy^2$$

This equation can be solved by assuming that molecular displacement (u) is dependent on the variable group (y + C × t) having units of centimeters. C has units of centimeters per second (cm/sec). The derivatives become $[d^2u/dt^2 = C^2 \times u'']$ and $[d^2u/dy^2 = u'']$

The equation becomes:

$$\text{Density} \times C^2 \times u'' = \text{stiffness} \times u''$$

Therefore, for *any* waveshape of u, the equation is correct if C^2 = (stiffness/density). In this equation, C^2 is positive, but the value of C can be either positive or negative, and is the speed of the ultrasound wave.

The following equation is an important relationship to remember for any longitudinal mechanical (sound) pulse or wave traveling through a material:

$$C = \sqrt{(\kappa/\rho)}$$

Of course, both stiffness and density depend on temperature; thus, C will vary with temperature.

The meaning of C is further understood by looking at Fig. 2. The wave has different locations at different times. As time advances (from top to bottom), the wave moves from left to right. The line marked "wave speed" shows a place on the wave near a crest where the value (y + C × t) is constant. In Fig. 2, C is negative; thus, as time increases, y must also increase to keep (y + C × t) constant. The expression (y + C × t) provides the relationship between advancing time and advancing location. That is speed. The wave period (T, or the time that it takes to change from one peak to the next) and the wavelength (λ, or the distance that it takes to change from one peak to the next) are related by C, the wave speed:

$$C = (\text{wavelength})/(\text{wave period}) = \lambda/T$$

in (seconds/cycle). Wave period (T) is the inverse of frequency (F) so that

$$C = \lambda \times F$$

Here are some important relationships to remember:

$$C = \lambda/T = \lambda \times F = \sqrt{(\kappa/\rho)}$$

You should also remember the speed of (ultra)sound in tissue (and water), 1.5 mm/μsec, and the speed of sound in air, 300 m/s, or 0.3 mm/μsec (1,000 ft/sec). These are determined by the density and stiffness of the materials. Typical sound and ultrasound wavelengths can be computed (Table 1). Sometimes, the speed will be written 1,500 m/s or 1,540 m/s. A review of *milli-*, *micro-*, and other prefixes is in Table 2.

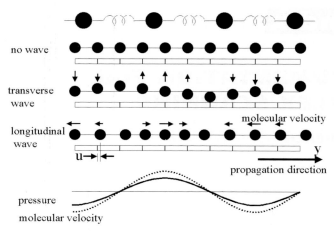

FIGURE 1. Mass and spring model for tissue mechanics. The ultrasound (and sound) transmission properties of tissue can be derived by considering the tissue to be assembled from masses (representing tissue density) and springs (representing tissue stiffness). *No wave*: At rest, with no wave present, the masses are equally distributed in the tissue. *Transverse wave:* If a transverse wave passes through the tissue, the sideways displacement of the tissues can be seen, like the sideways displacement as a wave passes along a rope. In tissue, transverse waves are attenuated in short distances converting all of the wave energy into heat. Ultrasound does not travel through tissue as a transverse wave. *Longitudinal wave*: Ultrasound passes through tissue as a longitudinal wave with regions of tissue compression and regions of tissue decompression. Although the pressure increase and decrease as an ultrasound wave passes can be several times atmospheric pressure, the motion of the tissue as the ultrasound wave passes is a few nanometers; the maximum molecular velocities are near 1 cm/sec and the accelerations are near 1,000 times the acceleration of gravity. *Pressure fluctuation and molecular velocity*: The pressure fluctuation and the molecular velocity are in phase, the ratio of pressure fluctuation to molecular velocity is the tissue impedance. The acceleration is one quarter cycle ahead of the molecular velocity and the displacement is a quarter cycle delayed.

WAVE PROPIGATION

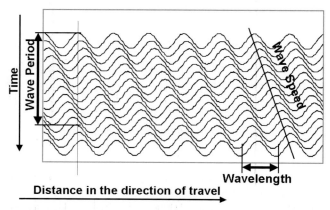

FIGURE 2. Wave propagation over time. As a wave travels through a medium, the wave length (λ) and the wave period (T=1/F) are related by the wave speed (C = λ/T = $\lambda \times$ F). The wave function is dependent on the variable (y −C×t) where y is the distance along the direction of travel and t is time.

TABLE 1. (ULTRA)SOUND WAVELENGTH FOR DIFFERENT FREQUENCIES

(Ultra)sound frequency	Wavelength in Air C = 300 m/s	Wavelength in tissue C = 1.5 mm/µs
20 Hz	15 M	75 M
1 KHz	30 cm	1.5 M
20 KHz	15 mm	7.5 cm
1 cy/µs = 1 MHz	0.3 mm	1.5 mm
10 cy/µs = 10 MHz	0.03 mm	0.15 mm

Ultrasound Frequencies and Wavelength

Frequency is measured in Hertz (after German physicist Heinrich Rudolf Hertz 1857–1894), which is an expression of cycles of compression and decompression per second. Medical ultrasound frequencies are measured in millions of cycles per second, or megahertz (MHz).

Wavelength is related to the resolution that is possible in an ultrasound image. Because your ears are 15 cm apart, you cannot tell where a 20-Hz sound (15-meter wavelength in air) is coming from, but you can identify where a 2-kHz sound (15 cm wavelength in air) is coming from. By using 5-MHz ultrasound in tissue (0.3-mm wavelength), it is possible to resolve objects that are a few millimeters apart.

It is useful to remember that the shape and properties of a wave in time and in distance along the propagation direction are intimately related. Time and distance are two views of the variable on which the waveshape is based. Therefore, a pulse in time will look like a pulse in distance along the propagation direction.

Impedance and Wave Speed

As a sound pulse (or wave) travels through tissue, there are zones of high pressure and low pressure. The high-pressure regions occur where the molecules are squeezed together, and the low-pressure regions occur where the molecules are spread apart. The pressure elevation or depression from atmospheric pressure (p) is called *pressure fluctuation*. Pres-

TABLE 2. UNDERSTANDING PREFIXES

Prefix	Symbol	Meaning	Examples
Giga	G or g	10^{+9}	Gigawatts
Mega	M	10^{+6}	Megahertz
Kilo	K or k	10^{+3}	Kilohertz, kilometers
		10^{0}	Hertz
Deci	d	10^{-1}	Decibels (dB)
Centi	c	10^{-2}	Centimeters (cm)
Milli	m	10^{-3}	Milliwatts (mW)
Micro	µ	10^{-6}	Micrometers (microns)
Nano	n	10^{-9}	Nanometers
Pico	p	10^{-12}	Picowatts
Femto	f	10^{-15}	

sure fluctuation is equal to the stiffness (κ) times du/dy, and because u is dependent on (y + C × t), du/dy = u'. As a sound pulse travels through tissue, the molecules jiggle in the direction of the sound wave. The instantaneous molecular velocity (v) of the jiggling molecules is du/dt, and because u is dependent on (y + C × t), du/dt = C × u' = v. Therefore, v/C = p/κ, or:

$$Z = p/v = \kappa/C = \sqrt{(\kappa \times \rho)} = \rho \times C$$

Z is called the *acoustic impedance* of the tissue. In physical terms, impedance is the ratio between the pressure fluctuation that the tissue feels as a wave passes and the molecular velocity of the molecules as the wave passes. Be sure to avoid confusing the molecular velocity of the molecules (v) with the wave speed (C). The molecular velocity (v) oscillates in the positive and negative directions during ultrasound wave passage at the ultrasound frequency; v is greater when the wave intensity is greater. C is the speed at which the wave passes and does not change with wave intensity, as long as the intensity is low. If the intensity is high, the "linear" model of springs and masses in Fig. 1 does not hold. The "nonlinear" waves at higher intensities cause harmonics. These harmonics are the basis of harmonic imaging.

An important note to remember:
Impedance (Z), like wavespeed (C), is dependent on the density and the stiffness (1/elasticity) of the tissue. As wave speed changes with temperature, so too does impedance change with temperature because temperature changes affect both stiffness and density. Tables in books usually list tissue density and the speed of ultrasound in tissue. (These are easy to measure.) Thus, to determine a value for impedance, it is easiest to compute it from the formula below:

$$Z = \rho \times C$$

Frequency and Period

It is common to mention ultrasound frequency measured in Hertz (cycles per second). The inverse of frequency is period measured in seconds (seconds per cycle).

Amplitude and Phase

In addition to the wavelength (in units of distance) and period (in units of time), each segment of the wave has two other properties: the amplitude and the phase (Fig. 3). All of the information in a wave is encoded in the amplitude and phase. Ultrasound B-mode imaging displays the echo amplitude, and Doppler velocity information is acquired from the phase. These two kinds of information are independent; one can change while the other remains constant.

The amplitude of a sound wave can be measured in many different ways, but each way measures properties experienced by the molecules of the material that the (ultra)sound is traveling through. Each molecule experiences a pressure fluctuation, which is a displacement back and forth along the direction of wave travel associated with a molecular velocity and acceleration. The displacement, velocity, and acceleration are like the displacement, velocity, and acceleration of a swing or pendulum.

Frequency and phase are closely related. When a 5-MHz Doppler looks at an approaching blood velocity of 75 cm/sec, the Doppler echo has a frequency of 5.005 MHz. The frequency is increased by 0.1% or 1/1,000 of the transmit frequency. Another way to think of this is that the phase becomes more advanced with every cycle; for every 1,000 cycles, the phase has advanced 1 cycle. After the first 10 cycles, the phase has advanced 1/100 of a cycle. Because one cycle is 360 degrees, after 10 cycles, the phase has advanced 3.6 degrees, and after 100 cycles, the phase has advanced 36 degrees. It is more convenient to think about the Doppler shift as a continuing change in phase rather than a frequency shift.

It is even more convenient to think as follows. Imagine the "ultrasound" frequency as a clock in the instrument running at 5 MHz (or some other frequency). The transmitted frequency is derived from that clock. The phase of each cycle of the received echo is measured from that clock. This is convenient because this allows the Doppler method of velocity measurement and the time domain method of velocity measurement to be unified into a single method. The two meth-

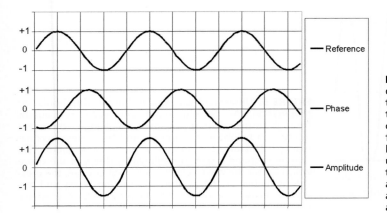

FIGURE 3. Wave phase and amplitude. Two parameters define a wave (or wave segment) of a particular frequency, the amplitude and the phase. The amplitude of a wave is taken as the peak difference of a parameter from ambient conditions. In ultrasound the parameter is usually pressure fluctuation from atmospheric pressure, but could be molecular velocity, acceleration or displacement. Amplitude of the ultrasonic echo is used for B-mode imaging. The phase is the time difference of a wave feature from the same feature on a reference wave. Therefore, phase is always represented as a difference. That difference could be in time or in distance along the propagation direction.

ods then differ only in the duration of the ultrasound transmit burst (there is a discussion of this later).

Pressure Fluctuation and Molecular Velocity, Displacement, and Acceleration

Molecular velocity, displacement, acceleration, and pressure are related to ultrasound intensity. These four measured values are ways to look at the mechanical "shaking" that the molecules feel as an ultrasound wave passes through the tissue. First of all, ultrasound intensity must be developed from energy.

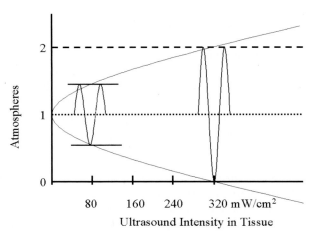

FIGURE 4. Medical ultrasound intensity versus maximum tissue pressure fluctuation. Intensity is equal to one-half times the square of the peak pressure fluctuation divided by the tissue impedance. Using the impedance of water which is near the impedance of human tissues, at an intensity (SPTP) of 320 mW/cm², the pressure fluction equals one atmosphere. 1 atmosphere, 1.01 bar, 1,013,250 barie, 1,013,250 barye, 406.78 in H_2O (inches of water), 760 mmHg (millimeters of mercury), 101,325 pascal, 101.33 pieze, 14.7 psi (pounds per square inch), 760 torr.

$$Energy = force \times distance$$
$$Power = energy/time = force \times distance/time$$
$$Intensity = power/area = force/area \times distance/time$$
$$= pressure\ fluctuation \times molecular\ velocity$$

The *pressure fluctuation* is the fluctuation of the pressure in the tissue due to the passing of an ultrasound wave; the *molecular velocity* is the velocity of molecules due to the passing of the ultrasound wave.

In the solution to Newton's equations, the ratio of tissue pressure fluctuation to molecular velocity fluctuation appears as a group, which is called tissue impedance (Z).

$$Z = (pressure\ fluctuation)/(molecular\ velocity)$$

By substitution:

$$Intensity = pressure\ fluctuation)^2/Z$$
$$= Z \times (molecular\ velocity)^2$$

This is important to remember:
If the ultrasound is continuous wave (CW), an average intensity is the average of the sine wave amplitude squared. That average is half of the maximum value.

$$Average\ intensity = (maximum\ pressure\ fluctuation)^2/2 \times Z$$
$$= Z/2 \times (molecular\ velocity)^2$$

for CW ultrasound. This is also true within a pulse. The temporal peak intensity is computed from this same expression.

A graph of the maximum and minimum pressure fluctuations versus CW intensity (Fig. 4) indicates that a physical problem occurs within the range of diagnostic ultrasound intensities: at temporal peak intensities greater than 320 mW/cm², the pressure fluctuation becomes greater than 1 atmosphere. Therefore, the minimum pressure theoretically becomes negative. This is impossible according to the physical laws of thermodynamics. Thus, the linear equation for compressibility, which is based on thermodynamics, does not apply for these conditions. The wave becomes nonlinear (Fig. 5), and gives rise to harmonics.

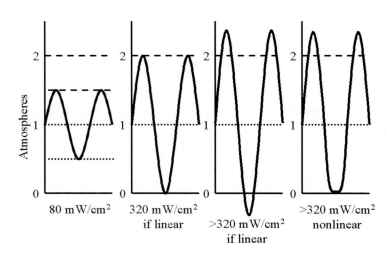

FIGURE 5. Ultrasound waveshape changes with nonlinear propigation. As an ultrasound sine wave propagates through tissue, the shape of the wave changes: the peaks increase in height and sharpness and the valleys become blunted. This effect is greater at greater intensities. This change in shape is due to nonlinear stiffness of the tissue which causes the wave velocity to be higher when the pressure is higher at the pressure fluctuation peaks and the wave velocity to be lower when the pressure is lower where the minimums are at or below zero pressure.

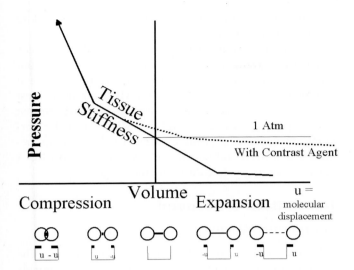

FIGURE 6. Nonlinear behavior of tissue stiffness. Near atmospheric pressure, the compressional force is linearly related to the change in dimension of the tissue, but at higher or lower pressures, deviations from the linear become large. The addition of an acoustic contrast agent consisting of bubbles expands the tissue and increases the nonlinearity.

Nonlinear Mechanics

With nonlinear mechanics, the equations above, which are linear, can no longer apply. The relationship between pressure and displacement, which is based on the nature of molecular bonds, does not hold for large fluctuations in pressure.

$$\text{Force} = \text{stiffness} \times \text{compression}$$

The nonlinear relationship between compression and force is shown in Fig. 6. In the central region, stiffness is linear where equation 2 holds, but when compression becomes too great (toward figure left) or too small (toward figure right), the effective stiffness changes. When the wave intensity is very large, during compression, the stiffness is increased, causing an increase in the wave speed and an increase in the wave impedance. Likewise, during decompression, the stiffness is decreased, causing decreases in both the wave "speed" and "impedance." Speed and impedance are in quotation marks in these cases because their definitions become less useful in these nonlinear conditions than in the linear conditions.

Harmonics and Ultrasound Contrast Agents

The flattening of the bottom of the waveshape in Fig. 5 (right), compared with the sine wave in Fig. 5 (left) and the enhancements of the peak, can be represented as a combination of sine waves (Fig. 7). In this example, only a sine wave at the original frequency and a sine wave at two times the frequency are shown. The wave at two times the frequency is called a *harmonic*; the wave at the original frequency is called the *fundamental*. The wave at two times the fundamental frequency is called by different names; it is called the "first harmonic" by some people and the "second harmonic" by others. Both groups agree on the name *first overtone* for that frequency. Harmonics may occur at 3 times, 4 times, or any integer multiple of the fundamental. Some people call the wave at 5 times the fundamental frequency the "fourth harmonic," whereas others call it the

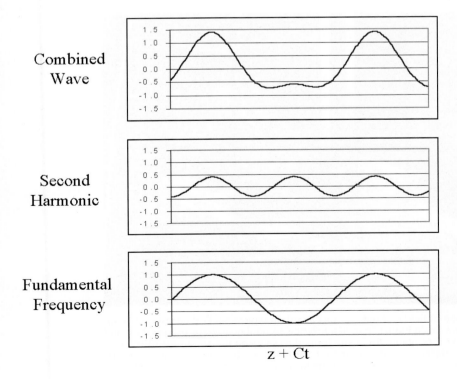

FIGURE 7. Harmonic components of nonsinusoidal waves. Fourier recognized that any periodic repeating wave could be represented by a series of sine waves starting with the fundamental and adding wave frequencies which were multiples of the fundamental. These waves are harmonics. The first harmonic is the fundamental, the second harmonic has a frequency twice the fundamental, etc. Each harmonic has unique phase and amplitude that it contributes to the combined wave. Here the 1.5 cycles of the fundamental **(bottom)** is added to 3 cycles of the second harmonic **(middle)** with a phase that causes the peaks to align to produce a wave with blunted minimums and enhanced maximums **(top)** which is similar to the wave in Fig. 5 which resulted from nonlinear propagation in tissue.

"fifth harmonic." Any periodic (repeating) waveshape can be formed from a series of sine wave harmonics of the fundamental by selecting the phase and the amplitude of each harmonic. This is the Fourier theorem (and is the basis of the Fourier transforms). The upper curve in Fig. 7 shows the combination of the fundamental and the harmonic.

Harmonics are present in all diagnostic ultrasound echoes. If the transmitted intensity is increased, the intensity of the harmonics increases as more of the power from the fundamental frequency is converted to the harmonics. The attenuation of ultrasound is proportional to frequency; thus, harmonics are attenuated more rapidly than the fundamental. Some of that attenuation is due to absorption (conversion to heat), so that if you double the ultrasound intensity, the amount of ultrasound converted to heat more than doubles, because of the conversion to harmonics and subsequent conversion to heat.

The subject of harmonics has been known for decades but was not often discussed until recently. Harmonic displays have only recently been included in diagnostic ultrasound instruments. Interest in the display of harmonics is primarily a result of a general desire to improve detection of ultrasound contrast agents. When ultrasound contrast agents were introduced, they were designed to increase the strength of the echo signals in ultrasound images. However, they did not produce the strong echoes on images that were hoped for. This led to the development of methods to display harmonics. The bubbles in ultrasound contrast agents will change the linear portions of the line in Fig. 6 and cause the generation of harmonics. Thus, displaying harmonic echoes was expected to show contrast agents more prominently. Surprisingly, tissues without contrast agents also reflect harmonic echoes back to the transducer (Fig. 8).

To generate a harmonic image using a 3-MHz transducer, it is logical to transmit at 3 MHz and receive at 6 MHz, but this cannot be done because a transducer is not sensitive at even multiples of the frequency. The 3-MHz transducer must have a "damping" material to make it "broad band," so that it will operate between 1.5 and 4.5 MHz. Then, for harmonic imaging, it is possible to reduce the transmit frequency to 2 MHz and raise the receive frequency to select 4 MHz echoes to generate the harmonic image.

Transmitted Ultrasound

Continuous Wave

CW ultrasound is used for Doppler applications. The instruments are generally inexpensive and often provide nondirectional audible output. However, CW Doppler instruments can be directional and have spectral waveform outputs. The transmitted ultrasound is "narrow band" because only one ultrasound frequency is transmitted. Because the transmission is continuous, no information about the depth of the detected flow is available; and because the wave is continuous, the temporal average intensity is equal to the temporal peak intensity.

Burst and Pulse

The terms pulse and burst have similar meanings. *Pulse* refers to the shortest burst of ultrasound that can be sent into tissue with the transducer available. *Burst* refers to an inten-

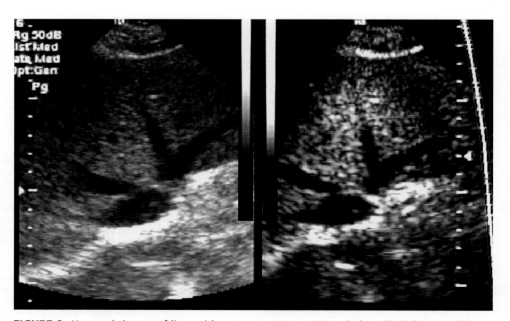

FIGURE 8. Harmonic image of liver without contrast agent. In typical medical ultrasound imaging, the SPTP intensities are much higher than 320 mW/cm^2 so nonlinear wave propagation and the formation of harmonics is common. An image formed by showing the amplitude of the fundamental frequency echo **(left)** looks different from an image of the same tissue formed by transmitting a lower frequency and forming an image based on the strength of the second harmonic of the transmitted frequency **(right)**.

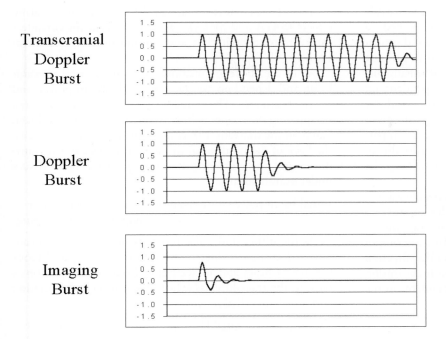

FIGURE 9. Burst length and band width of ultrasound pulses. For ultrasound B-mode imaging, short (broadband) ultrasound bursts are transmitted into tissue **(bottom)** to get the best depth resolution. For Doppler, medium length ultrasound bursts are transmitted into tissue **(middle)**. For transcranial Doppler, where the echoes are greatly attenuated and the transmitted burst energy must be high while limiting the SPTP intensity, long (narrow-band) ultrasound bursts are transmitted into tissue **(top)**.

tionally prolonged transmit oscillation. For most diagnostic imaging applications, the transmitted ultrasound pulse is on for a short period of time (Fig. 9), less than a microsecond, and off for 100 microseconds. For most pulsed Doppler applications, a burst of ultrasound lasting 1 microsecond is sent into tissue. For transcranial Doppler applications, the transmitted burst may last 15 microseconds. Long transmit bursts are narrow band because they define the Doppler frequency with precision, and they are resistant to noise. For B-mode imaging, a short (broad band) transmit pulse is used to ensure the best (smallest) depth resolution. This allows the visualization of small structures in the depth direction like the *intima–media thickness.*

During the off period, the receiver is accepting echoes from successively deeper locations. This period lasts between 40 and 400 microseconds. An ultrasound instrument computes the depth of the echo reflector by measuring the time from the transmit pulse to the echo, assuming a speed of ultrasound of 1.54 mm/μsec. Echoes from shallow structures (1 cm deep) return soon after the transmit pulse (about 13 microseconds); echoes from deeper structures (3 cm deep) return later after the transmit pulse (about 40 microseconds); echoes from the deepest structures (25 cm deep) return latest (about 325 microseconds) (Table 3).

Duty Factor

The duty factor (or duty cycle) is a measure of the fraction of time that the ultrasound instrument is transmitting. In a CW instrument, the system is always transmitting, and the duty factor is 1.0, or 100%. In a pulse-echo B-mode ultrasound instrument imaging a maximum depth of 19 cm, the transmit pulse is 1 microsecond, and the pulse repetition period (time between pulses) is 250 microseconds. Thus, the duty factor (DF) is 1/250, or 0.004, or 0.4%. The concept of duty factor also applies to your heating system at home. To heat your home on a cool day, the furnace might be on for 15 minutes out of every hour (DF = 25%), but on a cold day, the furnace might be on for 30 minutes out of every hour (DF = 50%).

The duty factor is an important part of the computation of ultrasound intensities.

Power and Intensity

There is a great deal of confusion in ultrasound physics literature about power and intensity. Here is the reason for the confusion. Power is a measure of energy per time and has units of watts. As an ultrasonic wave passes through tissue, the power is distributed over the cross-sectional area of the ultrasound beam pattern. Power divided by the cross-sec-

TABLE 3. TIME REQUIRED FOR AN ECHO TO RETURN FROM A KNOWN DEPTH

Depth (cm)	Time (Minimum possible PRI) (μs)	Maximum possible PRF (kHz)
1	13	60
2	26	40
3	39	20
5	65	12
10	130	6
15	195	5
20	260	4
25	325	3

PRI, pulse repetition interval; PRF, pulse repetition frequency.

tional area is equal to the intensity. The intensity is easily measured with an ultrasound transducer called a *hydrophone*, and determines whether the ultrasound propagation is linear or nonlinear. Intensity is related to pressure fluctuation and is therefore the quantity that is usually discussed in ultrasound physics. Intensity is dependent on both the ultrasound power in the beam pattern and the cross-sectional area of the beam pattern. Changes in intensity due to changes in cross-sectional area of the beam pattern can easily be confused with changes in intensity due to changes in ultrasound power. It is important to keep the two factors separate.

In tissue, ultrasound power decreases with distance as the wave propagates. The decrease in power is due to attenuation in the tissue. Attenuation has two factors: (a) conversion of the ultrasound power to heat, and (b) scattering of the ultrasound power in directions other than the direction of the ultrasound beam. The attenuation (both absorption and scattering) of ultrasound in tissue is dependent on the tissue type and the ultrasound frequency.

Measures of Ultrasound Intensity

Traditionally, there are six common measures of ultrasound intensity:

- Spatial average temporal average (SATA)
- Spatial peak temporal average (SPTA)
- Spatial average pulse average (SAPA)
- Spatial peak pulse average (SPPA)
- Spatial average temporal average (SATP)
- Spatial peak temporal peak (SPTP)

Between 1980 and 1990, the number of measures changed from four to six, and the naming of the measures changed. The new measures are *pulse average*, and they are the measures that were previously called *temporal peak*. Temporal peak now refers to an instantaneous peak value rather than a value averaged over the pulse. The values are related in Table 4.

Two of these measures are used for computing heating effects (SATA and SPTA); the rest are used for considering ultrasonic cavitation and nonlinear effects of ultrasound.

All of the above are measures of an ultrasound transmit beam and depend on two factors: (a) the beam power, and (b) the beam area. The initial power of the beam is selected by applying the proper voltage to the ultrasound transducer, based on the transducer thickness, the damping material on the back of the transducer, the area of the face of the transducer, and the efficiency of coupling to the body tissues under examination.

Initial beam power = (transducer voltage)^2 × (transducer area) × (coupling to tissue)/damping

As the ultrasound pulse proceeds into tissue, the beam power decreases, owing to absorption of ultrasound (conversion to heat) and to scattering (some of which comes back to the transducer as echo). Absorption and scattering combined are called *attenuation*.

Beam power = initial beam power × attenuation rate ^{depth}

The beam area is dependent on the focal character of the transducer. Intensity is the ratio of beam power divided by beam area:

Intensity = beam power/beam area = W/cm^2

The beam power can be expressed as a maximum or as a temporal average. Even these terms are not enough to complete the picture of tissue exposure. The factors relating to tissue exposure can be conveniently separated.

The six intensity measures are related by combinations of four factors: (a) duty factor or duty cycle (Fig. 10), (b) beam factor (Fig. 11), (c) pulse factor (Fig. 12), and (d) image factor (Fig. 13). The four factors all have the same range: maximum = 1, minimum = 0.

The most widely accepted method of measuring the ultrasound beam is to begin with a measurement of the total beam power. This is conducted by shining the beam onto a submerged weighing pan of a standard balance (or

TABLE 4. ABBREVIATIONS FOR ULTRASOUND EXPOSURE PARAMETERS

	Abbreviations	Multiplier Spatial average	*3 Spatial peak
Multiplier			
	Temporal average	SATA (>TI)	SPTA
*1/DF = 1	Pulse average	SAPA	SPPA
*2	Temporal peak	SATP	SPTP (>MI)

SATA along with tissue absorption and perfusion properties is used to compute the thermal index (TI).
SPTP along with tissue impedance and ultrasound frequency is used to compute mechanical index (MI).

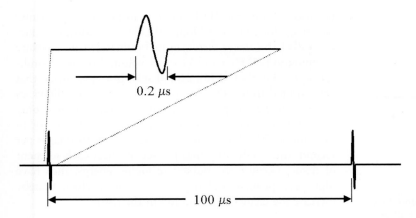

FIGURE 10. Duty factor. The duration of an ultrasound transmit burst is short compared to the time interval separating bursts. The ratio of burst length to interval is called the duty factor.

scale). When the ultrasound beam strikes the pan, a force appears. The force is equal to

$$Force = 2 \times power/C$$

In water, where the speed of sound is (C = 148,000 cm/sec), a 1-W temporal average ultrasound beam generates a force equal to the weight of a 1.38 mg mass. This force can be demonstrated by imaging a tank of water (a fish tank or dishpan will

do). By turning up the gain, particles suspended in the water can be seen. As the transmit power is increased, the suspended particles can be seen on the ultrasound image rushing away from the ultrasound scanhead because of the ultrasound force.

By exploring the ultrasound beam with a tiny ultrasound transducer called a hydrophone, the beam diameter and area can be determined. From these measurements, the SATA intensity can be determined:

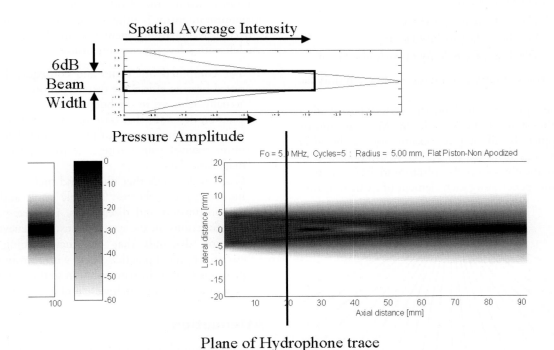

FIGURE 11. Beam factor. **Top:** A profile of the maximum pressure fluctuation taken across the beam at the transition zone between the Fresnel and Fraunhoffer zones shows the intensity peak. A flattened "box" shows the width of the central portions of the beam where intensities are at least 25% (above 6 db) of the peak. The spatial average intensity across that beam width is between half and a third of the central peak intensity. **Bottom:** The beam pattern of a flat circular transducer extends from the face of the transducer into tissue. Near the transducer in the Fresnel zone is a complex area of intensity formed by diffraction, which is the constructive and destructive interference of the waves from the transducer face. Far from the transducer in the Fraunhoffer zone, the beam pattern becomes much smoother.

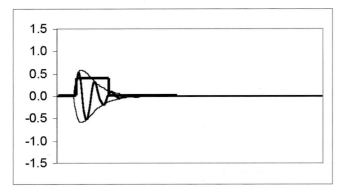

FIGURE 12. Pulse factor. Because of the gradual onset and decay of a transmit burst, the pulse average (PA) power of the pulse is about half of the instantaneous temporal peak (TP) power.

$$SATA = power/area$$

Using a hydrophone and an oscilloscope (which traces the voltage in time that is generated by the hydrophone), the factors shown in Figs. 10–13 can be determined. Then, the intensities can be computed:

SPTA = SATA/beam factor

SAPA = SATA/duty factor

SATP = SATA/duty factor/pulse factor

SPPA = SATA/beam factor/duty factor

SPTP = SATA/beam factor/duty factor/pulse factor

Different types of ultrasound result in different duty factors (Table 5).

These measures are based on the early types of ultrasound imaging systems, the A mode, the M mode, and the pulsed Doppler. In all of those examinations, the ultrasound beam was held stationary. Now, ultrasound scanheads automatically sweep the ultrasound beam across a plane of tissue, penetrating each element of tissue only once

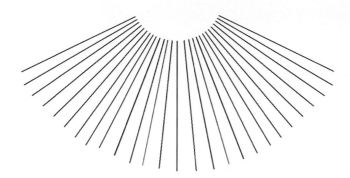

FIGURE 13. Image factor. The two-dimensional B-mode ultrasound image is formed from more than 100 pulse-echo lines. Therefore the average intensity exposure of tissue on any one line is equal to the exposure computed for repeat exposures if all pulses were delivered along a single line divided by the number of lines in the image.

per image frame for 2D B mode (and perhaps eight times per image for 2D color Doppler). Thus, an additional factor, called the *image factor*, must be included in exposure computations for a voxel (a small volume) of tissue, indicating the number of ultrasound scan lines per image that are acquired from other locations in tissue. This allows an increase in the energy in each transmit burst because only one ultrasound pulse passes through each voxel of tissue in each frame. The frame rate is usually about 30 images per second; thus, only 30 pulses per second heat each segment of tissue. Because the bursts are higher energy, they have high peak positive and negative pressures, which thereby increase the chance of cavitation in the tissue.

Theoretic Intensities versus Actual Intensities

Unknown factors, such as the attenuation of overlying tissue and refractive spreading of the ultrasound beam, make correct theoretic computations of the ultrasound intensities impossible. Experimental investigations of ultrasound intensities must be done if accurate values are to be known. Unfortunately, properly mimicking the conditions of an examination and then placing a calibrated hydrophone at the location of maximum intensity, a location that is unknown within the depths of tissue, to determine the maximum intensity, is either difficult or impossible. Almost any conceivable arrangement is seriously flawed. Thus, we are left with a few general conclusions:

1. The computed intensities and consequently the computed heating effects are certainly more severe than any actually achieved in the body tissues.
2. Caution demands that ultrasound examinations be limited to minimum transmit powers (and therefore maximum receiver gain settings) consistent with achieving diagnostic data.
3. Caution demands that ultrasound image acquisition be limited to the shortest possible time and that, for demonstrations and discussions, the freeze frame and cine functions on the system be used whenever possible.
4. Caution demands that examiner training, although essential to good practice, begin with learning about the proper use of the instrumentation so that training can be performed under guidelines 2 and 3.

Attenuation

As an ultrasound wave passes further and further into tissue, the energy in the ultrasound pulse decreases because of the conversion of that energy into other forms of energy, including heat, and into scattered ultrasound. Conversion can also occur from one ultrasound frequency into another, forming harmonics of the fundamental frequency. Attenuation computations can be easily understood by using the concept of the half energy layer (or half value layer). A *half energy layer* is a layer of tissue that is thick enough to con-

TABLE 5. TRANSMIT PARAMETERS FOR VASCULAR ULTRASOUND EXAMINATION METHODS

Method	F (MHz)	IF	PRF (KHz)	PRP (μs)	PD (μs)	DF
Continuous wave doppler	5	1.00	NA	NA	NA	1.00
Transcranial pulsed doppler	2	1.00	5	200	10.0	0.05
Cardiovascular pulsed doppler	5	1.00	10	100	1.0	0.01
M-mode imaging	5	1.00	1	1000	0.5	0.0005
2D RT B-mode imaging	5	0.01	5	200	0.5	0.000025
2D RT color flow imaging	5	0.05	5	200	1.0	0.00025

F, ultrasound frequency; IF, image factor (1/the number of ultrasound lines in an image); PRF, pulse repetition frequency (number of transmitted pulses per second); PRP, pulse repetition period (1/PRF); PD, pulse duration (length of transmit pulse or burst); DF, duty factor seen by tissue voxel; RT, real time.

vert half of the energy in an incoming ultrasound pulse into heat and scattered ultrasound, leaving the remaining half of the ultrasound energy in the pulse as it passes out of the layer. All other attenuation computations can be derived from this concept. Each tissue type has an attenuation rate that can be expressed as a half energy layer (Table 6). For most tissues, attenuation increases with ultrasound frequency, so that the half energy layer for 2-MHz ultrasound is half as thick as a half energy layer for 1-MHz ultrasound. The wavelength of 2-MHz ultrasound is half as long as the wavelength of 1-MHz ultrasound. Therefore, it is most convenient to express the thickness of the half energy layer in wavelengths. Attenuation measurements are difficult to obtain; thus, there is great variability in the results. For wavelength, a value near 3.5 mm/μsec can be used for bone; and for all other tissues, a value near 1.5 mm/μsec can be used. Differentiating the speed in muscle (1.58 mm/μsec) from the value in fat (1.45 mm/μsec) is not justified for attenuation purposes because the variability of values in the literature for different tissues is so great.

In the measurement of attenuation, several systems have been used; they are all based on the exponential curve, which is the mathematic function that describes the decay of the ultrasound power or energy as ultrasound passes through attenuating tissue. Methods have included the half value layer (in centimeters), the decibel, and the Neper. Half value layers and decibels are defined in units of energy, power, or intensity; Nepers are defined in units of amplitude. Here,

units of *half energy layers in wavelengths* (HELW) have been introduced to simplify understanding. An example can be used to explain this. It is easier to use binary numbers.

Imagine that a 15-MHz ultrasound burst with an energy of 64 ergs is sent into a layer of fat that is 0.5-cm thick. The wavelength of the 15-MHz ultrasound in fat is about 0.1 mm [(1.5 mm/μsec) / (15 cy/μsec)]. The fat layer is 50 wavelengths thick. That is 1-HELW thick. When the burst emerges from the other side, the remaining energy in the burst is 32 ergs. If the burst passes through another 1-HELW layer, the energy would be 16 ergs. After passing through a third 1-HELW layer, the burst contains energy of 8 ergs. Every HELW layer converts half of the energy into heat and scattered ultrasound, leaving half in the remaining beam. After 3 HELW layers, only $(1/2)^3$ of the energy remains. Thus, to compute the remaining energy in a burst,

$$\text{Remaining energy} = \text{initial energy} \times (1/2)^{T/\lambda/\text{HELW}}$$

where HELW is the number of half energy thickness that the ultrasound has passed through.

If the computation is done with attenuation and decibels, the equation is similar:

$$\text{Remaining energy} = \text{initial energy} \times (1/10)^{\alpha \times F \times T/10}$$

where α is in decibels per megahertz per centimeter, F is the ultrasound frequency, and T is the thickness of the tissue. The 10 in the denominator of the exponent converts decibels to Bels.

TABLE 6. HALF-ENERGY LAYERS IN WAVELENGTHS FOR DIFFERENT TISSUES

Tissue	Half-energy layer (λ)	Ultrasound speed (mm/μs)	Attenuation (dB/cm/MHz)
Plasma	700		
Blood	250	1.57	0.18
Brain	75		
Fat	50	1.45	0.63
Liver	30	1.55	
Kidney	20		
Muscle	15	1.58	
Muscle, longitudinal			1.2
Muscle, transverse			3.3
Cartilage		1.67	
Bone	0.1	3.2	20

A related equation can be written for Nepers:

Remaining amplitude = initial amplitude $\times (1/e)^{\gamma \times F \times T}$

where e is the exponent factor for 2.72, λ is the attenuation factor in Nepers per megahertz per centimeter.

The value of the exponent factor (e = 2.72) is a mathematic constant that can be found using calculus in the same way that pi (π = 3.14) is a mathematic constant that can be found using calculus. Amplitude must be converted into energy (or power) to compare with the other equations. Intensity is proportional to amplitude squared. This discussion assumes that the cross-sectional area of the ultrasound beam is constant. If it is not, the computations are correct for energy and power, but the computations for intensity and amplitude must be adjusted for the changes in beam cross-sectional area. For constant cross sction,

Remaining intensity = (remaining amplitude)^2
$$= (\text{initial amplitude} \times (1/e)^{\gamma \times F \times T})^2$$
Remaining intensity = (remaining amplitude)^2
$$= (\text{initial amplitude})^2 \times (1/e)^{\gamma \times F \times T \times 2}$$
Remaining intensity = initial intensity $\times (1/e)^{\gamma \times F \times T \times 2}$

If the beam cross section changes,

Remaining intensity $\times$ remaining beam area
$$= \text{initial intensity} \times \text{initial beam}$$
$$\text{area} \times (1/e)^{\gamma \times F \times T \times 2}$$

remembering that

Energy = time $\times$ power = time $\times$ intensity $\times$ area
Remaining energy = initial energy $\times (1/e)^{\gamma \times F \times T \times 2}$

The three equations can be compared by dividing both sides by initial energy.

Remaining energy/initial energy = $(1/2)^{\text{HELW}}$
$$= (1/10)^{(\alpha \times F \times T)/10}$$
$$= (1/e)^{\gamma \times F \times T \times 2}$$

Logarithmic conversions can be used to show these equations in another form.

Log(10) [(remaining energy)/(initial energy)]
$$= (-\alpha \times F \times T)/10$$
Log(e) [(remaining energy)/(initial energy)]
$$= -2 \times \gamma \times F \times T$$
Log(2) [(remaining energy)/(initial energy)]
$$= -T/\lambda/\text{HELW} = -T/\text{HVL(F)}$$

The half value layer is dependent on ultrasound frequency. These relationships indicate that a logarithmic plot of the ratio of the remaining to the initial energy versus distance will give a linear (straight line) graph (Fig. 14).

Some tables give attenuation rates in dB/cm/MHz (α), some in Nepers/cm/MHz (γ), and some in half value layers. The values in equations above show the logarithmic conversions can be related. Consider attenuation through a single half value layer:

$$-T = 10 \times [\text{Log(10) (0.5)}]/(\alpha \times F)$$
$$= [\text{Log(e) (0.5)}]/(2 \gamma \times F)$$
$$= [\text{Log(2) (0.5)}] \times \lambda \times \text{HELW}$$
$$= [\text{Log(2) (0.5)}] \times \text{HVL(F)}$$

Evaluating terms [−Log(10) (0.5)] = 0.301; [Log(e) (0.5)] = 0.693; [−Log(2) (0.5)] = 1 gives

$$-T = 3.01/(\alpha \times F) = 0.693/(2 \times \gamma \times F) = \lambda \times \text{HELW}$$
$$= \text{HVL(F)}$$

so that the attenuation values given in different tables can be compared.

Reflection and Scattering

The use of ultrasound in medicine spans the range from active tissue ablation to passive acoustic thermography. Between these extremes lies pulse-echo diagnostic ultrasound (Table 7). As ultrasound passes through tissue, it crosses boundaries between tissues having different impedances. At each boundary, some ultrasound is reflected, but most passes through the boundary. Cells are typical of these tissues; the boundaries are the cell walls. Typically, there are 1,000,000 cells in each voxel of tissue. A voxel is the smallest resolvable volume of tissue and must be analyzed as a single unit. The volume of a voxel is usually about a cubic millimeter. The reflections from each of the boundaries go off in a different direction. This is called *scattering*. Incident ultrasound is scattered in all directions from each voxel. The scattered ultrasound that goes back along the direction of the incident ultrasound beam to the transducer is called *backscatter*.

The backscattered ultrasound from each voxel along the ultrasound beam is the signal that is used to create the ultrasound image and Doppler waveform. That signal must be greater than the natural ultrasound noise emitted from the tissue. Tissues emit ultrasound because they are warm. The intensity of the "thermal noise" from tissue is about $10/1,000,000,000,000,000$ W/cm^2. This is more easily expressed in scientific notation as 10×10^{-15} Ws/ cm^2 or 10 femtowatts/cm^2. This can also be expressed in decibels. Decibels always need a reference value; in this case, the maximum SPTA transmit intensity 100 mW/cm^2 will be used as a reference. Thermal noise is 10^{-13} times the reference, or 13 Bels or 130 dB below the reference.

The backscatter reflectivity of most tissue voxels is less than 0.1% (30 dB) of the incident ultrasound. As an ultrasound burst travels into tissue to a voxel of interest, it may pass through 6.5 half value layers, which would attenuate the ultrasound to 1% (0.01) of the original energy in the burst. In the voxel containing liver or muscle cells, about 0.1% of the ultrasound will be reflected back to the transducer as backscatter. If the voxel contained the surface of a bone or a metal surgical clip, 100% (1.0) of the ultrasound would be returned as backscatter. If the voxel contained blood, 0.0001% (60 dB below bone) of the ultrasound would be

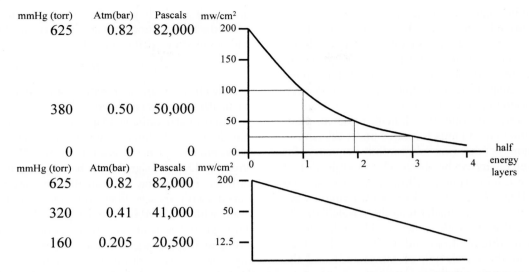

mmHg (torr)	Atm(bar)	Pascals	mw/cm²
625	0.82	82,000	200
380	0.50	50,000	
0	0	0	0

mmHg (torr)	Atm(bar)	Pascals	mw/cm²
625	0.82	82,000	200
320	0.41	41,000	50
160	0.205	20,500	12.5

FIGURE 14. Half energy layer. As ultrasound is attenuated by any tissue layer, a fraction of the incoming ultrasound is converted to heat. The fraction passing out of the layer is dependent on the thickness and the material. For any material, there is a thickness that will attenuate the ultrasound to half energy value. The decay in intensity is logarithmic *(upper curve)*. If the log of the energy is displayed on the vertical axis, then the decay forms a linear plot *(lower curve)*. In this figure, the vertical axis is plotted as intensity and associated pressure fluctuation amplitude. Intensity is only valid if the beam cross sectional area remains constant.

returned to the transducer as backscatter. As the backscatter passes back along the ultrasound beam pattern to the transducer, it will pass back through 6.5 half value layers attenuating the backscattered echo to 1% of the backscattered energy. Reviewing the path of the ultrasound from the voxel of interest: burst attenuation is 1% (0.01, or 20 dB), reflection from liver produces echo energy of 0.1% (0.001, or 30 dB), and backscatter attenuation is 1% (0.01, or 20 dB) for a total echo strength of (20 + 30 + 20) 70 dB (compared with the echo that would be produced by a metal plate in contact with the transducer backscattering all of the incident ultrasound). Summarizing for different possible tissues, in that voxel of interest, a bone surface echo is 40 dB down, liver is 70 dB down, and blood is 100 dB down.

For a good-looking ultrasound image, the strength of the backscattered echo must be about 100 times (20 dB) greater than the thermal noise. Therefore, if you want to see the moving speckles of blood in your image as brighter than the noise, you need a transmit intensity (100 + 20) 120 dB greater than thermal noise or (10^{-14} W/cm² × 10^{+12}) 10^{-2} W/cm² = 10 mW/cm². If you use a lower transmit intensity, blood in the voxel of interest will look like noise on the image, and the Doppler spectral waveform will look like noise. If the tissue between the ultrasound transducer is muscle, 6.5 HEL is about 133 wavelengths, 20 cm for 1-MHz ultrasound and 4 cm for 5-MHz ultrasound. If you want to see deeper with 5-MHz ultrasound, you must use a higher transmit intensity (power/area). The maximum recommended, 100 mW/cm², will permit imaging (also called penetration) to 6 cm with 5-MHz ultrasound.

Best Ultrasound Frequency for Doppler Evaluation of Blood Flow

The best choice of ultrasound frequency for imaging is a choice between obtaining the best lateral and depth resolu-

TABLE 7. ULTRASOUND INTENSITIES IN THE HUMAN BODY

Use	Comment	Intensities (mW/cm²)	Expected temperature increase
Arterial cautery	Pressures > systolic BP	>10,000,000	25°C rise per second
Surgical	Neurologic ablation	>10,000	46°–54°C 20 min
Medical	Metabolic injury	1,000	43°–44°C 60 min
Therapeutic	Heating	1,000	40°–45°C 10 min
Diagnostic	Transmitted	100	39°C 1 min
Diagnostic	Maximum echo	0.1	
Diagnostic	Minimum echo	10^{-8}	
Thermal	Acoustic noise	0.1* 10^{-10}	

tion and obtaining signals from the deepest tissues of interest. High ultrasound frequencies allow superior lateral and depth resolution but are strongly attenuated by tissue, limiting the ability to penetrate to great depths through tissue. As a general rule, those tissues that scatter ultrasound more strongly also attenuate ultrasound more strongly. In decreasing order of scattering and attenuation, we have calcium, muscle, fat, blood, and urine. It is difficult to obtain ultrasound echoes from fat and muscle located under calcium.

The selection of the best ultrasound frequency for Doppler measurements can be objectively determined. Red blood cells are 8 μm in diameter. Ultrasound waves are 300 μm long (5 MHz). When the reflectors scattering a wave (red blood cells) are much smaller than the wavelength, the scatterers are called *Reyleigh scatterers*. The relationship between the scattering of ultrasound by blood cells (which are smaller than the wavelength of ultrasound) and the ultrasound frequency is as follows:

$$R = B \times F^4$$

where R is the fraction of the ultrasound that is scattered back to the transducer by the red blood cells, B is a proportionality constant, and F is the ultrasound frequency. The penetration of ultrasound in tissue is as follows:

$$P = 10^{-2d(\alpha/10 \times T)}$$

where P is the fraction of the ultrasound energy that is still present after traveling through tissue of thickness, T. The power returning to the transducer is the fraction of power penetrating tissue going to the reflector (P) × the fraction of power scattered back toward the transducer (R) × the fraction of power penetrating tissue returning from the reflector (P), which equals

$$P \times R \times P \text{ or}$$
$$P \times R \times P = 10^{-2d(\alpha/10 \times T)} \times B \times F^4 \times 10^{-2d(\alpha/10 \times T)}$$

Using calculus, the ultrasound frequency that will give the greatest Doppler echo strength can be determined by setting the derivative with respect to frequency to zero and solving for frequency. The result shows the ultrasound frequency (F), which gives the strongest echo from blood when the blood is under an overlying tissue of thickness (T) and attenuation coefficient (α):

$$F = 2/T \times 1/\alpha/10 \times 1/\ln(10)$$

The effect on an examination of a blood vessel beneath particular tissues is tabulated in Table 8.

Intravascular catheter Doppler systems may penetrate 1 mm to 1 cm of blood to obtain the necessary signals. An ultrasound frequency greater than 50 MHz will give the strongest Doppler signal from blood using an intravascular catheter. Penetrating a 2-mm (0.2-cm) arterial wall from outside with muscle fibers transverse to the ultrasound beam with a 13-MHz Doppler gives the strongest signal. Through 0.2 mm of skull with transcranial Doppler, the strongest Doppler signal is achieved at 2.2 MHz. Examining a carotid artery through 2 cm of muscle and fat with a Doppler ultrasound frequency near 5 MHz gives the strongest signal. Examination of the aortic valve at a depth of 10 cm through 1 or 2 cm of muscle with fibers oriented transverse to the ultrasound beam requires 2- or 3-MHz ultrasound for the strongest signal.

Examination of the renal arteries or fetal arteries at a depth of 10 cm under muscle and fat may require an ultrasound frequency of 1 MHz to achieve the strongest signal. To date, ultrasound duplex scanners have been developed for transcutaneous applications in the heart and peripheral vascular applications with Doppler ultrasound frequencies ranging from 2 to 8 MHz. In the future, it is likely that intravascular duplex scanning will use higher ultrasound frequencies and that abdominal applications will use lower Doppler ultrasound frequencies than are currently available.

Depth Resolution

One goal in ultrasound B-mode imaging is the smallest depth resolution possible. To ensure that the depth resolution is as small as possible (able to resolve small structures), the shortest possible ultrasound transmit pulse is used (Fig. 9). One factor in resolution is that the burst-echo ultrasound path is

TABLE 8. ULTRASOUND FREQUENCY FOR THE STRONGEST DOPPLER SIGNAL FROM BLOOD IN VESSELS VIEWED THROUGH DIFFERENT TISSUES

| Overlying tissue attenuation | Blood 0.18 dB/cm/MHz | Fat 0.63 dB/cm/MHz | Muscle | | Bone 20 dB/cm/MHz |
			Longitudinal 1.2 dB/cm/MHz	Transverse 3.3 dB/cm/MHz	
Depth					
0.2 cm	241 MHz	69 MHz	36 MHz	13 MHz	2.2 MHz
0.5 cm	97 MHz	28 MHz	14 MHz	5 MHz	0.9 MHz
2 cm	24 MHz	7 MHz	4 MHz	1.3 MHz	0.2 MHz
5 cm	10 MHz	3 MHz	1.4 MHz	0.5 MHz	0.1 MHz
8 cm	6 MHz	2 MHz	0.9 MHz	0.3 MHz	
15 cm	3 MHz	1 MHz	0.5 MHz	0.2 MHz	

TABLE 9. ULTRASOUND WAVE SPEED IN DIFFERENT TISSUES

Tissue	Ultrasound speed (mm/μsec)
Bone	3.20
Cartilage	1.67
Muscle	1.58
Blood	1.57
Liver	1.55
Fat	1.45

folded, so that tissue voxels spaced at 1-mm intervals in depth add 2 mm per voxel to the roundtrip ultrasound path length, and the roundtrip path length is measured by the ultrasound system to determine depth. The ultrasound burst length is the smallest possible resolution division of the roundtrip ultrasound path. Therefore, the voxel dimension along the beam path should be equal to half of the burst length. If the burst length is 2 cycles of ultrasound, then the voxel length should be equal to the wavelength of the ultrasound. *Resolution* is defined as the closest that two objects can be and still be recognized as separate. Therefore, resolution is the distance between the centers of two bright voxels that have a third, dim voxel between them. The voxel between with low echo shows that the reflections are separate. Thus, the depth resolution is about equal to the burst length.

This is superior to the lateral resolution, which is about equal to the ultrasound beam pattern width. The beam pattern width is greater than the value of the wavelength times depth divided by aperture. Because depth is almost always greater than aperture, the lateral resolution is poorer than the depth resolution. In a typical case, the focal depth is 80 mm, and the transducer diameter (aperture) is 10 mm. The lateral resolution is greater than 8 times the wavelength of the ultrasound. The result is that a small reflecting sphere in the image, which should appear as a bright dot, instead appears as a horizontal dash. If imaged with 5-MHz ultrasound, the dash will appear to be about 0.3 mm deep and 3 mm wide.

Refraction

The single most common problem and confusion in ultrasound imaging is refractive distortion. The pulse-echo ultrasound imaging process assumes that the ultrasound beam passes into tissue and returns from a straight line along which the transducer is pointed. However, because of the range of speeds of ultrasound propagation, the ultrasound beam may bend, causing structures to appear in the wrong lateral location. This does not affect the depth location. The effect is most obvious when it results in double viewing of an object. This has been reported in early pregnancy (25% of women appear to have twins in the 5th week of gestation) and in the appearance of double aortic valves. The duplicate pregnancy images are due to refraction in the rectus abdominis muscles, and the duplicated aortic valve images are due to refraction in the parasternal cartilage. Refraction also distorts all other lateral measurements, including fetal bone length and the measured cross-sectional widths of blood vessels. Whenever ultrasound scan lines pass from a material with one ultrasound speed into another material with a different ultrasound speed (Table 9), the chance of refractive distortion is present. If the ultrasound beam is perpendicular to the interface, no deflection occurs, but if the ultrasound beam approaches the interface at a grazing angle, angular deflections of more than 45 degrees can occur, causing lateral displacement of the images of all objects deeper than that refracting interface.

The maximum refraction angle passing from one tissue to another and back can be computed from Snell's law of refraction, which can be found in almost any physics book (Table 10).

Length measurements in the depth direction may contain an error of 10% or less, depending on the speed of ultrasound in the tissue between the measurement lines. This error can be removed by substituting the proper speed into the measurement for the "average" soft tissue ultrasound speed of 154,000 cm/sec. The thickness of a layer of fat (speed = 145,000 cm/sec) that appears to be 1-cm thick on the ultrasound image, is actually 0.94-cm thick (1 × 145,000/154,000 = 0.94). In contrast, lateral measurements all have great uncertainty because of refractive bending of the ultrasound beams. The errors in lateral measurements cannot be removed or corrected because it is impossible to determine the refraction that has been introduced into the ultrasound beam by the tissue. Thus, lateral measurements and cross-sectional area measurements cannot be made with confidence from ultrasound images. An example is the dual aorta artifact (Fig. 15) when the aortic cross section is viewed through the fat and muscle prisms forming the abdominal midline.

TABLE 10. MAXIMAL ANGLE OF REFRACTION WITH SOUND PASSING FROM ONE TISSUE TO ANOTHER AND BACK

	Cartilage (1.67)	Muscle (1.58)	Blood (1.57)	Liver (1.55)	Fat (1.45)
Cartilage (1.67)	0 degrees	37 degrees	39 degrees	43 degrees	59 degrees
Muscle (1.58)	37 degrees	0 degrees	13 degrees	22 degrees	47 degrees
Blood (1.57)	39 degrees	13 degrees	0 degrees	18 degrees	45 degrees
Liver (1.55)	43 degrees	22 degrees	18 degrees	0 degrees	41 degrees
Fat (1.45)	59 degrees	47 degrees	45 degrees	41 degrees	0 degrees

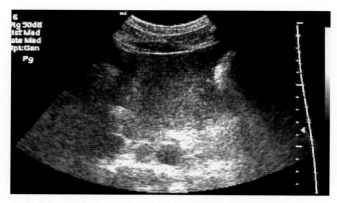

FIGURE 15. Aortic duplication due to refraction in the linea alba by fat. At a depth of 11 cm in this image, two aortas are visible separated by the inferior vena cava. This is not an anatomic anomaly, instead two images of the single aorta have been formed because some of the ultrasound beam patterns that are formed by the transducer are bent by an acoustic prism formed by the fat and rectus abdominus muscle to provide a second view of the aorta.

Reflection

Some tissue interfaces in the body are large and flat with great impedance changes, such as the diaphragm–pleura interface above the liver. Such interfaces act like mirrors, reflecting entire images into false locations. It is easy to see images of liver parenchyma, appearing to be located above the diaphragm where the lung is actually located, when viewed through the liver. It is also easy to view a mirror image of the subclavian artery reflected in the pleura, appearing to be at a depth in the lung. Vascular walls can cause such reflections as well. These reflected images are usually visible as lower echo intensity than a direct image would be. They are more likely to appear in color Doppler imaging than in B-mode imaging because color Doppler is designed to show full brightness even if the signal is weak, whereas B-mode brightness decreases if the echo is weak.

ULTRASOUND TRANSDUCERS AND SCANHEADS
PZT and PVDF

Ultrasound transducers are wafers of piezoelectric material that are coated on the top and bottom with an electrical conductor. The two materials commonly used for transducers are lead (Pb) zirconate (Z) titanate (Ti), which is a ceramic, abbreviated PZT, and polyvinylidene fluoride, which is a soft plastic, abbreviated PVDF. The two materials are similar in that they can have piezoelectric properties if polarized. *Piezoelectric* means that when a voltage is applied to the electrodes so that an electric field is present across the thickness, the transducer tends to expand (or if the polarity is reversed, the transducer tends to contract). This is the conversion of electrical energy to mechanical energy. Alternatively, if the transducer is squeezed or stretched in its thickness dimension, a voltage will appear between the electrodes. Conversion of

electrical to mechanical energy is used to transmit ultrasound, and conversion of mechanical to electrical energy is used to receive ultrasound.

The two materials differ in several respects. PZT is a brittle ceramic with very high acoustic impedance. When in contact with the body, which has low impedance, most of the ultrasound energy generated in the transducer is reflected back into the transducer, "trapping" the energy and making the transducer "ring" at a single frequency determined by the transducer thickness. An acoustic matching layer is required between the transducer and the body to allow efficient transmission of the ultrasound between the transducer and the body. This layer has an impedance midway between PZT and the body and a thickness of one fourth of a wavelength. In contrast, PVDF is a soft plastic with ultrasound impedance near that of tissue. When placed in contact with tissue, the ultrasound energy flows between the body tissues and the PVDF without reflection. Therefore, the PVDF does not resonate at a single frequency and is a broad-band transducer.

Thickness and Frequency

For a transducer to produce a vibration with a long duration and a narrow frequency band, it must retain the energy for many cycles, rather than transmitting the energy into tissue or into an absorbing material on the back of the transducer, called a *backing material*. It is therefore easy to make a narrow-band transducer with PZT, by not using a matching layer to couple it with tissue or backing material. Such a transducer is shown in Fig. 16. Notice that the PZT

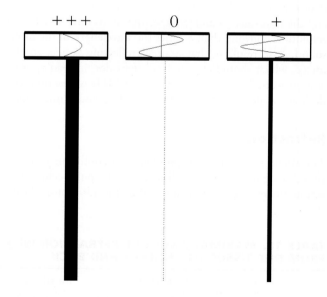

FIGURE 16. Sensitivity of ultrasound transducers. An ultrasound transducer is sensitive to odd harmonics of the fundamental frequency. Even harmonics **(center)** have a region of compression opposed by a region of decompression. The transducer has 1/3 of the voltage sensitivity to the third harmonic **(right)** as to the fundamental **(left)**.

transducer is most efficient at an ultrasound frequency at which the transducer thickness is equal to half a wavelength (in PZT). This is called the *fundamental frequency*. This frequency is a "natural" frequency of vibration because the impedance changes at the surfaces cause most of the ultrasound to reflect back into the transducer, trapping energy in the transducer for many cycles.

To create high-frequency ultrasound transducers, thin wafers of piezoelectric material are used; conversely, to create low-frequency ultrasound transducers, thick wafers of piezoelectric material are used. The thickness of the transducer is equal to half the wavelength of the ultrasound in the PZT material. A transducer that oscillates or rings at a single frequency is called a narrow-band transducer. This relationship is also true for PVDF transducers, but because of the impedance similarity between tissue and PVDF, energy is not trapped in the PVDF; thus, it does not oscillate like PZT. Therefore, PVDF transducers are not narrow band, they are *wide band*. In ultrasound, a wide-band transducer emits a short ultrasound burst if excited by a short electrical pulse.

The transducer is not sensitive (able to receive ultrasound) when the wavelength is equal to the thickness (twice the fundamental frequency) because the compression voltage of the first (positive) half cycle cancels the decompression voltage of the second (negative) half cycle (Fig. 16). At triple the fundamental frequency, the transducer is one third as sensitive because the voltage generated by the first (positive) half cycle of ultrasound is canceled by the second (negative) half cycle, leaving only the third (positive) half cycle to contribute to the voltage on the transducer not canceled. This is equally true for PZT and PVDF.

Nonpiezoelectric Transducers

New technologies may allow the creation of ultrasonic transducers of the future. One technology uses microelectromechanical systems (MEMS) methods, which were developed for electronic integrated circuits, to create electrostatic transducers that are smaller than 1 mm^2. Arrays of such transducers can be made in a single series of steps, with the electronics for the ultrasound scanner bonded to the back of the transducer array. These transducers use electrostatic attraction and repulsion across an air gap that is 1-μm thick to convert the electrical energy to ultrasound and use the change in capacitance with deflection to convert ultrasound to an electrical signal. Because of the small mass of the moving parts, these transducers promise to be broad band and efficient. The acoustic impedance of these transducers is entirely dependent on the associated electrical circuits, in contrast to the piezoelectric transducers, with acoustic impedance primarily depending on the transducer materials. Thus, impedance matching with electrostatic transducers may be easier than with piezoelectric transducers. Such technologies may allow an entire multipurpose 3D ultrasound scanner to be made in a package the size of a watch.

Single Element

From the earliest days of medical ultrasound in the 1950s to the advent of electronic switching in about 1985, pulse-echo ultrasound systems used a single transducer for both transmitting and receiving, whereas continuous wave Doppler systems used one transducer for transmitting and one for receiving. Single-element transducers can both transmit and receive because the transmit process (requiring between 10 and 400 V to create enough ultrasound intensity) is separated from the receive process (generating microvolts) by time. The transmit burst lasts less than 1 microsecond, and echoes are received for the following 100 microseconds (if the maximum depth of observation is 75 mm). It often takes a few microseconds for the transducer to settle down after transmitting to begin receiving well; this recovery period causes a blank zone in the shallowest few millimeters of the image.

Aperture Shapes

Each ultrasound beam pattern is determined by two design factors: (a) the ultrasound wavelength (determined by the ultrasound frequency and the tissue conducting the ultrasound beam), and (b) the shape of the aperture or transducer that is forming the ultrasound beam. The shape of the ultrasound beam pattern is determined by diffraction of the beam through the aperture. Most ultrasound systems use transducer apertures that are circular or rectangular in shape. However, other shapes sometimes are used, including multipointed stars.

Ultrasound Beam Patterns: Natural Focus, Fresnel Zone, and the Fraunhoffer Zone

The diameter or width of a diagnostic ultrasound transducer is always greater than several times the wavelength of ultrasound. When the echo from a point reflector located near the transducer face reaches the transducer face, some regions of the transducer face experience compression, and others experience decompression (rarefaction) (Fig. 17 left). The echo from a point reflector located far from the transducer face intersects the transducer surface with only a single compression or rarefaction zone at a time (Fig. 17 right). Reflectors that are near the transducer causing mixed compressions and rarefactions on the transducer face are in the Fresnel zone, or the near field; reflectors that are far from the transducer causing nearly uniform compression or expansion of the transducer are in the Fraunhoffer zone, or far field. There is a difference between the image speckle seen in the Fresnel zone and that seen in the Fraunhoffer zone. Speckle in the Fresnel zone has a fine structure in both the depth direction and the lateral direction; speckle in the Fraunhoffer zone has a fine structure in the depth direction but a course structure in the lateral direction, making the speckles look like transverse dashes.

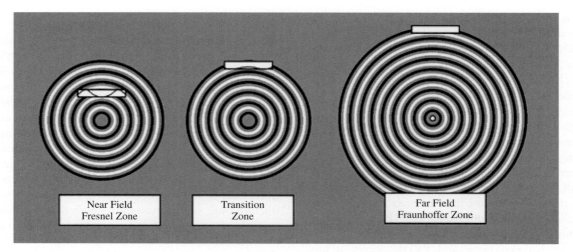

FIGURE 17. Near and far field of an ultrasound transducer. The Fresnel zone of a transducer is separated from the Fraunhoffer zone of a transducer by the transition zone which is the closest distance that the transducer can come to a point source of ultrasound and have times when the transducer face is subject to compression without decompression (or visa versa). The concentric rings show the expansion of spherical waves from a point origin. Not shown is that the intensity and pressure amplitude decrease with distance from the central origin of the waves.

Because an echo from the near field compresses a part of the transducer and expands another part, the resultant voltage, which is some average of the positive and negative effects, is less than it would be, had the transducer been expanded or compressed together because the negative portions "subtract" from the positive portions. At some positions, the net effect of an echo will be positive, and nearby, the net effect will be negative. A transition from a net positive voltage to a net negative voltage can occur if the reflector is moved a distance of one fourth of a wavelength. Either a net positive voltage or a net negative voltage causes a white spot (pixel) on the ultrasound image corresponding to the location of the reflector causing the voltage. If the magnitude is great (either positive or negative), the white pixel will be bright; if the magnitude is small (either positive or negative), the pixel will be dim. Only if the voltage is zero will the spot be black. Thus, one reflector in tissue may cause a bright pixel on the screen, and a similar reflector, located one fourth of a wavelength away, may cause a dark pixel on the screen. This process produces speckle on the ultrasound image. It is not tissue texture and cannot be used for identification of tissue type. The combining of positive and negative waves to cancel each other, providing a zero result, is called *destructive interference*; the combining of positive and positive waves or negative and negative waves to create a larger result is called *constructive interference*.

In contrast, an echo from a reflector in the far field serves to compress all points on the transducer surface in unison, causing improved sensitivity. Of course, the reflectors in the far field are so far away that the echoes are weak both because of attenuation and because the reflected ultrasound is spreading as it returns from the reflector.

At the boundary of the near and far fields, in the transition zone, there is a natural region of greatest ultrasound intensity and greatest transducer sensitivity. This zone is about half as wide as a flat transducer, with intensity and sensitivity dropping to near zero at the transducer radius from the axis. This is the natural focal zone of a flat transducer. This boundary between the Fresnel zone (near field) and the Fraunhoffer zone (far field) is called the *transition zone*. The smooth central lobe of the beam pattern in the Fraunhoffer zone (Fig. 11) differs markedly from the lumpy pattern in the Fresnel zone. The transition zone can be moved to a greater depth by increasing the width of the transducer. The transducer may be focused by making the transducer concave (or by placing a converging lens in the ultrasound beam path), which pulls the transition zone and far field closer to the transducer, thereby reducing the beam width at the focus.

Fixed Mechanical Focus

If the transducer is concave, a reflector at the center of curvature, equidistant from all points on the transducer surface, receives compression from the entire transducer surface at once. The transducer, in turn, can concentrate a compression or rarefaction on that point (Fig. 18), because of the principle of reciprocity. This is the focal zone of the transducer. To focus effectively, the focal zone must be within the Fresnel zone of an equivalent unfocused (planar) transducer.

Diffraction and Side Lobes

Every transducer generates side lobes because of wave diffraction. A flat disk sends most of the ultrasound energy along the central axis of the beam pattern. This axis is called the *central lobe* or *main lobe* of the beam pattern. The direction of the central lobe is not dependent on wavelength (or

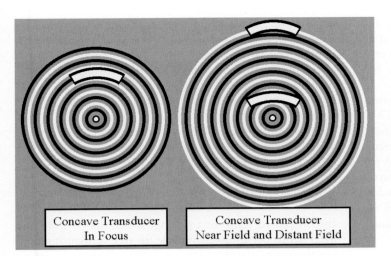

FIGURE 18. Concave focused transducer in focus; near and far zones. At the best focus of the transducer **(left)** there are times when the entire transducer face is exposed to maximum compression or decompression. This never happens to a flat transducer. There is a near field where the concave transducer is exposed to combined compression and decompression **(right,** near transducer). The concentric rings show the expansion of spherical waves from a point origin. Not shown is that the intensity and pressure amplitude decrease with distance from the central origin of the waves.

frequency). In addition to the central lobe, there are wavelength-dependent portions of the beam pattern formed by diffraction effects (Fig. 19). The side lobes are formed by constructive interference of the ultrasound waves coming from reflectors at an acute angle to the transducer face. According to reciprocity, the transducer also transmits power in the direction of side lobes.

Electronic Focus Annular Array

Although a transducer with a concave shape or a converging lens has a well-defined, fixed mechanical focus, to change the focus to a different depth requires constructing a new transducer. A transducer can be divided into elements (segments) that can be electronically controlled so that all

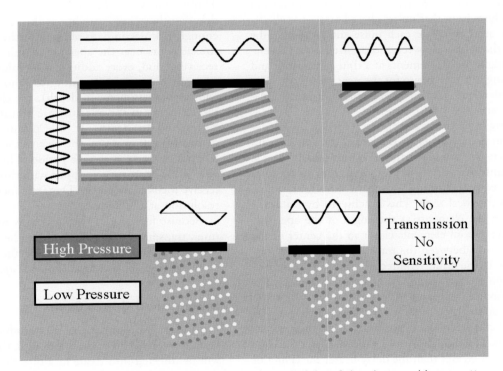

FIGURE 19. Side lobes from a flat transducer. The main lobe of the ultrasound beam pattern from a flat transducer is along the axis of the transducer **(upper left)**. For beam angles in which 3/2 cycles **(upper center)** or 5/2 cycles **(upper right)** intersect the transducer face, the transducer is also sensitive. The central axis main lobe of the beam pattern is called "n = 0", the upper center sidelobe is called "n = 1" and the upper right is called "n = 2". Between n = 0 and n = 1 is a null where the area of the transducer face under compression always equals the area of decompression as a wave travels from that angle toward the transducer **(lower left)**. A similar unsensitive angle is shown **lower right**. By the principle of reciprocity, the receive beam pattern sensitivity map and the transmit beam pattern intensity map are identical.

points on the transducer face no longer need to operate in unison. By operating the elements near the edge about a hundred nanoseconds early and the elements near the center a hundred nanoseconds later, the focal zone can be brought nearer to the transducer face.

One way to divide the transducer into elements is to form a series of concentric rings called an *annular array*. This transducer can be focused electronically, but the beam must be steered (pointed) electronically. The advantage of electronic focusing is flexibility. The focus can be changed in milliseconds by the ultrasound system. This allows the system to be focused at 3 cm deep 40 milliseconds after pulse transmission when echoes from 3 cm are returning, and to be focused at 6 cm deep 80 milliseconds after pulse transmission when echoes from 6 cm are returning.

Electronic Focus Linear Array

Another type of segmented transducer array used for electronic focusing is the linear phased array. This array has rectangular elements arranged in rows. Linear arrays and phased arrays are the extremes of a continuum of arrays. All consist of a straight row of rectangular transducers. Often, the array includes 64 or 128 transducers. Linear arrays use one transducer at a time to create an ultrasound pulse and receive the echoes from that pulse; phased arrays use all elements in the array to create each pulse and to receive the echoes from that pulse. Between those extremes, a 128-element array might use 16 elements at a time to transmit and receive, moving to a new group for the next pulse echo. The group of 16 elements is called an *aperture*. Individual transducers in the array are called *elements*.

In these arrays, mechanical focusing is used in the "thickness" direction perpendicular to the line of transducers, and electronic focusing is used in the direction parallel to the line of the transducers. Transmit focusing from an aperture of the array requires forming a concave wavefront, which converges on the focal zone. This is achieved by transmitting first from the elements at the edges of the aperture, then successively from elements closer to the center of the aperture. The time between the transmissions from successive elements is the time required for the ultrasound to travel a fraction of a wavelength from the prior element. For 5-MHz ultrasound, each cycle of the ultrasound takes 200 nanoseconds, so the time delay is a fraction of that, ranging from 0 to 40 nanoseconds, depending on the distance to the focal point. The time delay for elements nearer the edge of the aperture is greater than the delay nearer the center of the aperture because of the curvature of the focusing wavefront. On receive focus, the reverse process occurs.

Transmit Focusing

Because an ultrasound pulse is transmitted once for all depths along a particular ultrasound scan line, only one focal depth can be selected for transmission. Often, that focal depth is operator selectable. It is usually marked by a symbol "<" on the side of the ultrasound image. Some ultrasound instruments with electronic focusing allow multiple transmit focuses. In those cases, a separate pulse-echo cycle is used for each transmit depth. Multiple transmit depths are indicated by multiple "<" marks on the side of the ultrasound image. If three transmit zones are selected, and the same number of ultrasound scan lines is used, the image will take three times as long to form.

Receive Focusing

In contrast to transmit focusing, which allows only one focal depth per pulse-echo cycle, in receive focusing during the time intervals between depths, there is an ample amount of time to adjust the electronic focus. In a pulse-echo cycle, transmission typically lasts for 0.5 microseconds (2.5 cycles of 5-MHz ultrasound), but receive lasts between 40 and 200 microseconds (13 microseconds for each centimeter of depth). During the receive period, echoes consisting of curved wavefronts coming from a focal region arrive first at the center of the aperture and a few nanoseconds later at the margins of the aperture. Those echoes can be aligned in time by electronically delaying the echoes arriving at the central transducers by enough nanoseconds to align with the echoes arriving at the elements near the aperture margins. During a typical receive period, every additional 13 microseconds after the transmit pulse (corresponding to echoes coming from an additional centimeter in depth), the electronic delays for the elements in the aperture are adjusted to focus at the corresponding depth. If the ultrasound image spans depths from 0 to 8 cm, the receive focus will be adjusted 8 times during the receive period. This is called *dynamic focus*. In instruments equipped with this method, dynamic receive focus is always on. Dynamic focus improves lateral resolution at all depths.

Because focusing at deeper depths requires larger apertures, transducer elements will often be added to the aperture during the latter portion of the 200-microsecond receive period. This is called *dynamic aperture*.

Mechanical Beam Steering

If the diameter of an ultrasound transducer is much greater than the wavelength of the ultrasound, the ultrasound beam will be directed into tissue in a direction perpendicular to the face of the transducer. By tilting an ultrasound transducer so that its axis points in the desired direction, a particular line of tissue can be examined. Before 1975, most beam pointing was done by hand. The ultrasonographer would "scan" the ultrasound beam across a plane in tissue to form an image. However, around 1975, real-time 2D mechanical scanners were introduced, with the transducer driven by a motor to tilt the transducer in a sequence of directions to form a real-time sector scan automatically. Typically, an automatic scan takes 50 milliseconds to complete. After completing the scan, an image can be formed, 20 images per second, which is near the U.S. television frame rate of 30 frames per second, the European television frame rate of 25 frames per second, the sound movie frame rate of 24 frames per second, or the silent movie frame rate of 18 frames per second.

Within the mechanical scanhead, often, the transducer is mounted on a hinge pin and is motor driven to tilt to the left and right to sweep a sector scan. Manufacturers using this design included ADR, Diasonics, Interspec, Hofferel, and Honeywell. If the transducer is large and heavy, the oscillations cause vibrations in the scanhead. To avoid vibrations with a large transducer, Biosound used a fixed transducer and a mirror that directed the ultrasound beam to various angles. An alternative to angular oscillations is to mount transducers on a rotating wheel; both ATL and Pie Medical have used this design.

All of the above methods form a sector (fan-shaped) scan. A scan of parallel beams (raster scan) can also be formed mechanically. Rather than tilting the transducer, the transducer must be translated across the entire width of the field of view. The Picker Microview used this method. The scanhead was so cumbersome that, rather than moving the scanhead over the patient's body, the scanhead was mounted in a fixed location and the patient moved to it. The raster scan has

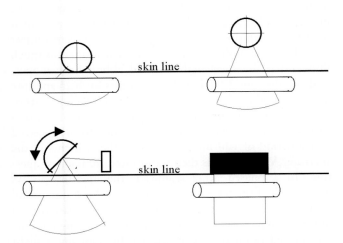

FIGURE 20. Sector and raster image formats. **Upper left:** Mechanical scanheads can create a large angle sector scan. **Upper right:** A standoff can be used to decrease the sector angle but retain a wider field of view. Such a sector scan can be achieved by mechanical scanning or phase array scanning. **Lower left:** A mechanical sector scan can be achieved by using an oscillating mirror rather than wobbling or rotating the transducer. **Lower right:** A raster scan can be generated by a linear array transducer. The layers of blood vessel walls can be easily seen if the ultrasound beams are perpendicular to the wall. Therefore a raster scan and a narrow beam sector scan provide superior images of vascular walls.

the advantage of using the superior depth resolution of ultrasound images to study the details of the superficial and deep vessel walls, which are parallel to the skin and therefore perpendicular to the ultrasound beam.

Several manufacturers have used a narrow sector scan to simulate a raster scan, thus using the superior depth resolution for vessel walls over a wider width of the image. To widen the field of view, a water path *standoff* is used between the transducer and the skin. Two examples of this are manufactured by Biosound and Diasonics (Fig. 20).

Linear Arrays: Electronic Beam Placing

Mechanical systems for scanning the ultrasound beam by moving a transducer from location to location or angle to angle are limited by inertia. To work well, the ultrasound beam pattern (scan line) must move from one location to another in a few microseconds, and it must be stable at the new location during the period of the pulse-echo cycle. An alternative is to use one transducer (or group of transducers) for every ultrasound scan line in the image and electronically switch on the appropriate transducer when needed. This allows rapid changing from one scan line to the next. There is no physical limit on how quickly the electronic switching can be done or how far the previous line is from the next. In today's world, electronic reliability is much greater than mechanical reliability; thus, the elimination of mechanical parts reduces the chance of future equipment failure. However, the cost of electronic systems is often greater than the cost of mechanical systems. The advantages of electronic scanheads over mechanical may be temporary. Methods of manufacturing both mechanical and electronic systems are evolving rapidly and converging in the new MEMS technologies.

Low-Density Linear Array

A raster scan can be obtained by placing a series of identical transducers in a line with the transducers aimed along parallel lines. This *linear array* scanhead must have a length equal to the width of the field of view of the image. To control each ultrasound beam, the width of each transducer must be much greater than the wavelength of the ultrasound. Thus, for 5-MHz (5,000,000 cycle/sec) ultrasound with a wavelength of 0.03 cm, the width of each transducer must be at least 0.15 cm; to form an image with 50 scan lines requires a scanhead 7.5 cm wide. The ADR obstetric scanners were of this design.

High-Density Linear Array

Lateral resolution is defined as the ability to see two closely spaced objects side by side in the image as separate objects. To achieve this, three ultrasound scan lines are required. In addition to two scan lines, one providing reflections from each of the two objects, a third ultrasound beam must pass between the objects without reflections to show the space between. Thus, with transducers spaced at 0.15 cm, the pair of objects must be separated by at least 0.3 cm to have one transducer receive a reflection from one, a second transducer pass an unreflected beam between them, and a third transducer get a reflection from the other. In addition, the ultrasound beam pattern of the middle scan line must be narrow enough to pass between the two objects without reflection.

To make the focal region of a beam pattern narrow, a large aperture is required. This aperture is often 10 times as wide as the focal region. Yet to image at the focal depth, the spacing between the beam patterns should be equal to the focal width. This requires overlapping the apertures for adjacent lines.

The newer linear array scanheads have divided the linear transducer into segments about 0.05-cm wide. These small apertures are too narrow to be able to point the ultrasound beam pattern to form a narrow focal zone (Fig. 21). To transmit and receive ultrasound along a single scan line, five or more elements are operated together, giving an effective aperture width of 0.25 cm and a narrowest beam (transition zone) at a depth of 0.5 cm while allowing the adjacent ultrasound lines to be spaced at 0.05 cm. If a larger group is selected, say 10 together, the transition zone occurs at a depth of 2 cm, near the depth of the carotid artery. If delays

are applied to the transducer elements in the aperture to focus the ultrasound beam in the near field, a narrow focus can be formed to improve the lateral resolution at depths near the focal region. A wide effective transducer aperture is required to achieve good focusing. The use of overlapping groups of transducer segments allows closely spaced scan lines and wide transducer apertures, which produce good ultrasound beam control and narrow focal zones. Most modern linear array ultrasound scanners use this method, including Acuson, Aloka, ATL, Hewlett Packard (HP) Quantum, and Unigon.

Curved Linear Array

A novel approach with the linear array is to locate the transducers on a curved line, convex to the ultrasound field. As adjacent groups of transducers are used, they not only originate from adjacent locations but also tilt in diverging directions, creating a sector scan rather than a raster scan. The Aloka and ATL color scanners use this method. An ultrasound scanner for venous research has been proposed implementing a concave linear array to obtain multiple views of the same structures. The scanhead surrounds the leg, and each transducer points inward. The ultrasound scan lines intersect in the leg.

Full Aperture Phased Arrays: Electronic Beam Pointing

Electronic methods can also be used to tilt the ultrasound beam originating from a single-segment transducer fixed in the scanhead. Electronic beam steering uses a segmented transducer with the segments aligned in a row as in a linear array. However, unlike a linear array, each segment is much thinner than the wavelength of sound, although when operated together, the 32, 64, or 128 segments form an aperture much wider than the wavelength of sound. In a linear array, ultrasound is transmitted from an aperture consisting of a part of the array; the echoes from all depths are received over a period of 100 microseconds by the elements in the aperture. A new pulse is then transmitted from a new aperture. In a phased array scanhead, the aperture always includes all of the transducers in the array. Each ultrasound scan line is formed by transmitting the beam pattern at a different angle from the same aperture. The angle of the transmitted beam pattern is selected by applying a slight time delay (nanoseconds) to each element in the array during the formation of the transmit burst. By applying similar delays to the echoes received by each element, the received beam pattern angle can also be selected to align with the transmitted pattern.

Suppose that a 5-MHz (0.03-cm wavelength) phased array scanhead has 128 segments, each 0.01 cm wide; the group is 1.28 cm wide. Transmitting from each segment in turn, starting with transducer element #1 and ending with

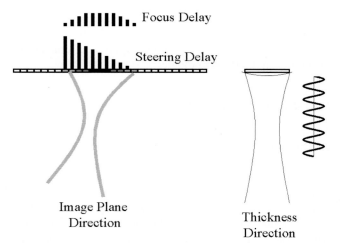

FIGURE 21. Phase-linear array transducer. This phase-linear transducer array is drawn with 28 elements in a row. The length of each element in the lateral image direction is half a wavelength, the length of the entire array is 14 wavelengths and the width of the active 10 element aperture is 5 wavelengths. The width of the elements in the array in the image thickness direction is 4 wavelengths. A set of electronic delays retard the cycles in the transmit and receive paths on the left side of the aperture to steer the ultrasound beam to the left. Focussing delays pull the focal zone close to the transducer array. In the image thickness direction, the fixed aperture and focus done by a lens provides a fixed focus in the thickness direction.

#128, waiting just 0.01 microsecond (millionth of a second) between transmissions, would take 1.28 microseconds to complete the transmission. The ultrasound transmitted from transducer element #1 has traveled just 0.197 cm (over six wavelengths) in that time (0.128 microseconds × 154,000 cm/sec = 0.128 microseconds × 0.154 cm/μsec). The result is to tilt the ultrasound beam toward the direction of element #128.

The angle of tilt, θ, can be determined by trigonometry:

$$\text{Sin } \Theta = 0.197 \text{ cm}/128 \text{ cm} \rightarrow\hspace{-0.3em}\rightarrow 9 \text{ degrees}$$

The transmission of the ultrasound burst (pulse) at this angle takes 1.28 microseconds. At 13 microseconds after the transmission, echoes will begin arriving from a depth of 1 cm. These echoes have traveled a total of 2 cm (1 cm down and 1 cm back) at a speed of 1.54 mm/μsec (20 mm /1.54 mm/μsec = 13 microseconds). At 39 microseconds, echoes will begin arriving from a 3-cm distance.

The echoes, coming from an angle of 9 degrees tilted toward element #128, reach element #128 first. It will take 1.28 microseconds for the echo wavefront to sweep from element #128 to element #1. If the receiving system is coordinated with the expected sweep of echoes from an angle of 9 degrees, echoes from that angle will be selectively enhanced; other echoes from other angles that do not progressively sweep across the elements at a rate of 0.01 microsecond/element will be suppressed. Thus, by properly timing the transmission, the outgoing ultrasound beam is directed, and by properly adjusting the incoming ultrasound for its timing (phase), the echoes from the chosen angle can be detected while ultrasound noise coming from all other angles is rejected.

It is difficult to manage the accurate timing of the transmission and reception, and this is particularly difficult with Doppler ultrasound. Thus, phased array scanheads are still in the development stage. One of the problems of a phased array system is that some of the ultrasound always propagates into tissue in the wrong direction. Some ultrasound goes straight into the tissue without being tilted; other parts of the ultrasound enter in selected directions dependent on the ultrasound wavelength and the spacing of the transducers. These unwanted (side-lobe) beams create ghost images of tissue structures that are displayed in the wrong location in the image screen. One way to control this problem is to use an array with more segments that are more closely spaced. Manufacturers have moved from 16 to 32 to 64 to 128 elements to improve beam steering and to suppress image ghosts. Each element requires a set of wires, a transmitter, and a receiver. This group (transmitter, wire, transducer, receiver) is called a *channel*. The more channels, the better control over beam pointing and the higher the cost and complexity.

Manufacturers have recently improved the method of cutting transducer blanks into elements and have also improved methods of attaching electronic matching circuits to the transducers and of applying backing materials to the back and matching layers to the front of the transducer array. Of greatest importance is the ability of the system electronics to operate 128 channels simultaneously. This means that if each transducer element is one fourth of a wavelength wide (allowing a broad beam pattern near 180 degrees from each element), the array aperture can be 32 wavelengths wide. Such an array can transmit at a range of angles up to 80 degrees from the central beam under electronic control.

Phased Linear Arrays

When the full aperture of an array is not needed for steering and beam control, the aperture origin of the ultrasound beam can be translated from location to location along the array, and the beam can be steered from that aperture to the available range of angles (Fig. 21). This allows flexibility in adjusting both the beam origin and angle. HP has used this method to create a trapezoidal image format, and ATL has used this method to perform compound real time imaging.

Modern Arrays

In recent years, the manufacture of transducer arrays has improved. Composite transducers have allowed the achievement of internal transducer damping with the associated improvement of depth resolution and have thus reduced the need for backing layers. One type of composite transducer is constructed from adjacent parallel rods of piezoelectric material crossing the thickness of the transducer, with the spaces between filled with a damping material. This construction controls unwanted vibrations in the array and allows the reduction of noise in the echo signal.

Rectangular Arrays (1.5-Dimensional Arrays) and Thickness Resolution

Some of the literature on evaluating vascular B-mode images suggests that the image is a tomogram providing a thin section that, if passed through the vessel in a longitudinal plane, would show only the superficial and deep portions of the vessel wall. Between the lines representing the wall, only intraluminal material would appear (Fig. 22). However, the most attractive ultrasound images of fetal faces are in conflict with this idea. The fetal images, taken in coronal section, show both the nose and the ears simultaneously. The nose and ears lie in quite different coronal planes. Thus, the image has considerable thickness.

In vascular imaging, the bright specular reflections from the superficial and deep portions of the arterial walls appear whenever those portions of the wall are within the image thickness. If the image is thick, the superficial and deep walls can be seen even if the scan plane is not parallel to the axis of the vessel. This makes vascular imaging easy. When

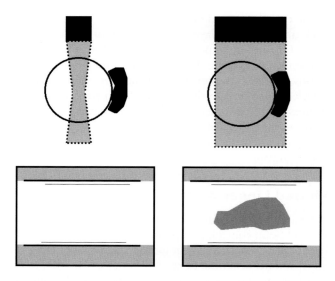

FIGURE 22. Effect of image thickness on the ultrasound image. A thin ultrasound image plane on the left images the superficial and deep arterial walls and the lumen between. An image of the same vessel done using a scanhead with a thick image plane includes objects in the image which are located in the lateral vessel walls. Some scanheads, at the depth of the thickness focus, form images 2 mm thick and other scanheads at depths farther from the depth of the thickness focus form images greater than 1 cm thick. Therefore it is possible to "see" objects which appear to be in the vessel lumen, which are actually on the lateral vessel walls. Looking at these structures in cross section may help to identify those that are not within the lumen.

viewing a curved vessel with a thin image, only a portion of the superficial and deep walls can be seen at a time, but with a thick image, the entire curve often lies within the image region. However, along with the attractive appearance and ease of examination using a thick image, there also comes a hazard.

Often, an extraluminal calcified region is present in the lateral arterial wall. This calcium is a good reflector of ultrasound and lies at a depth between the superficial and deep walls of the vessel in the image. The reflections from this extraluminal calcium structure will be excluded from a thin image but included in a thick image at a location between the deep and the superficial wall (Fig. 22). In addition, the reflector will move with the vessel. Thus, the scanhead generating the more attractive and easily acquired image with extended images of deep and superficial walls will show surface pathology as intraluminal echoes when they are in fact from extraluminal sources.

Thin images are generated by mechanical sector scanheads that have circular transducers. Circular annular array, electronic focused transducers generate the thinnest images. Fixed focused circular transducers generate thin images at the focal depth, but thicker images both shallow and deep to the focus. This is because the lateral focus and the thickness focus are identical with circular transducers. Thick

images can be generated by both linear array and phased array scanheads; lateral resolution and image plane thickness are completely independent with the rectangular apertures used in the linear and phased array scanheads.

To reduce the slice thickness of the ultrasound image, focusing must be applied in the slice thickness direction. With linear and phased arrays, a fixed lens is often used to focus the slice thickness at one depth. However, to allow dynamic receive focus and selectable transmit focus in the thickness direction, the transducer array must be divided in the thickness direction in addition to the divisions in the lateral direction. Because steering is not done in the thickness direction, only 5 or 7 elements are required in that direction.

The focusing is symmetric in the thickness direction; therefore, if 5 elements are present, only 3 wires are needed; elements on opposite sides from the center are hooked together. An array with 128 elements in the lateral direction and 3 channels (5 elements) in the thickness direction requires 3×128, or 384, channels, which is a number still challenging manufacturers.

Square Arrays (Two-Dimensional Arrays) for Three-Dimensional Imaging

For cardiac applications, there is interest in acquiring 3D ultrasound images at high volume rates. A volume rate is similar to a frame rate, except it is 3D rather than 2D. Workers at Duke University have produced a 3D real-time imaging system that is able to sweep an ultrasound beam in any direction from a 2D phase array transducer. With a square array divided into 32 elements in one direction and 32 elements in the other direction, there are 1,024 possible channels in all. If the elements are 1-mm wide, just attaching the wires becomes difficult. Consequently, the task of building such an instrument is heroic. One way to simplify the problem is by connecting to only half of the possible transducer elements, selecting them at random. This is called a *sparse array*. Such arrays will become more common as methods of shrinking electronics and mounting the transducer and electronics on a single structure are developed.

ULTRASOUND ECHO DEMODULATION AND IMAGING

The evolution of diagnostic medical ultrasound systems can be traced in Figs. 23 to 36. All pulse-echo ultrasound instruments from a simple A-mode system (Fig. 23) to a modern telesonography system (Fig. 36) are based on the same building blocks: a clock that can be used to determine the ultrasound frequency, a timer to select the maximum depth that times the pulse repetition interval (PRI) and therefore the pulse repetition frequency (PRF = 1/PRI), a

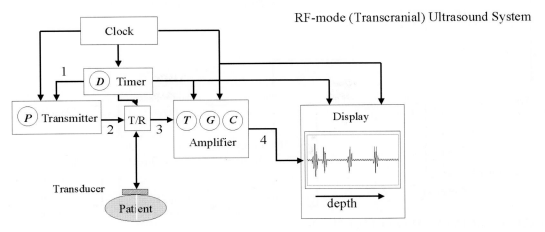

FIGURE 23. RF mode ultrasound system used in transcranial examination (c. 1960). This system displays the ultrasound echo in its most basic form. PRF was 1 KHz in these real time one-dimensional (depth) instruments that could show motion of structures. Faster PRF only would serve to make the display appear brighter.

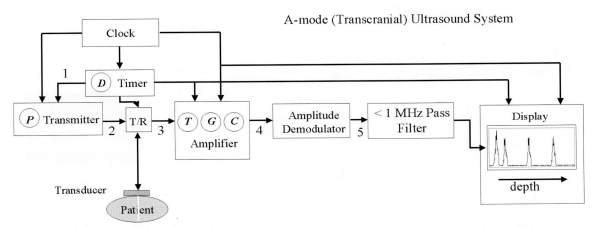

FIGURE 24. A-mode ultrasound system used in transcranial examination (c. 1960). This system added a demodulator but provided no new diagnostic information. RF was 1 KHz for the real time one-dimensional (depth) display.

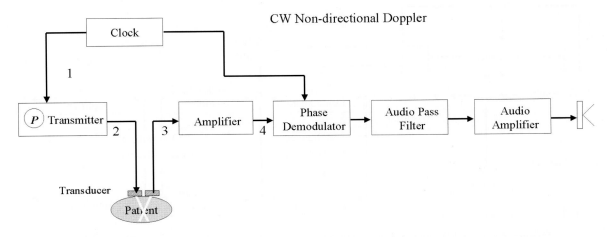

FIGURE 25. Nondirectional CW Doppler (Japan c. 1957 and US c. 1961). This system had an audio output. Pocket sized non-directional systems have been manufactured and used clinically since 1966.

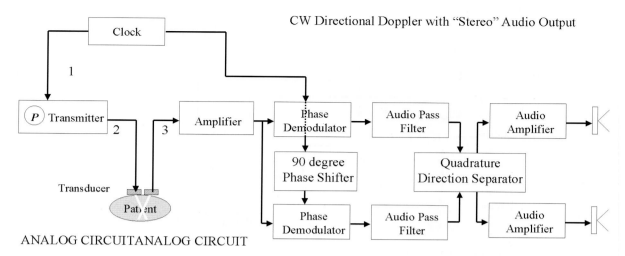

FIGURE 26. Directional CW Doppler (c. 1967). Tabletop directional systems have been manufactured and used clinically since 1970.

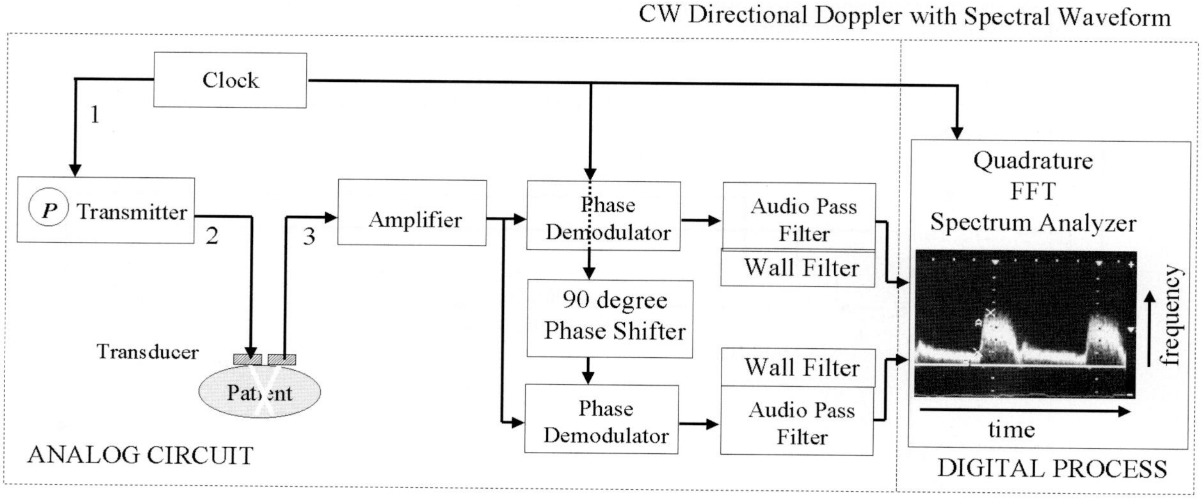

CW Directional Doppler with Spectral Waveform

FIGURE 27. Directional CW Doppler with spectral waveform display (c. 1980). Zero-crossing graphical displays were available by 1972 in tabletop Doppler systems. The spectral waveform provides more information about turbulence in the vessel and about mixed arterial and venous flow in the signal.

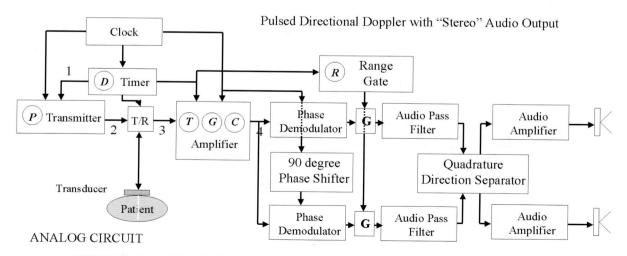

FIGURE 28. Pulsed Doppler (c. 1971). Pulsed Dopplers allow the selection of the depth of the sample gate which detects flow. Both pulsed and CW systems were also fitted with devices to track the position of the transducer to allow marking an image where flow was present to provide a map of the blood flow.

Pulsed Directional Doppler with Spectral Waveform

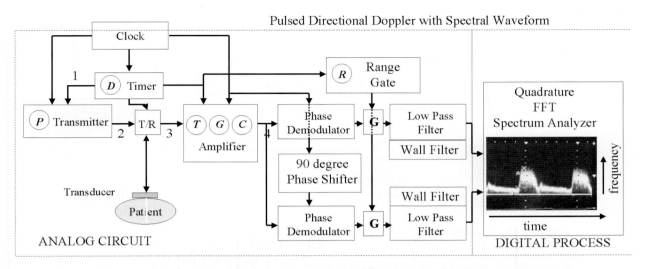

FIGURE 29. Pulsed Doppler with spectral waveform display (c. 1981). Pulsed Doppler systems can be fitted with spectral output displays.

M-mode (Cardiac) Imager

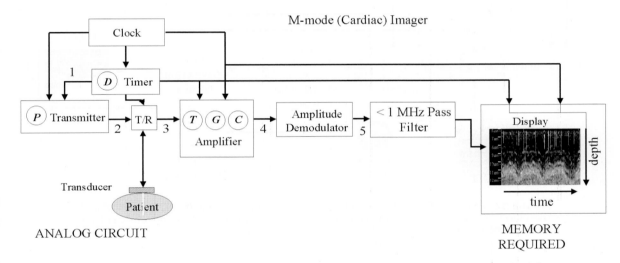

FIGURE 30. M-mode cardiac imager (c. 1970). The A-mode system (Fig. 24) can display the echo strength as gray levels on a two-dimensional image. In the M-mode (motion-mode), the vertical axis is depth in tissue and the horizontal axis is time. These displays can be used in cardiology to track the speed and excursion of moving heart structures during the cardiac cycle.

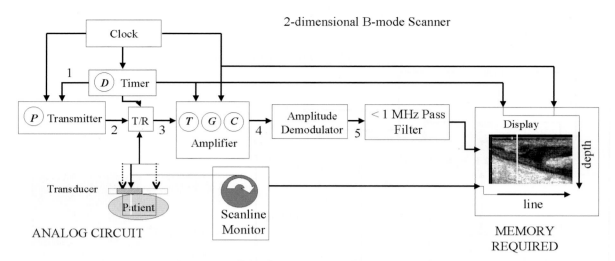

FIGURE 31. Two-dimensional B-mode manual "static" scanning (c. 1971). If the tissues under examination are not moving, then the horizontal dimension of the gray level image can be used for lateral dimension if the ultrasound beam pattern is moved in a plane through tissue and corresponding lines are drawn on the image plane.

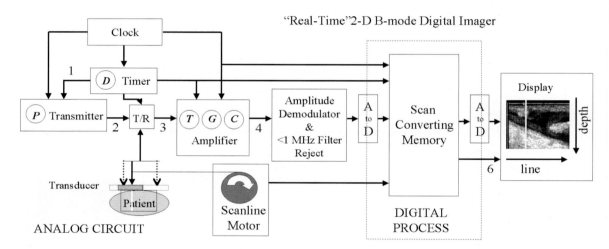

FIGURE 32. Real-time two-dimensional B-mode "automatic" scanning (c. 1971). By moving the transducer with a motor so that the beam pattern repeatedly is moved through a tissue plane, a series of images can be obtained which can be shown as a "real time" movie.

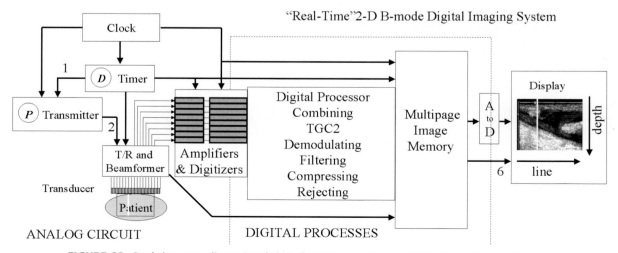

FIGURE 33. Real-time two-dimensional digital imaging system (c. 1985). The ultrasound beam can be moved electronically if the ultrasound scanhead has an array of transducers, and nearly all of the analog components of a system can be replaced by digital circuits or by digital software.

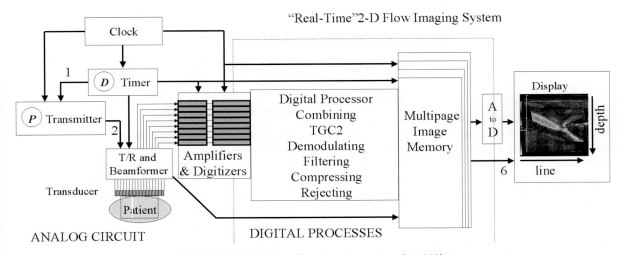

FIGURE 34. Real-time flow imaging system (c. 1990).

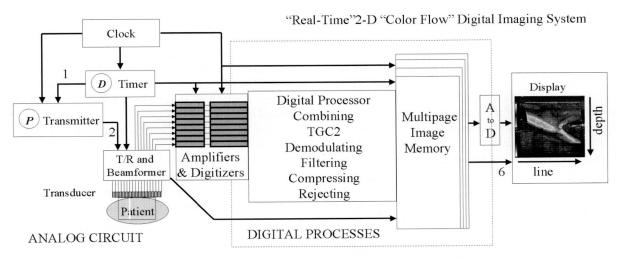

FIGURE 35. Real-time color Doppler imaging system (c. 1990).

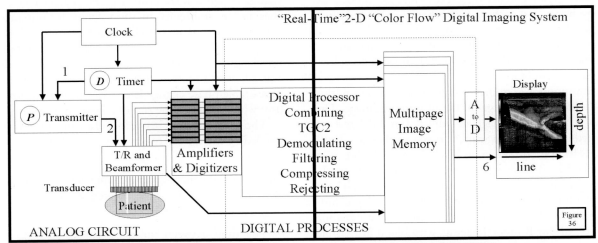

FIGURE 36. Telesonography ultrasound imaging system (c. 2005). By dividing the ultrasound scanner at the point in the data stream where the amount of information flow is the smallest to form two parts, one part of the system can be located next to the patient and the other, in the form of a desktop computer, can be in a consultant's office. The two pieces can be connected by a digital network.

transmit–receive switch, a transducer in contact with the patient, a time-gain compensation (TGC) system to adjust the signal amplitude to compensate for attenuation, and a demodulator-display system to provide the diagnostic information. Pulse-echo systems differ only in whether and how the ultrasound beam is moved across the body during an examination and how the echoes are demodulated (amplitude or phase) and assembled for display. Only the CW Doppler systems (Figs. 25–27) differ from this in that they have no timer, transmit–receive switch, or TGC system and have two transducers rather than one.

Two-Dimensional B-Mode Image

To create an amplitude-demodulated B-mode (brightness mode) image, a short pulse of ultrasound is transmitted into tissue. Echoes that return after 26.8 microseconds from a depth of 2 cm are amplified a small amount by the TGC system to compensate for the effects of ultrasound attenuation by 2 cm of tissue to and from the depth of the echo source. Echoes that return after 67 microseconds from a depth of 5 cm are amplified more by the TGC to compensate for the attenuation of the greater thickness of tissue traversed to obtain the echo. The amplified echo, in the form of an electrical oscillation, is then amplitude-demodulated by inverting the negative excursions and sending the result into a filter that selects the peaks for measurement of the amplitude.

The signal amplitudes are determined by the echogenicities of the corresponding tissues represented in the image. If attenuation has been properly compensated by the TGC, the image brightness corresponds to tissue type. The weakest echoes in the image are caused by clear fluid, the next brightest by blood; stronger echoes are generated by fat and muscle and organ parenchyma; the strongest echoes are caused by bone, metal clips, and other "hard" structures. The range of difference in echogenicity between blood and bone is 60 dB for 5-MHz ultrasound. This is the same as saying that calcium reflects 1,000,000 times more ultrasound energy than blood.

It is common for examiners to set the instrument to display a 40-dB dynamic range on the ultrasound image. The strongest echoes in the image are adjusted to 0 dB and are represented in the image as white; the echoes that are 40-dB weaker (1/10,000) are shown as black; blood, which generates echoes 55-dB weaker than the strongest, is also black. The echogenicity of the interior of muscular tissues, 45 dB below calcium, will also appear black if the display is limited to a range of 40 dB. Some examiners use a dynamic range of 60 dB for B-mode imaging, with blood just visible as the weakest noticeable echoes and calcium as the brightest echoes, which ensures that all echogenic tissues can be seen. At first, 60-dB dynamic range images are not pleasing to experienced examiners who have learned to use imaging systems that display only 30 or 40 dB of echo strength, but

with use, diagnostic detail in the images will become more easily distinguishable to the examiners.

Doppler Methods

In pulse-echo imaging, the brightness of each point on the 2D B-mode image screen is associated with the strength or amplitude of the echo returning from the corresponding depth in the direction that the ultrasound beam is pointed. Doppler data, corresponding to the speed of blood flowing through the tissue, use phase information (rather than amplitude information) in the echo (Fig. 3). Although the amplitude information obtained from a single pulse is sufficient to determine the echogenicity of the tissue (ability to generate a strong echo), the phase from a single pulse is not sufficient to determine the speed of moving blood. To determine the speed of the tissue, a series of pulse-echo cycles is required along the same ultrasound beam pattern. The change in phase from pulse to pulse corresponds to the change in distance from the reflector to the transducer; a change in phase of one fourth of an ultrasound wave represents a motion of one eighth of the wavelength of ultrasound in tissue.

If a new pulse of 5-MHz ultrasound is sent into the patient's body every 500 microseconds and if, during the interval between the pulses, the phase shifts by one fourth of a wave, corresponding to motion of the blood toward the transducer of 0.0393 mm, the speed at which the blood approaches the transducer can be computed:

$$\text{Speed of approach} = 0.00393 \text{ cm}/0.0005 \text{ sec}$$
$$= 7.85 \text{ cm/sec}$$

Phase changes that are much smaller or larger can also be measured. The maximum practical measurable phase change is half a wave (180 degrees). Larger changes cause aliasing, an ambiguity in the velocity measurement. The smallest practical measurable phase change is less than 1 degree (0.006 waves). Using 5-MHz ultrasound with a wavelength near 320 μm, the maximum phase change is equivalent to a motion of tissue of 80 μm, and the smallest measurable phase change is equivalent to a motion of 0.04 μm, which is about the size of a large molecule.

The phase change between pulses (measured in waves) divided by the time between pulses is called the *Doppler frequency.*

$$\text{Doppler frequency} = \text{phase change between pulses/} \\ \text{time difference between pulses} \\ = \text{Hertz}$$

The time between pulses is usually so short that the phase change is less than half of a wave or a cycle. The units are cycles per second, often called *Hertz.* A typical time between ultrasound pulses is 100 microseconds (0.1 millisecond). Using the numbers above for tissue motion, the maximum measurable speed is (80 μm /100 microseconds), or 0.8 m/sec; the smallest is (0.04 μm /100 microseconds), or 0.000 4 m/sec. This is the same as 80 cm/sec for the maximum and 0.04 cm/sec for the minimum speed detectable.

The expression above for Doppler frequency (f) is a form of the Doppler equation. The rate of phase change between pulses is equal to twice the speed at which the reflector approaches the ultrasound transducer (S) divided by the wavelength of sound (λ).

$$f = 2 \times S/\lambda = Hz = cycles/sec = cm/sec/cm/cycles$$

Unfortunately, the Doppler equation is rarely written like this. There seems to be a preference to compute the wavelength (λ) from the speed of ultrasound in tissue (C) and the ultrasound frequency (F):

$$\lambda = C/F = cm/cycle = cm/sec/cycles/sec$$

Substituting the wavelength into the Doppler equation yields the following:

$$f = 2 \times S \times F/C$$

To continue beyond this requires knowing the heading of the blood flow. Heading involves more than just direction. In Doppler, direction differentiates flow that is going away from the transducer from flow that is coming toward the transducer. Heading includes the angle of the velocity vector representing the blood flow. If the blood flow heading is known, the angle between the velocity heading and the ultrasound beam can be substituted (Fig. 37).

$$\cos \Theta = length\ of\ adjacent\ side/length\ of\ hypotenuse = S/V$$

yielding the conventional Doppler equation,

$$f = 2 \times F \times V \times \cos \Theta/C$$

which can be inverted to yield velocity, as follows:

$$V = f \times C/F \times 2 \times \cos \Theta$$

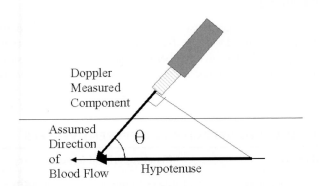

Doppler Measured Component

Assumed Direction of Blood Flow

θ

Hypotenuse

FIGURE 37. Doppler examination angle. The Doppler equation is written to describe the right triangle that is formed from the blood velocity vector and the Doppler ultrasound beam pattern. The blood velocity is the hypotenuse of the right triangle. A right triangle can be fitted into a circle with the hypotenuse as the diameter.

Testing the Doppler Equation

Although the substitution of ultrasound speed divided by frequency for wavelength is harmless, the substitution of (V × cos θ) for the speed of approach (S) introduces an unfortunate variability in the Doppler results. The final version of the Doppler equation suggests that the blood velocity magnitude (blood speed) can be determined if the Doppler angle is known. Blood speed would be useful for computing volume flow rates and for computing pressure differences. Examiners often substitute into this equation the angle between the axis of the blood vessel and the Doppler ultrasound beam pattern line measured on the ultrasound B-mode image during duplex scanning. This method is recommended by all manufacturers. Over a wide range of angles, this method should yield a single value of peak systolic velocity for a blood vessel. A simple attempt to validate this relationship in the common carotid artery yielded higher values of angle-adjusted velocity at an examination angle of 50 degrees than at an angle of 44 degrees (Fig. 38); the values measured at 60 degrees were even higher. The same result can be found in other arteries and with all electronic scanheads as well as other mechanical scanheads. Thus, for the same blood flow in the same vessel, changing the Doppler examination angle causes a change in the value of the velocity measurement. This Doppler angle–dependent variability is in addition to the physiologic variability. It occurs in most arteries and veins. This same problem occurs with all Doppler ultrasound systems in the same way. It does not depend on manufacturer or on whether the transducer is a single-element mechanical system or linear, phased, or linear phased array.

The reason for this problem does not rest in ultrasound physics. The problem lies with an incorrect assumption about the nature of blood flow. When blood or any fluid flows at (a) a constant rate along (b) a straight pipe (c) through long distances, the flow finally settles to a parabolic profile, with all velocity vectors parallel to the tube axis. However, blood flow in vessels is (a) pulsatile, not constant; (b) through curved vessels; and (c) divided in short segments rather than long and therefore does not flow along velocity vectors parallel to the vessel axis. In general, normal blood flow is helical and converges into stenoses. When a Doppler cursor is set parallel to the vessel axis, this does not mean that the cursor is parallel to the velocity vectors. Although the component of velocity parallel to the vessel axis is needed to compute the volume flow along the vessel, the magnitude of the velocity vector in the helical direction is needed to compute the kinetic energy if the Bernoulli equation is to be used. Thus, the meaning of velocity is obscure.

The effect of Doppler angle–dependent variability can be demonstrated by measuring the angle-adjusted velocity at a series of angles in two different arteries: the common

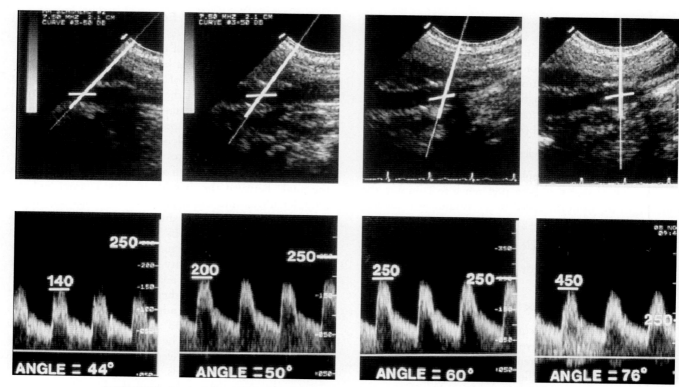

FIGURE 38. Angle adjusted blood velocity in the common carotid artery. A test of the Doppler equation in the carotid artery at different angles in the same blood vessel shows that the computed velocity is not independent of the Doppler examination angle used. Instead, the computed velocity is higher if the Doppler examination angle is closer to 90 degrees.

carotid artery and the distal superficial femoral artery (Table 11). The common carotid artery is short and curved proximal to the location of measurement; the distal superficial femoral artery is long and straight proximal to the location of measurement. The table demonstrates a nearly constant angle-adjusted velocity, in the distal superficial femoral artery, indicating velocities parallel to the vessel axis, but a progressive increase of measured velocity values at angles closer to 90 degrees in carotid arteries.

Because of this systematic progression of angle-adjusted velocity values with increasing Doppler examination angle, a consistent Doppler examination angle should be used in every examination to minimize this unnecessary source of variability; in addition, the examination angle should always be entered into data reports along with each measured Doppler frequency or velocity. In a long, straight vessel, far from a bifurcation, the effect does not occur; thus, in those cases, the conventional use of angle-adjusted velocities may be appropriate.

Aliasing

The phase changes between ultrasound pulses are used to determine the Doppler frequency. Phase changes that exceed one half of a wave between pulses cause confusion because a phase change increase of five eighths of a wave is

TABLE 11. MEASURED DOPPLER FREQUENCY AND ANGLE ADJUSTED VELOCITY IN DIFFERENT VESSELS

Doppler examination angle (degrees)	Common carotid artery		Distal superifical femoral artery	
	Doppler frequency	Velocity	Doppler frequency	Velocity
40	4.732 kHz	97 cm/s	3.561 kHz	73 cm/s
50	4.299 kHz	105 cm/s	2.906 kHz	71 cm/s
60	3.726 kHz	117 cm/s	2.292 kHz	72 cm/s
70	3.180 kHz	146 cm/s	1.524 kHz	70 cm/s

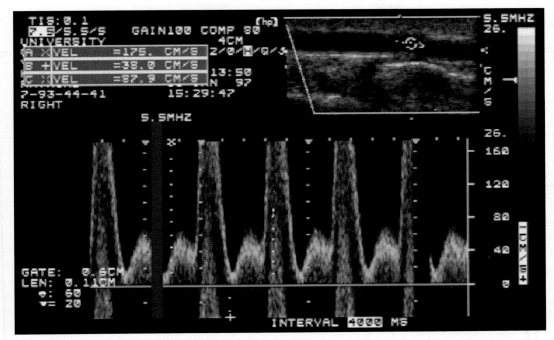

FIGURE 39. Aliasing of the arterial velocity waveform. This carotid arterial waveform shows peak systole disconnected from the onset of systole. This "aliased" peak systolic velocity display occurs because the Doppler pulse repetition frequency (PRF) sample rate was lower than half of the peak systolic Doppler frequency shift (Nyquist limit).

identical to a phase change decrease of three eighths of a wave (5/8 −1 = −3/8). If the phase change between pulses in the positive or negative direction is greater than one half of a wave, the smallest possible change is assumed to be correct in the absence of other evidence (Figs 39 and 40). This error in direction and magnitude of the frequency shift measurement is called *aliasing*. Aliasing can often be prevented by keeping the time between pulses short. If the data are being taken from great depths, the instrument must wait a long time after transmitting a pulse for the echo to return before transmitting a new pulse; therefore, the time between pulses may be long enough to introduce aliasing.

The aliasing frequency (Nyquist frequency) is determined by the maximum depth of Doppler analysis.

In most Doppler systems, the PRF and the Nyquist limit are lower than those listed in Table 12 to ensure spacing between the echoes from the deepest depths and the next transmit pulse.

If the speed of the blood is sufficient to produce Doppler signals that are of a higher frequency than the Nyquist limit, the frequency detected and displayed by a pulsed Doppler on a spectral waveform is in the wrong direction and of the wrong frequency. Thus, whenever possible, the highest PRF is used.

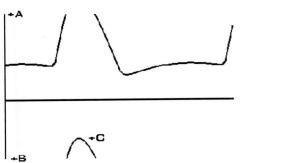

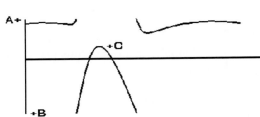

FIGURE 40. Computation of the peak frequency (PF) or velocity during aliasing. On the **left** note A is positive and B and C are negative. On the **right** note A and C are positive and B is negative. PF = A − B + C.

TABLE 12. TIME VERSUS DEPTH AND MAXIMUM PULSE REPETITION FREQUENCY FOR ULTRASOUND EXAMINATIONS AND NYQUIST (ALIASING) FREQUENCY FOR DOPPLER

Echo depth (cm)	Time for echo to return (μs)	Maximum pulse repetition frequency (kHz)	Nyquist frequency (kHz)
3	40	25.0	12.5
5	67	15.0	7.5
10	134	7.6	3.8
15	200	5.0	2.5
20	268	3.8	1.9

Color Doppler versus Spectral Waveform Doppler

Often, the phase measurement contains considerable noise; more than two pulse-echo cycles are required to average out the noise. The average phase change over a series of 8 to 32 pairs of pulse-echo cycles is used to determine the Doppler frequency in each sample volume in color Doppler instruments. Each color represents the average Doppler frequency shift from the corresponding sample volume in tissue. In conventional single-gate pulsed Doppler with spectral waveform analysis, each spectrum in the spectral waveform is generated using 256 pulse-echo cycles. This allows the data to be explored for the presence of more than one Doppler frequency. Each spectrum in the waveform includes data on the strength of each of the frequencies present, rather than reporting only a single average frequency. During the measurement of the spectral waveform, the highest frequencies are usually reported. Those are higher than the frequency resulting from the averaging process in the color image. Thus, velocity values reported from a conventional pulsed Doppler study are higher than the corresponding values reported from a color Doppler examination. If the lower color flow value were used for diagnosis, clinically significant arterial stenoses might be missed or underreported.

Doppler Systems: Continuous Wave Doppler

Doppler systems are often divided into CW systems and pulsed systems. It is useful to think of the CW Doppler and the pulsed Doppler as the extremes of a range of choices. All Doppler systems measure the speed of blood along the axis of the ultrasound beam. All Doppler systems can be used to measure the peak component of the velocity vector along the ultrasound beam axis. The differences between the pulsed and CW Doppler is the size of the active sample volume and the range of Doppler frequency shifts that can be measured without ambiguity.

Pulsed Doppler systems usually use a single ultrasound transducer for both transmitting and receiving. In the CW system, the transmitting transducer is always in use, so a second receiving transducer adjacent to the transmitting transducer is required. The width of the active Doppler sample volume is determined by the focal characteristics of the ultrasound transducer. The ultrasound transducer is designed to restrict the insonated region to a pencil-sized beam. The two transducers (transmitter and receiver) in CW Doppler each have a beam pattern. The active sample volume is the volume of overlap of the two beams. Because the two beam patterns are angled with respect to each other and cross at mid-depth, the active sample volume is widest at mid-depth and is narrow at both shallow and deep depths where the overlap is not so great. In pulsed Doppler, using a single transducer for both transmitting and receiving, the transmitting and the receiving beam patterns overlap throughout their length. Therefore, the width of the beam pattern is narrow at mid depths, where the narrow focal region is located.

In CW Doppler systems, the length (in the direction of the ultrasound beam) of the active sample volume within the beam is determined by the region of overlap between the beam patterns of the transmitting transducer and the receiving transducer (Figs. 25–27). In pulsed systems, the active sample volume is determined by the duration of the transmitted ultrasound burst and the duration of the receiver gate. The location of the sample volume is determined by the time between the transmit burst and the opening of the receiver gate to accept echo signals from the selected depth. Thus, CW Doppler systems have longer active sample volumes than do pulsed Doppler systems.

The highest blood velocity possible in humans can be computed by substituting the highest systolic blood pressure (225 mm Hg) into the Bernoulli equation:

$$p = 4 \times V^2$$

where p is pressure in mm Hg and V is velocity in m/sec, we find that the highest possible blood velocity in humans is 750 cm/sec (with systolic pressure of 144 mm Hg, V_{max} = 600 cm/sec). The maximum possible Doppler shift in humans can be calculated. Assuming a zero Doppler examination angle, the resultant Doppler shift is dependent on the ultrasound frequency. Using a 10-MHz Doppler, a blood velocity of 750 cm/sec produces a Doppler frequency shift of 100 KHz (f = 2 × S × F/C = 2 × 750 cm/sec × 10,000 KHz/150,000 cm/sec = 100 KHz). It is common to detect 450-cm/sec velocities at a Doppler examination angle of 60 degrees with a 5-MHz Doppler (= 2 × 450 × 5000/150,000/2) as an audible frequency of 15 KHz, or a 90-

cm/sec velocity as an audible frequency of 3 KHz. Of course, the limits of human hearing of the examiner must be considered when performing Doppler examinations (20 Hz to 20 KHz in young people; 30 Hz to 3 KHz in old people).

Electronic analysis of the frequencies can be performed over a wide frequency range. Most modern analyzers sample the audio signal to be analyzed and perform a digital frequency analysis. At a sample frequency of 50 KHz, the highest Doppler frequency that can be displayed without aliasing is 25 KHz. Thus, although the CW Doppler is capable of detecting the highest Doppler shifts possible in humans (100 KHz), those signals cannot be heard. In addition, if these signals are analyzed with a digital spectrum analyzer (most are digital), the resultant waveform will probably alias.

Doppler Systems: Pulsed Doppler

In pulsed Doppler, every time that the system transmits a burst of ultrasound and receives an echo back from the depth of interest, the phase of the echo is measured. This measurement is called a *sample*. In pulsed Doppler, the sample rate is equal to the PRF. The sample rate of a pulsed Doppler is limited by the depth to the selected Doppler sample volume because the Doppler ultrasound system must wait until the echo from the selected depth is received before transmitting again. If the system does not wait, the echo from the desired depth will arrive at the same time as stronger echoes from more recent transmissions reflecting from tissues at shallower depths. These shallow echoes will obscure the phase measurement from the depth of interest. Of course, when receiving the echo from the selected depth, echoes from deeper depths may also be present, but these have been attenuated and therefore are small enough to have little effect on the phase measurement. The depth of the expected Doppler sample volume (E) is found by the following equation:

$$E = C \times t/2$$

where t is the time between the transmit pulse and the receiver gate opening and C is the speed of ultrasound in tissue. Additional sample volumes along the ultrasound will be spaced at intervals of G from the shallowest volume:

$$G = C/(2 \times PRF)$$

The shallowest Doppler sample volume is located at a depth of less than G; thus, E < G because PRF is always selected to be below 1/t. In a typical example with a PRF of 12.8 KHz, the first Doppler sample volume must be at a depth of less than 6 cm [G = 6 cm = 154,000 cm/s/(2 × 12,800 cy/s)]. If the Doppler sample volume is set at a depth of 4 cm, other sample volumes will exist at 10 cm (4 + 6), 16 cm (10 + 6), 22 cm (16 + 6), and at deeper 6-cm intervals. The length (size) of the Doppler sample volume is often adjustable with the front panel controls on a duplex scanner. The sample volume length can be increased by increasing the duration of the transmit burst (Tt) or the

duration of the receiver gate (Tr). The sample volume length (Sl) is as follows:

$$Sl = C \times (Tt+Tr)/2$$

By increasing the ultrasound transmit duration and the receive duration, the length of the sample volume can become nearly equal to the depth of the sample volume.

Pulsed Doppler Aliasing

Sample volumes at deeper depths require lower PRFs because the system must wait for the return of the echoes. In Doppler, the low PRF may result in aliasing. As an example, if high Doppler shift frequencies are obtained from a sample volume at 9 cm, aliasing may occur. For the first sample volume to be located at 9 cm, a PRF as low as 8 KHz is required [PRF = C/(2 × depth) = 154,000 cm/sec/(2 × 9 cm) = 8.56 KHz]. Aliasing will occur at Doppler shift frequencies exceeding the Nyquist limit of 4 KHz (8 KHz/2) (Figs. 39 and 40).

Frequency Analyzer

During a Doppler examination, an experienced examiner can recognize the sounds of the high Doppler frequencies associated with stenoses and the hissing sounds associated with spectral broadening. Because of the need for paper documentation and quantitative measurement, images representing the Doppler signal can also be generated. The images are based on a frequency analysis of the Doppler shift. Although a few systems lump the Doppler data from systole with those from diastole, most Doppler frequency analysis systems display a waveform allowing analysis of the systolic frequencies separately from the diastolic frequencies. The displays can be divided into those that determine the complete spectrum of the Doppler frequencies representing all of the velocities in the sample volume and those that determine only a single characteristic Doppler frequency as representative of the blood velocities.

Spectrum Analyzer

There are a number of ways to determine rapidly the spectrum of Doppler frequencies in a signal and to display the successive spectra over time as a spectral waveform. The Fast Fourier Transform (FFT) method is the most popular; however, other methods, such as the time compression analyzer, the parallel filter analyzer, and the chirp Z analyzer work equally well. For the user, the difference between these systems rests in the cost and availability; the displays are identical. There are common features of the data analysis in these analyzers that will be discussed here.

The Doppler signal is analyzed in sections about 10-millisecond (0.01-second) long. Each analysis produces a spectrum, so that the spectral waveform consists of a display of 100 spectra per second. During each analysis of

10 milliseconds, the instrument records the Doppler signal and analyzes it. The recording is done in digital form (like the new high-fidelity compact disks or the digital audiotape systems), taking 25,600 samples per second. If the system takes 25,600 samples per second for 0.01 second, it has 256 samples to analyze. In the analysis, a test will be made for the strength of each of 128 frequencies in the signal (256/2). The number of samples is divided by 2 because of the Nyquist sampling theorem, which states that at least two samples are needed per cycle to identify the presence of a frequency in a signal. Harry Nyquist discovered this while working on trans-Atlantic telephone call transmission. (There is a more sophisticated version of the theorem that states that at least 4 samples must be present to determine correctly the power contained in a frequency that is present. A modern frequency analyzer is fast enough to ensure that tests for all 128 frequencies are completed in 10 milliseconds.) The results are then displayed, usually as a gray-scale spectrum. The number and choice of tested frequencies are determined by the time and sample rate. The lowest Doppler frequency in the display and the spacing between frequencies are equal to the number of spectra per second. A typical spectrum analyzer takes 0.01 second of Doppler data for each analysis: the lowest Doppler frequency is 100 Hz (cycles/sec). Other frequencies tested are 200 Hz, 300 Hz, 400 Hz, 500 Hz, 600 Hz, and so forth. The highest frequency tested is equal to half of the sample rate. If the Doppler sample rate is 25,600 Hz, the highest frequency tested is 12,800 Hz. Thus, a total of 128 frequency tests will be done on 256 data points.

Therefore, the frequency resolution of the spectrum analyzer is related to the time resolution of the spectrum analyzer; the frequency range is related to the Doppler sample volume depth. There is no agreement on the required or optimal frequency resolution. One manufacturer has a frequency resolution of 50 Hz because each spectrum takes 0.02 second; another has a poorer frequency resolution of 125 Hz because each spectrum takes 0.008 second. For the user, both look the same. In contrast, there is agreement that the highest sample frequency (or PRF) is the best to avoid aliasing. PRF, however, is determined by the depth of the vessel under examination rather than by the instrument manufacturer (Table 12).

With some instruments, it is possible to trick the instrument and perform the examination at a greater depth than the maximum examination depth. This is called *high pulse repetition Doppler*. The trick is to use a higher PRF than is allowed by the depth of the sample volume. The result is that the desired Doppler signal is not acquired from the shallowest active Doppler sample volume, but from a second or third sample volume in depth. Because of attenuation of ultrasound in tissue, the instrument is less sensitive to the deeper Doppler sample volumes than to the shallower. Thus, if moving blood is present in the associated shallow sample volume, the velocity in the shallow sample volume will dominate the signal.

Characteristic Frequency Analyzers

If the Doppler signal contains only a single frequency, that frequency can be determined in a number of ways. The first frequency analyzers used in ultrasonic Doppler diagnostic systems measured and displayed a single Doppler frequency as a function of time as a frequency (or velocity) waveform. These systems were used because they were electronically simple and thus inexpensive at the time.

The most popular system of this type of Doppler waveform display was the zero-crossing frequency detector. The system had difficulty separating noise from signal. Weak Doppler signals and Doppler signals resulting from turbulent flows produced erratic tracings. Such systems were not satisfactory for determining the maximum frequencies in Doppler signals. The characteristic frequency displayed was similar to the mode frequency or the frequency of greatest amplitude.

The frequency displayed by an analyzer is often called the *mean* or *average* frequency. The terminology causes a good deal of confusion. The definitions of the two terms are the same, but the definitions are incomplete. Two types of average frequency are used: (a) the instantaneous average over all frequencies and averaged over 0.01 second or less, and (b) temporal average frequency averaged over a full cardiac cycle, combining systole and diastole.

Three instantaneous characteristic frequencies could be used as the Doppler frequency: the mean, the mode, and the median. Often the term mean is used for any of these, but they are very different. The instantaneous average (properly called the mean) frequency is rarely used because the average is so sensitive to noise. If 90% of the Doppler power is between 500 and 600 Hz, the average should be near 550 Hz, but if 10% of the power is noise at 10,000 Hz, the average frequency is 1,495 Hz. The mode (most intense) frequency is resistant to noise; if 90% of the Doppler signal power is between 500 Hz and 600 Hz, the mode is likely to be present between 500 and 600 Hz. Noise at 10,000 Hz will not affect the mode. However, the exact value of the mode (is it 500 or 600 Hz?) is still subject to noise, and its resolution (in 100-Hz steps) is poor. The median also has poor resolution but is very resistant to noise. Half of the signal power is at frequencies lower than the median, and half of the power is at frequencies above the median. Each of these values is computed every 0.1 second. None of these is the value that is usually selected from the Doppler spectral waveform. The value selected from the Doppler spectral waveform for diagnostic purposes is selected as the highest value during systole from the upper envelope of the waveform. The upper envelope is the series of values from the spectra in the waveform: each value is about the highest frequency, with power at least $1/100$ of the mode frequency (20 dB down from the mode).

Sometimes, a time average velocity value is computed from the series of values of the mode, median, mean, or upper envelope value.

Color Doppler Imaging

In color Doppler imaging, each Doppler frequency is assigned a color. Once the Doppler shift is computed for a region in the image, the color corresponding to the Doppler shift is displayed at the corresponding image location. This allows only one frequency to be displayed for the Doppler signal in each Doppler sample volume. The color may represent the mode, the median, or the average instantaneous Doppler frequency.

The identification of the frequency for color Doppler at each depth is done by one of three methods: averaging the frequencies of an FFT spectrum, averaging the phase changes between pulses in the Doppler signal (lambda processor), and averaging the phase changes between pulses weighted by the strength of the signal (pulse pair covariance).

In a typical FFT analysis for color Doppler, the pulsed Doppler system acquires 16 phase samples in time from 16 pulse-echo cycles for each sample volume in depth. A Fourier transform is used to create a spectrum showing the intensity of eight frequency ranges in the forward direction and eight in the reverse direction. The ranges with low intensity are thought to contain noise and are set to zero. An average of the remaining adjacent frequencies is computed. A color is selected based on the result. Gathering the 16 pulse-echo cycles for a 4-cm depth takes less than 1 millisecond. This system was used in the Quantum color flow imager.

In a typical lambda processor, at each sample depth, the six phase changes occurring in the six intervals between seven pulse-echo cycles in sequence are averaged to determine the average frequency shift. If the sample volume is located in moving blood far from solid tissues, this system works well. If, however, there are strong echoes from nearby stationary solid structures mixed with the changing signals from moving blood, the lambda processor detects no Doppler frequency shift, even though an FFT analysis would. Thus, the lambda processor leaves gaps in the color display between the color, indicating blood flow in the center of an artery and the echogenic vascular wall. This system was used on the first duplex color Doppler imaging system.

In a typical pulse-pair covariance or autocorrelation processor, echoes from the first two (initializing) pulse-echo cycles of each sample volume are obtained to determine the phase and amplitude (intensity) of echoes from strong stationary reflectors. The phase and amplitude changes of subsequent echoes from each sample volume are compared to the initializing pulses, and the weighted average is taken; phase angle changes associated with strong differences from the initializing echo samples are weighted heavily since they are considered to be less likely to contain noise. Seven or eight pulse-echo cycles (taking about 0.5 millisecond) are required to determine the Doppler frequency and assign the appropriate color to the Doppler sample volume. This method is used in most color Doppler imaging systems.

In the color Doppler systems, about 64 Doppler sample volumes are processed at the same time along the length of a Doppler line. The number of samples is determined by the depth of the image and the size of the color Doppler pixels. In a typical image, each pixel (sample volume) represents 1 mm in depth, and the depth of the image is 6.4 cm—hence, 64 sample volumes are needed. Thus, data for all depths can be acquired as rapidly as data from a single depth. Because these systems are pulsed Doppler systems, all are subject to aliasing under the same conditions as conventional single-gate pulsed Doppler.

ULTRASOUND EXAMINATIONS

Examination Types

Early in this Appendix, the duration of the transmitted pulse was designated as 1 microsecond and the time allowed for the return of echoes was 500 microseconds; however, neither of these numbers is a fixed value. Although a Doppler transmit pulse typically lasts for 1 microsecond, an image transmit pulse varies with ultrasound frequency and transducer design. For best depth resolution, the B-mode image pulse is as short as possible.

The interval between pulses also varies. In a conventional M-mode imaging examination, the interval between ultrasound pulses is 1 millisecond; this is commonly described as a PRF of 1,000 cycles per second, or 1 KHz. For other types of imaging and Doppler, the highest possible PRF (shorter interval) is usually selected. The interval between pulses must be long enough for the echoes to return from the deepest depth of interest. Thus, the PRF is determined by the maximum depth of interest in the examination (Table 12).

Of all of the pulse-echo examinations, only the M-mode (motion-mode) examination is not limited by the PRF. The M-mode examination looks along only one ultrasound beam line in tissue; a full set of data about tissue echogenicity along the examination line is acquired from a single pulse-echo cycle. The M-mode examination was developed to study motions of the heart. Along the examination line, the motions of the heart structures are slow enough so that 1,000 samples per second are sufficient to characterize the motions. M mode is sometimes useful for looking at the pulsatile motions of arterial walls and the respiratory motions of venous valves.

2D real-time ultrasound B-mode imaging operates at the limits of image frame rate, image size, and image resolution. The 2D image must be formed in the 33 milliseconds available at the standard television frame rate of 30 frames per second. If the ultrasound image takes longer to acquire, the display frame rate is slower than the television frame rate, and the image looks jumpy. Although there is sufficient time to gather a high-resolution image consisting of 330 lines to a depth of 7.7 cm (PRF = 10 KHz), there is not enough time to form a high-resolution image consisting of 330 lines from a depth of 15.4 cm (PRF = 5 KHz).

The effects of increasing image depth can be tabulated for known depths. The increase in time between pulses combines with the wider base of the image in a sector scan to degrade lateral resolution due to ultrasound scan-line density. A 90-degree sector scan produces an image with a width of 10.8 cm at a depth of 7.7 cm, and a width of 21.6 cm at a depth of 15.4 cm. Because there is time to gather only 165 lines at the greater depth (waiting 200 microseconds for each echo), the line spacing at 15.4-cm depth is 1.3 mm, and the best possible resolution, based on line spacing, is twice that.

Because the time for each ultrasound scan line cannot be decreased (it is determined by the speed of ultrasound and the image depth), only two changes can be made to improve the lateral resolution at a depth of 15 cm: (a) decrease the image frame rate to give more time per image (a problem if the tissues are moving), and (b) decrease the width of the image by decreasing the sector angle.

The problem becomes more severe with a 2D color Doppler imaging system. If the image depth is 15.4 cm and 16 pulse-echo cycles are used for each image line, only 10 color Doppler image lines can be gathered in the 33 milliseconds available for the image. Each line would have 21 mm in width to fill. Thus, for color Doppler imaging, the number of ultrasound pulse-echo cycles per color Doppler image line is kept to a minimum (8 rather than 16), the frame rate is reduced (7.5 frames per second rather than 30), and a narrow color sector is displayed, all to keep the spacing between image lines small.

Reducing the number of pulse-echo cycles by a factor of 2 from 16 to 8 increases the noise in the signal by the square root of 2. Reducing the frame rate by a factor of 4 from 30 to 7.5 frames/sec creates serious problems, introducing image distortions due to motion during the image acquisition. Reducing the width of the sector is a small inconvenience. If the maximum depth could be reduced, an increase in the PRF would be possible, thus allowing a reduction in the spacing between the scan lines. These choices are all controlled by the ultrasound examiner. The examiner must choose between the color flow image size (lateral and depth), lateral resolution of the color Doppler data, and temporal resolution (frame rate). The depth resolution of the color Doppler data is selected by the manufacturer of the instrument. Logic suggests that using a higher-frequency ultrasound scanhead will improve depth resolution, but this might not be true of color Doppler data.

Scan Format

When forming a 2D ultrasound image, dimensions in the direction along the line of the ultrasound beam are estab-lished by measuring the time for the echo to return from a transmitted pulse (Table 12).

Data for the other dimension of the image, transverse to the direction of the ultrasound beam, can only be obtained by directing the ultrasound beam along a sequence of paths adjacent to each other. In early, "static" 2D imagers, the image was formed by "painting" the image by moving the ultrasound beam over a 2D field. The image could be properly formed only if the tissues or objects shown in the display were stationary during the scan across the image field. Both brightness mode (B-mode) and Doppler flow images were formed this way. When such images were formed, the direction of the ultrasound beam in any section of the image was determined by the examiner. This allowed the examiner to select a preferred perpendicular angle for imaging each tissue interface, or an angle nearly in line with the direction of blood flow for acquiring Doppler data. Static scanning provided the most *flexible* scanning format. However, it required that during the period of the scan (often lasting several minutes), the patient could not move even a few millimeters.

When real-time imagers were developed, the ultrasound beam was swept across the image plane automatically at high speed. 2D images were formed faster (in 33,000 microseconds), and the ultrasound scan lines conformed to a preselected, efficient pattern: *parallel* lines, called a *raster* scan; or a fan-shaped image called a *sector* scan (Fig. 20). Both of these formats are currently popular. The raster scan requires that the footprint of the scanhead on the patient be as broad as the image.

PULSE-ECHO ULTRASOUND ERRORS

The exact time for an echo to return cannot be determined from the depth of the reflector alone; the time also depends on the speed of travel of the ultrasound in tissue. In medical ultrasound examinations, 154,000 cm/sec is used as an average speed of ultrasound in soft tissue.

$$\text{Time} = \text{round trip distance/speed}$$
$$= 2 \times \text{depth/speed} = \text{cm/cm/sec} = \text{sec}$$

It is a common assumption that ultrasound travels at a speed of 1,540 m/sec in soft tissue (or 154,000 cm/sec, or 1.54 mm/μsec); however, the speed is quite variable:

- 1.45 mm/μsec in fat
- 1.55 mm/μsec in liver
- 1.57 mm/μsec in blood
- 1.58 mm/μsec in muscle
- 1.67 mm/μsec in cartilage

Thus, if the ultrasound passed only through fat on the way to and from the reflector, the reflector would appear to be 6% deeper than the actual depth because the echo returned 6% later than expected because the speed of ultrasound through the fat is 6% slower than the value assumed.

If the overlying tissue were muscle, the reflector would appear to be 3% shallower than the actual depth. When using a biopsy probe, part of the uncertainty of the expected location of the probe results from these errors.

TYPES OF ULTRASOUND INSTRUMENTS

Display Systems

Many types of tissue data can be obtained using pulse-echo ultrasound. Commonly displayed data include the echogenicity of structures at different locations under the transducer, the motions of tissue over time during the cardiac cycle, and the speed of blood during the cardiac and respiratory cycle. Conventional displays form a 2D static image showing the depth and lateral dimension of anatomy (2D B mode), depth versus time (M mode), and velocity versus time (spectral waveform), occasionally adding color to show blood velocity on anatomy. Quantitative dimensional and temporal measurements can be made from these displays. Lengths and areas can be measured from 2D B mode and M mode, and displacement over time can be measured from M mode. Velocity changes can be measured from spectral waveforms. These displays provide no convenient way to measure volumes, displacement in 2D or 3D space, or properties of tissue other than echogenicity. New displays under development include harmonic imaging, which shows whether the tissue deforms the ultrasound wave; imaging of ultrasound contrast agents, which shows tissue perfusion; 3D methods, which allow volume measurement; tissue velocity imaging, which shows myocardial viability; attenuation imaging, which shows ultrasound propagation through tissue; tissue compressibility imaging, which shows tissue stiffness; and tissue pulsatility imaging, which shows blood volume contained in tissue. Once each of these methods is developed, the clinical protocols must be developed, and the clinical utility of the methods must be assessed.

The five display systems common in conventional duplex scanning will be discussed in greater detail: (a) real-time 2D B-mode image, (b) real-time 2D B-mode image with superimposed Doppler sample volume, (c) gray-scale spectral waveform display, (d) real-time 2D color Doppler, and (e) differentiating color flow Doppler methods from color flow time-domain methods.

Real-Time Two-Dimensional B-Mode Image with Doppler Sample Volume

In the conventional ultrasound duplex scanner, an ultrasound B-mode tomographic image of the anatomy is formed, then a mark signifying the location of the Doppler sample volume in tissue is displayed as a cross on the image in the corresponding location. A line from the origin of the scanhead passing through the mark signifies the orientation of the ultrasound beam for the Doppler. The sample volume mark allows the examiner to position the Doppler sample volume in a blood vessel of interest by moving the mark into the image of the vessel while holding the ultrasound scanhead in a fixed location. Often, the image contains a longitudinal view of the vessel of interest. The examination angle between the image of the vessel and the Doppler line can be measured to standardize the examination method.

The length of the Doppler sample volume can be adjusted by changing the length of the Doppler transmit pulse or the duration of the receiver sample gate. The length of the Doppler sample volume can be shown by placing an adjustable-length bar on the Doppler line that extends to indicate the selected length of the Doppler sample volume. Because the lateral width of the Doppler sample volume is determined by the focusing of the ultrasound transducer, the width also varies with depth. Unfortunately, none of the Doppler display systems indicates the width of the Doppler sample volume by displaying a corresponding box width at the sample volume location on the screen.

Gray-Scale Spectral Waveform Display

The conventional spectral waveform displays show the Doppler frequency (representing a component of the blood velocity) on the vertical axis versus time on the horizontal axis, with the strength of the Doppler frequency shown as brightness. The frequency range of the display is equal to the PRF of the Doppler or the sample frequency of the spectrum analyzer. The earliest displays used a frequency range from PRF/2 to −PRF/2, allowing equal displays in the forward and reverse directions. High Doppler frequencies that exceed the Nyquist limit (PRF/2) in the positive or negative direction, leave one Nyquist limit of the display and reenter the display on the opposite Nyquist frequency limit, showing the wrong Doppler frequency in the wrong direction. This is called *aliasing*. By moving the improperly displayed portion of the waveform to a location adjacent to the other Nyquist limit, the waveform can be reconstituted. This maneuver is commonly called *baseline shift*.

Some Doppler instruments fail to show the full range of Doppler frequencies (e.g., Diasonics 400). Recognizing aliasing and correctly measuring peak frequencies with such systems is difficult. A method of measuring peak frequencies is shown in Fig. 40.

Although aliasing is easily recognized on the spectral waveform display, it will occur simultaneously in the audio signal and in the color Doppler display. If the "aliased" waveform is revised with a baseline shift, the audio display and the color display may not be automatically adjusted. Thus, aliasing may appear as flow reversal on the color display but not on the spectral waveform. Aliasing in the audio display is heard as a transient decrease in frequency during peak systole rather than an increase. The decision of whether to connect the spectral waveform display limits to the color Doppler display limits is made by the designer of the software in the ultrasound instrument. Because software is easily changed, this behavior of the system may be changed during a service call.

Real-Time Two-Dimensional Color Doppler

Real-time 2D color Doppler instruments allow the display of Doppler frequency shift at many locations in the image plane on the B-mode image. Although the displays are often attractive and interesting, the images may lead to diagnostic error. The problems with the display fall into three categories: (a) the apparent similarity to contrast angiography, (b) the effect of the Doppler angle on the color display, and (c) the disparity between the speed of data acquisition for the display and the speed of velocity wavefronts in the arterial system. If caution is used in the application of color Doppler systems, these displays can be used to increase examination efficiency.

1. The "contrast" that leads to color in the color flow image behaves quite differently from the "opacity" contrast that is seen in contrast angiography. There are several reasons for the differences. In a contrast angiogram, dye that is injected into the vascular system will stay in the image and move with the blood until it leaves through the edge of the image field. If the blood is moving or it is stopped, the contrast is still visible. In color Doppler, changes in direction and speed cause the color to appear and disappear. Portions of the vascular lumen may be dark in a color Doppler image, even though they contain moving blood. In angiography, when a region of contrast appears in one location in the first image frame and appears in a second location in the second image frame, this is evidence that the blood moved from the first location to the second. In color Doppler, no such relationship exists.

2. The angles between the ultrasound scan lines and the blood velocity vectors are different at every location in the image. A simple convergence into a stenosis and divergence back to a normal vessel, if viewed in end view, will not show a jet-like color streak. However, if the same stenosis is viewed from an angle of 60 degrees to the vessel axis, the velocity vectors that are more closely parallel to the ultrasound scan lines will create a high Doppler shift and therefore a bright color change. Conversely, the velocity vectors of the same magnitude on the opposite side of the vessel will be more perpendicular to the ultrasound lines and produce a low Doppler frequency shift and therefore have a dull color. Viewing such an image will give the false impression that a nonaxial jet exists. Some people call the edges of the bright color patch "streamlines" and believe that you should align the Doppler angle cursor with those lines. Unfortunately, those color streaks are not streamlines and do not represent the direction of blood flow.

3. There is a space–time distortion in color Doppler imaging (Fig. 41). A color Doppler imaging system that takes 1 millisecond to gather each color line and forms a 33-mm wide image in $^1/_{30}$ of a second from 33 color image lines should produce a good real-time image. In such an image, there is one line generated every millimeter and 10 lines per centimeter, taking 10 milliseconds or $^1/_{100}$ sec/cm. Thus, the color display sweeps across the image like a windshield wiper at a rate of 100 cm/sec. Each time the heart contracts, the onset of systole travels from the heart to the foot, a distance of more than 1 m, in just 0.06 second, with a pulse wave velocity of more than 16 m/sec.

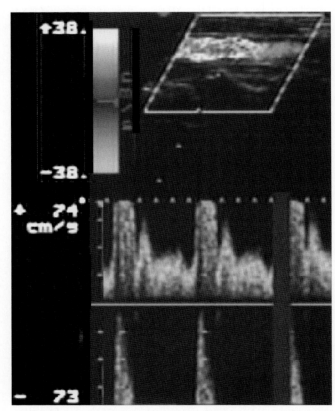

FIGURE 41. Comparison between two-dimensional color Doppler imaging and spectral waveform. The color flow display above ranges from +38 cm/sec to –38 cm/sec, the spectral waveform display ranges from +74 cm/sec to –74 cm/sec because the latter is adjusted by a factor of two for the 60 degree Doppler examination angle but the former is not. On the spectral waveform at the rightmost systole, a stripe of data is missing. The two-dimensional color Doppler image was acquired during this 200 millisecond blank period in the spectral waveform during the period of peak systole during which aliasing occurs. The blue aliased region in the center of the color flow image was taken during peak systole while the red region to the left was acquired prior to systole and the red region to the right was acquired after systole. The aliased region in the center of the color flow image might be mistaken for a stenosis because of the high velocity in that location, but the peak systolic velocity is uniform along the entire length of the vessel. This image demonstrates the space/time artifacts that can lead to errors in diagnosis.

Thus, pulse velocity (16 m/sec) is 16 times greater than image acquisition velocity (1 m/sec = 100 cm/sec). Systole begins at the ankle before it is finished at the heart; therefore, the length of the systolic bolus is more than 1 m. Arterial systole lasts 0.12 second, only one third as long as it takes to sweep the color display line across the image from the left to the right; thus, the entire systolic bolus extends only one third of the width of the image, appearing to be 1-cm long. This is much less than the 1-m length of the systolic bolus; although in actuality the systolic bolus is 1 m long, it appears in the image to be only 1 cm long.

POTENTIAL HAZARDS OF ULTRASOUND EXAMINATION

There are five commonly identified hazards of ultrasound examination:

1. Patient shock or electrocution
2. Patient contamination
3. Contact heating of patient tissues
4. Ultrasonic heating of deep tissues
5. Ultrasonic cavitation in deep tissues

Although these hazards are listed in approximate order of likelihood, the greatest attention in the literature is given to the fourth topic, followed by the third and the fifth; the second topic is receiving increasing attention; the first is rarely discussed. We will introduce these in the order that they are listed.

Electrical Hazards

The voltage applied to the ultrasound transducers during typical imaging procedures ranges from 40 to 400 V, values that often exceed the voltage in the power cord. The available instantaneous current may approach 1 amp. The transducer array is covered with a protective grounding plane on the anterior (patient) surface of the transducer, which in turn is covered by insulating plastic layers. During examination, the ultrasound transducer is placed against the poorly conductive cornified layer of the skin, which applies additional protection. Unfortunately, associated with ultrasound examinations, a series of deliberate and accidental events may occur that contribute to the breaching of the electrical isolation between the patient and the 100 V or more ultrasound transmit pulse.

The patient's skin may be shaved in preparation for the examination, damaging the cornified layer. A conducting ultrasound gel is usually placed between the ultrasound transducer and the patient's skin to increase the acoustic conductivity of the path, but this also increases the electrical conductivity of the path. (A less conductive material, such as mineral oil, may provide better electrical isolation of the patient than the commonly used water-based coupling mate-

rial.) The ultrasound transducer may be placed into a body cavity, such as the esophagus, rectum, vagina, peritoneum, urethra, or vascular space, where the protective cornified layer is not present. (Usually, when in such intimate contact with the body tissues, an electrically insulating sheath is placed between the transducers and the tissues for biologic protection, but this also provides some degree of electrical protection.) During cleaning or sterilization of the ultrasound scanhead, the protective plastic covering of the transducers may be damaged, or the connections to the protective grounding plane may deteriorate. Of course, defects in design and manufacture, as well as deterioration of ultrasound scanhead with age, will also contribute to the electrical hazard.

Of all ultrasound examinations, those with greatest risk for electrical hazards are interarterial examinations of the coronary arteries followed by transesophageal echocardiographic examinations. Both carry the risk for electrical effects to the heart. Electrical leakage from the ultrasound scanhead during other intracavity examinations are likely to result only in patient discomfort or local tissue injury.

Conventional electrical ground fault tests by the hospital safety department are not designed to detect electrical leakage from the scanhead, nor are scanhead leakage tests commonly done by ultrasound company service personnel. For assurance of electrical safety, testing for electrical leakage between a saline bath in contact with the face of the scanhead and the examination room grounding point should be done as part of regular quality assurance.

In addition to maintaining the ultrasound equipment in a safe condition, the examination should be designed to minimize electrical risk. At all times during an ultrasound examination, the ultrasound transmit power should be on only during essential imaging procedures; frozen images, or *cine loops*, should be used whenever possible for discussion. During examination, the transmit power control (which determines the transmit voltage) should always be set to the minimum value consistent with successful, noise-free imaging. Whenever possible, the ultrasound transducer should be covered in a protective sheath using mineral oil rather than ultrasound gel for ultrasound contact with minimum electrical conductance. Although ultrasound gel is not deliberately made with a conductive salt solution, unless designed for double service as an electrocardiograph conductive agent, the water base easily dissolves salt to make it conductive. Protective sheaths should never be cleaned and reused, nor used if damaged. Finally, if the patient complains of a sensation that might be due to electrical leakage, the ultrasound examination should be discontinued.

Patient Contamination

Ultrasound scanheads can never be sterilized in an autoclave. The high temperatures involved may destroy the piezoelectric properties of the transducer as well as damage the plastic materials in the scanhead. Some ultrasound scanheads can be cleaned with gas sterilization, although the manufacturer's recommendation should be obtained before attempting gas sterilization. Some solvents will damage the plastics and glue joints on the ultrasound scanhead, even if elevated temperatures are not used. A protective sheath can serve to protect the scanhead and the patient from contamination and can provide electrical and thermal protection of the patient.

Contact Heating of Patient Tissues

Ultrasound scanheads often generate significant amounts of heat during operation. The ultrasound transducers in all imaging scanheads are mechanically damped with an absorbing plastic material on the back of the transducer elements to absorb excess transducer vibrations and therefore improve the depth resolution of the ultrasound image. However, two deleterious consequences result: (a) excess electrical energy is required to generate transmit pulses of sufficient pulse energy for the examination, and (b) the sensitivity of the transducers to ultrasound echoes is reduced, thus requiring even more transmitted energy in each pulse to produce detectable echoes.

The result of the poor conversion efficiency is that more electrical energy (and thus a higher transmit voltage) is required for each ultrasound transmit pulse. The excess energy is converted to heat in the transducer assembly. Often, 80% of the electrical energy sent to the ultrasound transducer will be converted to heating the transducer, and only 20% will appear as ultrasound. Transducer heating can be a particular problem with transducers in the esophagus, rectum, urethra, or vagina, where no fluid flow is present to remove the heat. Intravascular transducers are cooled by the surrounding blood flow. Examinations should be designed to minimize the risk for heating.

An impression of the importance of scanhead heating can be obtained by simple experiments using new, thin, low-cost, liquid crystal thermometers available for measuring fish tank temperature, room temperature, and forehead temperature for fever. A room-temperature thermometer taped with double-face cellophane tape to the patient contact surface of an ultrasound scanhead may rise 5°C in 15 seconds, showing the capability of the scanhead to heat. A similar test can be done during a patient examination. By (double-face) taping a forehead thermometer to the patient's skin, the ambient skin temperature can be found. Then, by applying gel and the scanhead, an ultrasound scan can be done through the thermometer. The gel lowers the skin temperature markedly. During one test, even 5 minutes of stationary contact with the color Doppler on full power failed to return the skin temperature to normal. There are many problems with such a test. One problem is that the thermometer absorbs a great deal of ultrasound, which can be detected by comparing the brightness of the ultrasound image viewed through the adjacent skin to the brightness of the image viewed through the thermometer.

Again, at all times during an ultrasound examination, the ultrasound transmit power should be on only during essential imaging procedures; frozen images should be used whenever possible for discussion. During examination, the transmit power control (which determines the energy per pulse) should always be set to the minimum value consistent with successful, noise-free imaging. Whenever possible, the ultrasound transducer should be covered in a protective sheath to provide thermal insulation. Removal of heat by passing fluid around the transducer assembly should be considered. During intraperitoneal examinations, the transducer may not remain in continuous contact with tissues. Because tissues will often carry away the transducer heat, the transducer may reach a higher temperature during periods of noncontact. During such times, the ultrasound transmitter should be off. Finally, if the patient complains of a sensation that might be due to hot ultrasound transducers, the ultrasound examination should be discontinued. Consideration should be given to the possibility that nerves in some tissues may not be sensitive to temperature.

Ultrasound Heating of Deep Tissues

Most discussions of ultrasound safety and hazards are focused on the ultrasound heating of deep tissues. Heating is related to the ultrasound intensity and the duration of the examination. Potential damage to tissue depends on a combination of four factors: (a) temperature attained, (b) duration of elevated temperature, (c) type of tissue, and (d) susceptibility of tissue to damage. Some boundaries can be set for tissue temperatures:

- Normal body temperature, 37.0°C
- Safe higher temperature, 38.5°C
- Fetal hazard, 41.0°C for 15 minutes
- Adult proliferative cell damage, 42.0°C for 120 minutes (recovery expected)

Tissue temperature is dependent on the baseline temperature and the elevation resulting from ultrasound exposure. Thus, an ultrasound examination performed on a febrile patient will result in higher temperatures than a similar examination on an afebrile patient. As an ultrasound examination is performed, tissues exposed to ultrasound pass through two phases of temperature elevation: a transient phase and a steady-state phase. Initially, when the ultrasound is applied, the temperature of each voxel of tissue rises at a rate that depends on the power absorbed by the voxel and the heat capacity of the voxel. Later, as the temperature becomes elevated, heat is carried away from the voxel by two methods: (a) conduction through surrounding cooler tissues (if any), and (b) convection—the removal of heat by the blood flowing through the tissue. When the heat removed by conduction and convection equals the heat delivered by ultrasound absorption, a steady-state temperature is achieved, and no further temperature rise occurs.

TABLE 13. SPECIFIC MAXIMUM TRANSIENT RATE OF TEMPERATURE RISE

Tissue	Estimated heat capacity	Absorption coefficient	Specific rate of temperature rise (3 MHz, 1 W/cm²)
Muscle	4.0 J/cm³/°C	0.6 dB/MHz/cm	0.1°C/s
Fat	0.9 J/cm³/°C	1.5 dB/MHz/cm	1.2°C/s
Brain	1.0 J/cm³/°C	1.0 dB/MHz/cm	0.7°C/s
Cartilage	4.2 J/cm³/°C	4.0 dB/MHz/cm	0.7°C/s
Bone	3.7 J/cm³/°C	20.0 dB/MHz/cm	3.7°C/s

The computation of the rate of temperature rise during the transient period is easier (in theory) and more certain than computing the steady-state temperature. The rate of temperature rise depends only on the ultrasound intensity, the ultrasound absorption coefficient, and the tissue-specific heat capacity. The steady-state value depends on the temperature of the surrounding tissues (which is elevated in therapeutic ultrasound because of the broad ultrasound beam, but not in diagnostic ultrasound because of the focused ultrasound beam) and the blood perfusion rate (which may increase in response to elevated temperatures). Other documents have described methods of computing the steady-state temperature. Here, the rate of temperature rise during the transient period (Table 13) will be computed.

In theory, the computation is easy. However, finding correct values in the literature for tissue heat capacity is not trivial. Therefore, the values are often estimated from similar materials.

$$\text{Rate of temperature rise} = \text{intensity} \times \text{absorption/heat capacity}$$

Using the most severe assumptions, an upper boundary for temperature rise in tissue during different types of examinations can be computed.

Assumptions

- Minimum protective attenuation of overlying tissues
- Maximum absorption of ultrasound at the tissue exposed
- Minimum blood perfusion to carry away heat
- Minimum conduction to distribute heat to adjacent tissue
- Maximum time of beam on the tissue exposed

When commercial fixed beam pulsed Doppler systems are tested in a water tank at maximum ultrasound transmit power, SPTA intensity values as high as 5,000 mW/cm² can be detected at the focal zone. In one test of a 5-MHz transducer, the focal zone was about 2 cm from the transducer face. Thus, in an examination through 2 cm of muscle between the ultrasound transducer and the focal zone, the intervening muscle would absorb 75% of the transmitted power superficial to the focal zone, reducing the intensity in the tissue at the focal zone to 1,250 mW/cm². Such a beam striking bone (with the intervening muscle)

at the 2 cm depth for just 1 second will cause the temperature of the bone to jump 4°C, from 37° to 41°C in an afebrile patient; 41°C is close to a potentially harmful temperature. Had the overlying tissue been fat, 97% of the ultrasound power would be absorbed passing through 2 cm, and the 4° temperature rise in the bone would have taken 10 seconds.

Thermal Index

To provide a guide to the ultrasound examiner for avoiding heating of tissue, the modern indicator of tissue heating is called the thermal index (TI). This is a measure of the estimated temperature elevation in tissue due to prolonged exposure to ultrasound. A TI of 1 means that the temperature of tissue at the focal zone (or region of highest effect) will increase by 1°C during prolonged imaging of that location. The TI includes the effects of focusing, the attenuation of ultrasound in tissues superficial to the affected region, the absorption of ultrasound by the tissue, the thermal conductivity carrying heat away from the tissue, and the blood perfusion carrying heat away from the tissue. Only the heat capacity of the tissue is not included in the TI computation because heat capacity affects rate of temperature rise, but not the final temperature. As a rule, the TI is thought to predict the temperature rise within a factor of 2. The inclusion of the expected attenuation of ultrasound by superficial tissues, which makes the TI lower, is called *derating* the index.

Because bone is a strong absorber and strong reflector of ultrasound, the presence of bone in the ultrasonic image (and therefore the ultrasound exposure field) has a strong effect on heating. Therefore, separate TIs are computed for bone. Three TIs are now in frequent use: thermal index in soft tissue (TIS), thermal index in bone (TIB), and thermal index in transcranial examination (TIC).

The issue of heating has become more important in recent years as manufacturers and examiners have moved to use higher and higher ultrasound intensities for examination. The old limits of 100 mW/cm² SPTA were used out of tradition rather than objective analysis based on experimental evidence of bioeffects. Modern ultrasound instruments deliver intensities 8 times as high, and the TI is used to decide more objectively on safe limits.

Because of the ever-present potential for causing harm with ultrasound, even though harm is very unlikely, always use the lowest ultrasound transmit power consistent with performing a noise-free examination. Acquire data in the minimum possible time. Look for bone in the superficial portions of the ultrasound image where the intensities are highest. Remember that clear fluids such as urine, amniotic fluid, and the aqueous humor of the eye are poor attenuators of ultrasound. Limit ultrasound exposure to values "as low as reasonably achievable" (ALARA) while obtaining diagnostic data.

Ultrasonic Cavitation in Deep Tissues

During the insonication of tissue for an ultrasound examination, each element of tissue experiences compressions and decompressions. At intensities of 320 mW/cm^2, the amplitude of the pressure fluctuations equals the atmospheric pressure. This value is computed from the following equation:

Cycle average spatial peak temporal peak intensity = (pressure fluctuation)^2/(2 × Z)

During a typical M-mode ultrasound examination, with a PRF of 1 KHz, a pulse length of 1 microsecond, and a SPTA intensity of 10 mW/cm^2, the SPTP or at least the SPPA intensity will be 1,000 times greater than the temporal average intensity because the ultrasound is only on 1 of every 1,000 microseconds (PRF of 1 KHz means a PRI of 1,000 microseconds). Therefore, the SPPA intensity is 10 Ws/cm^2, and the pressure amplitude of the pulse is 5.5 atmospheres during the pulse. This means that during the compression portion of the ultrasound pulse, the tissue pressure is raised to 6.5 atmospheres; and during the decompression portion of the pulse, the tissue pressure is reduced below zero to −4.5 atmospheres for a period of a fraction of half a cycle, about 50 nanoseconds. Such negative pressures are impossible in equilibrium physics, but they can occur, at least theoretically, for very short periods. If the time is extended, the molecular forces that hold water and tissue together will fail, and a cavity will form. That cavity may survive or may collapse. If the cavity collapses, large amounts of energy are produced. In water, flashes of light can be seen as the cavities collapse. There is some concern that the heat and light generated could cause chemical reactions, including the disruption of chromosomes. Thus, cavitation should be avoided.

Mechanical Index

To predict the chance of cavitation, a numeric index called the *mechanical index* (MI) has been developed empirically. This index is larger when the peak negative pressure is higher and when the duration of the negative pressure is longer.

Mechanical index = peak negative pressure/ SQRT (ultrasound frequency)

Dividing by the square root of the ultrasound frequency accounts for the time duration of the negative pressure. As the ultrasound frequency goes down, the MI goes up. The term *peak negative pressure* is used in case the ultrasound pulse is shaped so that the positive part of the pressure oscillation is different from the negative part. Peak negative pressure means the value below atmospheric pressure, not the value below zero pressure. This is the choice that was made for the empiric index, although a better choice might be the negative pressure below zero. Then, if the sonic exposure were on a mountaintop where the ambient pressure is low or under sea where the ambient pressure is high, the index would work the same.

Cavitation does not occur below a threshold MI. Generally, a TI of 0.3 is considered safe in most examinations. However, the chance of cavitation is greatly increased by the presence of bubbles, including lung and ultrasound contrast agents, in the insonated field. At the surface of lung, diagnostic ultrasound intensities have created hemorrhage. In the presence of contrast agents, hemolysis of blood can occur at diagnostic intensities.

Therefore, careful attention to ultrasound safety issues is becoming more important as the field of ultrasound diagnostics continues to evolve.

SUBJECT INDEX